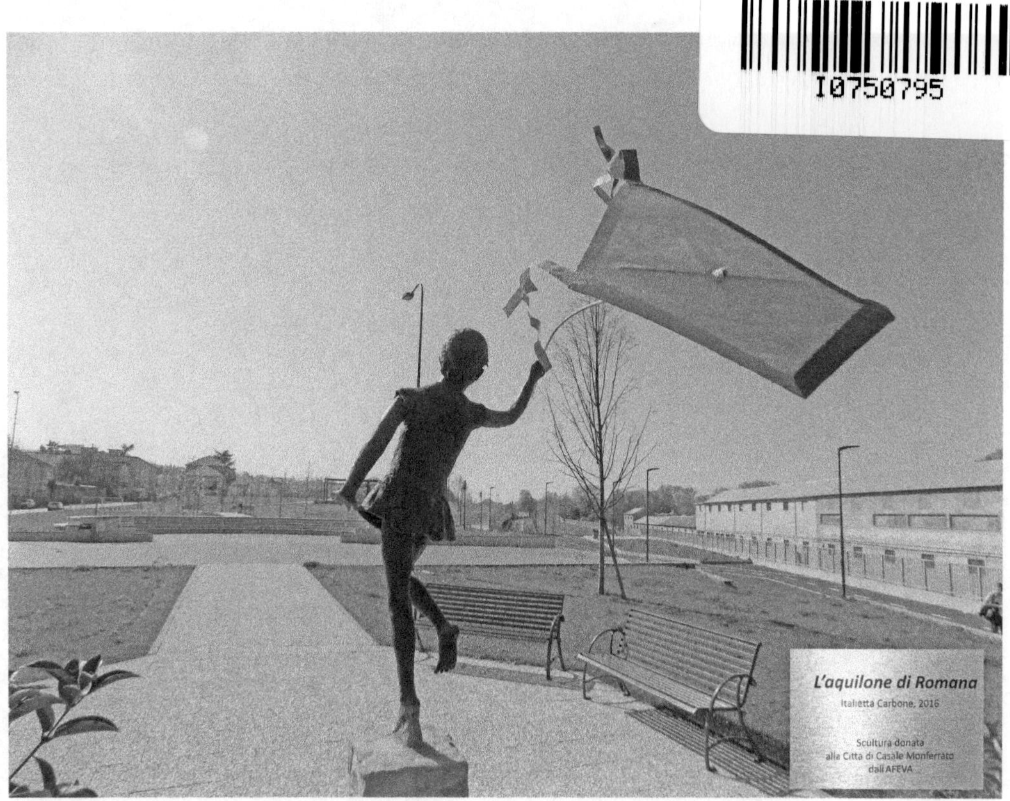

"Ethernot" Park, Science and Hope-A Real Life Human Experience Over Time with Asbestos.

RELEVANCE OF SCULPTURE TO CONTENT OF BOOK:

Ethernit, Casale Monferrato, Italy, was the largest asbestos manufacturer in Europe and has caused an ongoing epidemic of mesothelioma. The photo shows the "Ethernot" park that opened September 10, 2016. In the park, there is a children's playground and a sculpture.

This park has been built over the former factory that has been sealed in a sarcophagus of cement to prevent further exposure to the population. This park represents the ability of the human intellect to find a solution to a very difficult problem: how to safely get rid of many tons of asbestos. The beautiful sculpture of the girl flying a kite, represents the hope that preventive measures will result in a better future for the kids growing up in Casale who are now playing in the Ethernot park, the same place that caused so much pain to their parents and grandparents. Similarly, it is hoped that by having identified key mechanisms in the pathogenesis of mesothelioma and other malignancies, we will soon be able to develop novel and more effective therapies.

We think this photo shows a wonderful example of human ingenuity to prevent future deaths caused by asbestos, how to turn a negative (the Ethernit factory) into a positive (a park). It is a nice parallel with why research on mesothelioma and other asbestos induced diseases as well as preventing exposure to asbestos and potentially other elongated mineral particles is so important.

The sculpture was made and donated to the town of Casale Monferrato by the artist Italietta Carbone for the opening of the Ethernot park.

Asbestos

Asbestos: Risk Assessment, Epidemiology, and Health Effects offers a key text on the evolving information regarding asbestos and human health. Now in its third edition, this bestseller explores the pathological complexities of asbestos-related disease and examines how asbestos induces diseases in biological systems. The book also discusses the types of instruments and methods available for evaluation of the content of asbestiform minerals in products, air, water, surface areas, and tissue. It explains the relevance of each of these applications and gives readers the tools to evaluate data in the future.

Edited by leading authorities on the subject and with contributions from a team of international experts, this book takes a cross-disciplinary approach and an authoritative review of the history, pathology, epidemiology, sampling, and analysis of asbestos. Backed up with photos and numerous diagrams, tables, and photographs, it features case studies, methodologies, and sampling/analytical schemes that put learning into context. Fully up-to-date and featuring four brand new chapters covering asbestosis and immunity, asbestos litigation and surgical and non-surgical management of mesothelioma, this book remains the most comprehensive source of information on asbestos and the only guide the reader will ever need to own.

This essential text will appeal to any professional at any level who requires the latest expertise in dealing with asbestos. It suits researchers and practitioners alike, as well as those in the fields of law, health, education, hospitality, emergency response, building management and maintenance, construction, safety, insurance, and industrial hygiene.

Asbestos

Asbestos

Risk Assessment, Epidemiology, and Health Effects

Third Edition

Edited by

Michele Carbone, Ronald F. Dodson, Harvey Pass, and Haining Yang

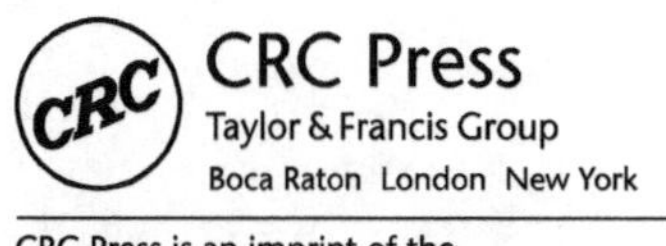

CRC Press is an imprint of the
Taylor & Francis Group, an informa business

Cover image: Michele Carbone, Ronald F. Dodson, Harvey Pass and Haining Yang

Third edition published 2025
by CRC Press
2385 NW Executive Center Drive, Suite 320, Boca Raton FL 33431

and by CRC Press
4 Park Square, Milton Park, Abingdon, Oxon, OX14 4RN

CRC Press is an imprint of Taylor & Francis Group, LLC

Second edition published by CRC Press 2012

Library of Congress Cataloging-in-Publication Data
Names: Carbone, Michele, editor. | Dodson, Ronald F., editor. | Pass, Harvey I., editor. | Yang, Haining, editor.
Title: Asbestos : risk assessment, epidemiology, and health effects / edited by Michele Carbone, Ronald Dodson, Harvey Pass and Haining Yang.
Description: Third edition. | Boca Raton : CRC Press, 2024. | Includes bibliographical references and index.
Identifiers: LCCN 2024009464 | ISBN 9781032521060 (hbk) | ISBN 9781032557175 (pbk) | ISBN 9781003431909 (ebk)
Subjects: LCSH: Asbestos--Toxicology. | Asbestosis.
Classification: LCC RA1231.A8 A74 2024 | DDC 615.9/2539224--dc23/eng/20240524
LC record available at https://lccn.loc.gov/2024009464

ISBN: 978-1-032-52106-0 (hbk)
ISBN: 978-1-032-55717-5 (pbk)
ISBN: 978-1-003-43190-9 (ebk)

DOI: 10.1201/9781003431909

Typeset in Times
by Deanta Global Publishing Services, Chennai, India

Contents

Asbestos III Edition, Preface

The third edition of the *Asbestos: Risk Assessment, Epidemiology, and Health Effects* textbook comes at a critical moment in the evolution of medical research on this topic. During the first 23 years of the 21st century research has:

- Uncovered the role of genetics in mesothelioma, pointing to the human body, not as a passive recipient of carcinogenic fibers, but rather as an active participant in the interaction in which genetics plays a key role in determining the outcome. The subsequent elucidation of the mechanisms of BAP1 tumor suppressor activity has led to clinical trials for early detection of mesothelioma in carriers of germline *BAP1* mutations. Most importantly, several patients carrying *BAP1* germline mutations have survived mesothelioma, while asbestos-induced mesothelioma is uniformly fatal, as discussed in Chapter 10;
- Led to the development of novel and more specific diagnostic markers to distinguish malignant from benign mesothelial growths and to distinguish mesothelioma from other malignancies, increasing the accuracy of diagnosis, as discussed in Chapter 11;
- Elucidated some of the key mechanisms of asbestos carcinogenesis, as discussed in Chapter 5;
- Led to a significant reduction in the incidence of asbestos-related mesothelioma/100,000 persons in the USA, as discussed in Chapter 6. This is evidence that the measures enacted in the 1980s and 1990s to ban or significantly limit the use of asbestos products in the Western world (USA, Europe, Australia, and a few other countries) are working. We, the editors, hope that these important results will motivate developing countries—where unfortunately the use of asbestos has increased exponentially in the recent past—to introduce a similar asbestos ban to save many lives from mesothelioma;
- The research in the recent past demonstrated that elongated particles other than asbestos are associated with risks of disease and mesothelioma, like those induced by "asbestos". The list of carcinogenic fibers, including natural fibers and man-made fibers is constantly expanding. Exposure includes work-related exposure as well as environmental exposure, as discussed in Chapter 7.

The book starts with an historical review of asbestos exposure, Chapter 1, followed by a critical analysis of the methods and criteria used to verify asbestos exposure, Chapters 2-4. This is a critical issue, as determining asbestos exposure is of utmost importance to implement remediation and preventive measures, and for medical-legal considerations. We may all have been exposed to asbestos or asbestos-like fibers because carcinogenic fibers, including asbestos, are present in the natural environment of some geographic areas. Humans and other species are able to deal with background levels of fibers in their lungs as there is no evidence that they cause disease. However, when the air concentration of these fibers is above background levels, people inhale high amounts of fibers that are deposited in the lungs where they cause inflammation. Fibers, via lymphatic drainage, can also reach other organs. Over the course of several years, the chronic inflammatory process caused by deposition of fibers in tissues leads to fibrosis, pleural plaques and in some individuals causes mesothelioma and lung cancer, as discussed in Chapters 6, 7, 10, and 15.

Although the incidence of mesothelioma/100,000 persons is declining, the overall number of mesotheliomas in the USA has remained constant. This is because of several reasons:

First the population has significantly increased in recent decades, and in particular the fraction of people older than 70 is increasing. Cancer is a genetic disease that largely affects old people as they inevitably accumulate genetic damage during aging: as the overall number of old people increases, cancers increase, including mesothelioma.

Secondly, we are developing rural areas, often inhospitable areas, where human settlements were rare, for example the Mojave desert in Nevada, and the Badlands in Montana, North and South

Dakota. Here, developers inadvertently used and/or built roads and towns over terrain-containing various types of mineral fibers including asbestos, antigorite and erionite: all of them are carcinogenic to humans and may cause mesothelioma upon prolonged exposure, as discussed in Chapter 7. The imaging findings associated with asbestos exposure are discussed in Chapter 8.

Thirdly, we have seen a significant increase of post-radiation therapy-induced mesotheliomas. Radiation therapy has been used in the past decades to treat lymphomas, seminomas and gynecological tumors, often in young patients. This therapy is very effective and cured most of these cancer patients. However, therapeutic radiation causes widespread genetic damage in normal cells within the irradiation field. Five or more years later some of these patients developed various types of sarcomas, including pleura and peritoneal mesothelioma as the pleural and the peritoneum are inevitably within the area that receives therapeutic radiation.

Finally, approximately 12–16% of mesotheliomas are now attributed to germline mutations of *BAP1* or less frequently of other tumor suppressor genes. These mesotheliomas, especially when there is no evidence of asbestos exposure, have unique clinical characteristics that set them apart from other mesotheliomas:

For the most part they occur in people younger than 55, in contrast to asbestos-induced mesotheliomas that occur usually in older individuals.

The M:F ratio is 1:1, in contrast to asbestos-induced mesothelioma where the M:F ratio is 4:1 to 9:1. The pleural-to-peritoneal ratio is 1:1, in contrast to asbestos-induced mesothelioma where the pleural-to-peritoneal ratio is 4:1 to 9:1.

Most importantly median survival is 6-7 years and several patients were cured and died 20+ years later of other diseases/old age. This is in contrast to the 6–18 months survival for asbestos-induced mesotheliomas which, sadly, is uniformly fatal. Discussed in Chapter 10.

The additional diseases and malignancies that have been linked to asbestos exposure are critically reviewed in Chapter 15. The effects of asbestos on immunity are discussed in Chapter 8 and the developing findings related to the new multi-omics tissue and bioinformatic analyses are discussed in Chapter 12.

Chapter 16 deals with the medical-legal issues related to mesothelioma in the USA, a litigation that moves each year billions of dollars. This chapter has been written together by three of the most experienced and respected lawyers that work on opposite sides of this litigation.

All the complexities of these issues and more are discussed in depth in the various chapters of the book that were written by some of the top international experts in the field. It is our intent that the content of the book will provide informational awareness of the issues of exposure to elongated mineral particles and through this awareness minimize exposures and subsequent risks of fiber-induced diseases.

As for the future, recent clinical trials questioned the value of immunotherapy and surgery for patients with mesothelioma. It is likely that in coming years these therapeutic modalities will be used for a selected group of patients rather than for all patients with this malignancy. This is discussed in Chapters 13 and 14. On the bright side, we hope that the findings about the mechanisms that underlie asbestos carcinogenesis and mesothelioma will lead to the development of targeted therapies to interfere with the process and prevent/delay tumor growth.

We are hopeful and optimistic that studying the paradox that carriers of germline mutations on the one hand are susceptible to mesothelioma and on the other hand are able to effectively fight mesothelioma growth, may result in new effective therapies for this deadly cancer. There are now two ongoing clinical trials at the Bethesda NCI Medical Center to study exactly that. Will mesothelioma patients carrying germline mutations provide a new approach to mesothelioma therapy? We shall see, and we very much hope so.

Michele Carbone
Ronald F. Dodson
Harvey Pass
Haining Yang

Editors

Michele Carbone is Director of Thoracic Oncology at the University of Hawaii Cancer Center, USA. With degrees from the Medical School of Rome, University of Rome and University of Chicago, Dr. Carbone specializes in pleural pathology and mesothelioma. Dr. Carbone discovered that heterozygous germline BAP1 mutations modulate susceptibility to asbestos and cause mesothelioma. Carbone's research is a combination of fieldwork in the third world and in remote areas of the USA, sophisticated molecular genetics work in his laboratory, and vital clinical-diagnostic work.

Ronald F. Dodson's research interests include the use of light and transmission electron microscopy in identification and/or effects of particulates in tissue and other biological environments. He retired from academia in 2005 and established his own company, Dodson Environmental Consulting in Tyler, Texas, USA. He continues to conduct research in this role as well as write scientific and biomedical publications and serve as an expert in his field as requested by the private sector, academia, federal agencies, and international agencies/scientific organizations. Dr. Dodson's research/academic career included serving as a reviewer for scientific journals and serving as an Advisory Board Member on the Texas Department of Health's committee that was charged with developing the State Law governing asbestos-related activities in public buildings in Texas.

Harvey Pass is Professor in Thoracic Oncology in the Department of Cardiothoracic Surgery at NYU Langone Health's Perlmutter Cancer Center. He serves as Chief of the Division of Thoracic Oncology at NYU and oversees a laboratory at Bellevue Hospital where much important research work funded by the National Cancer Institute takes place, including the new Mesothelioma Pathogenesis Program Project. Dr. Pass has held numerous positions in professional associations, has served as a guest reviewer for major medical journals and publications and has served as a consultant to private companies as well as public agencies and foundations.

Haining Yang is Professor in the University of Hawaii Cancer Center at the University of Hawaii at Mānoa, USA. Her research work focuses on the pathogenesis of mesothelioma, a malignancy often related to exposure to asbestos or other carcinogenic mineral fibers. She discovered that a protein called high mobility group box 1 protein (HMGB1) kickstarts the growth of mesothelioma cancer cells once the individual is exposed to asbestos. As a result, Dr. Yang explored targeting these proteins as a therapy method for mesothelioma. She was one of the recipients of the American Association for Cancer Research (AACR)–Landon Foundation INNOVATOR Award for International Collaboration in Cancer Research in 2008. She also received the iMig Research Award in 2018.

Contributors

Francine Baumann
University of New Caledonia
Nouméa, New Caledonia

Elena Belluso
University of Turin
Turin, Italy

Barbara Bertoglio
University of Pavia
Pavia, Italy

Chandra Bortolotto
University of Pavia
Pavia, Italy

Alan Brayton
Brayton Purcell LLP
Novato, CA, USA

Silvana Capella
University of Turin
Turin, Italy

Michele Carbone
Unit of Thoracic Surgery
San Camillo Forlanini Hospital
University of Hawaii Cancer Center
Honolulu, HI, USA

Giuseppe Cardillo
Unit of Thoracic Surgery
San Camillo Forlanini Hospital
Unicamillus-University of Health Science
Rome, Italy

Stephanie Chang
NYU Langone Health
New York, NY, USA

David B. Chapel
University of Michigan – Michigan Medicine
Ann Arbor, MI, USA

Claudio Colosio
University of Milan
Milan, Italy

Steven P. Compton
MVA Scientific Consultants
Duluth, GA, USA

Ronald F. Dodson
Dodson Environmental Consulting, LLC
Tyler, TX, USA

Cristina Favaron
University of Pavia
Pavia, Italy

Nobukazu Fujimoto
Okayama Rosai Hospital
Okayama, Japan

Giovanni Gaudino
University of Hawaii Cancer Center
Honolulu, HI, USA

Lydia Giannakou
University of Hawaii Cancer Center
Honolulu, HI, USA

Delia Giovanniello
University of Rome, La Sapienza
Rome, Italy

Steven G. Gray
Trinity St James's Cancer Institute, St James's Hospital
Dublin, Ireland

Douglas W. Henderson
Flinders University, SA Pathology
Adelaide, SA, Australia

Aliya N. Husain
University of Chicago
Chicago, IL, USA

Sonja Klebe
Flinders University, SA Pathology
Adelaide, SA, Australia

Thomas Krausz
University of Chicago
Chicago, IL, USA

Sara Kryeziu
NYU Langone Health
New York, NY, USA

James Leigh
University of Sydney
Sydney, NSW, Australia

Alessandra Marrocco
University of Pavia
Pavia, Italy

Tomer Meirson
Davidoff Cancer Center, Rabin Medical Center-Beilinson Hospital
Petah Tikva, Israel

James R. Millette
Millette Technical Consulting
Stone Mountain, GA, USA

Yosuke Miyamoto
Okayama Rosai Hospital
Okayama, Japan

Luciano Mutti
University of L'Aquila
L'Aquila, Italy

Yasumitsu Nishimura
Kawasaki Medical School
Kurashiki, Japan

Harvey Pass
NYU Langone Health
New York, NY, USA

Sara Ricciardi
San Camillo Forlanini Hospital
Rome, Italy

Emanuela Taioli
Icahn School of Medicine at Mount Sinai
New York, NY, USA

Ellen Tenenbaum
Perago Law PLLC
New York, NY, USA

Silvia Damiana Visonà
University of Pavia
Pavia, Italy

Haining Yang
University of Hawaii Cancer Center
Honolulu, HI, USA

Craig Zimmerman
Perago Law PLLC
New York, NY, USA

Alicia A. Zolondick
University of Hawaii Cancer Center; University of Hawaii at Manoa
Honolulu, HI, USA

1 The History of Asbestos Utilization and Recognition of Asbestos-Induced Diseases

Sonja Klebe, James Leigh, and Douglas W. Henderson

1.1 WHAT IS "ASBESTOS"?

"Asbestos"—derived from the Greek for *inextinguishable* or *unquenchable*—is a commercial term applied to a variety of hydrated fibrous silicates that have: (i) the capacity to add tensile strength when added to other materials (such as cement to produce asbestos-cement); (ii) resistance to fire; (iii) poor thermal conductivity (insulating properties); and (iv) resistance to corrosion by acids and alkalis (especially the amphibole varieties of asbestos). Because of these properties, it was once regarded as a "magic mineral" (1)—used in about 3000–4000 different products—but it is now regarded as a deadly threat to health ("killer dust" (1)) and has been banned in more than 60 nations, although its use continues, most notably in the "developing world" and especially in Asia.

Asbestos is conventionally divided into two broad groups (Table 1.1) (2): (i) the serpentine group that contains only a single member, namely chrysotile (the name of which is derived from the Greek for gold (chrysos) and fiber (tilos); and (ii) the amphiboles, which include crocidolite, amosite and the (usually) non-commercial amphiboles namely tremolite, actinolite and anthophyllite (the last of these being mined at the Paakkila mine in Finland until it was closed, and at a few other sites). The serpentine chrysotile is characterized by curly fibers that tend to matt together, whereas the amphiboles are characterized by straight needle-like fibers with a capacity for longitudinal splitting (2–4).

1.2 PRE-INDUSTRIAL HISTORY OF ASBESTOS

Accounts of past and continuing use of asbestos can be found in many standard texts and journal articles (3–7). One of the best-documented and referenced accounts of its pre-industrial usage can be found in Rachel Maines' book *Asbestos and Fire: Technological Trade-offs and the Body at Risk* (7), although her argument in later sections of the book is open to dispute (see later discussion).

The occasional and sometimes colorful use of asbestos has extended from Neolithic times until the 21st century. In this setting, asbestos (anthophyllite) has been found in Neolithic pottery in Finland from about 2500 BCE (3)—apparently added to confer tensile strength when added to clay—and its use has also been recorded in other Neolithic sites, including Central Russia, Norway and Lapland (8). However, in the Western literature the earliest known documented reference to what might have been asbestos has been attributed by some to Theophrastus (ca. 372–287 BCE)—a student of Aristotle and his successor at the Lyceum in Athens (8). In his book *De Lapidibus* [On Stones] (9), compiled around 300 BCE, in chapter II.17, he wrote:

> In the mines at Scapte Hyle a stone was once found which was like rotten wood in appearance. Whenever oil was poured on it, it burnt, but when the oil had been used up, the stone stopped burning, as if it were itself unaffected.

DOI: 10.1201/9781003431909-1

(Scapte Hyle was a mining district in Thrace opposite the island of Thasos in the Northern Aegean (9).) In commentary on this description, Theophrastus' 20th-century translators/editors Caley and Richards (9) set forth the following commentary:

> Moore [in *Ancient Mineralogy,* p. 153] thought that Theophrastus was really referring to asbestos. The color of the stone makes this unlikely, though its structure makes it less improbable, since some forms of decayed wood do have a fibrous structure like asbestos. We know from statements of various early authors that asbestos was known in antiquity, and that it was mainly used for the manufacture of incombustible cloth, though evidently wicks for oil lamps were also made of it. Moreover, direct evidence of the use of asbestos by the ancients has been obtained in modern times by the discovery of ancient garments woven from this mineral. It is, however, unlikely that Theophrastus is alluding to asbestos, since the mineral does not occur in the locality mentioned. There were only two known sources of asbestos in Greece and its vicinity in ancient times: Karystos at the southern extremity of the island of Euboea, and a place to the southeast of Mt. Troodos on Cyprus, where the abandoned workings are still to be seen today.
>
> It is much more probable that Theophrastus [was] referring to the well-known brown fibrous lignite, which in appearance and in other respects very often closely resembles rotten wood. Lignite of various kinds is known to occur in the region named by Theophrastus. … Lignite of the kind to which he apparently refers often contains in its natural state as much as 20 per cent of water; thus it cannot readily be ignited.

Maines (8) refers to Chinese, Singhalese and Indian sources concerning the use of asbestos in antiquity. She (8) mentions Lih-tsze who wrote near the end of the 5th century BCE concerning a fireproof cloth that was cleaned by fire. It is also claimed that Herodotus recorded the use of asbestos in a cremation shroud (5, 10, 11).

Gaius Plinius Secundus (23/24–79 CE), better known as Pliny the Elder, certainly refers to asbestos in book XXXVI.xxi of his *Natural History* where he commented (12):

> Asbestos looks like alum and is completely fire-proof; it also resists all magic potions, especially those concocted by the Magi.

Maines (8) refers to book XIX.iv:

> Chapter IV. Also a linen has now been invented that is incombustible. It is called 'live' linen, and I have seen napkins made of it glowing on the hearth at banquets and burnt more brilliantly clean by the fire than they could be by being washed in water. This linen is used for making shrouds for Royalty, which keep the ashes of the corpse separate from the rest of the pyre.

Having stated this, it appears that Pliny thought that asbestos was a plant that grew,

> in the deserts and sun-scorched regions of India where no rain falls, the haunts of deadly snakes, and it is habituated to living in burning heat; it is rarely found, and is difficult to weave into cloths because of its shortness. … The Greek name for it is asbestinon, derived from its peculiar properties.

It is sometimes claimed that Pliny had warned of the dangers of asbestos and that slaves who worked with the material wore masks to protect against the dust (6). However, Maines (8) asserts that no reference can be found to the wearing of masks by "slaves" who worked with this material—so that the often-repeated claim on this issue appears to be in error. It seems more likely that the masks were worn by artisans who worked with cinnabar, not asbestos, and Pliny apparently does not state that the artisans were slaves (Book XXXIII.xli) (8).

It is said that Pausanias (ca. 175 CE) recorded a gold lamp made by Callimachus of Athens for the goddess Minerva, which had a wick made of Carpasian linen—"the only linen which is not consumed by fire" (10). Over a thousand years later, in *The Travels*, Marco Polo (13) described cloths used by Tartars in the Khanate Province of Ghinghintalas, during the Yüan dynasty:

> When the stuff found in this vein … has been dug out of the mountain and crumbled into bits, the particles cohere and form fibres like wool … Then this wool-like fibre is carefully spun and made into cloths. When the cloths are first made, they are far from white. But they are thrown into the fire and left there for a while; and there they turn as white as snow. And whenever one of these cloths is soiled or discoloured, it is thrown into the fire and left there for a while, and it comes out as white as snow … One of these cloths is now at Rome; it was sent to the Pope by the Great Khan as a valuable gift.
>
> **(pp 89–90)**

Marco Polo's account clearly indicated that asbestos is mineral in character as opposed to the hair of a mythical fire-resistant salamander as widely supposed in Medieval superstition.

It has been claimed that the Emperor Charlemagne (?742–814 CE) had a tablecloth made of asbestos, thrown into the fire after dinner, to the amazement of his guests, but this story seems apocryphal (8). However, Maines (8) refers to an account by Ibn al-Fatiq, who recorded that 10th-century Christian pilgrims to Jerusalem were sold small pieces of what appears to have been asbestos, claimed to have been fragments of the True Cross, the divine and magical properties of which were proven by their incombustibility.

Benjamin Franklin, when he found himself broke in London, paid his bills by selling an asbestos purse to a curiosity-collector. Earlier letters suggest that he sought out the collector, but later in life he wrote (14):

> I had brought some curiosities with me from America; the principal of which was a purse made of the asbestos, which fire only purifies. Sir Hans Sloane hearing of it called upon me and invited me to his house in Bloomsbury-square, where, after showing me everything that was curious, he prevailed on me to add this piece to his collection; for which he paid me very handsomely.

Either way, asbestos at that time, was a cherished and desirable curiosity.

Much later, the chevalier Jean Albini (1762–1834)—nephew of Galvani and a professor of physics at the University of Bologna—used asbestos cloth to make a fire-resistant suit that he exhibited in several European cities and at the Royal Institution in London in 1829 (15).

1.3 ASBESTOS FROM THE BEGINNING OF THE INDUSTRIAL ERA

A useful account of the modern history of asbestos has been set forth by Frank (16) and by Hammar and Dodson (3). By about 1850, chrysotile deposits had been found around Thetford in Canada and at about that time the fire-resistant properties of asbestos were demonstrated by a forest fire in the mid-1870s, where the rocky outcrops of asbestos deposits did not burn, unlike the trees (16). According to Frank (16), about 50 tons of asbestos were mined in Quebec by 1876, and by the 1950s over 900,000 tons were mined each year (16). In the early 19th century, asbestos was noted in South Africa, particularly in the North-West area of Cape Province, and the name crocidolite was assigned to the blue-grey stone ("wooly stone") (16). According to Frank's account (16), serious production of asbestos in South Africa did not get underway until the early 20th century, with production far less than in Canada, and below about 10,000 tons each year until 1940. In the Transvaal area, amosite (reportedly an acronym for *Asbestos Mines of South Africa*) (3, 16) was mined, and about 80,000 tons of amosite were produced each year by 1970.

Other nations with significant production of asbestos include Russia, where chrysotile was discovered in 1720 in the region of the Ural Mountains near the Tagyl River (17). The deposit was soon mined, and an asbestos cloth produced therefrom was presented to Peter the Great in 1722 (17). However, by 1735 production was discontinued "due to lack of practical importance of the deposit" (17). In 1765, an anthophyllite deposit was discovered south of Ekaterinburg, in a hill subsequently called Asbestoyaya (17). Still later, the Bazhenovskoye chrysotile deposit was found in late 1884 and mining began in 1886(18) (the Vosnessenskiy mine) (17, 18)—where production of chrysotile still continues around the *monogorod* town of Asbest.[1] Other chrysotile deposits were later found in the middle and southern Urals (17).

Major chrysotile asbestos production continues in Kazakhstan, Zimbabwe (initially the Shabata deposits and then the Shabani mine from about 1950 (3)), and since 2019 the King Mine where asbestos production from old tailings commenced in 2019, Brazil and, more recently, China (16, 19). Curiously, exports from Brazil continue despite a 2017 ban. In July 2019, the government of the State of Goias authorized the extraction of asbestos for export purposes. The effect of a ruling from August 2021, by the Federal Court of Uruacu that the mining must be suspended immediately remains to be seen (19). Figure 1.1 shows worldwide production from 1920 to 2022.

Asbestos was also mined in Italy (e.g., chrysotile at the Balangero mine). In the USA, small deposits of asbestos were mined in Vermont, Arizona and California, as well as even smaller deposits of anthophyllite in North Carolina and Georgia (16). The use of asbestos in the USA (20) is shown in Table 1.2 for the years 1920–2022.

In Australia, approximately 47 tonnes of amphiboles were mined at Jones' Creek, near Gundagai, New South Wales, between 1880 and 1889, and about 35 tonnes of chrysotile were mined at Anderson's Creek, Tasmania, between 1890 and 1899. South Australia was the first State to mine crocidolite, in a very small mine at Robertstown in 1916. During the 20th century there was a gradual increase in asbestos production, with more chrysotile than amphiboles mined until 1939. After commencement of mining at Wittenoom in Western Australia (WA) (21) in 1937, crocidolite dominated production until final closure in 1966. New South Wales, the first State to mine asbestos, also produced the largest tonnages of chrysotile (until 1983) as well as smaller quantities of amphiboles (until 1949). With the closure of the crocidolite mine at Wittenoom in 1966, Australian asbestos production declined to a pre-1952 level. Exports declined from 1967. Imports of chrysotile also began to decline. The earliest records of asbestos imports date from 1929: the main sources of raw asbestos imports were Canada (chrysotile) and South Africa (crocidolite and amosite). About twice as much chrysotile was imported as was mined, and half as much crocidolite was imported than was mined. After Wittenoom was closed, a small amount (122 tonnes) of crocidolite was mined in South Australia. In New South Wales, the chrysotile mine at Baryulgil continued production. In 1971, the chrysotile deposits at Woodsreef near Barraba, New South Wales began to be exploited and exports of asbestos fiber expanded as production increased; this operation was open-cast with dry milling.

Australian production of asbestos decreased in 1981 because of the drop in world demand for asbestos and the increased operating costs at the Woodsreef mine. This mine ceased production in 1983 when the dry milling plant could not meet dust control regulations. Tables 1.3. and 1.4 set forth data for the production, importation and consumption of asbestos in Australia.22

In this context, it has been asserted by some authors such as Price and Ware (23) and Kelsh et al. (24) (with no cited supporting evidence)—that "the Australian high rates of [malignant mesothelioma] are not unexpected due to widespread environmental exposures to high levels of amphibole asbestos including crocidolite" (23). In reality in Australia, most mesotheliomas are attributable to specifically identifiable asbestos exposure, especially amphibole-containing exposures, whether occupational (direct and bystander) or non-occupational, and including low-"dose" exposures from identified point sources of exposure (25). Studies on airborne asbestos fiber concentrations in the general urban environment have not demonstrated environmental exposures significantly in excess of those recorded for other nations. For example, a 1990 report from the *Western Australian Advisory Committee on Hazardous Substances* (26), found that among schools in WA—mainly schools in Perth, the capital city of the Australian State where the Wittenoom Blue Asbestos Industry was located—the airborne concentrations of asbestos fibers were less than 0.002 fiber/mL, perhaps even less than that figure by one order of magnitude (i.e., below the working detection limit).[2] These fiber levels in the "general environment" are comparable to those recorded in other nations—e.g., see references (27) and (28). However, if there is damage to the building materials, increased fiber concentrations of up to 4 fiber/mL are described (29). Abatement activities can be a source of exposure (30). JC Wagner in his foreword to the author's 1992 book *Malignant Mesothelioma* comments that

"The wholesale removal of chrysotile from buildings is absurd" (31). However, more recent publications suggest that the presence of asbestos in the build environment can affect air quality in some instances (32).

Major producers of asbestos now include Russia, Kazakhstan and China (19). Russian production in 2021 was about 700,000 tonnes followed by 250,000 tonnes in Kazakhstan, 120,000 tonnes in China and 110,000 tonnes in Brazil (see Table 1.5 for data for 2021). In 2000, the worldwide production of asbestos was 2,130,000 tonnes, mostly chrysotile from Canada, Russia and China, with a sharp decline in production thereafter (see Figure 1.1). As mentioned in the first paragraph of this chapter, over 60 nations (including the UK, Europe (33), Scandinavian countries, Australia and Japan) have now banned the use of all forms of asbestos, apart from a few special applications for which no substitute is available.

It appears that on average the largest importers of asbestos in 2019 were India (374,649 tons), Indonesia 122,142 tons) China (127,551,000 tons) and Uzbekistan (94,167,700 tons). Among countries with no asbestos bans in place the USA is among those with the lowest per capita consumption (16) (https://dataweb.usitc.gov/trade/search, accessed August 31, 2023). The U.S. International Trade Commission for 2022 reports a total of 232 tons of raw chrysotile imports, the bulk of which came from Brazil (https://dataweb.usitc.gov/trade/search, accessed August 31, 2023). Those imports are driven by the chlor-alkali industry. In contrast, whilst the European Union introduced a ban on the use of *all* asbestos products in 2005 (noting that many of its member nations had implemented bans much earlier), in 2019, 1252 tons of asbestos were imported into the European Union (https://wits.worldbank.org/, accessed August 31, 2023).

Japan has been an importer of asbestos as opposed to a significant producer. Little asbestos was used in Japan during World War II because of the Allies' blockade, but its use steadily increased after 1945. In 1960, 77,000 tons of asbestos were imported into Japan, reaching a peak of 352,316 tons in 1974. The amount of raw asbestos imported between 1930–2005 totaled 9,879,865 tons (34, 35) and as a consequence there was a rise in asbestos-related diseases, similar to Western industrialized nations. This led to a governmental decision toward a ban in 2002, and since 2006, zero tons of asbestos have been imported.

The major uses of asbestos have included (16):

- The use of asbestos (both chrysotile and commercial amphiboles)—as an insulating and fire-resistant material in a variety of circumstances that include commercial buildings, ships (naval vessels including submarines, merchant ships and passenger liners[3]), power stations, locomotives, as insulation around steam pipes and in boilers of all types and furnaces and ovens, and the list goes on.
- The use of both chrysotile or crocidolite or amosite in differing proportions in asbestos-cement building materials, including asbestos-cement walls; the use of thick asbestos blocks in wet areas of houses, and in the roofs of houses, for example, in the eaves; and as corrugated asbestos-cement roofing material itself. Such high-density asbestos products were based on the capacity of asbestos fibers to add tensile strength to such materials, their lightness in terms of weight, and their fire-resistance and insulating properties.
- The use of chrysotile in particular for brake blocks/linings and gaskets.
- Asbestos textiles (chrysotile) for the production of asbestos blankets, fire-resistant and insulating suits, for example, for firemen and workers in foundries, as well as asbestos rope.
- The use of asbestos filters, for example, in gas masks and as a filter for wine.
- Other occasional or idiosyncratic uses such as blue asbestos mattresses; the use of asbestos in fire-resistant paints; and the production of asbestos paper (asbestos was also used in the production of "ordinary" paper).

The use of asbestos in ships is particularly noteworthy. Ships of all types are particularly vulnerable to fire at sea with problems in the evacuation of passengers and crew from vessels on fire (7). One of the most notorious examples concerned the *Morro Castle* in 1934, when it appears the captain was murdered by a member of the crew who then set fire to the focsle of the ship (7). The first mate, who had assumed command, appears to have been very inexperienced and steered the ship toward the nearest port, but in doing so headed the ship into the wind, which then blew the fire back along the vessel, resulting in the deaths of some 137 people (7).

1.4 EVOLUTION OF KNOWLEDGE CONCERNING ASBESTOS-RELATED DISEASES

1.4.1 Asbestosis

By definition, *asbestosis* refers to diffuse interstitial fibrosis affecting lung parenchyma, induced by the inhalation and deposition of asbestos fibers (40–43).

Castleman(6) refers to mention by the Viennese physician Netolitzky of the "emaciation and pulmonary problems in asbestos weavers" in his *Handbuch der Hygiene* (1897), and in Great Britain the first reference to the injurious effects of asbestos seems to have been made by the Lady Inspectors of Factories in 1898. Castleman (6) sets forth the following quotation concerning their observations:

> In the case of one particular asbestos works … far from any precaution having been taken, the work (sifting, mixing, and carding) appeared to be carried on with the least possible attempt to subdue the dust.

Reportedly, an inspection in 1906 revealed a "thick, foglike atmosphere of dust … the atmosphere is of a thick whitey-yellow consistency" (6).

The first patient with asbestosis for whom a record seems to exist was a 33-year-old man seen in 1899 by Dr H. Montague Murray at the Charing Cross Hospital in London (5). Before his death in 1900, the patient was the sole survivor of 10 men who had worked together in the carding room of an asbestos factory (all the others had died at around 30 years of age). Murray's case was never published in detail in the mainstream medical literature, but in evidence to the Departmental Committee on Industrial Diseases in 1906, Murray referred to the presence of spicules of asbestos in sections of the lung (5).

Germany never produced raw asbestos on a significant scale, perhaps explaining why fatalities from asbestosis were not reported there until 1914, but products manufacture did take place (44). Alexander von Humboldt in 1797 reported on the presence and properties of serpentinite (serpentine rock) within veins of asbestos in certain mines, in his role as mining inspector in the Kegelgebirge (45). According to Proctor (44), asbestos at about that time was often called *Bergflachs* in Germany ("mountain flax"), and asbestosis was known as *Bergflachslunge*. In 1914, Fahr recorded the presence of crystals in the lung tissue of German patients with asbestosis.

In 1918, a statistician with the Prudential Insurance Company referred to premature mortality among asbestos workers, after which those workers were refused life insurance (6).

In 1924, Cooke (46) published the first account of asbestosis in the English language literature. Detailed descriptions followed in 1927 (10, 47), complete with high-quality photomicrographs of asbestos bodies (then referred to as "curious bodies" (47)). Cooke's case appears to have been that of Nellie Kershaw who worked for Turner Brothers Asbestos Company from the age of 13 and intermittently after she was aged 26, until her total disability at 31 and her death at the age of 33(6). It seems that a doctor's certificate referred to her having sustained "asbestos poisoning," but Turner and Newall (T&N) Industries repudiated that diagnosis and noted that no such condition was listed among the compensable diseases in the Workmen's Compensation Act (6) (one of the first in a long litany of denial and suppression of information, and then derisory *ex gratia* payments to the partners of those who had died—vividly described in Tweedale's book *Magic Mineral to Killer Dust: Turner & Newall and the Asbestos Hazard* (1)—subject to an undertaking that there would be no further claim against the company for a particular case.) Castleman's book *Asbestos: Medical and Legal Aspects* (6) discusses further reports on asbestosis in the medical literature in Great Britain.

In 1930, Merewether and Price completed an investigation into the asbestos textile industry in the UK (6). They found that about 26% of workers examined had asbestosis and a further 21 of 363 cases had "precursive signs" of the disease. They also found that the severity of the asbestosis and its speed of development appeared to correlate with the intensity of the exposure.

A memorable publication was that by Wood and Gloyne (48) in 1934. These authors reviewed 100 cases of asbestosis and outlined the circumstances in which asbestosis was encountered:

> The picture of pulmonary asbestosis is that of a pneumonoconiosis occurring in a factory in which few precautions have been taken to protect the workers from a danger, the gravity of which was not realised. Happily these conditions are now a thing of the past. … There is thus good reason to believe that the disease is now under control [*sic!*].

It is also worth pointing out that one of the asbestosis cases reported by Wood and Gloyne (48) concerned an 18-year-old van boy who mixed asbestos in an open yard for a period of about 2.5 years.

In 1938, Dreessen et al. (49) published an extensive study of asbestosis in the asbestos textile industry in Charleston, South Carolina, where Canadian commercial chrysotile was used almost exclusively (in this regard, chrysotile appears to be less potent for the induction of almost any asbestos disease than the amphiboles, with the exception of the asbestos textile industry). Dreessen et al. (49) suggested that an airborne asbestos dust concentration under 5 million particles per cubic foot (mppcf) would probably prevent the development of asbestosis. However, as acknowledged by Dreessen et al. (49) themselves, their study was flawed, because about 150 workers in the factory had been replaced by other workers "with little or no previous asbestos exposure" about 15 months before the study began (apparently, many of the 150 workers who left did so because they had asbestosis, and although efforts were made to trace them, less than half could be examined). Accordingly, there was an "abnormally large percentage of workers with less than five years' employment" in that industry at the time of the study. Nonetheless, Dreessen et al. (49) suggested their standard of 5.0 mppcf or less was appropriate until better data could be derived, and it became a widely used standard (it was introduced into Victoria in Australia in about 1945). In this regard, in order to convert mppcf into asbestos fibers per mL of air, a conversion factor of about 3 is generally used, so that 5.0 mppcf corresponds to about 15 fibers/mL (50), but a number of studies have used a variety of different conversion factors, so there are problems in extrapolating from counts expressed as mppcf to airborne asbestos fiber concentrations in terms of fibers/mL (33, 50). In fact, *The Dreessen Standard* did *not* prevent the development of asbestosis in many workers exposed to airborne asbestos fibers at a level of 5.0 mppcf or even substantially less.

On pages 43–44 of their report, Dreessen et al. (49) also recommended the following:

- Control of dust at the point of origin with dust-removal devices.
- Replacement of dust-laden air by clean air, by the use of exhaust systems attached to the equipment.
- The use of "approved types of respirators."
- "Periodic studies of the condition of the working environment … to determine whether the control methods adopted are constantly adequate. This requires the dust concentrations to be determined for each operation."

It is notable that in many work situations—in both industry and especially at various points of end-use of asbestos-containing materials such as work in the building construction industry—no systematic measurements of airborne dust/fiber concentrations were carried out.

In 1968, the British Occupational Hygiene Society (BOHS) proposed a limit of 2 fibers/mL of air for amosite and chrysotile (immediately introduced by government) to reduce the incidence of asbestosis in a workforce to 1% (1, 51). In 1970, a British government-issued note advised workplace inspectors that no action was required when fiber levels were below 2 fibers/mL; that for fiber concentrations ranging from 2 to 12 fibers/mL further readings should be taken; and only when the levels were above 12 fibers/mL over a 10-minute average should the use of exhaust ventilator and respirators be advised (1). The BOHS did not attempt to set a standard for control of mesothelioma or lung cancer. Flaws in the proposed standard were apparent in the published report (e.g., failure to include ex-workers causing bias, and taking clinical findings on trust) (51). The whole BOHS process in 1966–1968 has since been critically evaluated and the standard shown to have been too high by a factor of about ten (51).

1.4.2 Asbestos-Related Lung Cancer

In 1938 three German papers and a review from Austria reported evidence of a link between asbestosis and lung cancer (44), and Nordmann (52) referred to this occurrence as *der Berufskrebs der Asbestarbeiter* (the occupational cancer of asbestos workers). In his book *The Nazi War on Cancer,* Proctor (44) comments in the chapter on *Occupational Carcinogenesis* that the German reports were the most convincing at that time, although anecdotal autopsy reports of lung cancer in patients with asbestosis had been reported earlier, beginning in the mid-1930s (53–56). Proctor (44) mentions that Franz Koelsch noted in 1938 that the 12 cases of asbestosis-related lung cancer reported by that time "while suggestive, did not prove the link," whereas Ludwig Teleki in Vienna expressed greater confidence ("extremely likely"). Nordmann thought that about 12% of asbestosis patients would develop lung cancer. In 1939, Wedler stated that "there was not the slightest doubt ('*kaum ein Zweifel daran*') that asbestos in the lungs could cause cancer" (44), and a 1942 review remarked on the reluctance ("*grosse Zurückhaltung*") of English and American scientists to acknowledge the link. In 1941, Nordmann and Sorge (57) induced lung tumors in mice subjected to inhalation of chrysotile asbestos (*Chrysotilasbest*): a photograph of the apparatus used for this experiment is reproduced on page 112 of Proctor's book (44). In 1943, the German government designated lung cancer in association with any degree of asbestosis as a compensable disease (44, 58). In a world preoccupied with other issues, no attention seems to have been given to this matter, and the analysis of the association between asbestos/asbestosis and lung cancer languished until 1955 when it was further revived by Doll (59).

In 1991, Enterline (58) commented on the gap of about 12 years between the recognition of the link between asbestos in Germany, and the publication of Doll's paper in 1955:

> A lack of experimental and epidemiological evidence played a major role in delaying a consensus [on asbestos and lung cancer]. Other important factors included a rejection of science conducted outside of the U.S. during this period, particularly a rejection of German scientific thought during and after WWII, and a rejection of clinical evidence in favor of epidemiological investigations. Individual writers rarely changed their minds on the subject of asbestos as a cause of cancer.

During the 1930s and 1940s, assessment of causation of cancer was approached largely from a clinical (e.g., case series) and experimental approach, whereas epidemiologic investigations were in their infancy (including studies on the role of tobacco smoke in the causation of lung cancer).

In opening his 1955 paper, Doll (59) stated that some 61 cases of lung cancer had been recorded in association with asbestosis: the "large number" of cases was considered suggestive but did not prove that "lung cancer is an occupational hazard among asbestos workers." He placed stronger emphasis on: (i) Merewether's 1949 observation that lung cancer was found at autopsy in 31 of 235 cases of asbestosis (13.2%) but only 91 out of 6,884 cases of silicosis (1.3%); and (ii) Gloyne's finding at autopsy of lung cancer in 17 of 121 cases of asbestosis (14.1%) in comparison to 55 out of 796 cases of silicosis (6.9%). In Doll's study, lung cancer was found at autopsy in 18 cases among 105 deceased workers at one asbestos factory, 15 of the cases being associated with asbestosis. In addition (59).

> One hundred and thirteen men who had worked for at least 20 years in places where they were liable to be exposed to asbestos were followed up and the mortality among them compared with that which would have been expected on the basis of the mortality experience of the whole male population. Thirty-nine deaths occurred in the group whereas 15.4 were expected. The excess was entirely due to excess deaths from lung cancer (11 against 0.8 expected)[4] … All the cases of lung cancer were confirmed histologically and all were associated with presence of asbestosis.
> … the average risk among men employed for 20 or more years has been of the order of 10 times that experienced by the general population. The risk has become progressively less as the duration of employment under the old dusty conditions has decreased.

Causation of lung cancer by asbestos is discussed elsewhere.

1.5 ASBESTOS EXPOSURE AND MESOTHELIOMA: HISTORICAL KNOWLEDGE

The causal relationship between asbestos and mesothelioma had been well established by the late 1960s, and at that time it was recognized that mesothelioma could follow exposures to asbestos that were non-occupational in character—brief, transient and low-"dose"—including, for example, the development of mesothelioma from asbestos exposures related to "handyman"-type work on asbestos-cement building materials; and the development of mesothelioma from bystander, environmental and neighborhood-type exposures was described in 1965 (60, 61).

Two cases of mesothelioma were described by Wedler in 1943 (62, 63), two by Cartier in Canada in 1952 (64) and three by van der Schoot in Holland in 1958 (65). However, the relationship between asbestos exposure (most notably crocidolite [blue asbestos] exposure) and pleural mesothelioma was more firmly established in 1960 in the seminal paper by Wagner et al. (66).[5]

Of the 33 cases comprising that series of mesotheliomas (66), several did not involve *direct* occupational exposures to asbestos but rather *indirect/environmental* exposures. For example, Case 3 involved a 53-year-old woman who "lived her whole life in a location near an asbestos mill." Cases 5, 6, 8 and 9 also involved patients who lived in the vicinity of mines. Case 15 was a 42-year-old woman whose mother also had mesothelioma and who "lived at mine until age of 20; went to school near cobbing sheds." Case 20 concerned a 53-year-old woman who "spent [her] whole life in village on wagon route to Kimberley." Case 21 was a 44-year-old man "who lived in the vicinity of mines until the age of 16; often on dumps as a child." Case 23 was a 63-year-old woman who "lived in the vicinity of the mines until the age of 30." Case 24 was a 35-year-old man who "lived in the vicinity of a mill from the age of 1–7; played on the dumps as a child." Case 25 was a 50-year-old woman who "lived in a mining area from the age of 10 to 18 years; after 1918 spent whole life in same town as case 24" (the 35-year-old man referred to above).

Smither et al. (76) and McCaughey et al. (77) recorded further cases of asbestos-related mesothelioma in 1962 in the *British Medical Journal*, and the comment was made that the asbestos exposures for some cases of mesothelioma had been "minimal."[35] The first case of asbestos-related mesothelioma in Australia was published in 1962 in the *Medical Journal of Australia* (78). In the same year, Wagner et al. (79) published studies on the mucin histochemistry of mesothelioma (80) and on the induction of mesothelioma in experimental animals by asbestos (in the journal *Nature*). In 1962, the third edition of Hunter's *The Diseases of Occupations* referred to the remarkable association of mesothelioma with asbestos, citing the Wagner 1960 study. At that time there were no clear distinctions between the potency of different asbestos fiber types for the induction of mesothelioma.[6]

In the USA, Selikoff and his coworkers documented the risks of cancer, and specifically mesothelioma, from asbestos exposure in 1964 and 1965 in the *Journal of the American Medical Association* (*JAMA*) (92) and in the *New England Journal of Medicine* (93) as well as the induction of mesothelioma in hamsters by asbestos, including amosite (94).

In their 1964 paper in *JAMA* dealing with neoplasia and asbestos exposure among insulation workers, Selikoff et al. (92) also commented:

> A particular variety of environmental exposure may be of even greater concern. Asbestos exposure in industry will not be limited to the particular craft that utilizes the material. The floating fibers do not respect job classifications. Thus, for example, insulation workers undoubtedly share their exposure with their workmates in other trades: intimate contact with asbestos is possible for electricians, plumbers, sheet-metal workers, steamfitters, laborers, carpenters, boiler makers, and foremen; perhaps even the supervisory architect should be included.

In 1965, Newhouse and Thompson (60, 61) described the occurrence of mesotheliomas as a consequence of: (i) *domestic (household contact) asbestos exposure* among the wives who shook out and laundered the asbestos-contaminated work clothes of their partners; and (ii) *neighborhood exposures* to asbestos. For example, these authors (61) referred to the following in relation to neighborhood exposures:

> The factory where more than a fifth of the series were employed opened in 1913, having been situated nearer the City of London for the previous seven years. There were three affected female patients living within half a mile of the factory during the seven years it was in production at its first site. At the time it opened, they were children between five and seven years old. At the present site, there were eight patients living with a half mile radius of the factory. One, a male, was born within a quarter of a mile of the factory in 1922 and remained at the same address for 16 years. The other seven were females and aged between six and 13 when the factory opened. They remained in the area for only between three and seven years, except for one who remained at the same address until she died 48 years later. …
>
> Thus, among those with no occupational or domestic exposures to asbestos there are 11 (30.6%) of the patients in the mesothelioma series and five (7.6%) in the control series who lived within half a mile of the factory at its present and previous sites ... The difference in the proportion of patients in the two series who lived in the vicinity of the factory and had no other exposure to asbestos is statistically significant (χ^2 = 7.85, *P* < 0.01).
>
> Including the 11 patients who lived near the asbestos factory there are 51 who had been exposed to asbestos. In 39, exposure first occurred before 1930, in the remaining 12 before 1943. The interval between first exposure and onset of symptoms varied between 16 and 55 years (mean 37.5). The duration of exposure also varied widely, ranging from five weeks to over 50 years.

In the same paper, Newhouse and Thompson (61) commented:

> There seems little doubt of the risk of both occupational and domestic exposure of asbestos. Wagner *et al.* (1950) [*sic*: it should have been 1960] described patients with no other exposure except living as a child in the vicinity of the asbestos mines.

They[44] also referred to mesotheliomas as a consequence of household contact exposure:

> among the women [with mesothelioma] only 10 worked in the asbestos factories and a further 17 had nonindustrial exposures, seven in the home and 10 living near asbestos factories [p 586] … The group of nine, seven women and two men, whose relatives worked with asbestos, are of particular interest. The most usual history was that of the wife who washed her husband's dungarees or work clothes. In one instance we were told that the husband, a docker, came home 'white with asbestos' every evening for three or four years and she brushed him down. The two men in the group, when boys of eight or nine years old, had sisters who were working at the asbestos factory where others of this series were employed. One of these girls worked as a spinner from 1925 to 1936. In 1947 she died of asbestosis. The press report of the inquest states, "she used to return home from work with dust on her clothes." Her brother had no other exposure to asbestos.
>
> **(p. 584).**

In a 1968 review on the *Geographic Pathology of Pleural Mesothelioma* published in the monograph *The Lung* by the International Academy of Pathology, Churg and Selikoff (95) commented as follows:

The tumor [mesothelioma] is more often seen in workers who have only moderate or small amount of asbestos in their lungs, and who show little, if any, clinical or radiologic evidence of pulmonary fibrosis. This amount of asbestos may be inhaled not only by professional asbestos workers, but also by those who handle products containing only a small proportion of asbestos, those who do not handle asbestos at all but merely work alongside asbestos workers such as craftsmen employed in the building industry—carpenters, electricians, etc.—those who have relatives who carry asbestos home in their work clothes and those who live close to asbestos plants. Taken together, this is a large group which can contribute significantly to the incidence of mesothelioma. Beyond that is the general population, particularly the urban population, which, as has been recently been demonstrated, inhales small amounts of asbestos. Reports from Cape Town, South Africa, Miami and Pittsburgh, United States, London, England, and areas of Finland indicate that at least a few asbestos bodies are present in the lungs of 20 to 57% of adults dying in these locations. Because the minimal carcinogenic dose of asbestos has not been established, the significance of this slight exposure is not known. However, the use of asbestos is increasing very rapidly both in quantity (from 500,000 tons per year in 1930 to nearly 4 million in 1965) and in diversity of applications (over 3000 applications now known). The current cases of mesothelioma due to asbestos must be ascribed to the dust inhaled some 30 years ago. The 8-fold increase in asbestos production over these 30 years suggests that there may be an appreciable prevalence of mesothelioma in the years to come, not only among those occupationally exposed but perhaps also among the general population.

1.6 TRADE-OFFS (COST-BENEFIT ARGUMENTS): A DEFENSE OF ASBESTOS?

One of the defenses of the asbestos industry and its apologists is that human life in all its complexity involves the balancing of myriad benefits versus risks: e.g., treatment of diseases with almost any pharmaceutical drug involves probabilistic assessment of the benefit expected for the treatment in question versus non-responsiveness and, more importantly, the risk and severity of side effects (a drug that causes bone marrow aplasia only rarely would clearly require more critical assessment than another drug that caused most of those who take it to sneeze once or twice only) (33). In the case of asbestos, the argument is advanced that the benefits from its past (and in some nations continuing) use far outweighed the disadvantage of the diseases that it caused among a minority of those exposed to it (at older ages than other competitive risks such as fire (7))—even taking into account the fact that lung cancer has a poor prognosis overall and the mortality rate for malignant mesothelioma approaches 100%.

The trade-off argument is sometimes buttressed by specific examples, some apocryphal. A few eclectic quasi-anecdotal examples follow:

- Maines (7) quotes Morgan and Gee (96) to the effect that "the Challenger [space shuttle] disaster was a consequence of substituting a non-asbestos-containing putty … to seal the O-rings of the craft." However, this seems to be an urban myth adduced to emphasize the allegedly baleful consequences of non-use of asbestos. It seems that the *O-rings never contained asbestos and weren't 'putty'*. The late quantum physicist Richard Feynman was a member of the commission appointed by President Ronald Reagan to investigate the Challenger disaster and he pointed out that the cause appeared to be loss of resilience of the *rubber* O-rings at low temperatures. Accordingly, in his biography of Feynman, *Genius: Richard Feynman and Modern Physics* (97), James Gleick wrote:

Feynman noted that there were well-known problems with the rubber O-rings that sealed the joints between sections of the tall solid-fuel rockets … they were *ordinary rubber rings,* thinner than a pencil yet thirty-seven feet long, the circumference of the rocket. They were meant to take the pressure of hot gas and form a seal by squeezing tight into the metal joint. … Feynman pressed Molloy on why resiliency was crucial: a soft metal like lead, squeezed into the gap, would not be able to hold a seal amid the vibration and changing pressure. "If this material weren't resilient for say a second or two," Feynman said, "that would be enough to be a very dangerous situation?" … [emphasis in italics added] …

'Dr Feynman: … I took this stuff that I got out of your seal and I put it in ice water, and I discovered that when you put some pressure on it for a while and then undo it it doesn't stretch back. It stays the same dimension. In other words, for a few seconds at least and more seconds than that, there is no resilience in this particular material when it is at a temperature of 32 degrees [Fahrenheit]. … I believe that has some significance for our problem.' …

When … tests were finally performed on behalf of the commission … they showed that failure of the cold seals had been virtually inevitable—not a freakish event, but a consequence of the plain physics of materials.

- The terrorist attack on the World Trade Center in New York on September 11, 2001, is cited as another example: one of the World Trade Towers had asbestos insulation up to the 40th floor (about half later replaced), whereas the other did not. The fire generated by 90,000 L of aviation fuel would have burned at about 1000°C, and the lightweight structural steel used for construction of the Towers (a "perimeter tube" design) would have softened at about 450°C, losing half its tensile strength at about 650°C. Eagar and Musso (98) commented that:

the building was not able to withstand the intense heat of the jet fuel fire. While it was impossible for the fuel-rich diffuse-flame fire to burn at a temperature high enough to melt the steel, its quick ignition and intense heat caused the steel to lose at least half its strength and to deform, causing buckling or crippling. This weakening and deformation caused a few floors to fall, while the weight of the stories above them crushed the floors below, initiating a domino collapse.

Taking into account these circumstances and the structural damage inflicted by the initial impact of the aircraft, it seems that nothing would have prevented or significantly delayed the collapse of the towers. Conversely, there has been concern about the possible potential health hazards from the asbestos in the dust created when the buildings collapsed (99). A follow-up study of 57 402 rescue workers 14 years after the collapse of the twin towers identified nine mesothelioma cases, resulting in Standardized incidence ratios of 1.38 (0.63–2.62) to 1.51 (0.65–2.98), depending on the method of analysis used.

At a less anecdotal level, Maines' book *Asbestos & Fire: Technological Trade-offs and the Body at Risk* (7) seems to argue that the health consequences were worthwhile as a trade-off against deaths from fire. For example, she states:

In 1948, of the approximately 10,000 Americans who died from fire every year,[7] almost 40% were children—about 10 deaths per day of children of elementary school age or younger. In 1999, the latest year for which the Centers for Disease Control (CDC) have published statistics, 2,355 persons died of mesothelioma and 449 of asbestosis, none of whom were under the age of 15. More *children* died every year from fire, before we built the fire safety system that includes asbestos, than *adults* are now dying from asbestos-related disease.

She also comments that asbestos building materials and fire safety systems for which asbestos materials were an important component "successfully reduced the annual rate of fire deaths in the US from 9.1 per 100,000 in 1913 to 1.0 in 1998." Yet in Table 1.2 where she lists the fire deaths—including the rate per 100,000 people *versus* asbestos use—it is evident that the fire death rate fell from 6.2 down to 3.3 during the years 1947–1970, and for each of those years the use of asbestos was at its peak, at over one billion pounds weight for each of those years, with peak use of almost 1.59 billion pounds in 1965 and 1.47 billion for 1970 (the two years when the use was maximal). Subsequently, between 1975 and 1990, asbestos use declined from 197,308,000 pounds down to 91,156,736 pounds, but during those years of declining use, the fire death rate per 100,000 *declined further* from 2.9 to 2.0—so that the reduction in fire deaths appears to have been explicable at least in part by factors other than asbestos use (e.g., general improvements in building construction and less use of inflammable materials such as wood, as well as fire detectors, sprinkler systems, more efficient fire brigade systems, and so forth).

The "trade-offs" defense is beset with a number of problems from the perspective of history and ethics (discussed in some detail by Smith (100) in the 1992 book *Malignant Mesothelioma*):

- As discussed by Smith (100), there are significant ethical problems in justifying trade-offs in human life—which can essentially involve a pricing of life—although such trade-offs obviously do occur (as examples he cites skyscraper construction, rescue of humans from life-threatening situations where the rescuers' lives are put at risk, and decision-making on resource allocation in medicine). He states (100):

> We can deduce … that to argue that the benefits of asbestos to society outweigh any harm caused to a "small" number of workers is fallacious, because it attempts to equate *incommensurable* values on some imaginary scale of utility.[8] That even a small number of workers die for the benefit of the production of certain consumer products [even if those products save lives] does not make this situation morally right. At best, it is a socially necessary evil that should [be] eliminated as soon as possible by technical advances.

- As shown clearly in Castleman's (6) and Tweedale's (1) books, the asbestos industry was aware of the capacity of asbestos to cause serious disease in the form of asbestosis since the 1930s. Yet the record was one of denial or suppression of the information then available, which was usually not communicated to the workers—raising the issue of consent of the workers to be put at risk by their employment. As Smith states:

> Where there is uncertainty about the risks to health of workers, or a possible threat to the environment, workers and society have an *unqualified, unconditional* right to be informed of those risks in an impartial and understandable way.

Maines (7) comments on what she calls *The Conspiracy of Silence Hypothesis* (p. 160):

> It is an article of faith in the anti-asbestos literature that the dangers of asbestos disease were deliberately kept from all but a privileged few, thus preventing workers from understanding the risks they took in the workplace. … A conspiracy of silence that results in seven hundred publications surely cannot be considered a success, as a spokesman from Johns-Manville pointed out in 1978. … Anyone with an interest in the subject, which apparently did not often include the staff or elected representatives of the insulators or building trades unions, could have learned about these risks as workers in other occupations learned about lead, mercury, gasoline, and other known hazards. An hour in a public library at any time after 1926 would have revealed all of the 'secrets' the asbestos products manufacturers were allegedly trying to conceal.

Of course, there was (and continues to be) a serious imbalance between the resources and information available to individual workers and their union representatives *versus* the employing corporations. If such corporations were in possession of such information, there was (and still is) an over-riding and unbreakable obligation for them to communicate that information to those potentially affected by their products.

Smith (100) comments:

> Governments, whose role is the protection of their citizenry, have a moral obligation to ensure safe working conditions, and even in the worst-case scenario, where there are unavoidable dangers, they are obliged to monitor industrial activities closely and to eliminate dangers whenever possible. One can argue that *all* participants in industrial activity (corporations, governments at all levels, and union organizations) have a responsibility to address these issues. Even so, failure to fulfill the most fundamental role of government—the protection of human life—has no bearing on the moral responsibility

of asbestos (or other) mine operators. X's failure to fulfill one obligation cannot excuse Y from fulfillment of another obligation. Thus, one of the strongest arguments advanced by the asbestos industry in its own defence is logically unsound and morally fallacious.

- An exposure standard designed to prevent asbestosis had been developed by 1938 (49), even though it was flawed and did not prevent the development of this disease (but adherence to the standard would have reduced the frequency and severity of asbestosis). Dreessen et al. (49) had set forth various steps to be taken to reduce exposure to comply with the standard (which included monitoring of airborne dust levels). But in many industries, including the building construction industry and some shipyards, no such measurements were ever carried out. Here, one can comment that enforcement of occupational standards is as strong an obligation of government as compliance is for industry.
- Of course, another defense that has been raised in relation to the causation of mesothelioma is that industry could not have been aware of this risk before 1960 and even for some time thereafter. In response to this claim, one can comment: (i) by 1962 it had been recognized that mesotheliomas had been recorded in those whose exposures seemed to have been "minimal"; and (ii) as stated in footnote on page 367 of *Malignant Mesothelioma* (100):

> an industry cannot reasonably claim immunity for blame or moral accountability for its failure or inability to anticipate a hitherto unforeseen form of occupational disease X, if its control measures have been inadequate to prevent known occupational diseases Y or Z resulting from its activities or products. This is because the industry is already culpable on the basis of prevailing knowledge and it cannot realistically expect absolution simply because its actions (or inactions) have some unpredictable consequences.

1.7 THE GLOBAL BURDEN OF ASBESTOS-RELATED DISEASES

The greatest concern over asbestos-related diseases in industrialized nations now focuses on cancer, especially malignant mesothelioma—including concern over likely future cases of asbestos-induced cancer for developing nations where asbestos use continues and where there are few controls on occupational dust exposures (or a failure to enforce existing standards) and also where there are few restrictions on tobacco smoking (relevant to lung cancer). Asbestos was responsible for 63% of the 349,000 (95% uncertainty interval 269,000 to 427,000) deaths in 2016 that were due to occupational carcinogens. Lung cancer accounted for 86% and mesothelioma for 7.9% of all occupational deaths. The highest mortality rates were seen in high-income regions, likely reflecting the quality of data (101). Despite this limitation, those 218,827 (165,455–274,682) deaths due to asbestos in 2016 alone are much higher than previous estimates of 90,000–100,000 annual deaths from asbestos-related diseases worldwide and the final estimated total in the order of 5–10 million (102).

Predicting the burden of disease is extremely difficult (103). It had been estimated that there are approximately 6000 deaths annually from mesothelioma in the USA (104), but the most recent CDC report identified 62,550 deaths from mesothelioma between 1989 and 2018, suggesting about 3000 deaths/year. Between 2017 and 2019 a total of 2394 deaths from mesothelioma were recorded in the UK.[9] The *incidence* of mesothelioma in these countries (Table 1.6, and illustrated in Figures 1.2 and 1.3) has remained stable between 1990 and 2019, with no or relatively small decreases over the past 30 years in deaths of mesothelioma per 100,000 of population (Figure 1.3). However, the *age-standardized incidence rates* have declined in some countries (106), related to bans of asbestos (Figure 1.4) (107, 108). In Australia, age-standardized rates have declined since the early 2000s (peaking in males at 5.9/100,000 and in all persons at 3.2/100,000) (109). Most mesotheliomas continue to be identified in the Western world even though the use of asbestos is increasing exponentially in the developing world (106). This may be related to a lack of recording and the limited reliability of the diagnosis of mesothelioma. Even in developed countries, changes in diagnoses, including benign to malignant or vice versa are reported in 3–9% of cases that are referred for expert opinion or submitted to review panels for compensation (110–112). The long latency period of 30 to 60 years between exposure and mesothelioma diagnosis is also relevant.

As of 1 November 2022, 722 cases of mesothelioma diagnosed in 2021 had been reported to the Australian Mesothelioma Register (AMR). The number of new cases of mesothelioma reported annually has continually increased between 1982 and 2021—from 135 to 577 for men and from 22 to 145 for women. The year in which the highest overall number of cases (824) were diagnosed is 2017, and it is important to note that the apparent fall in cases in 2021 is likely due to delays in notifications to the AMR, in no small part due to COVID-19. Particularly notable is the increase in the number of cases in women, from 22 in 1982 to 112 in 2005 and 145 in 2021 (113) (107). A similar trend for a rising incidence of mesothelioma in women has been recorded in the UK (114) and the USA (115, 116). In Israel, between 1978 and 1980 and between 1993 and 1996 the incidence among females increased from 0.33 to 2.56 per million/year, paralleling the use of asbestos (117). The shifting of mesothelioma from a mostly male disease to a disease that also affects females in substantial numbers is supported by large international studies (116). This trend indicated that the claim advanced by some authors (118)—that the mesothelioma rate in women has remained unchanged over decades, despite increased use of asbestos, and that this unchanging rate is the "background" (environmental) rate and is evidence of a "threshold" level of asbestos exposure for mesothelioma induction—is wrong. There is general agreement that mesothelioma induction by asbestos is governed by a cumulative dose–response relationship *with no identified threshold* (e.g., see the World Health Organization Monograph *Environmental Health Criteria 203: Chrysotile Asbestos* (28) and Hodgson and Darnton (91)).

Based on data for Britain, France, Germany, Italy, the Netherlands and Switzerland, Peto et al. (119) predicted in 1999 that the number of men who would die from mesothelioma in Western Europe each year would almost double over the ensuing 20 years, from about 5000 in 1998 to about 9000 around 2018. The numbers would then decline, but they predicted a total of about 250,000 deaths in men for the period 1995–2029. Subsequently, Pelucchi et al. (120) suggested the total number of deaths is likely to be less than the estimate of 250,000. The Global Burden of Disease (GBD) Study for 2019 reports an estimated 29,251 cases of mesothelioma caused by asbestos in that one year alone worldwide (upper and lower estimates 31,006 and 26,668), suggesting that the total number of deaths is higher than what was predicted. Furthermore, the GBD data may also underestimate total numbers, owing to the continuous underrecognition and lack of reporting and recording in many countries.

Because of the long latency interval between first exposure to asbestos and the subsequent diagnosis of the disorder, mesothelioma cases and deaths are expected to continue until 2030–2050, even in those countries that have implemented bans on all forms of asbestos. There have been calls on global bans, but to date this has not been achieved (102, 121). Some countries, such as Brazil, continue mining of asbestos (Figure 1.1 and Table 1.5) beyond the time when national bans were implemented in 2017. In 1998, Canada lodged a complaint with the World Trade Organization (WTO) against the French ban on asbestos that had occurred in 1997, based on a claim that the ban violated free-trade principles. Asbestos thus became the subject of a so-called international trade dispute. Without waiting for the conclusion of this dispute, the European Commission adopted Directive 1999/77/EC to prohibit asbestos beginning January 1, 2005. The WTO made its final decision in 2001: It rejected the Canadian complaint (33) and concluded that "it is undisputed that WTO Members have the right to determine the level of protection of health that they consider appropriate in a given situation." The WTO response agreed that the ban "protects human life or health" and upheld that the ban was justified. The impact on incidence rates after bans is starting to become noticeable in some countries, most pronounced in those countries with high rates of mesothelioma (122), and is visualized in Figure 1.4.

1.8 SUMMARY

Asbestos-related diseases have imposed significant morbidity and mortality across industrialized nations approximately for the last 80 years and will continue to do so for decades to come, as a consequence of past exposures to asbestos during the 1950s to the 1980s and beyond—in part because of the latency interval between exposure and subsequent disease such as asbestosis, lung cancer and malignant mesothelioma. In addition, the use of chrysotile asbestos continues, especially in developing and now Asian nations (chrysotile is still mined in and exported from Russia, Brazil (despite a ban), Kazakhstan, China and Zimbabwe, and some of these countries also mine for domestic usage. The nations that continue to import asbestos include India, Sri Lanka and Indonesia, among others. Many of the nations to which asbestos is exported have poor surveillance and controls on occupational exposures (123), limited recording disease incidence, and in many such countries the situation is compounded by the high frequency of cigarette smoking. Asbestos-related diseases will continue to plague mankind for the foreseeable future.[10]

NOTES

1. A monogorod town is one based upon and exists because of a single industry, such as Togliatti in the former Soviet Union, which came into existence for the specific purpose of automobile production.
2. All but one of the 13 schools inspected had asbestos-cement (AC) roofs; a visual inspection was carried out and samples were taken from each of the roofs and samples were also taken from gutters, downpipes and soil. The condition of the roofs was assessed and ranked on a scale of 1–5, with the score of 1 indicating that the condition was virtually as good as new and a score of 5 corresponding to extensive deterioration. The roofs ranged in size from small to very large and they had been in place for 10–34 years. Only one achieved a ranking of 1 (time of construction unknown); all others had scores of 2–5, and the highest scores correlated with the longest times since construction. The percentage asbestos content for the roof samples ranged from zero, to 40% in one sample, and most samples contained 10–20%. Crocidolite was detected in six of 18 roof samples (only in roofs 30 or more years old), and amosite was identified in 14 out of 18; all samples contained chrysotile. High-volume air sampling (about 10 m^3) was carried over 24 hours out at three sites whenever possible at each of seven schools—a classroom, a verandah and a remote open site such as a sports field—using a vertical elutriator/37 mm cassette/vacuum pump and was studied by both phase-contrast light microscopy and scanning electron microscopy (SEM). Despite more than 100 hours of scanning, not a single fiber was found in 20 samples; a single amosite fiber attached to a 3.25 µm non-fibrous particle and assessed as non-respirable was found at one school. Not one fiber was found on air sampling either in central Perth or in a rural town some 100 km east of Perth (York). Air sampling carried out in 1989 in a railways workshop in Perth—where there were more than "8 acres" of AC roofing more than 60 years old—revealed a concentration of more than 0.01 fibers/mL in one sample from the "asbestos shed" used for asbestos removal (as assessed by phase-contrast light microscopy: PCLM); two other samples with fiber concentrations of 0.05 and 0/02 fibers/mL (PCLM) from the same "shed" were then assessed by SEM: in one of these samples, only one of 16 fibers was asbestos, and there were no asbestos fibers in the other.
3. The present authors' files include cases of mesothelioma among workers involved in the dismantling of German U-boats after World War II, in Barrow-in-Furness (36).. The health issues associated with the ship-breaking which typically occurs in places with little occupational health measures are increasingly being recognized (3738–39).
4. Some notable aspects of Doll's paper include the following: (i) for the 18 lung cancers in "… a large asbestos works …," there were eight deaths in the first half of the period 1935–1952, all associated with asbestosis, whereas there were 10 deaths during the second half, seven associated with asbestosis and three without; (ii) the consistent association with asbestosis in the follow-up study is unsurprising, given that all the workers were involved in "scheduled areas" (dusty trades) for at least 20 years; and (iii) there was no adjustment for smoking. In addition, at that time there was no way to estimate how much the risk of lung cancer would decline with reducing exposures (i.e., it is obvious that the follow-up for the second half of the period studied was substantially shorter than for the first half). Tweedale G. *Magic Mineral to Killer Dust: Turner & Newall and the Asbestos Hazard.* Oxford: Oxford University Press (2000) has given a graphic account of the industry's attempts to prevent publication of Doll's paper.

5. In 1991/1992, Wagner set out the story of how he came to discover the relationship between asbestos and mesothelioma (31, 67). He commented on the fiber types implicated in the causation of mesothelioma (31):
   1990: There is overwhelming evidence that crocidolite is the main fiber associated with mesotheliomas. Amosite has been associated with a few mesotheliomas in South Africa and a few more in the United States, but these cases are minimal when compared with those caused by crocidolite.
   In fact, by 1990 amosite had been implicated in the causation of mesothelioma in the USA (68–71) and is now recognized as the most common fiber type implicated in mesothelioma causation in the USA, especially in insulation workers (72–75).
6. The Amphibole Hypothesis was developed later during the 1980s and published most clearly in the paper by Mossman et al. (81) in the journal *Science* in 1990. It has been the subject of debate in the literature during the 1990s (82–89). But most authorities (including the authors of this chapter) now recognize the differential potency of the amphiboles (crocidolite; amosite; non-commercial amphiboles, notably tremolite) versus chrysotile for the causation of mesothelioma in particular (4, 33, 90).
7. In her Table 1.2, she gives a figure of 7688.
8. It also begs the question: who decides?
9. See: https://www.cdc.gov/cancer/uscs/about/data-briefs/no27-incidence-malignant-mesothelioma-1999-2018.htm; Takala J. ILO's role in the global fight against asbestos. European Asbestos Conference, 2003. http://www.hvbg.de/e/asbest/konfrep/konfrepe/repbeitr/takala_en.pdf and https://www.cancerresearchuk.org/health-professional/cancer-statistics/statistics-by-cancer-type/mesothelioma/mortality.
10. On the 18th March 2024 the US Environmental Protection Agency s banned chrysotile asbestos. There is a transition periods of up to 12 years for some chlor-alkali plants using asbestos to complete the transition because of the need to construct new facilities and obtain new permits, and the gaskets used to protect workers from radiation during the disposal of nuclear materials remain exempt.

REFERENCES

1. Tweedale G. *Magic Mineral to Killer Dust: Turner & Newall and the Asbestos Hazard*. Oxford: Oxford University Press; 2000.
2. Craighead JE, Gibbs A, Pooley F. Mineralogy of asbestos. In: Craighead JE, Gibbs AR, editors. *Asbestos and Its Diseases*. Oxford: Oxford University Press; 2008. p. 23–38.
3. Hammar SP, Dodson RF. Asbestos. In: Tomashefski JFJ, editor. *Dail and Hammar's Pulmonary Pathology*, 3rd edition, vol. 1. New York: Springer; 2008. p. 950–1031.
4. Hammar SP, Henderson DW, Klebe S, Dodson RF. Neoplasms of the pleura. In: Tomashefski JFJ, editor. *Dail and Hammar's Pulmonary Pathology*, 3rd edition, vol. 2. New York: Springer; 2008. p. 558–734.
5. Henderson DW, Shilkin KB, Whitaker D. Introduction and historical aspects: With comments on mesothelioma registries. In: Henderson DW, Shilkin KB, Langlois SL, Whitaker D, editors. *Malignant Mesothelioma*. New York: Hemisphere Publishing Corporation; 1992. p. 1–22.
6. Castleman BI. *Asbestos: Medical and Legal Aspects*, 4th edition. New York: Aspen; 1996.
7. Maines R. *Asbestos & Fire: Technological Trade-Offs and the Body at Risk*. New Brunswick: Rutgers University Press; 2005.
8. Maines R. Asbestos before 1880: From natural wonders to industrial material. In: *Asbestos & Fire: Technological Trade-Offs and the Body at Risk*. New Brunswick: Rutgers University Press; 2005. p. 24–44.
9. Caley ER, Richards JFC, editors. *Theophrastus on Stones*. Columbus, OH: Ohio State University; 1956. p. C–300 BCE.
10. Cooke WE. Pulmonary asbestosis. *British Medical Journal*. 1927;2(3491):1024–5.
11. Cooke WE. Asbestos dust and the curious bodies found in pulmonary asbestosis. *British Medical Journal*. 1929;2(3586):578–80.
12. Pliny the Elder. *Natural History. A Selection*, Healy JF, Trans. Harmondsworth: Penguin Classics; 1991, p. 360.
13. Polo M. *The Travels*, Latham R, Trans. Harmondsworth: Penguin; 1979. p. 89–90 (c. 1299).
14. Sweet JM. Benjamin Franklin's purse. *Notes and Records of the Royal Society of London*. 1952;9(2):308–9.
15. Murray R. Asbestos: A chronology of its origins and health effects. *British Journal of Industrial Medicine*. 1990;47(6):361–5.
16. Frank AL. The history of the extraction and uses of asbestos. In: Dodson RF, Hammar SP, editors. *Asbestos: Risk Assessment, Epidemiology and Health Effects. Boca Raton: CRC*. Taylor & Francis; 2006. p. 1–8.

17. Kashansky SV. A 300-year history of the discovery of asbestos in the Urals. In: Peters GA, Peters BJ, editors. *Sourcebook on Asbestos Diseases*, vol. 20. Charlottesville: Lexis; 1999. p. 129–44.
18. Zorina LI, Kashansky SV. The Bazhenovskoye chrysotile asbestos deposits. In: Peters GA, Peters BJ, editors. *Sourcebook on Asbestos Diseases*, vol. 19. Charlottesville: Lexis; 1999. p. 193–204.
19. Flanagan D. Asbestos. In: *Mineral Commodity Summaries*. Reston: Us Geological Survey; 2022.
20. Larson T, Melnikova N, Davis SI, Jamison P. Incidence and descriptive epidemiology of mesothelioma in the United States, 1999–2002. *International Journal of Occupational and Environmental Health*. 2007;13(4):398–403.
21. Layman L. The blue asbestos industry at Wittenoom in Western Australia: A short history. In: Henderson DW, Shilkin KB, Langlois SL, Whitaker D, editors. *Malignant Mesothelioma*. New York: Hemisphere Publishing Corporation; 1992. p. 305–27.
22. Leigh J, Driscoll T.. Malignant mesothelioma in Australia, 1945–2002. *International Journal of Occupational and Environmental Health*. 2003;9(3):206–17.
23. Price B, Ware A. Asbestos exposure and disease trends in the 20th and 21st centuries. In: Craighead JE, Gibbs AR, editors. *Asbestos and Its Diseases*. Oxford: Oxford University Press; 2008. p. 375–96.
24. Kelsh MA, Craven VA, Teta MJ, Mowat FS, Goodman M. Mesothelioma in vehicle mechanics: Is the risk different for Australians? *Occupational Medicine (Oxford, England)*. 2007;57(8):581–9.
25. NOHSC. *The Incidence of Mesothelioma in Australia 1997 to 1999: Australian Mesothelioma Register Report 2002*. Canberra: National Occupational Health and Safety Commission; 2002.
26. Multiple Authors. *Asbestos Cement Products*. Report by the Western Australian Advisory Committee on Hazardous Substances. Perth; 1990.
27. HEI-AR. *Asbestos in Public and Commercial Buildings: A Literature Review and Synthesis of Current Knowledge*. Cambridge, MA: Health Effects Institute - Asbestos Research; 1991.
28. Authors M. *Environmental Health Criteria 203: Chrysotile Asbestos*. Geneva: World Health Organization; 1998.
29. Ganor E, Fischbein A, Brenner S, Froom P. Extreme airborne asbestos concentrations in a public building. *British Journal of Industrial Medicine*. 1992;49(7):486–8.
30. Scarselli A, Corfiati M, Di Marzio D. Occupational exposure in the removal and disposal of asbestos-containing materials in Italy. *International Archives of Occupational and Environmental Health*. 2016;89(5):857–65.
31. Wagner JC. Foreword. In: Henderson DW, Shilkin KB, Langlois SLP, Whitaker D, editors. *Malignant Mesothelioma*. New York: Hemisphere; 1992. p. xvii–xxv.
32. Pawełczyk A, Božek F. Health risk associated with airborne asbestos. *Environmental Monitoring and Assessment*. 2015;187(7):428–.
33. Various Authors. *World Trade Organization (WTO). European Communities -- Measures Concerning Asbestos and Asbestos-containing Products*. Geneva: WTO; 2000.
34. Morinaga K, Kishimoto T, Sakatani M, Akira M, Yokoyama K, Sera Y. Asbestos-related lung cancer and mesothelioma in Japan. *Industrial Health*. 2001;39(2):65–74.
35. Furuya S, Takahashi K. Experience of Japan in achieving a total ban on asbestos. *International Journal of Environmental Research and Public Health*. 2017;14(10).
36. Edge JR, Choudhury SL. Malignant mesothelioma of the pleura in Barrow-in-Furness. *Thorax*. 1978;33(1):26–30.
37. Beckett WS. Shipyard workers and asbestos: A persistent and international problem. *Occupational and Environmental Medicine*. 2007;64(10):639–41.
38. Wu WT, Lin YJ, Li CY, Tsai PJ, Yang CY, Liou SH, et al. Cancer attributable to asbestos exposure in shipbreaking workers: A matched-cohort study. *PLOS One*. 2015;10(7):e0133128.
39. Singh R, Cherrie JW, Rao B, Asolekar SR. Assessment of the future mesothelioma disease burden from past exposure to asbestos in ship recycling yards in India. *International Journal of Hygiene and Environmental Health*. 2020;225:113478.
40. Churg A. Nonneoplastic disease caused by asbestos. In: Churg A, Green FHY, editors. *Pathology of Occupational Lung Disease*, 2nd edition. Baltimore: Williams & Wilkins; 1998. p. 277–338.
41. Mossman BT, Churg A. Mechanisms in the pathogenesis of asbestosis and silicosis. *American Journal of Respiratory and Critical Care Medicine*. 1998;157(5 Pt 1):1666–80.
42. De Vuyst P, Gevenois PA. Asbestosis. In: Hendrick DJ, Burge PS, Beckett WS, Churg A, editors. *Occupational Disorders of the Lung: Recognition, Management, and Prevention*. London: Saunders; 2002. p. 143–62.
43. Sporn TA, Roggli VL. Asbestosis. In: Roggli VL, Oury TD, Sporn TA, editors. *Pathology of Asbestos-Associated Diseases*, 2nd edition. New York: Springer; 2004. p. 71–103.

44. Proctor RN. *The Nazi War on Cancer.* Princeton: Princeton University Press; 1999. p. 73–119.
45. von Humboldt A. Ueber den polarisirenden Serpentinstein. In: *Chemische Annalen für die Freunde der Naturlehre, Aerzneygelahrtheit, Haushaltungskunde und Manufacturen*, vol. 1; 1797. p. 99–112.
46. Cooke WE. Fibrosis of the lungs due to the inhalation of asbestos dust. *British Medical Journal.* 1924;2(3317):147.
47. McDonald S. Histology of pulmonary asbestosis. *British Medical Journal.* 1927;2(3491):1025–6.
48. Wood WB, Gloyne SR. Pulmonary asbestosis: A review of 100 cases. *Lancet.* 1934;2:1383–5.
49. Dreessen WC, Dallavalle JM, Edwards TI, Miller JW, Sayers RR. *A Study of Asbestosis in the Asbestos Textile Industry.* US Treasury Department, Public Health Service: Public Health Bulletin No 241. Washington, DC: United States Government Printing Office; 1938. p. 1–126.
50. Henderson DW, Rödelsperger K, Woitowitz H-J, Leigh J. After Helsinki: A multidisciplinary review of the relationship between asbestos exposure and lung cancer, with emphasis on studies published during 1997–2004. *Pathology.* 2004;36(6):517–50.
51. Greenberg M. The 1968 British occupational hygiene society chrysotile asbestos hygiene standard. In: Peters GA, Peters BJ, editors. *Sourcebook on Asbestos Diseases: Medical, Technical, and Historical Aspects*, vol 14. Charlottesville: Michie; 1997. p. 219–57.
52. Nordmann M. Der Berufskrebs der Asbestarbeiter. *Zeitschrift für Krebsforschung.* 1938;47:288–302.
53. Lynch KM, Smith WA. Pulmonary asbestosis III: Carcinoma of lung in Asbesto-silicosis. *American Journal of Cancer.* 1935;24(1):56–64.
54. Gloyne SR. Two cases of squamous carcinoma of the lung occurring in asbestosis. *Tubercle.* 1935–1936;17:5–10.
55. Egbert DS, Geiger AJ. Pulmonary asbestosis and carcinoma. Report of a case with necropsy findings. *American Review of Tuberculosis.* 1936;34:143–50.
56. Gloyne SR. A case of oat cell carcinoma of the lung occurring in asbestosis. *Tubercle.* 1936–1937;18:100–1.
57. Nordmann M, Sorge A. Lungenkrebs durch Asbestsatub im Tierversuch. *Zeitschrift für Krebsforschung.* 1941;51:170.
58. Enterline PE. Changing attitudes and opinions regarding asbestos and cancer 1934–1965. *American Journal of Industrial Medicine.* 1991;20(5):685–700.
59. Doll R. Mortality from lung cancer in asbestos workers. *British Journal of Industrial Medicine.* 1955;12(2):81–6.
60. Newhouse ML, Thompson H. Mesothelioma of pleura and peritoneum following exposure to asbestos in the London area. *British Journal of Industrial Medicine.* 1965;22(4):261–9.
61. Newhouse ML, Thompson H. Epidemiology of mesothelial tumors in the London area. *Annals of the New York Academy of Sciences.* 1965;132(1):579–88.
62. Wedler HW. Uber den Lungenkrebs bei asbestose. *Deutsches Archiv für Klinische Medizin.* 1943;191:189–209.
63. Wedler HW. Asbestose und Lungenkrebs. *DMW – Deutsche Medizinische Wochenschrift.* 1943;69(31/32):575.
64. Cartier P. In Smith WE. Survey of some current British and European studies of occupational tumor problems. *Archives of Industrial Hygiene and Occupational Medicine.* 1952;5:242–63 (a contribution to the discussion, p. 62).
65. Van der Schoot HC. Asbestosis en pleuragezwellen. *Nederlands Tijdschrift Voor Geneeskunde.* 1958;102(23):1125–6.
66. Wagner JC, Sleggs CA, Marchand P. Diffuse pleural mesothelioma and asbestos exposure in the North Western Cape Province. *British Journal of Industrial Medicine.* 1960;17(4):260–71.
67. Wagner JC. The discovery of the association between blue asbestos and mesotheliomas and the aftermath. *British Journal of Industrial Medicine.* 1991;48(6):399–403.
68. Omenn GS, Merchant J, Boatman E, Dement JM, Kuschner M, Nicholson W, et al. Contribution of environmental fibers to respiratory cancer. *Environmental Health Perspectives.* 1986;70:51–6.
69. Otte KE, Sigsgaard TI, Kjaerulff J. Massive exposure to asbestos and malignant mesothelioma, familial accumulation. *Ugeskrift for Laeger.* 1990;152(41):3013–4.
70. Barnes R, Rogers AJ. Unexpected occupational exposure to asbestos. *Medical Journal of Australia.* 1984;140(8):488–90.
71. Morinaga K, Kohyama N, Yokoyama K, Yasui Y, Hara I, Sasaki M, et al. Asbestos fibre content of lungs with mesotheliomas in Osaka, Japan: A preliminary report. *IARC Scientific Publications.* 1989;90(90):438–43.
72. Dodson RF, O'Sullivan M, Corn CJ, McLarty JW, Hammar SP. Analysis of asbestos fiber burden in lung tissue from mesothelioma patients. *Ultrastructural Pathology.* 1997;21(4):321–36.

73. Langer AM, Nolan RP. Asbestos in the lungs of persons exposed in the USA. *Monaldi Archives for Chest Disease*. 1998;53(2):168–80.
74. Levin JL, McLarty JW, Hurst GA, Smith AN, Frank AL. Tyler asbestos workers: Mortality experience in a cohort exposed to Amosite. *Occupational and Environmental Medicine*. 1998;55(3):155–60.
75. Roggli VL, Vollmer RT. Twenty-five years of fiber analysis: What have we learned? *Human Pathology*. 2008;39(3):307–15.
76. Smither WJ, Gilson JC, Wagner JC. Mesotheliomas and asbestos dust. *British Medical Journal*. 1962;2(5313):1194–5.
77. McCaughey WTE, Wade OL, Elmes PC. Exposure to asbestos dust and diffuse pleural mesotheliomas. *British Medical Journal*. 1962;2(5316):1397.
78. McNulty JC. Malignant pleural mesothelioma in an asbestos worker. *Medical Journal of Australia*. 1962;2:953–4.
79. Wagner JC. Experimental production of mesothelial tumours of the pleura by implantation of dusts in laboratory animals. *Nature*. 1962;196:180–1.
80. Wagner JC, Munday DE, Harington JS. Histochemical demonstration of hyaluronic acid in pleural mesotheliomas. *Journal of Pathology and Bacteriology*. 1962;84:73–8.
81. Mossman BT, Bignon J, Corn M, et al. Asbestos: Scientific developments and implications for public policy. *Science*. 1990;247(4940):294–301.
82. Mossman BT. Mechanisms of asbestos carcinogenesis and toxicity: The amphibole hypothesis revisited. *British Journal of Industrial Medicine*. 1993;50(8):673–6.
83. Cullen MR. The amphibole hypothesis of asbestos-related cancer--Gone but not forgotten [editorial]. *American Journal of Public Health*. 1996;86(2):158–9.
84. Stayner LT, Dankovic DA, Lemen RA. Occupational exposure to Chrysotile asbestos and cancer risk: A review of the amphibole hypothesis. *American Journal of Public Health*. 1996;86(2):179–86.
85. Cullen MRMD. Asbestos-related cancer and the amphibole hypothesis: 5. Cullen responds. *American Journal of Public Health*. 1997;87(4):690–1.
86. Langer AMP, Nolan RPP. Asbestos-related cancer and the amphibole hypothesis: 3. The amphibole hypothesis: Neither gone nor forgotten. *American Journal of Public Health*. 1997;87(4):688–9.
87. Mossman BT, Gee JBL. Asbestos-related cancer and the amphibole hypothesis. 4: The hypothesis Is still supported by scientists and scientific data. *American Journal of Public Health*. 1997;87(4):689–90.
88. Stayner LT, Dankovic DA, Lemen RA. Asbestos-related cancer and the amphibole hypothesis: 6. Stayner and colleagues respond. *American Journal of Public Health*. 1997;87(4):691.
89. Stayner LT, Dankovic DA, Lemen RA. Asbestos-related cancer and the amphibole hypothesis: 2. Stayner and colleagues respond. *American Journal of Public Health*. 1997;87(4):688.
90. Wagner JCMDFF. Asbestos-related cancer and the amphibole hypothesis: 1. The first documentation of the association. *American Journal of Public Health*. 1997;87(4):687–8.
91. Hodgson JT, Darnton A. The quantitative risks of mesothelioma and lung cancer in relation to asbestos exposure. *Annals of Occupational Hygiene*. 2000;44(8):565–601.
92. Selikoff IJ, Churg J, Hammond EC. Asbestos exposure and neoplasia. *Journal of the American Medical Association*. 1964;188:22–6.
93. Selikoff IJ, Churg J, Hammond EC. Relation between exposure to asbestos and mesothelioma. *New England Journal of Medicine*. 1965;272:560–5.
94. Smith WE, Miller L, Churg J, Selikoff IJ. Mesotheliomas in hamsters following intrapleural injection of asbestos. *Journal of the Mount Sinai Hospital*. 1965;32:1–8.
95. Churg J, Selikoff IJ. Geographic pathology of pleural mesothelioma. In: Liebow AA, Smith DE, editors. *The Lung. International Academy of Pathology Monograph No. 8*. Baltimore: Williams & Wilkins; 1968. p. 284–97.
96. Morgan WKC, Gee JBL. Asbestos-related diseases. In: Morgan WKC, Seaton A, editors. *Occupational Lung Diseases*. Philadelphia: Saunders; 1994. p. 308–73.
97. Gleick J. *Genius: Richard Feynman and Modern Physics*. London: Abacus; 1992.
98. Eagar TW, Musso C. Why did the World Trade Center collapse? Science, engineering and speculation. *JOM*. 2001;53(12):8–11. http://www.tms.org/pubs/journals/JOM/0112/Eagar/eagar-.html.
99. Landrigan PJ, Lioy PJ, Thurston G, Berkowitz G, Chen LC, Chillrud SN, et al. Health and environmental consequences of the world trade center disaster. *Environmental Health Perspectives*. 2004;112(6):731–9.
100. Smith JW. The asbestos industry: A perspective on the bioethics of industrial activity and disasters. In: Henderson DW, Shilkin KB, Langlois SL, Whitaker D, editors. *Malignant Mesothelioma*. New York: Hemisphere; 1992. p. 351–61.

101. Collaborators GBDOC. Global and regional burden of cancer in 2016 arising from occupational exposure to selected carcinogens: A systematic analysis for the Global Burden of Disease Study 2016. *Occupational and Environmental Medicine*. 2020;77(3):151.
102. LaDou J, Castleman B, Frank A, Gochfeld M, Greenberg M, Huff J, et al. The case for a global ban on asbestos. *Environmental Health Perspectives*. 2010;118(7):897–901.
103. Furuya S, Chimed-Ochir O, Takahashi K, David A, Takala J. Global asbestos disaster. *International Journal of Environmental Research and Public Health*. 2018;15(5):1000.
104. Lemen RA. Epidemiology of asbestos-related diseases and the knowledge that led to what is known today. In: Dodson RF, Hammar SP, editors. *Asbestos: Risk Assessment, Epidemiology, and Health Effects*. Boca Raton, FL: CRC Press /Taylor & Francis; 2006. p. 201–308.
105. Bianchi C, Bianchi T. Malignant mesothelioma: global incidence and relationship with asbestos. *Industrial Health*. 2007;45(3):379–87
106. Huang J, Chan SC, Pang WS, Chow SH, Lok V, Zhang L, et al. Global incidence, risk factors, and temporal trends of mesothelioma: A population-based study. *Journal of Thoracic Oncology: Official Publication of the International Association for the Study of Lung Cancer*. 2023;18(6):792–802.
107. AIHW. Mesothelioma in Australia 2021. In: *AIHW*. Canberra: AIHW; 2023.
108. Zhai Z, Ruan J, Zheng Y, Xiang D, Li N, Hu J, et al. Assessment of global trends in the diagnosis of mesothelioma from 1990 to 2017. *JAMA Network Open*. 2021;4(8):e2120360.
109. Walker-Bone K, Benke G, MacFarlane E, Klebe S, Takahashi K, Brims F, et al. Incidence and mortality from malignant mesothelioma 1982–2020 and relationship with asbestos exposure: The Australian mesothelioma Registry. *Occupational and Environmental Medicine*. 2023;80(4):186–91.
110. Dixon DL, Griggs KM, Ely M, Henderson DW, Klebe S. The usefulness of expert opinion in medicolegal referrals of malignant mesothelioma. *Pathology*. 2013;45(5):523–5.
111. Klebe S, Griggs KM, Ely M, Henderson DW. Is there a need for expert opinion for biopsy diagnosis of difficult cases of malignant mesothelioma? *Pathology*. 2012;44(6):562–3.
112. A GSI, SD, CG, S AD, S CS, A DQ, et al. Bulletin épidémiologique hebdomadaire (BEH) (n° 3-4, 2015/01/20). *Bulletin épidémiologique hebdomadaire (BEH)*. 2015;3–4:17–28.
113. Australia SW. *Mesothelioma in Australia: Incidence 1982 to 2005; Deaths 1997 to 2006*. Canberra: Commonwealth of Australia; 2009.
114. Peto J, Rake C, Gilham C, Hatch J. *Occupational, Domestic and Environmental Mesothelioma Risks in Britain: A Case-Control Study*. London: HSE Books; 2009.
115. Strickler HD, Goedert JJ, Devesa SS, Lahey J, Fraumeni JFJ, Rosenberg PS. Trends in US pleural mesothelioma incidence rates following Simian Virus 40 contamination of early poliovirus vaccines. *Journal of the National Cancer Institute*. 2003;95(1):38–45.
116. Alpert N. Gerwen MV, Taioli E. Epidemiology of mesothelioma in the 21st century in Europe and the United States, 40 years after restricted/banned asbestos use. *Translational Lung Cancer Research*. 2019:S28–S38.
117. Ariad S, Barchana M, Yukelson A, Geffen DB. A worrying increase in the incidence of mesothelioma in Israel. *Israel Medical Association Journal: IMAJ*. 2000;2(11):828–32.
118. Price B, Ware A. Mesothelioma trends in the United States: An update based on surveillance, epidemiology, and end results program data for 1973 through 2003. *American Journal of Epidemiology*. 2004;159(2):107–12.
119. Peto J, Decarli A, La Vecchia C, Levi F, Negri E. The European mesothelioma epidemic. *British Journal of Cancer*. 1999;79(3–4):666–72.
120. Pelucchi C, Malvezzi M, La Vecchia C, Levi F, Decarli A, Negri E. The mesothelioma epidemic in Western Europe: An update. *British Journal of Cancer*. 2004;90(5):1022–4.
121. van Zandwijk N, Rasko JEJ, George AM, Frank AL, Reid G. The silent malignant mesothelioma epidemic: A call to action. *The Lancet Oncology*. 2022;23(10):1245–8.
122. Chimed-Ochir O, Rath EM, Kubo T, Yumiya Y, Lin RT, Furuya S, et al. Must countries shoulder the burden of mesothelioma to ban asbestos? A global assessment. *BMJ Global Health*. 2022;7(12):e010553.
123. Choi Y, Lim S, Paek D. Trades of dangers: A study of asbestos industry transfer cases in Asia. *American Journal of Industrial Medicine*. 2013;56(3):335–46.

TABLE 1.1
Chemical Composition of Asbestos Fiber Types

Asbestos type	Chemical formula
Serpentine	$Mg_3Si_2O_5(OH)_4$
Chrysotile	
Amphiboles: commercial	$Na_2(Fe_3^{2+})(Fe_2^{3+})Si_8O_{22}(OH)_2$
Crocidolite	$(Fe, Mg)_7Si_8O_{22}(OH)_2$ Fe > 5
Amosite	
Amphiboles: non-commercial	$Ca_2Mg_5Si_8O_{22}(OH)_2$
Tremolite	$(Mg, Fe)_7Si_8O_{22}(OH)_2$ Mg > 6
Anthophyllite	$Ca_2(Mg, Fe)_5Si_8O_{22}(OH)_2$
Actinolite	

TABLE 1.2
Asbestos Production, Imports and Consumption for the USA, 1920–2020, by 10-Year and 5-Year Intervals, with Data for 2022

Year	Production	Imports	Exports	Consumption
1920	1500	151,000	600	152,000
1930	4000	189,000	700	192,000
1940	17,000	224,000	4000	237,000
1950	38,000	640,000	17,000	660,000
1960	41,000	607,000	5000	643,000
1970	114,000	589,000	35,000	668,000
1975	89,000	489,000	33,000	545,000
1980	80,000	327,000	49,000	359,000
1985	57,000	142,000	46,000	154,000
1990	20,000	41,000	29,000	32,000
1995	9000	22,000	17,000	15,000
2000	5000	15,000	19,000	1000
2005	–	2	–	100
2010	–	171	–	100
2015	–	358	–	358
2020	–	300	–	450
2022	–	232	–	100

Data are from U.S. Geological Survey (USGS), available online at http://www.usgs.gov/pubprod, and The U.S. International Trade Commission (https://dataweb.usitc.gov/trade/search, accessed August 31, 2023) .
See also Larson et al.[18]
All data are in metric tons. Apparent consumption calculated as production + imports minus exports, with no adjustment to account for changes in government and industry stocks: negative values indicate shipments from stocks.
Figures in the USGS are stated to be reasonably accurate to the first three digits, so that the numbers listed above have been rounded off to the nearest 50 tonnes for figures < 1000, to 500 for figures in the range of 1000–10,000 and to the nearest 1000 tones for numbers > 10,000: this being so, some of the figures do not add up exactly.

TABLE 1.3
Production and Imports of Asbestos in Australia, 1930–1983

	Chrysotile		Crocidolite		Amosite	
Years	Production	Imports	Production	Imports	Production	Imports
1930–1939	1200	–	400	–	50	–
1940–1949	3000	–	5600	–	750	–
1950–1959	11,500	314,100	63,250	2800	1	107,500
1960-1969	8850	329,000	86,550	–	–	81,450
1970–1979	394,350	388,000	–	–	–	87,900
1980–1983	160,400	64,650	–	–	–	8500

Based on data from the Bureau of Mineral Resources and modified from Leigh and Driscoll.[22]
Data have been rounded off to the nearest 50 tonnes.

TABLE 1.4
Production, Imports, Exports and Apparent Consumption in Tonnes of Asbestos (All Types) for Australia, 1930–1985

Year	Production	Imports	Exports	Apparent Consumption
1930–1939	1600	51,550	1200	52,000
1940–1949	9350	140,000	2400	146,900
1950–1959	74,750	314,100	51,400	337,400
1960–1969	95,400	434,700	44,700	485,400
1970–1979	394,350	555,600	45,500	704,450
1980–1985	160,400	104,300	109,800	154,950
Totals	740,300	1,602,800	450,000	1,888,000

Based on data from the Bureau of Mineral Resources and modified from Leigh and Driscoll.[22]
Figures have been rounded off to the nearest 50 tonnes and therefore may not add up exactly.

TABLE 1.5
Major Producers of Asbestos in 2021, Plus Estimated Reserves

World Mine Production and Reserves	Mine Production 2021 (Tons)	Reserves
USA	–	Small
Brazil	110,000	11,000,000
China	120,000	95,000,000
Kazakhstan	250,000	Large
Russia	700,000	110,000,000
Zimbabwe	1000	Large
World total (rounded)	1,200,000	Large

Data are from US Geological Survey (USGS) 2022.

TABLE 1.6
Estimates of Mesothelioma Incidence in 30 Nations

Country	Incidence Rate*	Country	Incidence Rate*	Country	Incidence Rate*
Australia	32**	France	10–13	Austria	5.6
Great Britain	30	Finland	>10	Poland	4
Belgium	29	Canada	9	Slovakia	4
Netherlands	23	Cyprus	9	Slovenia	4
Italy	17	USA	9	Spain	4
Norway	16	Hungary	8	Estonia	3
New Zealand	15	Turkey	7.8	Israel	3
Denmark	13	Croatia	7.4	Latvia	3
Germany	13	Japan	7	Lithuania	3
Sweden	12	Romania	6	Macedonia	3

Modified from estimates in Bianchi and Bianchi, 2007.[105]
*Incidence rate = Estimated crude incidence rate per million of the population per year.
**For 2003.
Also refer to Figure 1.2.

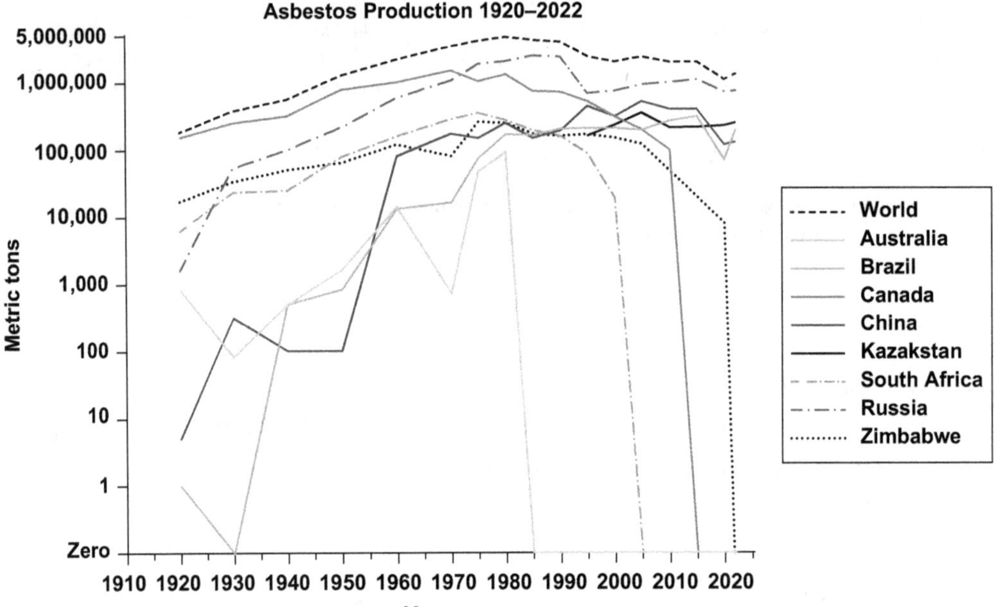

FIGURE 1.1 Production of asbestos worldwide from 1920 to 2022.

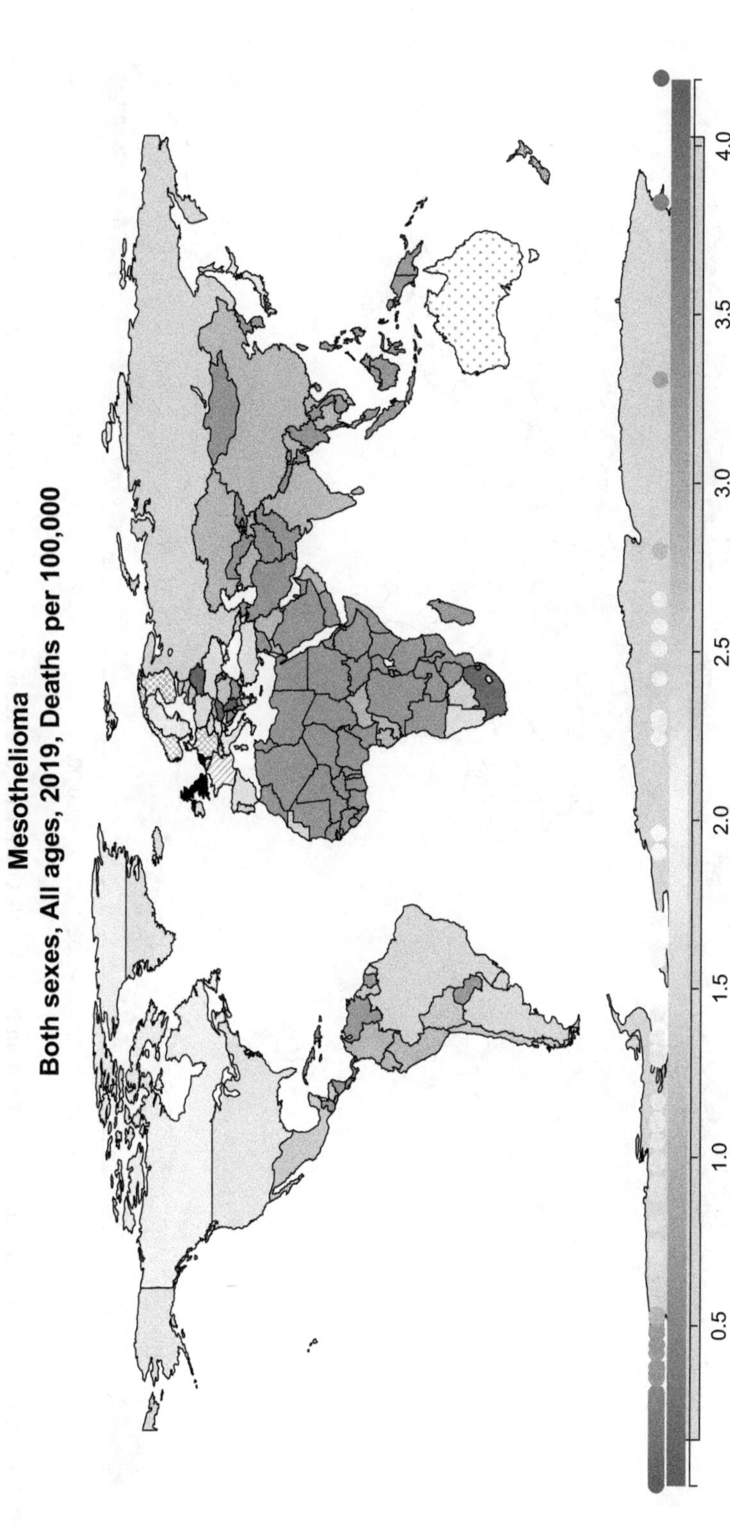

FIGURE 1.2 Number of deaths from mesothelioma per 100,000 worldwide. Data obtained from: Institute for Health Metrics and Evaluation (*IHME*). *GBD* Compare. Seattle, WA: *IHME*. University of Washington, 2023.

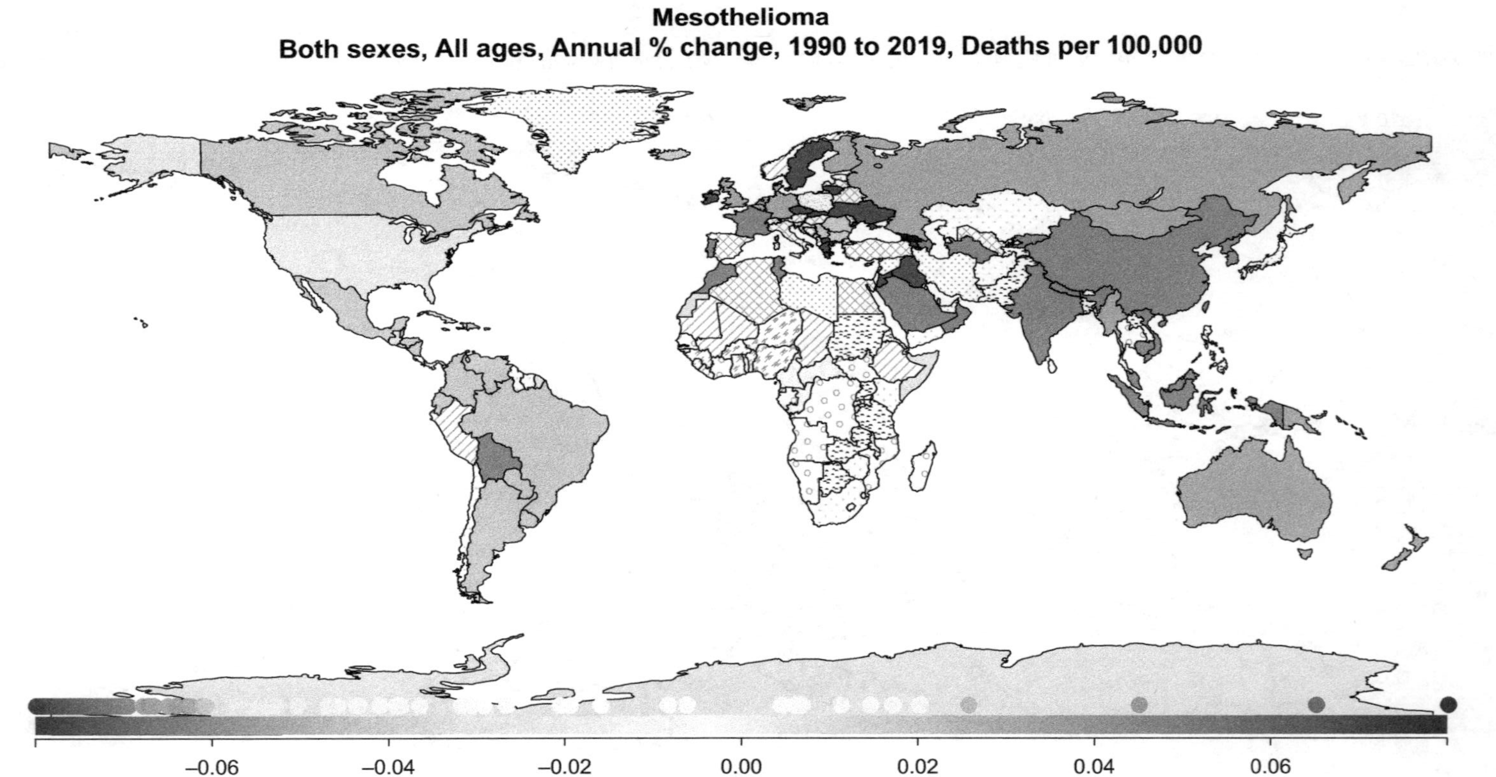

FIGURE 1.3 Percent change in deaths per 100 000 from 1990 to 2019. Overall, the changes in incidence of mesothelioma in many regions in the world over the past 30 years have been minor. Data obtained from: Institute for Health Metrics and Evaluation (*IHME*). *GBD* Compare. Seattle, WA: *IHME*, University of Washington, 2023.

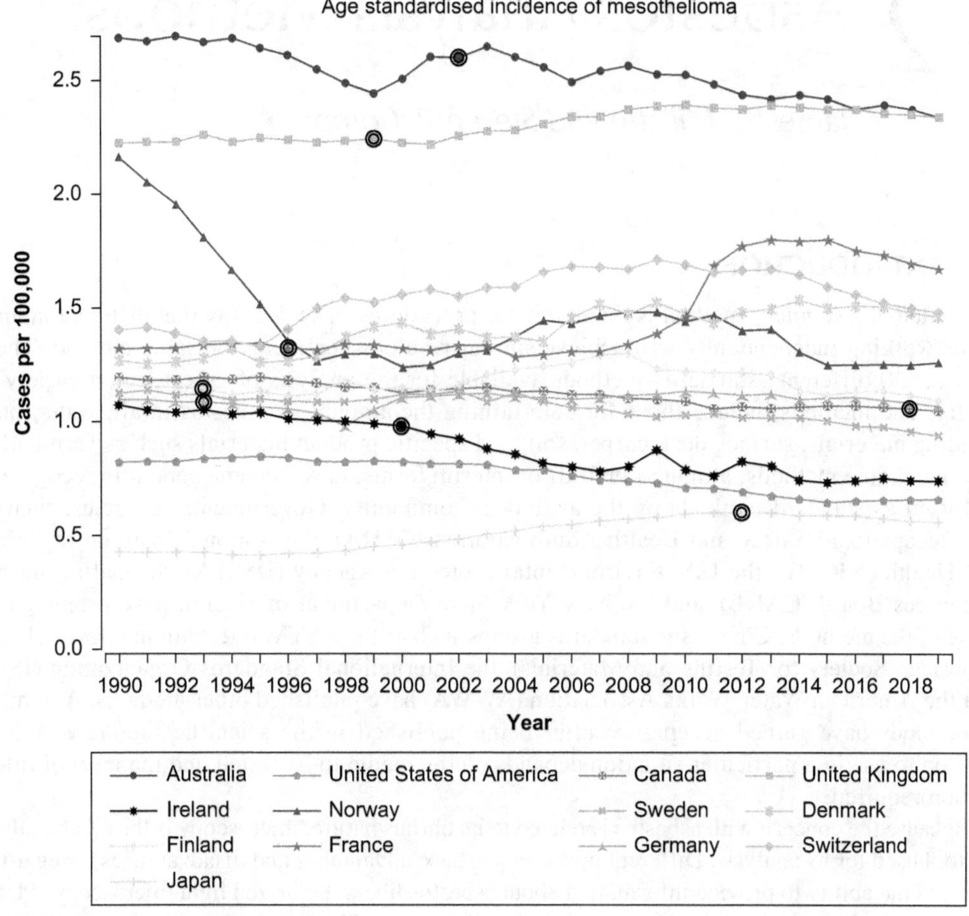

FIGURE 1.4 Age-standardized incidence of mesothelioma in selected countries with/without bans. Data from the IHME global burden of disease from 1990 to 2019 were analyzed (Institute for Health Metrics and Evaluation (*IHME*). *GBD* Compare. Seattle, WA: *IHME*, University of Washington, 2023.) The year a particular country banned the use of asbestos is circled on the graph (◎). The USA has not instituted a complete ban to date, and Norway, Sweden, Denmark and Switzerland instituted bans before 1990.

2 Asbestos Analysis Methods

James R. Millette and Steven P. Compton

2.1 INTRODUCTION

The value of a standard method is that it defines procedures in such a way that different laboratories working independently will achieve similar results when using the same method. There are over 30 different "standard" methods available for the analysis of asbestos in a variety of media. The methods include those for determining the amount of asbestos in air, water, bulk building materials, surface dust, carpet, soil, and specific product materials such as vermiculite and talc. Some methods, although in draft or interim forms, have become generally recognized and used as standard methods by the analytical community. Governmental agencies, such as the Occupational Safety and Health Administration (OSHA), the National Institute of Safety and Health (NIOSH), the U.S. Environmental Protection Agency (USEPA), the California Air Resources Board (CARB), and the New York State Department of Health, have promulgated some of the methods. Consensus standards groups such as the ASTM International (formerly the American Society for Testing and Materials), the International Standards Organization (ISO), and the American Water Works Association (AWWA) have published other methods. A number of methods have gained acceptance after being published in the scientific literature. Which method to use in a particular situation depends on the media to be tested and the level of information required.

Because the concern with asbestos is related to its fibrous nature, microscopy is the chief analytical tool used for its analysis. Different microscopes have advantages and disadvantages in regard to cost and the ability to provide information about asbestos fibers. Polarized light microscopy (PLM) is the standard way to analyze for asbestos in bulk materials. Phase-contrast microscopy (PCM) is the instrumental technique used for many occupational air sample analyses. Transmission electron microscopy (TEM) and, in some cases, scanning electron microscopy (SEM) are used for all types of samples when small fibers are involved or specific identification of individual asbestos fibers is desired.

2.2 SAMPLE COLLECTION

The collection of samples for analysis depends on the media to be tested and the specific procedures for sample collection are usually provided in the particular analysis method. In general, air samples are collected on membrane filters, water samples in glass or plastic bottles, surface dust by microvacuum or wipe samplers, and solid materials such as building materials, soil and specific products in plastic bags, or rigid plastic containers. Air samples are collected on either mixed cellulose ester (MCE) or polycarbonate (PC) filters using either 25 or 37 mm diameter air cassettes. To be quantitative, air samples must be collected with a measured amount of air volume and surface dust samples must be collected from measured areas of a surface.

2.3 POLARIZED LIGHT MICROSCOPY

A polarized light microscope (Figure 2.1) is a compound light microscope, which contains a piece of polarizing material in the light path below the sample and another in the light path above the

DOI: 10.1201/9781003431909-2

sample. The "polarized light microscopy (PLM) method" uses a stereo light microscope (Figure 2.2) to help in taking apart a bulk sample and a polarizing light microscope to identify the fibers among the binders and fillers. Work in the 1980s by McCrone established the procedures for asbestos fiber identification by PLM.[1, 2] The PLM identification of asbestos fibers depends on several optical crystallographic properties: refractive indices, dispersion staining, birefringence, sign of elongation, and extinction angle.

The *refractive index* of a substance is numerically equal to the ratio of the velocity of light in a vacuum to its velocity in a substance.[1] The velocity (of light) in any given substance depends on composition; in general, the higher the atomic number of the atoms involved, the lower the velocity and the higher the index.[1] *Dispersion staining* produces its color, not by any chemical interaction but by virtue of the difference between the dispersion of refractive index for a particle and the liquid medium in which the particle is immersed.[1] *Birefringence* refers to the difference between the two refractive indices at right angles to the axis of the microscope.[2] Elongate particles are said to have a positive *sign of elongation* when they have a greater refractive index in the parallel direction than in the perpendicular direction.[1] *Extinction* refers to the behavior on the rotation of the microscope stage when a crystalline substance is observed between crossed polarizing sheets. Each particle will show alternate brightness (polarization colors) and darkness (extinction). The particle shows parallel extinction when a prominent direction, for example, length of the fiber, is oriented parallel to the polarizer or analyzer vibration direction in its darkness position.[2]

Because of the size of the wavelength of light, PLM methods of identification are limited to fibers approximately 1 μm in diameter (Figure 2.3).

2.4 BULK ASBESTOS METHODS

The USEPA has defined the term "asbestos-containing material" or ACM as any material or product that contains more than 1% asbestos.[3, 4] The bulk analysis procedure most often specified is the "Method for the Determination of Asbestos in Bulk Building Materials (EPA-600/R-93/116)" published in 1993.[5] In the analytical industry it is referred to as "EPA R-93". Although it is generally accepted as an improvement over the USEPA "Interim Method for the Determination of Asbestos in Bulk Insulation Samples (EPA-600/M4-82-020)" published in December 1982,[6] the 1993 method has never been formally adopted by the USEPA. NIOSH Method 9002 and OSHA Method ID-191 involve similar procedures as the EPA R-93 bulk method.[7, 8]

Bulk asbestos analysis performed by PLM methods involves identifying the type of asbestos present on the basis of optical properties and then estimating the relative amount of asbestos in relation to the rest of the bulk sample. The estimates are given in terms of volume percents or, in some cases, area percents. PLM analysts practice with samples of known asbestos percentages until they can visually estimate the known values on a consistent basis. The PLM visually estimated asbestos percent values do not necessarily correspond to the weight percent of asbestos in a product. When all components of a bulk material have similar densities, the volume percent value is expected to be similar to the weight percent value. However, if the sample contains 12% chrysotile asbestos by weight in a binder of a denser material such as calcium carbonate (limestone), then the PLM analytical result may show 30–40% asbestos by volume. Similarly, if a sample contains 45–50% chrysotile asbestos by weight in a material that contains the same weight of a less dense component such as cellulose (paper fibers), then the PLM analytical result may show 5–10% asbestos by volume. In most asbestos-containing materials, the precise determination of the percent of asbestos by weight is not of great importance, because once a material is shown to contain over 1% asbestos, it is considered a regulated asbestos-containing building material. In most products such as insulation, fireproofing, acoustical plasters, friction products, asbestos-cement pipe, and pipe covering where asbestos was intentionally added; the amount of asbestos present is above 1%. Products containing 1% or less asbestos are still regulated under some OSHA requirements.[9]

In some materials such as ceiling tiles, floor tiles, caulks, paints, and joint compounds, the amount of asbestos added may have been in the low range, around 1%. For these materials, special procedures should be used. One special procedure is called "point counting."[10] In this procedure, the particles of the sample material are dispersed on a microscope slide and 400 nonempty points on the slide are randomly selected for examination. If, on one of the points, an asbestos fiber happens to line up with the center of the microscope eyepiece crosshairs, the fiber is counted. The percentage of asbestos is calculated based on the number of positive "hits" during the count. Counting three asbestos fibers out of 400 nonempty points, for instance, corresponds to an asbestos percentage of 0.75%. A stratified point-counting method is available as a method in the Certification Manual of the New York State Department of Health Environmental Laboratory Approval Program (ELAP).[11, 12] The New York State point-count method states "For samples containing high amounts of asbestos the stratified point-count technique invokes labor-saving semi-quantitative counting rules. The stratified method is based on the premise that accurate quantitation is unnecessary for materials that contain substantial amounts of asbestos. In contrast, extensive analytical effort is still required for samples that contain positive but small amounts of asbestos."[11] Although more quantitative, the point-count technique has been criticized as not being statistically valid at the 1% level.[13] For a sample in which a value of exactly 1% was determined by the 400 point-count procedure, repeated point-count analyses would be expected to fall variously within the range of 0.27–2.6% asbestos on the basis of Poisson statistics. To provide a more statistically valid analysis when low levels of asbestos may be present, matrix reduction is used to concentrate the asbestos fibers. When possible, combustible material is ashed away, acid-soluble material is dissolved away, and density separation is used to prepare the sample of bulk material so that low levels of asbestos fibers can be readily found. Electron microscopy can also be used to help provide quantitative values for low levels of asbestos. The USEPA 1993 bulk method, the NIOSH 9002, the OSHA ID-191, and ELAP Item 198.4 all contain some discussion of matrix reduction and use of electron microscopy.[7, 8, 14] A bulk microscopy method that incorporates various forms of matrix reduction for particular sample product types and use of electron microscopy has been developed, balloted and published by ISO. This method is designated as ISO 22262. [15–17] A comparison of several of the bulk methods is shown in Table 2.1.

2.5 PHASE-CONTRAST MICROSCOPY (PCM): AIR ANALYSIS

The phase-contrast microscope (Figure 2.4) is a compound light microscope, which illuminates a specimen with a hollow cone of light. The cone of light is narrow and enters the field of view of the objective lens. Within the objective lens is a ring-shaped device, which introduces a phase shift of a quarter of a wavelength of light. This illumination causes minute variations of refractive index in a transparent specimen to become visible. The phase-contrast mode pushes the ability of the light microscope to see fibers as thin as 0.2 μm in diameter, but it does so at the expense of identification. PCM is not used to identify asbestos fibers.

The most commonly used PCM method, NIOSH 7400, requires a positive phase (dark) contrast microscope with green or blue filter, an adjustable field iris, ×8–10 eyepieces, and a ×40–45 phase objective (total magnification is about ×400).[18] Most PCM analysts use binocular PCMs. Within one of the eyepieces, there is a Walton-Beckett-type graticule, which forms a circular analysis area of approximately 0.00785 mm^2 at the specimen plane. The other U.S. government-promulgated PCM method, OSHA ID-160, has similar requirements.[19] Under the PCM methods, fibers are counted when they are greater than 5 μm in length and have an aspect ratio (AR) (length to width) of at least 3:1. The NIOSH 7400 method "A" counting rules used for counting asbestos fibers have no upper limit on the diameter of the fiber counted. A fiber that appears to be partially obscured by a particle is counted as one fiber. If the fiber ends emanating from a particle do not seem to be from the same fiber and each end meets the length and AR criteria, they are counted as separate fibers. Results of the PCM methods are given in terms of fibers per cubic centimeter of air.

2.6 TRANSMISSION ELECTRON MICROSCOPY

The TEM (Figure 2.5) uses electromagnetic coils as lenses to form magnified images with an electron beam in the same way that a light microscope uses glass lenses and a light beam to form images. Electrons can be accelerated with high potential energies, which produce a beam with a very small wavelength and thus allow much higher magnifications than can be achieved with the wavelengths of light. The commonly used TEM methods call for a TEM that can operate at an accelerating potential of 80,000 to 120,000 volts (80–120 kV). If operating properly at 80–120 kV, a TEM is easily capable of obtaining a direct screen magnification of about ×100,000 with a resolution better than 10 nm. This allows the smallest asbestos fibers, which are approximately 20 nm (0.02 μm) in diameter, to be examined. In addition to the analysis of fiber morphology by TEM (Figure 2.6), selected area electron diffraction (SAED) and energy dispersive X-ray spectroscopy (EDS or EDX) can be used to gain information about a particle's crystal structure and elemental composition, respectively. Measurements of the distances and angles between spots (indexing) of an electron diffraction pattern provide information about crystal zone axes that can be compared with known crystallographic data to identify the mineral name of an individual fiber. Indexing an SAED pattern is often used when classifying amphibole asbestos fibers. A more complete discussion of this technique is available in the published papers of Dr Shu-Chun Su.[20, 21] A link on the McCrone Research Institute website provides access to the whole comprehensive suite of d-θ look-up tables for indexing Zone-Axis SAED patterns of amphibole asbestos and related minerals generated by Dr Su.[20] The tables currently include d-θ data for the following minerals: actinolite, anthophyllite, cummingtonite, grunerite, richterite, riebeckite, talc, tremolite, and winchite. Tables for additional minerals may be added in the future. An analysis performed on a TEM with SAED and EDS is referred to as analytical electron microscopy (AEM). Examples of a chrysotile SAED pattern and EDS spectra from reference asbestos minerals are shown in Figures 2.7 and 2.8.

The NIOSH 7402 method is the complementary TEM method for the PCM method 7400.[18, 22] NIOSH 7402 provides the identification of fibers counted under NIOSH 7400. With 7402, fibers greater than 5 μm in length and having an AR (length to width) of at least 3:1 and a width of at least 0.25 μm are characterized by SAED and EDS. These fibers are then classified as non-asbestos or asbestos based on the crystal structure (SAED) and elemental composition (EDS). The type of asbestos is also determined. A value of percent asbestos is determined and this percentage is applied to PCM results of "the same filter or on other filters for which the TEM sample is representative."[22] No concentration of fibers per cubic centimeter is reported under Method 7402. The ASTM method for the PCM analysis of workplace exposures, D4240, has been removed from official ASTM practice and has been replaced with ASTM D7201.[23, 24]

Early TEM measurements of airborne asbestos such as those used by Nicholson involved the collection of fibers on a membrane filter followed by an indirect-transfer method.[25, 26] In the TEM specimen procedure known as the "rubout" method, air samples collected using MCE filters were ashed in a low-temperature plasma asher and the residual ash was dispersed in a solution of nitrocellulose. The dispersion was "rubbed out" or spread as uniformly as possible on an optical microscope slide. After the solvent had evaporated, a portion of the film containing the particles from the filter residue was mounted on a TEM grid for examination. The value of asbestos was reported in terms of nanograms per cubic meter of air. The values were determined by summing the masses of the fibers that were calculated from the TEM dimensions of each fiber and an appropriate density for the type of asbestos found.

In 1978, Samudra et al. published the first methodology for the determination of the numerical concentration of asbestos fibers in ambient atmospheres using a direct preparation method.[27] This provisional methodology developed under contract for the USEPA recommended air sampling using a 0.4 μm pore size PC filter and preparation of TEM specimen grids by carbon coating followed closely by chloroform extraction to remove the filter polymer. The Samudra methodology was never taken beyond the provisional status.

In the early 1980s, Yamate at the Illinois Institute of Technology Research Institute (IITRI) was asked under contract to USEPA to take the methods that were being used by various labs and put together a TEM method for airborne asbestos.[28] His document, circulated in draft form in 1984, was never officially adopted by USEPA. It has always remained in draft form. As a fiber definition, it used the minimum AR of 3:1 from the NIOSH and OSHA methods but had no minimum fiber length. However, fibers less than 1 mm at the fluorescent screen magnification level were characterized as being 1 μm. At the analysis magnification of ×20,000, the 1 mm size corresponded to 0.5 μm. In addition to asbestos fibers, the method classified asbestos-containing objects as bundles, clusters, and matrices; see Table 2.2 for a comparison of fiber definitions used by several airborne asbestos analysis methods. Yamate also included the concept of levels of analysis because he realized that analytical tools available with the AEM provided progressively more specific identification of asbestos fibers depending on the amount of time devoted to the task. The method's levels are known among the TEM asbestos analytical community as Yamate level 1, level 2, and level 3. Level 1, requiring the least amount of identification, was designed for those situations where the airborne particulate was well characterized. If a particular process was known to emit only chrysotile, level 1 permitted identification based on morphology alone. For level 2, asbestos identification was determined by morphology and visual diffraction characteristics for chrysotile. For amphiboles, level 2 included some X-ray elemental information. Asbestos identification in Yamate level 3 began with the identification steps in level 2 and added diffraction pattern indexing to more specifically identify the amphibole mineral.

The draft Yamate method also contained a section for the situation when an air filter was overloaded. The preparation was an indirect procedure where a portion of the filter was ashed and the ash was suspended in water. A second filter was prepared with a portion of the suspension and then processed using the same direct procedures described in the main method. The concepts proposed in the indirect section of the draft Yamate method were used by ISO 13794 (indirect air—TEM) which was published in 1999.[29] ISO 13794 is more fully discussed in a later section.

On October 22, 1986, President Reagan signed into law the Asbestos Hazard Emergency Response Act (AHERA).[30] The Act required that USEPA describe the methods used to determine completion of response actions such as the abatement of school buildings. Following the deliberations of a panel of asbestos analysis experts, the "Interim TEM Analytical Methods" were published in the Federal Register on October 30, 1987, as Appendix A to Subpart E of the USEPA's "Asbestos-containing Materials in Schools; Final Rule and Notice." Following an asbestos abatement and before the protective plastic barriers are removed, leaf blowers and fans are used to aggressively stir the air and resuspend any settled dust while five area air samples are collected. For abatement clearance, the five area air samples collected inside the containment were to be compared with five or more area air samples collected outside the containment. No aggressive disturbance of the air outside the containment was to be done. If there was no statistical difference between the two sets of samples, the abated area was cleared and prepared for re-occupancy. A simplified version of the Yamate draft method was needed to create a rapid method for the clearance of school buildings. The AHERA method maintained many of the method particulars of the Yamate method but simplified the counting and recording for a rapid clearance procedure. As in the Yamate method, structures were counted. A structure was defined as a microscopic bundle, cluster, fibers, or matrix which may contain asbestos. A matrix was defined as a fiber or fibers with one end free and the other end embedded in or hidden by non-fibrous particulate. The exposed fiber must meet the fiber definition. Under the AHERA method, an asbestos fiber was defined as a structure greater than or equal to 0.5 μm in length with an AR (length to width) of 5:1 or greater and having substantially parallel sides. Individual dimensions of structures or fibers are not recorded under the AHERA method but information about the fiber length is classified as either between 0.5 and 5.0 μm or greater than/equal to 5.0 μm. The size data are not used to determine compliance with the AHERA regulations but are included so if an area does not pass, the Project Manager might infer something about the source of the contamination. Many large structures found in the air would suggest improper cleaning, while small structures could have come from a source external to the cleaning effort. During the deliberations of the expert panel, the question was raised about whether all ten samples needed to be analyzed if no asbestos structures were found on the five inside-the-containment samples. On the basis of the experience of some of the panel in finding occasional asbestos fibers on blank (unused) PC filters, it was decided a sample was clearly above the blank filter level if it had a filter loading greater than 70 structures per millimeter square (str/mm^2). In the real-world abatement industry, the 70 str/mm^2 became the generally recognized clearance level and contractors were and still are normally instructed to reclean if the average of the five inside samples exceeded that value. Only rarely today is the comparison made of the five inside and five outside samples. Those few cases are usually where a contractor believes that asbestos contamination outside the containment area is contributing to the air within the abatement area.

2.7 SCANNING ELECTRON MICROSCOPY

Like TEM, the scanning electron microscope (SEM) uses a beam of electrons; however, the SEM generally operates at lower voltages than TEM and it scans the beam across the surface of a sample rather than passing through individual particles as in the case with TEM (Figure 2.9). As such, the SEM is capable of providing surface images analogous to stereomicroscopy, but with higher resolution and depth of field (Figure 2.10). The SEM can also be adapted to collect elemental composition data (EDS). There is research currently under development for crystal structure analysis similar to SAED using an electron backscatter diffraction detector although this approach is not currently validated or generally accepted and was not implemented historically in connection with asbestos testing methodologies. In 1987, when the AHERA method mandated the use of TEM, the scanning electron microscope was determined to be inadequate for building clearance. The reasons given in the AHERA document were (1) currently available methodologies were not validated for the analysis of asbestos fibers, (2) SEM was limited in its ability to identify the crystalline structure of a particular fiber, (3) the National Bureau of Standards found that the image contrast of the microscopes was difficult to standardize between individual scanning electron microscopes, and (4) no current laboratory accreditation program existed for accrediting SEM laboratories.[30] NBS had determined that the only SEM method recognized at that time, the Asbestos International Association (AIA) protocol,[31] had inherent difficulty when examining certain types of asbestos. In 2023, there are still no laboratory accreditation programs for SEM laboratories analyzing for asbestos in the USA. In the USA, no standard SEM method is in use for asbestos, although it is mentioned in the OSHA ID-160 method. However, there is interest internationally and the ISO method 14966 for SEM analysis of inorganic fibrous particles that includes asbestos, ceramic fibers, and glass fibers in air was approved in 2002[32].

2.8 TEM BEYOND AHERA

In 1987, when the AHERA method was published in the Federal Register as an interim method, it contained a provision that the method would be updated by the National Institute of Standards and Technology (NIST). As of 2023, no updated version of the method has been published by NIST or any other federal agency. The AHERA method became the generally accepted TEM method for the analysis of asbestos in the air. However, its lack of a requirement to report specific size data for individual asbestos structures was considered a deficiency in some situations. A Yamate level 2 analysis was occasionally requested when information about fiber size was needed. In March 1988, the CARB issued Method 427 for the determination of particulate asbestos emissions from stationary sources using stack sampling, light microscopy, and electron microscopy.[33] Although the NIOSH 7400 PCM method may be used with the CARB Method 427, it is evident that the TEM portion is the focus of the method. Fiber size data is recorded according to the classifications described in the draft Yamate method.

In 1995, the ISO released a more comprehensive TEM airborne asbestos analysis procedure, largely developed by Dr Chatfield of Chatfield Technical Consulting.[34] The International Standard 10312 contains counting rules which expand on the Yamate and AHERA concept of asbestos structures. Clusters and matrices are subdivided into dispersed and compact structures. A dispersed cluster or matrix contains asbestos fibers that can be measured and reported separately, while a compact cluster or matrix has fibers and other particles too intertwined to report each fiber individually. In this method, cluster and matrix components are identified, measured, and recorded separately up to a maximum of nine substructures. The ISO 10312 method was followed in 1998 by the ASTM International Standard Test Method D6281-98, which was a translation of the ISO 10312 method into ASTM format with the same fiber counting rules.[35] The major difference between ISO 10312 and ASTM D6281 is that precision data for D6281 was validated by inter-laboratory testing and included in the method. For samples that contain any appreciable amount of asbestos, analysis using either ISO 10312 or ASTM D6281 takes more time and is thus more expensive than an AHERA analysis. The data produced by ISO 10312/ASTM D6281 was designed to allow another analyst to review the data of the original analyst and understand how the asbestos structures were present on the filter grid. The method of data recording was designed with future re-evaluations in mind. This allows for updates in interpreting the fiber data as new medical evidence or regulatory requirements become available. From the results of an ISO 10312 (or ASTM D6281) analysis, it should be possible to determine several different airborne asbestos structure concentration values based on a number of fiber size classifications. For instance, it should be possible to extract what a structure per cubic centimeter concentration would have been if the sample had been analyzed by AHERA counting rules. Both ISO 10312 and ASTM D6281 have an annex, which describes procedures for the determination of concentrations of asbestos fibres (international spelling of fiber) and bundles longer than 5 μm, and of PCM-equivalent (PCME) asbestos fibers (fibers bundles longer than 5 μm with aspect ratios equal to or greater than 3:1). To improve analytical sensitivity and statistical precision, the analyst counts larger fibers at lower magnifications, which allows for examination of a greater filter area. A comparison of four common asbestos methods for the analysis of air samples is shown in Table 2.3.

In 1999, ISO 13794 (indirect air) was published.[29] The asbestos structure and fiber counting procedures in this method are the same as those presented in ISO 10312 and ASTM D6281. ISO 13794 provides an indirect-transfer procedure so overloaded filters can be analyzed. The filter preparation methods described in both ISO 10312 and ASTM D6281 are direct-transfer procedures. For the indirect preparation in ISO 13794, a portion of the original filter is ashed and the ash is suspended in water that is mixed in a mild ultrasonic bath. A second filter is prepared with a known portion of the suspension and then processed using the same direct procedures described in ISO 10312 and ASTM D6281. Although the method states "This International Standard is applicable to measurement of airborne asbestos in a wide range of ambient air situations, including the interior atmospheres of buildings, and for detailed evaluation of any atmosphere," the user is cautioned that comparison of results using this indirect-transfer procedure with those from a direct-transfer procedure should not be made presumptively.[29] The best study of the differences between direct and indirect air sample preparation remains the study by Chesson and Hatfield.[36] Their findings supported the generally accepted opinion that TEM analysis of air samples using indirect-transfer methods provides estimates of the total airborne asbestos structure concentration that are higher than those using direct-transfer methods. They concluded that no single factor can be used to convert measurements made by one method to a value that is comparable with measurements made by the other. They also concluded that the breakdown of larger structures into smaller ones during indirect preparation does not appear to be sufficient to explain the difference in measured concentrations. Interference by debris and association of unattached structures may also be important. They recommended that additional research was needed to determine which transfer method more accurately reflects biologically meaningful airborne asbestos concentrations.

2.9 WATER ANALYSIS

There are three standard methods available for the analysis of drinking water for asbestos: USEPA 100.1, USEPA 100.2, and the AWWA 2570.[37–39] These methods are all TEM methods and are compared in Table 2.4.[40] The USEPA has set a maximum contaminant level of 7 million fibers longer than 10 μm per liter of drinking water and has listed both the 100.1 and 100.2 methods as acceptable for the analysis of waterborne asbestos. The USEPA 100.1 method is a research report produced in 1984 before the USEPA drinking water regulations and describes counting procedures that include asbestos fibers longer than 0.5 μm. USEPA 100.2 describes counting only those fibers longer than 10 μm. Guidance as to the modifications of USEPA 100.1 necessary to comply with the USEPA drinking water regulations was published by Feige et al.[41] The Environmental Laboratory Accreditation Program (ELAP) Certification Manual Item 198.2 describes a modification to Method 100.2 required for New York State Department of Health compliance.[42] In the modification, the ozone generator is considered optional *only* if all samples are filtered within 48 h.

2.10 SURFACE DUST ANALYSIS

In 1989, the ASTM subcommittee D22.07 began work on methods for the analysis of asbestos in settled dust.[43] Two ASTM methods are currently available for the analysis of surface dust for asbestos. These methods include one microvacuum method: ASTM D5755-22[44] and one wipe method: ASTM D6480-19[45] Both methods report a numerical concentration of asbestos on the sample surface based on asbestos fiber structure counts. The precision data for D5755 was validated by inter-laboratory testing and included in the method.[46] The precision data for D6480 was also validated by inter-laboratory testing and included in the method.[47] ASTM also developed a third dust method, D5756[48] a microvacuum collection method similar to D5755 that reported results based on the mass of asbestos fibers detected. Unfortunately, no acceptable inter-laboratory validation testing was ever done for D5756 and the method was withdrawn as a standard method from the ASTM International suite of asbestos in dust methods. A USEPA carpet method, EPA/600/J-93/167, was developed during a research study that was published as an article in 1993.[49] The USEPA number was assigned in 2001. The two ASTM methods are nondestructive, while the carpet method requires that a piece be cut from the carpet and sent to the laboratory. A comparison of the methods is shown in Table 2.5.

Because dust particles can be arranged in layers of more than one particle thick, direct preparation techniques are of limited value for TEM because the electron beam must be able to penetrate the sample. Indirect preparation procedures are used for all three of these settled dust methods. The results of the analysis are expressed in numbers of asbestos structures per square centimeter of surface sampled. The number count methods were originally designed with an analytical sensitivity of about 1000 str/cm^2 but can achieve much better sensitivities on clean surfaces. There are no federal government levels with which to compare the results of the surface dust methods and there is some disagreement on how to interpret the data.[50–58] Because the amount and type of dust collected by each method differ, it is clear that the results of one method cannot be necessarily compared directly with data from another. For instance, the bulk carpet method, EPA/600/J-93/167, is an analysis of the total amount of dust in a carpet. Because carpets are known to be excellent traps for dust and dirt, the amount of asbestos in the carpet may be considerably higher than that collected from the surface of the same carpet using the D5755 microvacuum method. It is not appropriate to compare bulk carpet values with the results of the D5755 method, although both are given in terms of structures per square centimeter. In one set of tests, the EPA/600/J-93/167 results were found to be about 100 times higher than that of the D5755 type analysis, because the bulk carpet method involves all dirt trapped in the carpet and the microvacuum method only analyzed the top, readily releasable dust.[58] Asbestos in dust deep in the carpet may not be releasable under normal activities and may only be of concern when the carpet is being removed. Asbestos fibers that are in a sticky film on a surface and therefore not readily releasable are collected by the D6480 wipe method. The wipe method gives an index of all the asbestos fibers on a surface regardless of how much they are stuck, whereas the microvacuum method gives an index of the readily releasable fibers.

2.11 SOIL ANALYSIS

Soil is a difficult medium for the analysis of asbestos because soil minerals are not easily separated from the asbestos fibers. In a method used by the USEPA Region 1 in 1997, sieving was used to enhance the ability to find asbestos fibers that were then identified using essentially the standard PLM bulk analysis procedure.[59] In 2013, ASTM International issued the Standard Test Method D7521 for the Determination of Asbestos in Soil.[60] This test method describes the gravimetric, sieve, and other laboratory procedures for preparing the soil for analysis as well as the identification and quantification of any asbestos detected. Pieces of collected soil and material embedded therein that pass through a 19-mm sieve become part of the sample that is analyzed and for which results are reported. Asbestos is identified and quantified by polarized light microscopy (PLM) techniques including analysis of morphology and optical properties. Optional transmission electron microscopy (TEM) identification and quantification of asbestos is based on morphology, selected area electron diffraction (SAED), and energy dispersive X-ray analysis (EDS). The sample is dried and sieved with sieves arranged from top to bottom: 19 mm, 2 mm, 106 μm, and collection pan. The sieve fractions are designated coarse fraction (<19 to >2 mm), medium fraction (<2 mm to >106 μm), and fine fraction (<106 μm). Weight for each fraction is measured and recorded. Objects greater than 19 mm may be analyzed using stereomicroscopy and polarized light microscopy (PLM) and reported separately but are not considered part of this method. Any building material debris collected from the field along with the soil sample may also be analyzed and reported separately. The coarse, medium, and fine fractions are all analyzed by stereomicroscopy and PLM visual area estimation (VAE) in terms of a percentage. The final result of the PLM portion of D7521 is a summation of the three sieve fractions: coarse, medium, and fine. If asbestos is detected at less than 1% in the fine fraction, then a point count is performed by preparing eight separate slide mounts and examining at 100× following EPA 600/R-93/116 until 400 points are counted. Additional points may be counted to improve the analytical sensitivity. In addition, if PLM results indicate none detected, then the fine fraction of the sample may be analyzed for asbestos using transmission electron microscopy (TEM) drop mount. If the TEM drop mount is negative or a quantitative result is desired, then it is recommended that the sample be gravimetrically reduced by ashing in a muffle furnace, treated with concentrated hydrochloric acid, and the ash placed in ultrapure water. The suspension is filtered and the filters are prepared for TEM examination using a direct method consistent with ASTM Test Method D6281. Analysis follows ASTM Test Method D6281 with results reported in total structures per microgram of sample. TEM results of the fine fraction in which the percent of asbestos is visually estimated on the TEM screen can be expressed as a weight percent if the weight measurements have been recorded.

A more complicated procedure that looks at the airborne asbestos fibers that might be released from the soil is called the Superfund method. [61, 62] The soil sample is placed in a rotating drum and air samples collected in a vertical elutriator. The samples are analyzed by TEM according to procedures based on the ISO 10312 method. The counting procedure may be modified to count "protocol" fibers. Protocol fibers are asbestos fibers with certain length and width characteristics as determined by studies in biological systems. At one point in time, fibers longer than 40 μm were thought to be of greatest interest and the method was modified to count more grid openings at a lower magnification for better counting statistics.

The fluidized bed aerosol segregator (FBAS) is a newer sample preparation instrument that utilizes air elutriation to separate asbestos structures and other fine particles from heavier matrix particles in soil and deposit these structures onto a filter which can then be analyzed by transmission electron microscopy (TEM) or other appropriate microscopic techniques.[63] Tests with reference samples containing known percentages of asbestos have shown that there is an approximately linear relationship between the concentration of asbestos in the soil (as mass percent) and the mean airborne concentration estimated by the TEM analysis following preparation by FBAS, expressed as asbestos structures captured on the filter per gram of test material (str/g). There are several advantages of the FBAS over the Superfund method equipment. The FBAS unit is compact, fitting into a standard laboratory fume hood, and components of the unit are relatively easy to decontaminate. Some components are disposable.

2.12 VERMICULITE ANALYSIS

Vermiculite is a special case for bulk asbestos analysis. Just using the USEPA bulk asbestos PLM method was deemed not sufficient for the analysis of the asbestos fibers that were associated with vermiculite.[64, 65] Without special sample preparation to separate the asbestos fibers from the books of vermiculite, undercounting of fibers is a problem. A history of the development of analytical methods for asbestos in vermiculite and a summary of various methods was published in 2015.[65] The New York State Department of Health Environmental Laboratory released a specific Test Method, 198.8, in 2014 for identifying and quantitating asbestos in sprayed-on fireproofing containing vermiculite.[66] Method 198.8 only uses polarized light microscopy (PLM) techniques for fiber identification but requires density separation to separate the asbestos fibers from the vermiculite before analysis. Heavy liquid centrifugation (using an aqueous solution of either lithium metatungstate or sodium polytungstate) is used to separate particles with densities exceeding 2.75 g/mL that include any of the amphibole minerals. The method also involves preparation steps of gravimetric matrix reduction by ashing for 10 hours at 485°C to remove the organic materials and acid treatment to remove acid-soluble components such as gypsum. Analysis is done by PLM and point counting (400 points). The method states that reliable and routine discrimination between the various calcium-containing amphiboles present in vermiculite from Libby is not possible by PLM; therefore, the fibers are identified as "amphibole asbestos." Under NYS DOH 198.8, amphibole asbestos includes the minerals richterite and winchite.

Sometimes referred to as "The Cincinnati Method," the USEPA research method EPA/600/R-04/004 for the sampling and analysis of fibrous amphibole in vermiculite attic insulation (VAI) uses a flotation step to separate the vermiculite from the more dense amphiboles.[64] The fibrous amphiboles found in the Libby, MT vermiculite can be hand-picked from the "sinks" using a stereomicroscope and weighed to get a direct weight percent estimate. The method also includes a TEM portion for the analysis of amphibole fibers that might be present in the "suspended particle" fraction of the water used in the flotation step. Criteria for examination of the TEM specimens are specified in ASTM D6281, ISO 10312 or ISO 13794. Matrix reduction steps (ashing and acid dissolution) for the preparation of vermiculite sprayed products are provided in the International Standards Organization Method 22262-2.[16] ISO 22262-2 allows for analysis of the residue for amphiboles by both PLM and TEM which allows for analysis of all the amphibole fibers that are not seen by PLM alone.

Early in 2004, USEPA held a day and a half workshop for a panel of experts to meet and propose a quicker, simpler method specific to the determination of whether Libby amphibole is present in a sample of vermiculite attic insulation (VAI). The objective of the method was to be accurate with respect to identifying Libby amphibole, affordable to the average homeowner, and adaptable to most current commercial fiber analysis laboratories. Working Groups within ASTM International D22.07 are currently tasked with developing a "quick" TEM analysis method for Libby vermiculite and a more robust vermiculite method for use with research efforts.

2.13 TALC ANALYSIS

The asbestos minerals chrysotile, tremolite, actinolite, and anthophyllite are known to occur as potential accessory minerals in talc deposits. The purity of talc that has been mined and processed for use in personal hygiene, cosmetic, or pharmaceutical powders has been under scrutiny since the 1960s with investigations by independent labs using a variety of approaches dominated by X-ray diffraction (XRD), optical microscopy, and electron microscopy.[67–81] In 1973, the U.S. Food and Drug Administration proposed a PLM method for talc that claimed to achieve a detection limit of approximately 0.01% to 0.1% asbestos. The FDA proposed method was met with criticism by the talc industry and an alternative method, developed by the Cosmetic, Toiletry, and Fragrance Association (CTFA) industry group, was proposed.[82]

The CTFA method, J4-1, requires an initial analysis of the talc sample for amphibole minerals by XRD with a stated detection limit of 0.5%.[83] Because XRD does not involve microscopy, a second step requires examination by PLM only if any of the amphibole mineral types were detected by XRD. The PLM examination requires reporting of "asbestiform fibrous amphibole minerals" based on five criteria. First, the particle must appear to be fibrous rather than as crystals or slivers. Reported fibers must exhibit a diameter no greater than 3 μm, length no greater than 30 μm, and a minimum AR of 5:1. The fifth criteria is rather confusing as it requires fibers to exist in bundles, "unless they are at a nondivisible stage." The CTFA method has never been updated and is still one of two commonly referenced methods for talc analysis by the industry.

The second non-regulatory method, proposed by the non-profit U.S. Pharmacopeia, was developed in the 1980s for pharmaceutical talc. Similar to the cosmetic talc method J4-1, the USP "talc monograph" required an initial analysis using either XRD or infrared spectroscopy (IR), both of which are now admitted by USP to lead to false-negative results.[84] Only if a positive result was obtained by either XRD or IR, was some level of optical microscopy performed to confirm whether mineral fibers were present. The reference to optical microscopy was minimal, consisting almost entirely of a restatement of a set of criteria proposed by Wylie in 1990 (discussed in detail in section 2.17); however, the use of polarized light was optional. In 2010, the FDA submitted a request to USP "to modernize the high-priority USP Talc monograph."[84] In May of 2022, USP proposed two new chapters to complement the updated talc monograph: "<901> Detection of Asbestos in Pharmaceutical Talc"[85] and "<1901> Theory and Practice of Asbestos Detection in Pharmaceutical Talc."[86] The new chapters describe the use of XRD and PLM as recommended previously; however, PLM is now mandatory. The two chapters are scheduled to become official in December 2023 and the talc monograph is anticipated to be updated in December 2025.[87] An electron microscopy method is under consideration by USP, but has yet to be proposed at this time.

Several approaches to talc analysis have been proposed in peer reviewed journals as well. In 1984, Paoletti et al. published an approach for evaluation of talc using electron microscopy.[76] In this method, samples of industrial, cosmetic, and pharmaceutical grade talc were suspended in a Formvar/dichloroethane suspension and deposited onto freshly cleaved mica. The resulting film was then transferred onto TEM grids and carbon coated. The 1991 publication by Blount titled, "Amphibole Content of Cosmetic and Pharmaceutical Talcs" describes a sample preparation approach which takes advantage of the differences in density between talc and some of the amphibole minerals associated with asbestos (namely, tremolite and actinolite).[77] A heavy liquid sedimentation was used to extract the heavier amphibole particles and analyze them using PLM. In 2015, Millette published the "Procedure for the Analysis of Talc for Asbestos," which recommended a combination of PLM and TEM, with the possible use of XRD as a potential screening step.[88] The recommendations proposed by Millette make use of decades of research and method validation for asbestos analysis by TEM using the counting rules established in methods discussed previously, like ISO 10312 and ASTM D6281. Millette also references the EPA R93 method as "a good description of the light microscopy techniques available." but cautions against using the Wylie criteria listed in the glossary of R93 for differentiation of asbestos fibers from "cleavage fragments." The concern over application of the Wylie criteria and its reference to a 20:1 mean aspect ratio to mineral powders or soil samples is shared by the USEPA, which states that "[t]he building material analytical method is designed to detect commercially processed asbestos in items like floor tiles, roofing tiles, paper insulation, paints, and mastics, not naturally occurring asbestos on air filters or in soil samples."[89]

The incorporation of PLM and TEM for talc analysis was also endorsed by the Interagency Working Group on Asbestos in Consumer Products (IWGACP) White Paper in 2021 and considers TEM in particular "to play an indispensable role in the analysis of cosmetic products containing talc and for talc intended for use in cosmetics for asbestos and other amphibole particles."[90] The IWGACP is comprised of a panel of 38 experts from the Food and Drug Administration, National Institute for Occupational Safety and Health, National Institutes of Health/National Institute of Environmental Health Sciences, Environmental Protection Agency, Consumer Product Safety Commission, and the Department of Interior's U.S. Geological Survey. The IWGACP proposal to the FDA is possibly the most inclusive method to date and advocates reporting of all amphibole mineral fibers, not just those which were mined commercially and fall under current regulatory definitions of asbestos. Further, the approach described requires reporting of chrysotile and amphibole fibers meeting a minimum length of 0.5 μm and a minimum aspect ratio of 3:1. The IWGACP also discourages discriminatory counting approaches and "advises against categorizing particles using terms such as 'cleavage fragment,' 'bladed,' or 'acicular' to imply these are not asbestiform when there is ambiguity as to a particle's habit of growth."[90] Appendix J to the IWGACP White Paper provides a detailed discussion on the benefits of various sample preparation steps that may be performed prior to PLM or TEM analysis including ashing, acid dissolution, water separation, fluidized bed separation (discussed previously), and heavy liquid separation. Ashing, acid dissolution, water separation, and fluidized bed separation have all been addressed in detail previously in this chapter. Heavy liquid separation is typically not required for most asbestos samples (since they do not often contain mixed mineral assemblages); however, the technique for mineral separation has been utilized in mineralogy since the 1800s and was specifically investigated for the presence of asbestos in talc as early as the 1970s.[90] Heavy liquid separation was also referenced in the previously discussed 1991 Blount paper and in 2014 was incorporated into the suite of sample preparation techniques described by ISO 22262-2 (2014).[16]

2.14 METHODS FOR ASBESTOS ANALYSIS IN OTHER MEDIA

In addition to media such as bulk materials, air, water, soil, and dust, methods for analyzing asbestos in clothing and biological specimens have appeared in the scientific literature.[91, 92, 93] Only two of the many scientific papers that contain descriptions of asbestos analysis methods are referenced here. Sample preparation procedures are generally different for each type of sample matrix, but the type of microscopy to be used and the counting rules are usually borrowed from one of the standard methods described earlier.

2.15 ASBESTOS DEFINITIONS AND TERMINOLOGY

The term 'asbestos' is a commercial term rather than a scientific one. This has led to different definitions for asbestos in different analytical methods. Some use the mineralogical term "asbestiform" in an attempt to clarify what is meant by "asbestos." This can cause some confusion. For instance, the definition in the ISO Standard 10312 for "asbestiform" is listed as a "specific type of mineral fibrosity in which the fibres and fibrils possess high tensile strength and flexibility." This definition may seem helpful to a person without knowledge of asbestos analysis until it is understood that no method of asbestos analysis exists that measures the tensile strength or flexibility of individual fibers. While the definition involving tensile strength is true for hand samples of the highest grades of commercial chrysotile asbestos materials such as for weaving, the characteristics of tensile strength and flexibility are not universally true for all forms of asbestos.[94] More importantly, they cannot be determined by a microscopist and are not used in the analysis for asbestos for public health policy. Since the analyst cannot measure the tensile strength or flexibility of individual fibers, they look to the method counting rules and definition of "fiber" to be counted (e.g., ISO 10312 definition 3.22 or ASTM D6281 definition 3.2.23) for the key of how to use a standard method to analyze a sample for asbestos.

For some methods it is explicit. For instance, in the USEPA AHERA method for bulk asbestos analysis published in the U.S. Federal Register,[3] under the heading "1.7.2.4 Quantitation of Asbestos Content" it states, "For the purpose of this method, asbestos fibers are defined as having an aspect ratio greater than 3:1 and being positively identified as one of the minerals in Table 1–1." The minerals identified in Table 1-1 of the AHERA method are chrysotile, amosite, crocidolite, anthophyllite, and tremolite-actinolite. Therefore, for example, under this U.S. government-authorized method a particle identified by microscopy as being an amphibole mineral of the tremolite species with an aspect ratio (length divided by width) of 4:1 would be counted as an asbestos fiber. A particle with a 2:1 aspect ratio identified as tremolite could be reported as an amphibole particle but could not be reported as an asbestos fiber because its aspect ratio is below 3:1.

The definition of a "Federal Asbestos Fiber" depends on the federal agency involved. The Occupational Safety and Health Administration (OSHA) uses a definition of a fiber that is at least 5 μm long with an AR (length to width) of 3:1. The USEPA uses a definition of a fiber that is at least 0.5 μm long with a 5:1 AR. The ISO 10312 and ASTM D6281 methods use the same 0.5 μm length with a 5:1 AR definition in their main procedures and provide an annex that describes counting fibers greater than 5 μm long with an AR of 3:1. References to average ARs such as 10:1 and 20:1 are found in the PLM bulk method EPA R-93 but are not found in standard air methods that use PCM or TEM.

From the microscopical analyst's point of view, an asbestos fiber is defined by the counting method being used. Under the AHERA counting rules, a fiber is a structure having a minimum length greater than 0.5 μm and an AR (length to width) of 5:1 or greater and substantially parallel sides. The appearance of the end of the fiber, that is, whether it is flat, rounded, or dovetailed, is to be noted. However, AHERA does not use this information about fiber ends, nor does it say whether to record this information. Under Section 3.22 of the ISO 10312 counting rules (and a similar section in ASTM D6281), a fiber is defined as an "elongated particle that has parallel or stepped sides."

Individual chrysotile fibers, called fibrils, are too thin to be seen by the light microscope during the PCM analysis by NIOSH 7400. The fibers of chrysotile that are seen in the light microscope are actually bundles of fibrils. During the analysis by TEM using the NIOSH 7402 method that considers only elongate particles longer than 5 μm in length, greater than 0.25 μm in width, with a minimum 3:1 AR, the chrysotile "fibers" are more correctly listed as bundles. As stated in the ISO 10312 method: "For chrysotile, PCME fibres will always be bundles."[34] During the analysis by TEM using the AHERA method, chrysotile fibrils are listed as fibers. These AHERA chrysotile "fibers" (actually fibrils less than 0.05 μm in diameter) are not visible with the light microscope. Similar terminology is used in the water methods and in the dust methods. With the exception of the NIOSH 7402 method, all TEM chrysotile fibers are actually fibrils and not visible with the light microscope.

The ASTM D6281 and ISO10312 air methods both use the minimum fiber size of ≥0.5 μm in length and aspect ratio of ≥5:1 found in the AHERA method. The AHERA method was designed for the clearance of school buildings after an asbestos abatement. The rule to count all diameters including those smaller than can be seen with the light microscope and fibers less than 5 μm in length was included to get a more complete picture of the true asbestos fiber concentration. The aspect ratio of 5:1 was a compromise between scientists and health professionals who wanted to use the 3:1 aspect ratio of the PCM counting methods and a 10:1 or greater aspect ratio that was wanted by other scientists. Although there is general agreement that the longer, thinner asbestos fibers are more hazardous than the shorter, thicker ones, there have been no human or animal studies that have authoritatively established the aspect ratio above which is hazardous, and below which is not hazardous. Similarly, there is no general agreement regarding a "safe" fiber length. The choice of 0.5 μm as a cutoff for TEM fiber counting rules was intended to be more inclusive than the PCM limitation of 5.0 μm; however, the minimum length of 0.5 μm specifically was not driven by health studies. Rather, it reflected an analyst's ability to produce reliable, consistent, comparable results using a TEM microscope.

In the conclusions of the White Paper published by the Interagency Working Group on Asbestos in Consumer Products (IWGACP), it is stated "Reporting of particles >0.5 μm in length is consistent with the rules for identification and counting established by the global standard for TEM sampling and analysis, ISO 10312, and by the 1987 Federal AHERA standards for protecting children from asbestos in public and private elementary and secondary school buildings.[90] Many studies indicate that asbestos and other mineral particles <5 μm in length could pose a health concern." The asbestos experts from seven U.S. government agencies are in agreement with the reporting of fibers less than 5 μm in length. The IWGACP also concluded that TEM results should be reported by tabulating each particle to facilitate an estimate of the number of particles per unit mass of sample analyzed (particles/gram), rather than as weight percent. The IWGACP concluded that reporting as weight percent can be misleading and weight percent does not necessarily correlate with the number of particles.

2.16 PCM FIBER COUNT EQUIVALENCY

The U.S. NIOSH Standard Method 7400 uses PCM and involves counting only those fibers that can be seen with the light microscope (i.e. thicker than 0.25 μm) and longer than 5 μm. The TEM companion method NIOSH 7402 considers the same fiber characteristics as the 7400 method but because the TEM can resolve thin asbestos fibers, 7402 analysis is restricted to fibers greater than 0.25 μm in width. The TEM fibers analyzed under NIOSH 7402 are then assumed to be those which would be counted by PCM. However, the NIOSH 7402 method was not established to provide concentrations of asbestos fibers. The reportable value from 7402 is a percentage of asbestos fibers of all fibers in the PCME size range in the sample. This percentage can thereby be applied to 7400 values to determine asbestos fiber concentrations in fibers/cm^3. Other TEM methods (primarily ISO 10312, D6281, and also occasionally AHERA) have been used to determine PCME concentrations. It is important when interpreting the data to understand the differences in counting rules between methods. Appendix C of method NIOSH 7400 contains a description of the asbestos fiber counting rules (referred to as "A" Rules) as they apply to labeled objects in Figure 2 of the 7400 method. For Object 3 in Figure 2, the method states: "Although the object has a relatively large diameter (>3 μm), it is counted as a fiber under the rules. There is no upper limit on the fiber diameter in the counting rules." The ISO 10312 and ASTM D6281 Methods define a PCME fiber as "any particle with parallel or stepped sides, with an aspect ratio of 3:1 or greater, longer than 5 μm, and which has a diameter between 0.2 and 3.0 μm." Using the ISO 10312 method for PCME counting will therefore not provide a count of PCM fibers equivalent to the NIOSH 7400 method unless it is modified so that fibers of all diameters are included.

There are important cautions to consider when attempting to use AHERA counts to estimate PCME concentrations. It is important to realize that the NIOSH 7400 method includes fibers associated with other particles. For Object 6 in Figure 2 of the method, the NIOSH 7400 method states: "A fiber partially obscured by a particle is counted as one fiber. If the fiber ends emanating from a particle do not seem to be from the same fiber and each end meets the length and AR criteria, they are counted as separate fibers." The AHERA method counts all asbestos objects as structures. Objects that contain one or more fibers partially obscured by a non-asbestos particle are counted as matrices. Under the NIOSH PCM method, several fibers meeting the length and AR criteria, which are overlapping but do not seem to be part of the same bundle, would be counted as separate fibers. Under the AHERA TEM method, these would all be counted as one cluster. If an analyst attempts to use the AHERA data to estimate a PCME fiber count and chooses only those structures identified as bundles greater than 5 μm, they will miss PCME fibers that are parts of matrices or clusters. Because AHERA uses a 5:1 aspect ratio while the PCM method uses a 3:1 ratio, an AHERA count would not have included a fiber over 5 μm with only a 3:1 aspect ratio. Considering the differences in the two methods, it does not seem appropriate to attempt to estimate PCME fiber concentrations from AHERA data. However, an AHERA analysis in which no asbestos structures are found is considered to be consistent with the detection of no PCME fibers. It would be a most unusual sample to have no AHERA countable asbestos structures but still have some large fibers with ARs between 3:1 and 5:1.

2.17 CLEAVAGE FRAGMENTS

It is generally acknowledged that elongated amphibole particles (amphibole fibers) can be generated by two mechanisms. They can be formed as fibers in the ground as a result of the geological process called metamorphism or can be generated by an industrial process, such as crushing in mining operations where more massive amphibole mineral crystals are cleaved along crystal cleavage planes to form cleavage fragment particles. For an individual fiber that fits the length, width, and aspect ratio designated in an asbestos regulation, it is not possible to definitively determine how it was formed. Although a number of ideas have been suggested to differentiate between amphibole cleavage fragment fibers and amphibole geologically "formed" fibers, none of these have been accepted and included in government-promulgated methods or methods that have been validated, balloted, and accepted by consensus-method development groups such as ASTM International or ISO.

In the glossary of the 1993 USEPA method[5] for the analysis of bulk samples, asbestos is described as a population of fibers observed as having the asbestiform habit that is generally recognized by several characteristics. These include mean aspect ratios in the range from 20:1 to 100:1 or higher for fibers longer than 5 μm. Asbestos is further characterized by very thin fibrils, usually less than 0.5 μm in width, and two or more of the following:

- Parallel fibers occurring in bundles
- Fiber bundles displaying splayed ends
- Matted masses of individual fibers
- Fibers showing curvature

This description was adopted from the mineralogical rationale published by Dr Ann Wylie, a mineralogist at the University of Maryland, in 1990 based on her work with Siegrist in 1980.[95, 96] The EPA R-93 document did not explain why the asbestiform characteristic "fibers in the form of thin needles" that appeared in the Wylie 1990 rational was not included.[95] The aspect ratio value of 20:1 which appears in the Glossary description of asbestiform contradicts the statements stated earlier in the R-93 method in Table 2-2 that the asbestiform properties of amosite (grunerite), crocidolite (riebeckite), anthophyllite, tremolite, and actinolite are "straight to curved, rigid fibers with aspect ratios typically >10:1."

Aspect ratio values as a way to discriminate between asbestos and non-asbestos fibers run the gamut in the published literature from 5:1 used by Van Orden in his flow chart showing the various characteristics that can be used to determine if a particle is asbestos or non-asbestos,[97] to 10:1 in Table 2-2 of the EPA R-93 bulk method, to 20:1 proposed by Wiley, to 35:1 for fibers less than 10 μm in length determined by Chatfield from his studies of fiber sizes used in animal toxicology studies.[98]

It is not possible to classify individual fibers as "asbestiform" because individual fibers do not exhibit all the characteristics of a population. With the exception of the requirements that the asbestos fibers have substantially parallel or stepped sides, there is little specific information given in the TEM standard methods that allows an analyst in a reproducible, scientifically acceptable way to classify individual fibers that fit the counting rules as asbestos or non-asbestos. Research has shown that a population of cleavage fragment particles has a smaller mean AR than a population of commercial asbestos fibers. However, the AR distributions of the two populations can overlap, and without strict adherence to a method, on an individual basis, some fibers could be classified either way. In Figure 2.11 the ARs of tremolite fibers found in an industrial talc sample are compared with the ARs determined from the National Institute for Standards and Technology (NIST) standard reference tremolite asbestos sample SRM 1876. The population of tremolite fibers in the industrial talc sample could be considered by some to be non-asbestiform because the mean AR is less than 20:1 as stated as a defining characteristic in some published articles. However, some individual tremolite fibers in the talc sample like the one shown in Figure 2.12 would be counted as an asbestos fiber under standard methods if found by itself. The use of population statistics such as an average AR for classification presumes that the sample is either entirely "asbestiform" or not and does not consider the possibility that the population of fibers could be composed of both "asbestiform" and "non-asbestiform" fibers. The use of population statistics based on bulk sample characteristics such as an average AR is not appropriate for the classification of individual fibers when present in air samples. Air sample filters produced from standard reference amosite asbestos fibers contain many fibers but very few parallel fibers occurring in bundles, fiber bundles displaying splayed ends, matted masses of individual fibers, or fibers showing curvature. Even when applied to bulk samples, such discrimination may be misleading since a single sample of amphibole particles may include fibers formed both through geologic metamorphism and through mechanical alteration.

A method to discriminate between asbestos fibers and cleavage fragments on the basis of fiber width was published in the scientific literature in 2012 by Dr Martin Harper of the Exposure Assessment Branch of the National Institute for Occupational Safety and Health (NIOSH).[99] After extensive inter-laboratory testing, Dr Harper found the width of the fiber to be the best discriminator for the classification of fibers as "asbestos" or "non-asbestos." The Harper paper concluded that using a criterion of width that is less than or equal to 1 μm provides the least number of false negatives, that is falsely classifying a fiber as non-asbestos when it actually is asbestos.

The question of whether or not standard asbestos methods should include discrimination between asbestos fibers and cleavage fragments is controversial. NIOSH believes that they should be counted even if they are derived from the non-asbestiform analogs of the asbestos minerals while OSHA does not agree.[100–102] The conclusions of the Finnish Institute of Occupational Health report of 2019 and the French ANSES opinion of 2015 support the opinion that regardless of whether the mineral fibers have been formed as a result of geological metamorphism or in an industrial process, such as in mining operations, mineral fibers within the dimensions specified by governmental health agencies should be considered when assessing asbestos exposures.[103, 104]

2.18 AMPHIBOLES

For most standard asbestos methods, "asbestos" means chrysotile and the five amphibole varieties: crocidolite (riebeckite), amosite (cummingtonite–grunerite), anthophyllite, tremolite, and actinolite. Other amphiboles can also exhibit asbestiform or fibrous habits. The difference between non-regulated fibrous amphiboles and those that are regulated is the amount of elemental substitution that has occurred when the mineral was formed on the Earth. The different amphibole names are defined by different elemental compositions and have been refined or modified over time. Two generally accepted nomenclature recommendations were published in Leake et al.[105] in 1997 and more recently by Hawthorne et al.[106] in 2012. Among the amphiboles present in the vermiculite from the Libby area of Montana are tremolite, richterite, and winchite.[107–110] The specific mineralogical determinations were made after extensive mineralogical studies. It is difficult to distinguish between tremolite, richterite, and winchite by PLM due to their very similar optical properties. Figure 2.8 shows examples of elemental spectra produced by NIST reference asbestos materials using TEM–EDS methodology. As seen in Figures 2.13 and 2.14, the elemental spectra from several Libby amphibole fibers are similar to tremolite or actinolite reference materials but differ in small amounts of sodium and potassium.

The association of amphibole fibers with some chrysotile ores has been noted in the scientific literature.[111, 112] Addison and Davies reported finding 28 of 81 samples of chrysotile positive for tremolite and Ilgren stated that chrysotile from the Jeffrey Mine in Quebec, Canada contained amphiboles but the chrysotile from the deposit in Coalinga, California did not.[113, 114] Williams-Jones et al. reported that the bulk of the amphibole in the Jeffry Mine in Quebec, Canada, is in the form of tremolite and actinolite, and is found mainly in serpentinite adjacent to or included within felsic dikes.[115]

Because the levels of asbestos that contaminate chrysotile are generally low compared to chrysotile (less than 1%) it is necessary to concentrate the possible amphibole material for analysis. To do this, an acid/base digestion procedure is used to eliminate the chrysotile and acid-soluble fractions.[16, 113, 116, 117] A portion of the sample is ashed and the residue remaining is transferred to a 100 mL round-bottom flask containing 80 mL of acid (2N H_2SO_4) and fitted with a reflux condenser. The suspension is boiled for one hour. The residue is collected by centrifugation, and the reflux procedure is repeated with sodium hydroxide (4N). The residue was then suspended in water, and a known aliquot is extracted and filtered through a 0.2 µm pore size polycarbonate filter. The filter is dried and can be analyzed by PLM or grids can be prepared following standard direct TEM preparation procedures for analysis by TEM using ASTM D6281 or ISO 10312. A study of 140 samples of finished products containing chrysotile asbestos using this acid/base reduction technique found amphibole asbestos fibers in 99% the products in the range from approximately 0.00005% to 0.5% in terms of weight percent and between 540,000 and 2.7 billion amphibole fibers per gram of product.[117]

2.19 METHODOLOGIES FOR TESTING THE FIBER RELEASE OF ASBESTOS-CONTAINING PRODUCTS

In addition to asbestos test methods for the analysis of bulk materials, air, water, dust, and tissue; there are also controlled testing procedures for gathering information about asbestos fiber exposure while various activities are performed with asbestos-containing materials. Activity-based sampling (ABS) is used by the USEPA during Superfund exposure assessments to determine the appropriateness of different types of personal protective equipment.[118–120] ABS, chamber studies and glove box testing are used by industrial hygienists during work practice studies to investigate historical exposures. All of these studies rely on the proper collection and analyses of air samples while investigators are performing an asbestos-related activity in a controlled setting. As summarized in a 2021 paper by Compton and Underwood,[121] there are several published papers and government documents which describe asbestos fiber release testing methodologies using glove boxes[122–125] and room-size containments.[126–139]

2.20 ACKNOWLEDGMENTS

The authors would like to thank Bryan Bandli, Randy Boltin, Pronda Few, Al Harmon, Whitney Hill, Bill Turner, Beth Wortman, Melissa Holman, Matthew Underwood, and Patrick Millette for their help in providing figures and editing assistance for this chapter.

REFERENCES

1. McCrone, WC. *The Asbestos Particle Atlas*, Ann Arbor Science Publishers Inc., Ann Arbor, MI, 1980, p. 21.
2. McCrone, WC. *Asbestos Identification*, McCrone Research Institute, Chicago, IL, 1987.
3. AHERA (Asbestos Hazard Emergency Response Act). Asbestos-Containing Materials in Schools, *Federal Register*, 52(210), 41846, 1987.
4. NESHAP (National Emission Standards for Hazardous Air Pollutants). Asbestos NESHAP Revision, Final Rule, *Federal Register*, 55(224), 48405, 1990.
5. EPA-600/R-93/116. *Method for the Determination of Asbestos in Bulk Building Materials*, U.S. Environmental Protection Agency, Washington, DC. 1993.

6. EPA-600/M4-82-020. *Test Method: Interim Method for the Determination of Asbestos in Bulk Insulation Samples*, U.S. Environmental Protection Agency, Washington, DC. 1982.
7. NIOSH Method 9002, Issue 2. *Asbestos (Bulk) by Polarized Light Microscopy (PLM), NIOSH Manual of Analytical Methods*,4th ed., National Institute of Occupational Safety and Health, Cincinnati, OH. 1994, p. 94.
8. OSHA ID. 191, 1915.1001 App K. Polarized Light Microscopy of Asbestos --Non-mandatory. Occupational Safety and Health Standards for Shipyard Employment, Subpart Z: Toxic and Hazardous Substances, *Federal Register*, 59 (113), 40964, Occupational Safety and Health Administration, Salt Lake City,UT. 1994.
9. Fairfax, RE. United States Department of Labor. Compliance Requirements for Renovation Work Involving Material Containing Less Than 1% Asbestos, *Occupational Safety and Health Administration*, 24 November 2003. https://www.osha.gov/laws-regs/standardinterpretations/2003-11-24-0.
10. Perkins, RL. Point-Counting Technique for Friable Asbestos-Containing Materials, *Microscope*, 38, 29–39, 1990.
11. ELAP Item 198.1. *Polarized-Light Microscope Methods for Identifying and Quantitating Asbestos in Bulk Samples*, New York State Department of Health Environmental Laboratory Approval Program Certification Manual, New York State Department of Health, Albany, NY, 2003.
12. Webber, JS, Janulis, RJ, Carhart, LJ, Gillespie, MD. Quantitating Asbestos Content in Friable Bulk Samples: Development of a Stratified Point-Count Method, *American Industrial Hygiene Association Journal*, 51(8), 447–452, 1990.
13. Chatfield, EJ. A Validated Method for Gravimetric Determination of Low Concentrations of Asbestos in Bulk Materials, in *Advances in Environmental Measurement Methods for Asbestos, ASTM STP 1342*, Beard, ME and Rook, HL, eds., American Society for Testing and Materials, West Conshohocken, PA, 2000, pp. 90–110.
14. ELAP Item 198.4. *Transmission Electron Microscope Method for Identifying and Quantitating Asbestos in Non-friable Organically Bound Samples. Environmental Laboratory Approval Program Certification Manual*, New York State Department of Health, New York State Department of Health, Albany, NY, 1997.
15. ISO 22262-1. *Air Quality - Bulk Methods Part 1: Sampling and Qualitative Determination of Asbestos in Commercial Bulk Materials*, International Standards Organization, Geneva, Switzerland, 2012.
16. ISO 22262-2. *Air Quality - Bulk Methods - Part 2: Quantitative Determination of Asbestos by Gravimetric and Microscopical Methods*, International Standards Organization, Geneva, Switzerland, 2014.
17. ISO 22262-3. *Air Quality - Bulk Methods - Part 3: Quantitative Determination of Asbestos by X-ray Diffraction Method*, International Standards Organization, Geneva, Switzerland, 2016.
18. NIOSH Method 7400. *Asbestos and Other Fibers by Phase Contrast Microscopy (PCM). NIOSH Manual of Analytical Methods*,5th ed., no. 3, U.S. Department of HHS, National Institute of Occupational Safety and Health, Cincinnati, OH, 2019.
19. Crane, D. Occupational Safety and Health Administration, OSHA ID-160, *Asbestos in Air*, July 1997.
20. Su, S. Comprehensive Suite of d-θ Look-Up Tables for Indexing Zone-Axis SAED Patterns of Amphibole Asbestos and Related Minerals, *The Microscope*, 68(3–4), 99–110, 2020.
21. Su, S. Indexing and Interpretation of Zone-Axis SAED Patterns of Amphibole Asbestos Minerals in the Asbestos Analysis by Transmission Electron Microscopy, in *Asbestos and Other Elongate Mineral Particles—New and Continuing Challenges in the 21st Century, STP 1632*, Millette, JR and Webber, JS, eds., ASTM International, West Conshohocken, PA, 2021, pp. 471–499.
22. NIOSH Method 7402. *Asbestos Fibers by Transmission Electron Microscopy (TEM). NIOSH Manual of Analytical Methods*,5th ed., U.S. Department of HHS, National Institute of Occupational Safety and Health, Cincinnati, OH, 2022, pp. 94–126.
23. ASTM D4240-83. *Standard Test Method for Airborne Asbestos Concentration in Workplace Atmosphere*,ASTM-International, West Conshohocken, PA, 1989.
24. ASTM D7201-06. *Standard Test Method for Airborne Asbestos Concentration in Workplace Atmosphere by Phase Contrast Microscopy (with an Option of Transmission Electron Microscopy)*, ASTM-International, West Conshohocken, PA, 2020.
25. Nicholson, WJ, Rohl, AN, Ferrand, EF. Asbestos Air Pollution in New York City, in *Proceedings of the Second International Clean Air Congress*, Englund, HM and Beery, WT, eds.,Washington, DC., December, 1970, Academic Press, New York, NY, 1971, pp. 136–139.
26. EPA 450/3-76-004. *Asbestos Contamination of the Air in Public Buildings*, U.S. Environmental Protection Agency,Research Triangle Park, NC. 1975.

27. Samudra, A, Harwood, CF, Stockham, JD. *Electron Microscope Measurement of Airborne Asbestos Concentration: A Provisional Methodology Manual*, Office of Research and Development, Washington, DC, EPA 600/2-77-178, 1978.
28. Yamate, G, Agarwall, SC, Gibbons, RD. *Methodology for the Measurement of Airborne Asbestos by Electron Microscopy*, EPA Draft Report Contract #68-02-3266, 1984.
29. ISO 13794. *Ambient Air: Determination of Asbestos Fibers -- Indirect Transmission Electron Microscopy Method*, International Standards Organization, Geneva, Switzerland, 2019.
30. AHERA. Appendix A to Subpart E — Interim Transmission Electron Microscopy Analytical Methods, U.S. EPA, 40 CFR Part 763, Asbestos-Containing Materials in Schools, Final Rule and Notice, *Federal Register*, 52(210), 41857–41894, 1987.
31. AIA Recommended Technical Method 2 (RTM2). *Method for the Determination of Airborne Asbestos Fiber and Other Inorganic Fibers by Scanning Electron Microscopy*, AIA Health and Safety Publication. Asbestos International Association, London, England, 1982.
32. ISO 14966. *Ambient Air: Determination of Numerical Concentration of Inorganic Fibrous Particles -- Scanning Electron Microscopy Method*, International Standards Organization, Geneva, Switzerland, 2002.
33. CARB 427. *Determination of Asbestos Emissions from Stationary Sources*, California Air Resources Board. Sacramento, CA, 1988.
34. ISO 10312. *Ambient Air: Determination of Asbestos Fibres -- Direct-Transfer Transmission Electron Microscopy Procedure*, International Standards Organization, Geneva, Switzerland, 1995.
35. ASTM D6281-15. *Standard Test Method for Airborne Asbestos Concentration in Ambient and Indoor Atmospheres as Determined by Transmission Electron Microscopy Direct Transfer*, ASTM International,West Conshohocken, PA, 2004.
36. Chesson, J, Hatfield, J. *Comparison of Airborne Asbestos Levels Determined by Transmission Electron Microscopy Using Direct and Indirect Transfer Techniques*, EPA 560/5-89-004, 1990.
37. EPA 600/4-84-043. *Method 100.1, Analytical Method for the Determination of Asbestos Fibers in Water*, U.S. Environmental Protection Agency, Washington, DC, 1984.
38. Brackett, KA, Clark, PJ, Millette, JR. *U.S. Environmental Protection Agency, Method 100.2, Determination of Asbestos Structures Over 10 µm in Length in Drinking Water*, EPA/600/R-94/134, 1994.
39. AWWA 2570. *Asbestos, Standard Methods for the Examination of Water and Wastewater*, 18th ed., American Public Health Association, American Water Works Association, Washington, DC, 1994.
40. Millette, JR, Few, P, Krewer, JA. Asbestos in Water Methods: EPA's 100.1 and 100.2 and AWWA's Standard Method 2570, in *Advances in Environmental Measurement Methods for Asbestos, ASTM STP 1342*, Beard, ME and Rook, HL, eds., American Society for Testing and Materials, Conshohocken, PA, 2000, pp. 227–241.
41. Feige, MA, Clark, PJ, Brackett, KA. Guidance and Clarification for the Current U.S. EPA Test Method for Asbestos in Drinking Water, *Energy and Environment Technology Supply*, 13–14(Fall), 1993, 13–14
42. ELAP Item 198.2. *Revision to Waterborne Asbestos Analysis, New York State Department of Health Environmental Laboratory Approval Program Certification Manual*, New York State Department of Health, Albany, NY, 1997.
43. Beard, ME, Millette, JR, Webber, JS. Developing ASTM Standards, Monitoring Asbestos, Standardization News, *American Society for Testing and Materials*, 32(4), 26–29, 2004.
44. ASTM D5755-02. *Standard Test Method for Microvacuum Sampling and Indirect Analysis of Dust by Transmission Electron Microscopy for Asbestos Structure Number Surface Loading*, ASTM-International, West Conshohocken, PA, 2002.
45. ASTM D6480-19. *Standard Test Method for Wipe Sampling of Surfaces, Indirect Preparation, and Analysis for Asbestos Structure Number Concentration by Transmission Electron Microscopy*, ASTM-International, West Conshohocken, PA, 2019.
46. Millette, JR. Use of the ASTM Inter-laboratory Studies (ILS) Program in Developing Precision Data for ASTM D5755 – Asbestos in Dust by Microvacuum Sampling, *Journal of ASTM International*, 8(8), 1–5. On-line: JAI (Journal of ASTM International) 103509. July 2011. Also published in ASTM STP 1533, pp. 177–186, Eds: M. Brisson and K. Ashley. 2011.
47. Ehrenfeld, FE III. ASTM International Research Report and Inter-laboratory Study for Development and Validation of ASTM D6480-10, Standard Test Method for Wipe Sampling of Surfaces, Indirect Preparation, and Analysis for Asbestos Structure Number Surface Loading by Transmission Electron Microscopy, in *Asbestos and Other Elongate Mineral Particles—New and Continuing Challenges in the 21st Century, STP, 1632*, Millette, JR and Webber, JS, eds., ASTM International, West Conshohocken, PA, pp. 500–512, 2021.

48. ASTM. D5756-95. *Standard Test Method for Microvacuum Sampling and Indirect Analysis of Dust by Transmission Electron Microscopy for Asbestos Mass Surface Loading*, ASTM-International, West Conshohocken, PA, 2002. Note: No Longer a Standard Method Maintained by ASTM;Withdrawn as of 2017.
49. Millette, JR, Clark, PJ, Brackett, KA, Wheeles, RK. Methods for the Analysis of Carpet Samples for Asbestos, U.S. Environmental Protection Agency, EPA/ 600/J-93/167, *Environmental Choices Technologies Supply*, 1(2), 21–24, 1993, (21–24 March/April).
50. Millette, JR, Hays, SM. *Settled Asbestos Dust: Sampling and Analysis*, Lewis Publishers, Boca Raton, 1994.
51. Hatfield, RL, Krewer, JA, Longo, WE. A Study of the Reproducibility of the Micro-vac Technique as a Tool for the Assessment of Surface Contamination in Buildings with Asbestos-Containing Materials, in *Advances in Environmental Measurement Methods for Asbestos, ASTM STP 1342*, Beard, ME and Rook, HL, eds., American Society for Testing and Materials, West Conshohocken, PA, 2000, pp. 301–312.
52. Lee, RJ, VanOrden, DR, Stewart, IM. Dust and Airborne Concentrations — Is There a Correlation? in, *Advances in Environmental Measurement Methods for Asbestos, ASTM STP 1342*, Beard, ME and Rook, HL, eds., American Society for Testing and Materials, West Conshohocken, PA, 2000, pp. 313–322.
53. Ewing, WM. Further Observations of Settled Asbestos Dust in Buildings, in *Advances in Environmental Measurement Methods for Asbestos, ASTM STP 1342*, Beard, ME and Rook, HL, eds., American Society for Testing and Materials, West Conshohocken, PA, 2000, pp. 323–332.
54. Fowler, DP, Price, BP. Some Statistical Principles in Asbestos Measurement and Their Application to Dust Sampling and Analysis, in *Advances in Environmental Measurement Methods for Asbestos, ASTM STP 1342*, Beard, ME and Rook, HL, eds., American Society for Testing and Materials, West Conshohocken, PA, 2000, pp. 333–349.
55. Crankshaw, OS, Perkins, RL, Beard, ME. An Overview of Settled Dust Analytical Methods and Their Relative Effectiveness, in *Advances in Environmental Measurement Methods for Asbestos, ASTM STP 1342*, Beard, ME and Rook, HL, eds., American Society for Testing and Materials, West Conshohocken, PA, 2000, pp. 350–365.
56. Millette, JR, Mount, MD. Applications of the ASTM Asbestos in Dust Method D5755, in *Advances in Environmental Measurement Methods for Asbestos, ASTM STP 1342*, Beard, ME and Rook, HL, eds., American Society for Testing and Materials, West Conshohocken, PA, 2000, pp. 366–377.
57. Chatfield, EJ. Correlated Measurements of Airborne Asbestos-Containing Particles and Surface Dust, in *Advances in Environmental Measurement Methods for Asbestos, ASTM STP 1342*, Beard, ME and Rook, HL, eds., American Society for Testing and Materials, West Conshohocken, PA, 2000, pp. 378–402.
58. Hays, SM. Incorporating Dust Sampling into the Asbestos Management Program, in *Advances in Environmental Measurement Methods for Asbestos, ASTM STP 1342*, Beard, ME and Rook, HL, eds., American Society for Testing and Materials, West Conshohocken, PA, 2000, pp. 403–410.
59. Clifford, S. *The Protocol for Screening Soil and Sediment Samples for Asbestos Content Used by the U.S. Environmental Protection Agency*, U.S. Environmental Protection Agency Region 1, Lexington, MA, 1997.
60. ASTM D7521. *Standard Test Method for Determination of Asbestos in Soil*, ASTM-International, West Conshohocken, PA, 2016.
61. Berman, DW, Chatfield, EJ. *Interim Superfund Method for the Determination of Asbestos in Ambient Air*, EPA 540/2-90/005a, May. EPA, Washington, DC, 1990.
62. Berman, DW, Kolk, AJ. *Superfund Method for the Determination of Releasable Asbestos in Soils and Bulk Materials, (Interim Version) prepared for U.S. EPA*, Office of Solid Waste and Emergency Response, Washington, DC, Contract, 68-W9-0059, July 1995.
63. Januch, J, Brattin, W, Woodbury, L, Berry, D. Evaluation of a Fluidized Bed Asbestos Segregator Preparation Method for the Analysis of Low-Levels of Asbestos in Soil and Other Solid Media, *Analytical Methods*, 5(7), 1658–1668, 2013.
64. EPA/600/R-04/004. *Research Method for Sampling and Analysis of Fibrous Amphibole in Vermiculite Attic Insulation,Cincinnati Method*, U.S. Environmental Protection Agency, Washington, DC, 2004.
65. Millette, JR, Compton, S. Analysis of Vermiculite for Asbestos and Screening for Vermiculite from Libby, Montana, *The Microscope*, 63(2), 55–70, 2015.
66. ELAP Test Method 198.8. *Polarized-Light Microscope Method for Identifying and Quantitating Asbestos in Sprayed-On Fireproofing Containing Vermiculite - Bulk Samples. Environmental*

Laboratory Approval Program Certification Program (NY ELAP), New York State Department of Health, Albany, NY, 2014.
67. Cralley, J. Fibrous and Mineral Content of Cosmetic Talcum Products, *American Industrial Hygiene Association Journal* (July–August) , 29(4), 350–354, 1968.
68. Lewin, S. Letter and Final Analytical Results from S. Lewin (New York University) to A. Weissler (U.S. Dept Health and Human Services), Dated 3 August 1972.
69. Snider, D, et al. Asbestosform Impurities in Commercial Talcum Powders, *The Compass of Sigma Gamma Epsilon*, 49(2), 65–67, 1972.
70. Dement, JM, et al. *Preliminary Report: Fiber Exposure During Use of Baby Powders. Environmental Investigations Branch, Division of Field Studies and Clinical Investigations*, National Institute for Occupational Safety and Health: Cincinnati, OH, July 1972.
71. Langer, A. Aspects of Mineralogy of Talc, Proceedings of the Symposium on Talc, Washington, DC, 5 August 1973, pp. 82–88.
72. Rohl, AN. Asbestos in Talc, *Environmental Health Perspectives*, 9, 129–132, 1974.
73. Rohl, AN, Langer, AM. *Fibrous Mineral Content of Consumer Talc-Containing Products*, Pathotox Publishers, Inc. of Park Forest South, Illinois, 393–403, 1979.
74. Rohl, AN, Langer, AM. Identification and Quantitation of Asbestos in Talc, *Environmental Health Perspectives*, 9, 95–109, 1974.
75. Rohl, AN, et al. Consumer Talcums and Powders: Mineral and Chemical Characterization, *Journal of Toxicology and Environmental Health*, 2(2), 255–284, 1976.
76. Paoletti, L, et al. Evaluation by Electron Microscopy Techniques of Asbestos Contamination in Industrial, Cosmetic and Pharmaceutical Talcs, *Regulatory Toxicology and Pharmacology*, 4(3), 222–235, 1984.
77. Blount, AM. Amphibole Content of Cosmetic and Pharmaceutical Talcs, *Environmental Health Perspectives*, 94, 225–230, 1991.
78. Mattenklott, M. Asbestos in Talc Powders and Soapstone – The Present State, (Translation of) Asbest in Talkumpudern und Speckstein – heutige Situation, *Gefahrstoffe – Reinhaltung der Luft*, 67(7/8), 287–291, 2007. (translation courtesy of Springer- VDIVerlag, Düsseldorf).
79. Gordon, R, et al. Asbestos in Commercial Cosmetic Talcum Powder as a Cause of Mesothelioma in Women, *International Journal of Occupational and Environmental Health*, 4, 318–332, 2014.
80. Steffen, J, et al. Serous Ovarian Cancer Caused by Exposure to Asbestos and Fibrous Talc in Cosmetic Talc Powders—A Case Series, *Journal of Occupational and Environmental Medicine*, 62(2), e65–e77, 2020. doi: 10.1097/JOM.0000000000001800.
81. Moline, J, et al. Mesothelioma Associated with the Use of Cosmetic Talc, *Journal of Occupational and Environmental Medicine*, 62(1), 11–17, 2020.
82. Rosner, D, et al. Nondetected: The Politics of Measurement of Asbestos in Talc, 1971-1976, *Public Health Then and Now, AJPH*, 109(7), 969–974, July 2019.
83. CTFA Method J4-1. *Asbestiform Amphibole Minerals in Cosmetic Talc*, Cosmetic, Toiletry, and Fragrance Association, Washington, DC, October 1976.
84. Block, L, et al. Modernization of Asbestos Testing in USP Talc, *U.S. Pharmacopeial Convention, Stimuli to the Revision Process*, 40(4), 455–4722014.
85. USP 48(2) <901>. General Chapter: <901>. *Detection of Asbestos in Pharmaceutical Talc*, United States Pharmacopeia and National Formulary, Rockville, MD, 22 May 2022.
86. USP48(2) <1901>. General Chapter: <901>. *Theory and Practice of Asbestos Detection in Pharmaceutical Talc*, United States Pharmacopeia and National Formulary, Rockville, MD, 22 May 2022.
87. Talc, <901> Detection of Asbestos in Pharmaceutical Talc, <1901> Theory and Practice of Asbestos Detection in Pharmaceutical Talc. *USP*, 26 May 2023, www.uspnf.com/notices/talc-official-dates-20230601.
88. Millette, JR. Procedure for the Analysis of Talc for Asbestos, *The Microscope*, 63(1), 11–20, 2015.
89. Response to the November 2005 National Stone,Sand & Gravel Association Report Prepared by the R J. Lee Group, Inc. *Evaluation of EPA's Analytical Data from the El Dorado Hills Asbestos Evaluation Project*,U.S. Environmental Protection Agency, Region, IX, San Francisco, CA, 20 April 2006.
90. Interagency Working Group on Asbestos in Consumer Products (IWGACP). Scientific Opinions on Testing Methods for Asbestos in Cosmetic Products Containing Talc. White Paper, December 2021.
91. Chatfield, E. Analytical Protocol for Determination of Asbestos Contamination of Clothing and Other Fabrics, *Microscope*, 38, 221–222, 1990.
92. Krewer, JA, Millette, JR. Comparison of Sodium Hypochlorite Digestion and Low-Temperature Ashing Preparation Techniques for Lung Tissue Analysis by TEM, Proceedings of the Microbeam Analysis 1986, 21st Conference on Microbeam Analysis Society, San Francisco Press, Inc., Albuquerque, NM, August 1986.

93. Vos, MA Asbestos in Ontario: Industrial Mineral Report 36, Ontario Department of Mines and Northern Affairs, 1971.
94. Dodson, RF, et al. Usefulness of Combined Light and Electron Microscopy: Evaluation of Sputum Samples for Asbestos to Determine past Occupational Exposure, *Modern Pathology*, 2(4), 320–322, 1989.
95. Wylie, AG. Discriminating Amphibole Cleave Fragments from Asbestos: Rationale and Methodology, Proceedings of VII International Pneumoconiosis Conference, 1990.
96. Siegrist, HG Jr, Wylie, AG. Characterizing and Discriminating the Shape of Asbestos Particles, *Environmental Research*, 23(2), 348–361, 1980.
97. Van Orden, DR, Allison, KA, Lee, RJ. Differentiating Amphibole Asbestos from Non-asbestos in a Complex Mineral Environment, *Indoor and Built Environment*, 17(1), 58–68, 2008.
98. Chatfield, EJ. Measurement of Elongate Mineral Particles: What We Should Measure and How Do We Do It?, *Toxicology and Applied Pharmacology*, 361, 36–46, 2018.
99. Harper, M, Lee, EG, Slaven, JE, Bartley, DL. An Inter-laboratory Study to Determine the Effectiveness of Procedures for Discriminating Amphibole Asbestos Fibres from Amphibole Cleavage Fragments in Fibre Counting by Phase-Contrast Microscopy, *Annals of Occupational Hygiene*, 56(6), 645–659, 2012.
100. DHHS (NIOSH) Publication Number 2011-159. *Current Intelligence Bulletin 62: Asbestos Fibers and Other Elongate Mineral Particles: State of the Science and Roadmap for Research*, National Institute for Occupational Safety and Health (NIOSH), Washington, DC, April 2011.
101. Final Asbestos Standard, Intro to 29 CFR Parts 1910 and 1926, Occupational Exposure to Asbestos, *Tremolite, Anthophyllite and Actinolite, Section 4 - Mineralogical Considerations*, 57(110), 219 -246, Occupational Safety and Health Administration, Washington, DC. 1992.
102. Tran, TH, Egilman, DS, et al. The Definition of Asbestos – A Manufactured Defense to Avoid Regulation and Victim Compensation, Medical Research, *Archives*, 10(6), 2022. doi: 10.18103/mra. v10i6.2778.
103. Agence Nationale de Sécurité Sanitaire (ANSES). Opinion of the French Agency for Food, Environmental and Occupational Health & Safety, in: *Health Effects and the Identification of Cleavage Fragments of Amphiboles from Quarried Minerals*, Request No. 2014_SA_0196, Agence Nationale de Sécurité Sanitaire (ANSES): Paris, France, 2015.
104. Finnish Institute of Occupational Health. *Asbestos Risk Management Guidelines for Mines*, vol. 6, Finnish Institute of Occupational Health: Helsinki, Finland, 2019.
105. Leake, BE, et al. Nomenclature of the Amphiboles: Report of the Sub-committee on Amphiboles of the International Mineralogical Association, Commission on New Minerals and Mineral Names, *Canadian Mineralogist*, 35, 219–246, 1997.
106. Hawthorne, FC, et al. Nomenclature of the Amphibole Supergroup, *American Mineralogist*, 97(11–12), 2031–2048, 2012.
107. Wylie, AG, Verkouteren, JR. Amphibole Asbestos from Libby, Montana: Aspects of Nomenclature: Table, *American Mineralogist*, 85(10), 1540–1542, 2000.
108. Bandli, BR, Gunter, ME. Identification and Characterization of Mineral and Asbestos Particles Using the Spindle Stage and the Scanning Electron Microscope: The Libby, Montana, U.S.A. Amphibole-Asbestos as an Example, *Microscope*, 49, 191–199, 2000.
109. Meeker, GP, et al. The Composition and Morphology of Amphibole from the Rainy Creek Complex, near Libby, Montana, *American Mineralogist*, 88(11–12), 1955–1969, 2003.
110. Bandli, BR, et al. Optical, Compositional, Morphological, and X-ray Data on Eleven Particles of Amphibole from Libby, Montana, U.S.A., *Canadian Mineralogist*, 41(5), 1241–1253, 2003.
111. Gibbs, GW, LaChance, M. Dust Exposure in the Chrysotile Mines and Mills of Quebec, *Archives of Environmental Health*, 24(3), 189–197, 1972.
112. Nayebzadeh, A, Dufresne, A, Case, B, Vali, H, Williams-Jones, AE, Martin, R, Normand, C, Clark, J. Lung Mineral Fibers of Former Miners and Millers from Thetford-Mines and Asbestos Regions: A Comparative Study of Fiber Concentration and Dimension, *Archives of Environmental Health*, 56(1), 65–76, 2001.
113. Addison, J, Davies, LST. Analysis of Amphibole Asbestos in Chrysotile and Other Minerals, *Annals of Occupational Hygiene*, 34(2), 159–175, 1990.
114. Ilgren, E, Chatfield, E. Coalinga Fibre- A Short, Amphibole-free Chrysotile, *Indoor and Built Environment*, 7, 18–31, 1998.
115. Williams-Jones, AE, Normand, C, Clark, JR, Vali, H, Martin, RF, Dufresne, NA. Controls of Amphibole formation in Chrysotile Deposits: Evidence from the Jeffery Mine, Asbestos, Quebec. The Health Effects of Chrysotile Asbestos: Contribution of Science to Risk-Management Decisions, *Canadian Journal Specifications Publishing*, 5, 89–104, 2001.

116. Millette, JR, Harmon, A, Few, P, Turner, WL Jr, Boltin, WR. Analysis of Amphibole Asbestos in Chrysotile-Containing Ores and a Manufactured Asbestos Product, *Microscope*, 57(1), 19–22, 2009.
117. Compton, SP, Millette, JR. Quantification of Amphibole in Chrysotile Asbestos-Containing Products, in *Asbestos and Other Elongate Mineral Particles—New and Continuing Challenges in the 21st Century, STP, 1632*, Millette, JR and Webber, JS, eds., ASTM International, West Conshohocken, PA, 341–361.
118. EPA OSWER Directive No. 9200.0-68. *Framework for Investigating Asbestos-Contaminated Superfund Sites, U.S.* Environmental Protection Agency, Washington, DC, 2008.
119. EPA SERAS SOP No. 2084-rl.1. *Activity-Based Air Sampling for Asbestos,* U.S Environmental Protection Agency, Washington,DC, 2017.
120. ASTM D7886-14. *Standard Practice for Asbestos Exposure Assessments for Repetitive Maintenance and Installation Tasks*,ASTM International, West Conshohocken, PA, 2019.
121. Compton, SP, Underwood, MR. Asbestos Fiber Release Studies Using a Constructed Simulation Chamber, in *Asbestos and Other Elongate Mineral Particles—New and Continuing Challenges in the 21st Century*, Millette, JR and Webber, JS, eds., ASTM International: West Conshohocken, PA, 2021, pp. 91–115.
122. Geraci, C, Baron, P, Carter, J, Smith, D. *Testing of Hair Dryers for Asbestos Emissions, Interagency Agreement*, NIOSH with U.S. CPSC, IA-79-29, Cincinnati, OH, September 1979.
123. Rock, A. *Report on the Results of the Asbestos Product Fiber Release Testing, U.S.*, Consumer Product Safety Commission, 13 October 1985.
124. Falgout, D. *Environmental Release of Asbestos from Commercial Product Shaping*, U.S. EPA, 600/S2-85/044, August 1985.
125. Millette, JR. Microscopical Studies of the Asbestos Fiber Releasability of Dryer Felt Textiles, *Microscope*, 47(2), 93–100, 1999.
126. Fleming, RM. *Asbestos – Burlap Bags, Environmental Investigations Branch*, NIOSH, Cincinnati, OH, 14 January 1972.
127. Millette, JR, Mount, MD. A Study Determining Asbestos Fiber Release During the Removal of Valve Packing, *Applied Occupational and Environmental Hygiene*, 8(9), 790–793, 1993.
128. Millette, JR, Mount, MD, Hays, SM. Releasability of Asbestos Fibers from Asbestos-Containing Gaskets, *EIA Technical Journal*, 10–15(Fall), 1995.
129. Fowler, D. Exposures to Asbestos Arising from Bandsawing Gasket Material. *Applied Occupational and Environmental Hygiene*, 15(5), 404–408, 2000.
130. Boelter, F, Crawford, G, Podraza, DM. Airborne Fiber Exposure Assessment of Dry Asbestos-Containing Gaskets and Packings Found in Intact Industrial and Maritime Fittings, *AIHA Journal: A Journal for the Science of Occupational and Environmental Health and Safety*, 63(6), 732–740, 2002.
131. Longo, W, Egeland, WB, Hatfield, RL, Newton, LR. Fiber Release During the Removal of Asbestos-Containing Gaskets: A Work Practice Simulation, *Applied Occupational and Environmental Hygiene*, 17(1), 55–72, 2002.
132. Mowat, FF, Bono, M, Lee, RJ, Tamburello, S, Paustenbach, D. Occupational Exposure to Airborne Asbestos from Phenolic Molding Material (Bakelite) During Sanding, Drilling, and Related Activities, *Journal of Occupational and Environmental Hygiene*, 2(10), 497–507, 2005.
133. Mowat, F, Weidling, R, Sheehan, P. Simulation Tests to Assess Occupational Exposure to Airborne Asbestos from Asphalt-Based Roofing Products, *Annals of Occupational Hygiene*, 51(5), 451–462, 2007.
134. Sheehan, PF, Mowat, F, Weidling, R, Floyd, M. Simulation Tests to Assess Occupational Exposure to Airborne Asbestos from Artificially Weathered Asphalt-Based Roofing Products, *Annals of Occupational Hygiene*, 54(8), 880–892, 2010.
135. Compton, SP, Millette, JR. Airborne Asbestos Exposure from Gooch Fiber Use, *The Microscope*, 60(4), 165–170, 2012.
136. Millette, JR, Compton, SP, DePasquale, C. Microscopical Analyses of Asbestos-Cement Pipe and Board, *The Microscope*, 66(1), 2–20, 2018.
137. Millette, JR, Compton, SP, DePasquale, C. Microscopical Analyses of Asbestos-Containing Dental Tape, *The Microscope*, 67(3), 99–109, 2019.
138. Millette, JR, Compton, SP, DePasquale, C. Microscopical Analyses of Asbestos-Containing Fibrous Adhesive, *The Microscope*, 68(2), 71–79, 2020.
139. Millette, JR, Compton, SP, DePasquale, C. Microscopy in the Investigation of Asbestos-Containing Friction Products, *The Microscope*, 68(3/4), 111–131, 2020.

TABLE 2.1
Comparison of Standard Microscopy Methods for the Analysis of Bulk Materials

	EPA-600/M4-82-020 1982	EPA-600/R-93/116 1993	NIOSH 9002	OSHA ID-191	ISO 22262-1 ISO 22262-2
Instrument	Stereo, PLM, XRD	Stereo, PLM, TEM	Stereo, PLM	Stereo, PLM mention of SEM, TEM	Stereo, PLM, TEM
Sample Preparation	As is Some matrix reduction	As is Some matrix reduction	As is Some matrix reduction	As is Some matrix reduction	As is Detailed matrix reduction
Minimum Fiber diameter	Approximately >1 μm	PLM: approx. >1 μm TEM: approx. >0.002 μm	Approximately >1 μm	Approximately >1 μm	PLM: approx. >1 μm TEM: approx. >0.002 μm
Aspect Ratio	>3:1	Generally >10:1	Not addressed	>3:1 with mention of 100:1	Not addressed for PLM 5:1 by TEM
Measurement	Volume or areal estimation	Visual estimation	Areal estimation	Areal estimation	Volume estimation Weight
Identification	PLM: refractive indices, dispersion staining, birefringence, sign of elongation, and extinction angle	PLM: refractive indices, dispersion staining, birefringence, sign of elongation, and extinction angle TEM: morphology, crystal structure, elemental composition	PLM: refractive indices, dispersion staining, birefringence, sign of elongation, and extinction angle	PLM: refractive indices, dispersion staining, birefringence, sign of elongation, and extinction angle. SEM: morphology, elemental composition TEM: morphology, crystal structure, elemental composition	PLM: refractive indices, dispersion staining, birefringence, sign of elongation, and extinction angle TEM: morphology, crystal structure, elemental composition
Reporting	% Asbestos	% asbestos and possible weight %	% asbestos	% asbestos	Volume or areal % asbestos Weight % or weight % range

TABLE 2.2
Comparison of Fiber Definitions Used in Measuring Asbestos in Air

Term	Method	Definition
Fiber	NIOSH 7400 (PCM)	Longer than 5 μm with a length-to-width ratio equal to or greater than 3:1
Fiber	NIOSH 7402 (TEM)	All particles with a diameter greater than 0.25 μm that meet the definition of a fiber (AR greater than or equal to 3:1, longer than 5 μm) [AR = Aspect ratio]
Fiber	OSHA ID-160 (PCM)	A particle that is 5 μm or longer, with a length-to-width ratio of 3:1 or longer
Fiber	Draft Yamate (TEM)	Particle with an AR of 3:1 or greater and with substantially parallel sides
Fiber	AHERA (TEM)	A structure greater than or equal to 0.5 μm in length with an AR (length-to-width) of 5:1 or greater and having substantially parallel sides
Fiber (Fibre)	ISO 10312 and ASTM D6281 (TEM)	An elongated particle which has parallel or stepped sides. For the purposes of this international standard, a fiber is defined to have an AR equal to or greater than 5:1 and a minimum length of 0.5 μm
Bundle	NIOSH 7400 (PCM)	Not defined in method, but counted as a fiber
Bundle	NIOSH 7402 (TEM)	Not defined in method
Bundle	OSHA ID-160 (PCM)	Not defined in method
Bundle	Draft Yamate (TEM)	Particulate composed of fibers in a parallel arrangement, with each fiber closer than the diameter of one fiber
Bundle	AHERA (TEM)	A structure composed of three or more fibers in a parallel arrangement with each fiber closer than one fiber diameter
Bundle	ISO 10312 and ASTM D6281 (TEM)	A structure composed of parallel, smaller diameter fibers attached along their lengths. A fibre bundle may exhibit diverging fibers at one or both ends
Cluster	NIOSH 7400 (PCM)	Not defined in method, but counted individually as fibers if not originating from the same bundle
Cluster	NIOSH 7402 (TEM)	Not defined in method
Cluster	OSHA ID-160 (PCM)	Not defined in method
Cluster	Draft Yamate (TEM)	Particulate with fibers in a random arrangement such that all fibers are intermixed and no single fiber is isolated from the group
Cluster	AHERA (TEM)	A structure with fibers in a random arrangement such that all fibers are intermixed and no single fiber is isolated from the group. Groupings must have more than two intersections
Cluster	ISO 10312 and ASTM D6281 (TEM)	A structure in which two or more fibers, or fibre bundles, are randomly oriented in a connected grouping
Matrix	NIOSH 7400 (PCM)	Not defined in method, but counted as fibers
Matrix	NIOSH 7402 (TEM)	Not defined in method
Matrix	OSHA ID-160 (PCM)	Not defined in method
Matrix	Draft Yamate (TEM)	Fiber or fibers with one end free and the other end embedded or hidden by a particulate
Matrix	AHERA (TEM)	Fiber or fibers with one end free and the other end embedded in or hidden by a particulate. The exposed fiber must meet the (AHERA) fiber definition
Matrix	ISO 10312 and ASTM D6281 (TEM)	A structure in which one or more fibers, or fibre bundles, touch, are attached to, or partially concealed by, a single particle or connected group of non-fibrous particles

TABLE 2.3
Comparison of Standard Methods for Measuring Asbestos in Air

	NIOSH 7400	NIOSH 7402	AHERA	ASTM 6281 and ISO 10312
Instrument	PCM	TEM	TEM	TEM
Filter Preparation	Direct	Direct	Direct	Direct Indirect—ISO 13794
Magnification	400–450×	10,000×	~20,000×	~20,000×
Fiber Length	>5 µm	>5 µm	>0.5 µm	≥0.5 µm PCME >5 µm
Fiber Width	Any observed by PCM	>0.25 µm	No minimum, approx. >0.002 µm	No minimum, approx. >0.002 µm PCME >0.2 to <3 µm
Aspect Ratio	≥3:1	≥3:1	≥5:1	≥5:1 PCME ≥3:1
Counting	Fibers	Fibers	Structures	Structures PCME—fibers
Identification	None	Morphology, crystal structure, elements	Morphology, crystal structure, elements	Morphology, crystal structure, elements
Reporting	Fibers/cm^3 (F/cc)	% Asbestos	Asbestos structures/cm^3 (str/cc)	Asbestos structures/cm^3 (str/cc) PCME—asbestos F/cc

TABLE 2.4
Comparison of Standard Methods of Measuring Asbestos in Water

	EPA 100.1	EPA 100.2	AWWA 2570
Instrument	TEM	TEM	TEM
Filter preparation	Indirect Polycarbonate filter	Indirect Polycarbonate filter or mixed cellulose ester filter (MCE)	Indirect Polycarbonate filter or mixed cellulose ester filter (MCE)
Magnification	~20,000×	~20,000×	~20,000×
Fiber length	>0.5 µm	≥10 µm	≥0.5 µm
Fiber width	Approx. >0.002 µm	Approx. >0.002 µm	Approx. >0.002 µm
Aspect ratio	≥3:1	≥3:1	≥5:1
Counting	Asbestos structures	Asbestos structures	Asbestos structures
Identification	Morphology, crystal structure, elements	Morphology, crystal structure, elements	Morphology, crystal structure, elements
Reporting	Millions of asbestos fibers/L (MFL)	Millions of asbestos fibers >10 µm/L	Millions of asbestos fibers/L (MFL)

TABLE 2.5
Comparison of Standard Methods of Measuring Asbestos in Settled Dust

	ASTM D5755 Microvacuum	ASTM D6480 Wipe	EPA/600/J-93/167 Carpet
Surface	Any dry surface	Hard Non-porous	Piece of carpet
Instrument	TEM	TEM	TEM
Filter preparation	Indirect	Indirect	Indirect
Magnification	~20,000×	~20,000×	~20,000×
Fiber length	≥0.5 µm	≥0.5 µm	>0.5 µm
Fiber width	Approx. >0.002 µm	Approx. >0.002 µm	Approx. >0.002 µm
Aspect ratio	≥5:1	≥5:1	≥5:1
Counting	Asbestos structures	Asbestos structures	Asbestos structures
Identification	Morphology, crystal structure, elements	Morphology, crystal structure, elements	Morphology, crystal structure, elements
Reporting	Asbestos str/cm^2	Asbestos str/cm^2	Asbestos str/cm^2 of carpet

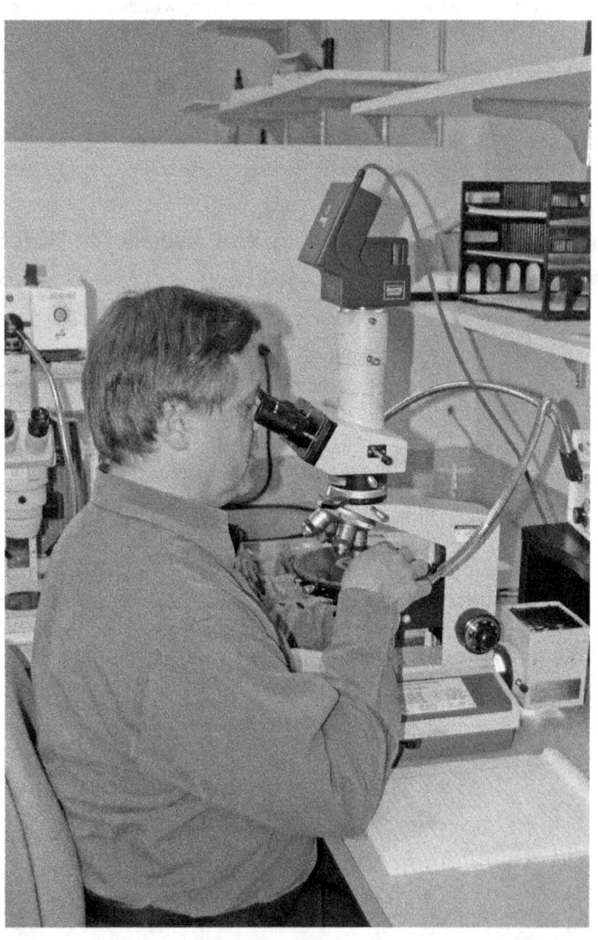

FIGURE 2.1 Analyst using a PLM for asbestos analysis.

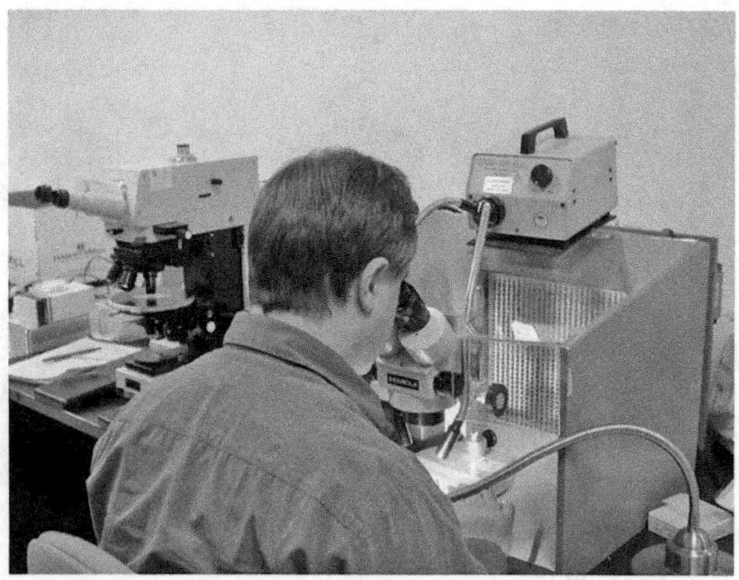

FIGURE 2.2 Analyst using a stereo-binocular microscope in a HEPA-filtered hood to examine a bulk sample for asbestos.

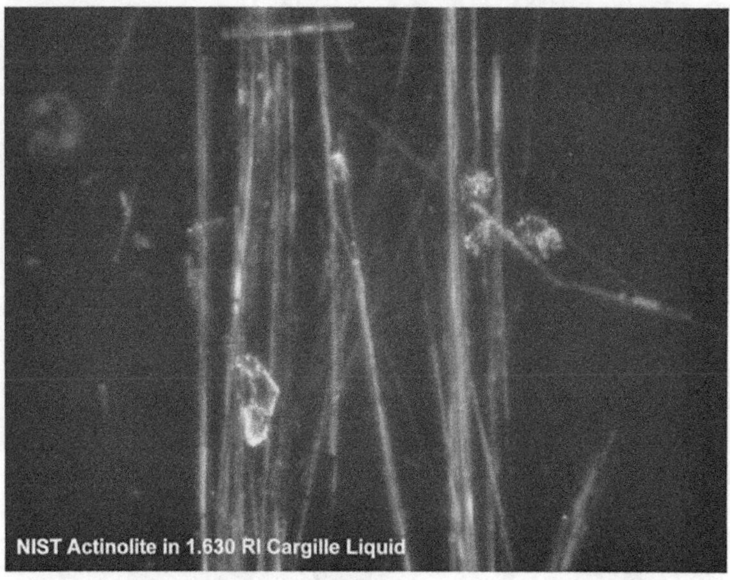

FIGURE 2.3 Image of asbestos as seen with a PLM.

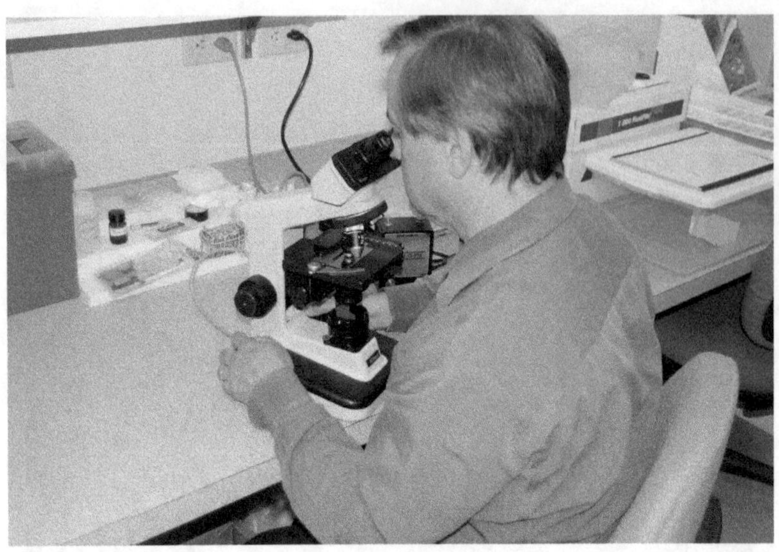

FIGURE 2.4 Analyst using a PCM for asbestos analysis.

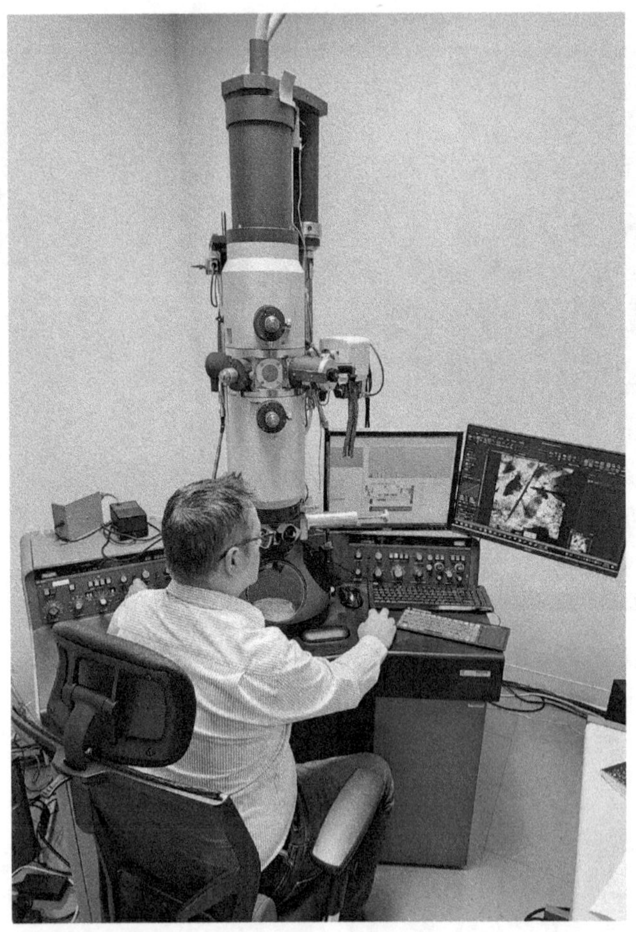

FIGURE 2.5 Analyst using a TEM for asbestos analysis.

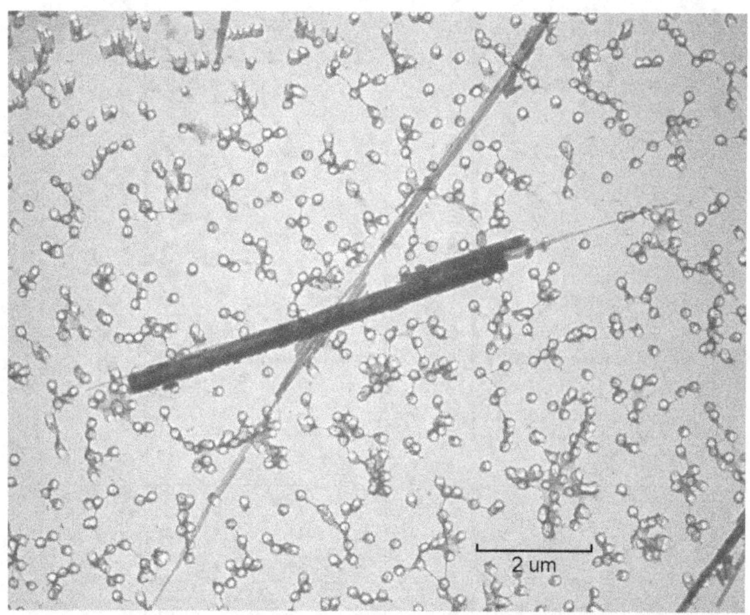

FIGURE 2.6 Image of crocidolite and chrysotile asbestos fibers as seen with a TEM. Crocidolite is the thicker fiber; chrysotile is longer and thin. The circles are carbon replicas of the PC filter.

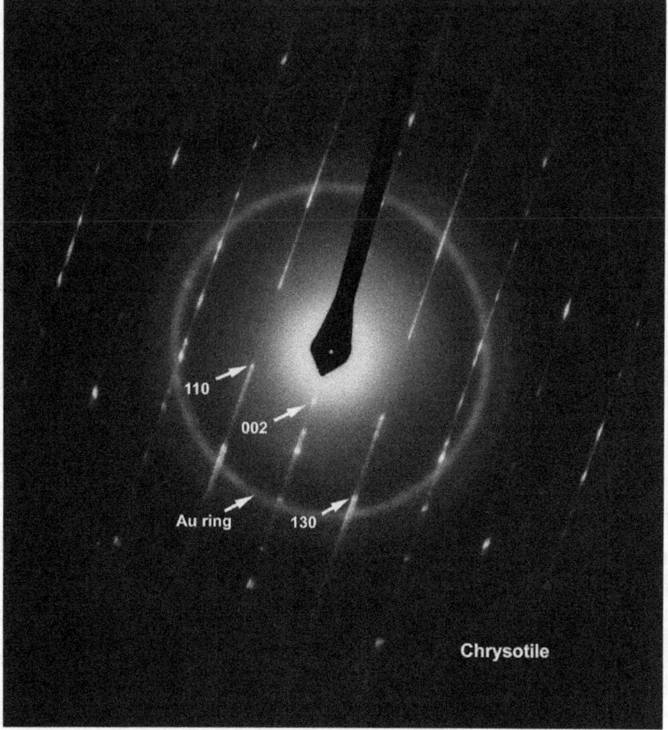

FIGURE 2.7 Chrysotile SAED pattern. The gold ring results from coating the fiber with a thin layer of gold and is used for calibration.

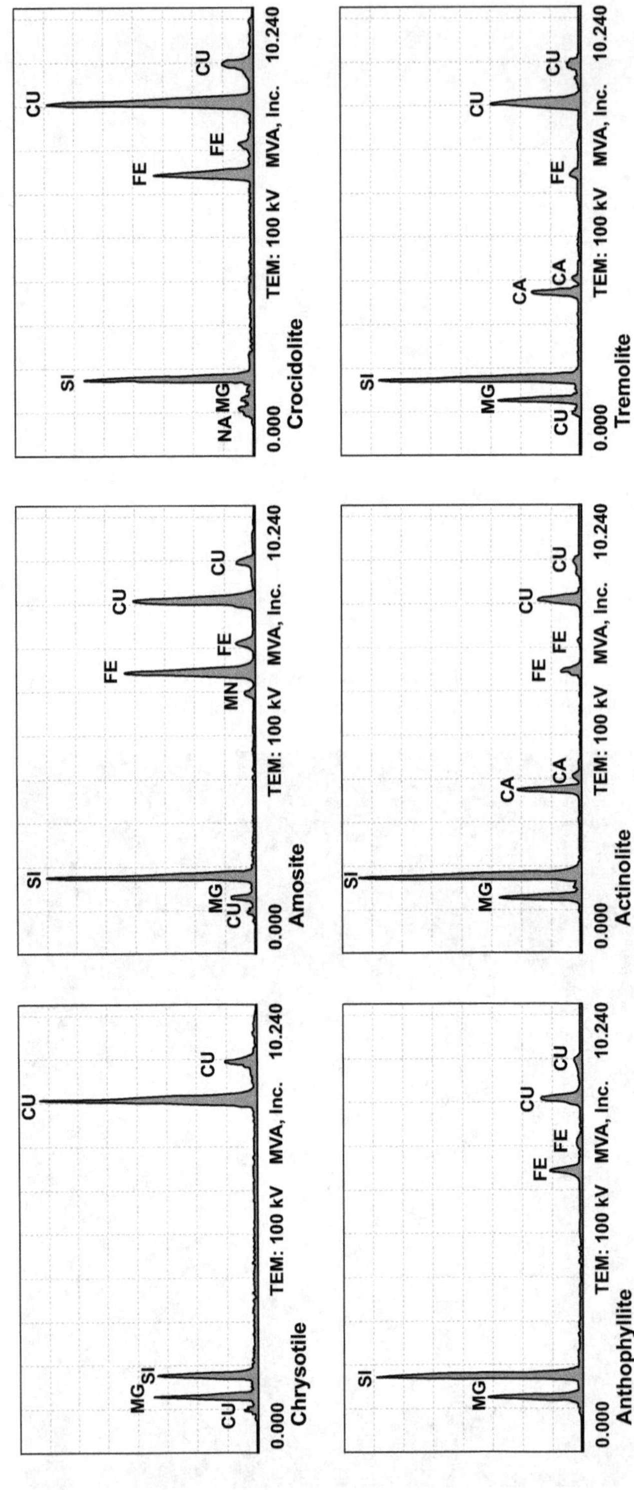

FIGURE 2.8 EDS X-ray spectra for NIST reference asbestos fibers.

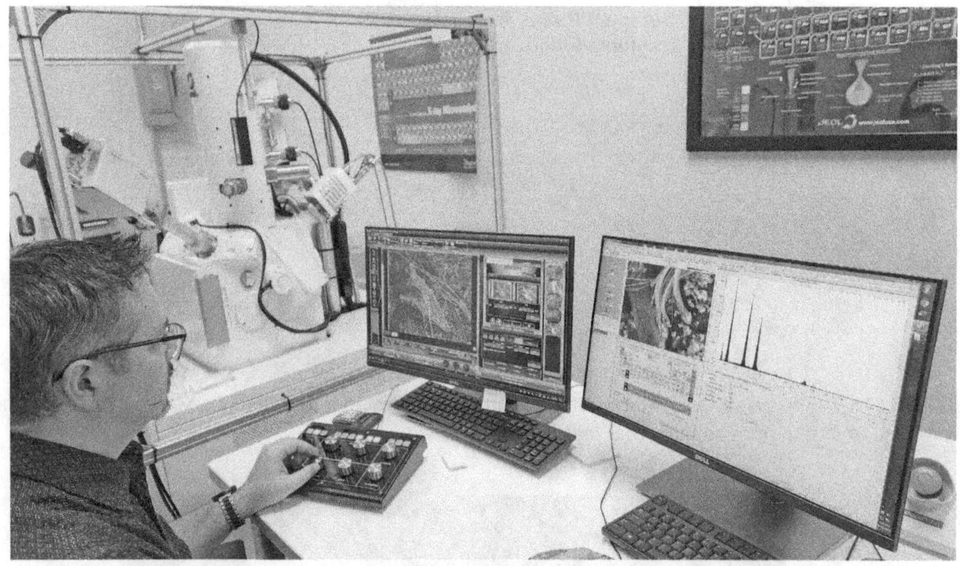

FIGURE 2.9 An example of an SEM that is used for asbestos analysis.

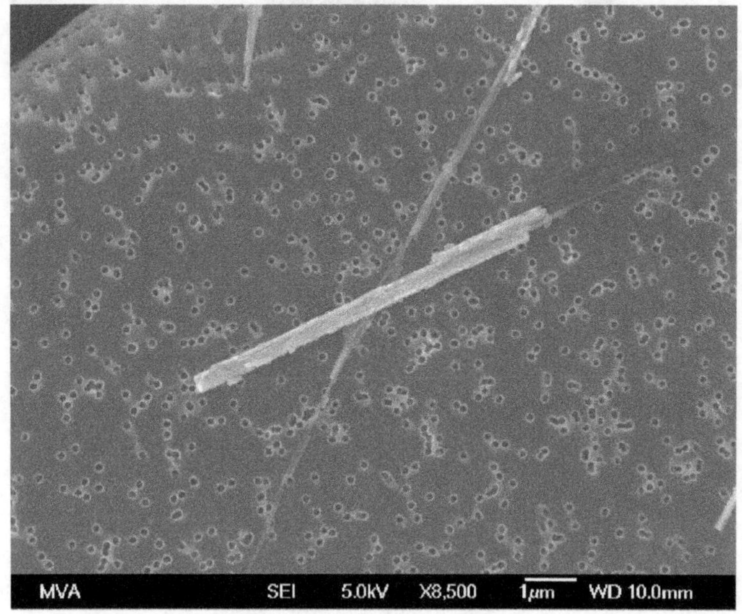

FIGURE 2.10 Image of crocidolite and chrysotile asbestos fibers as seen with an SEM. Same fibers as shown in Figure 2.6.

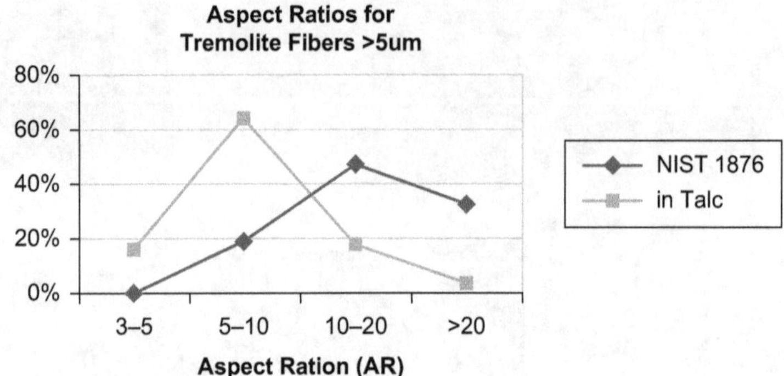

FIGURE 2.11 Comparison of ARs for tremolite fibers from the Standard Reference Material 1876, tremolite asbestos and tremolite from an industrial talc sample.

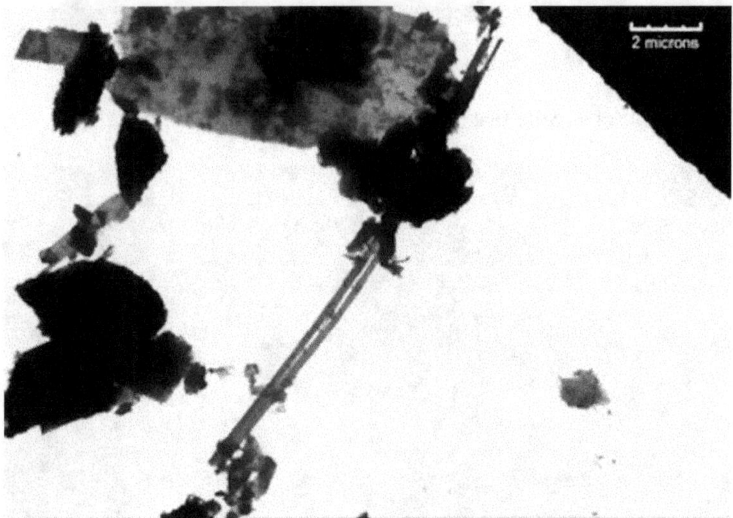

FIGURE 2.12 TEM image of a tremolite fiber found in an industrial talc sample.

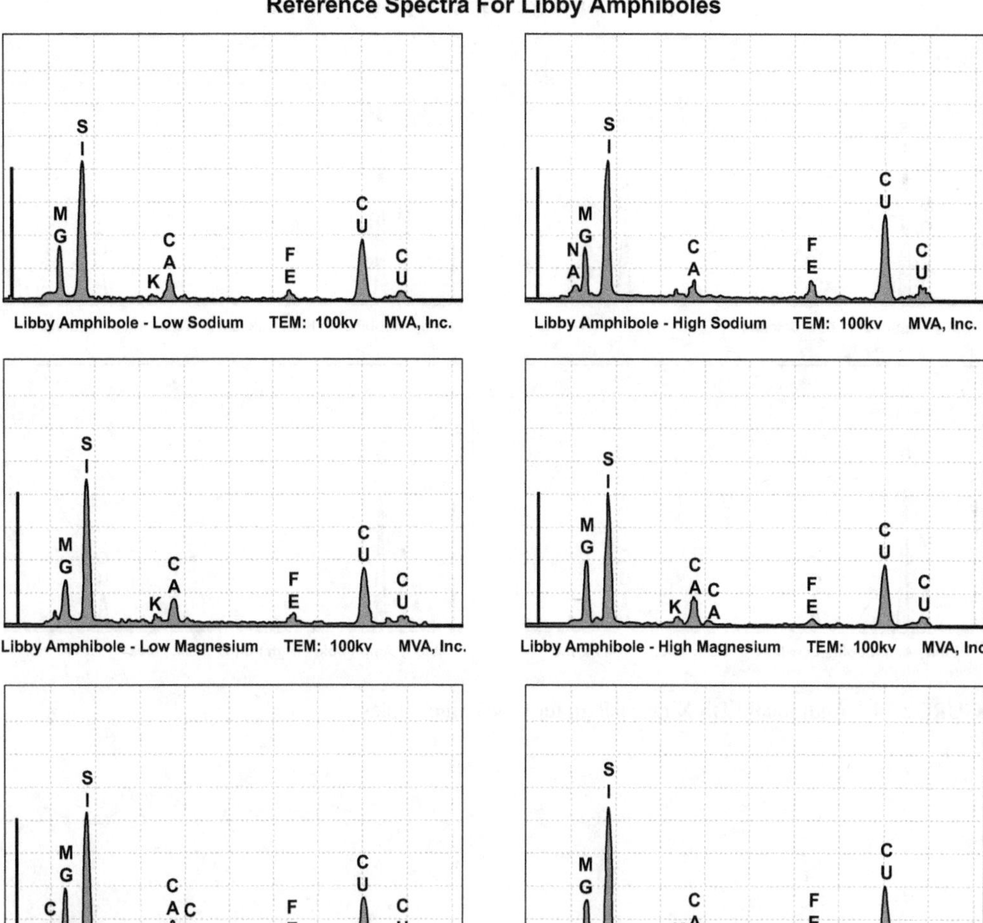

FIGURE 2.13 EDS X-ray spectra for Libby amphiboles.

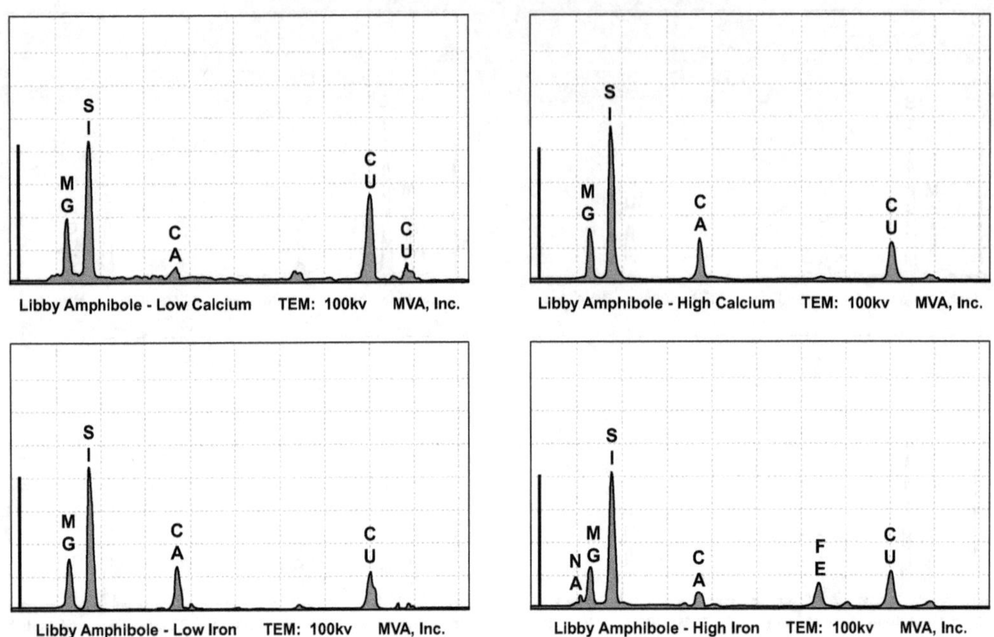

FIGURE 2.14 Additional EDS X-ray spectra for Libby amphiboles.

3 Analysis and Relevance of Asbestos Burden in Tissue

Ronald F. Dodson

3.1 RESPIRATORY SYSTEM AND WHY IT IS VULNERABLE TO INHALED DUST

To appreciate the significance of asbestos in body tissues, it is first relevant to understand how it got there and the normal functioning of the major portal of entry for dust into the body-the respiratory system. The design of the respiratory system has evolved into highly functional anatomical regions. The upper airways are designed to warm, moisten, and filter the incoming air. These can be thought of primarily as conducting tubes or conduits for two-directional airflow. In the ideal situation, the first contact with the external air is as it passes through the nasal cavity. As with the other conducting passageways, the nasal chambers create directional changes in airflow (via the angular changes in the passages) and are provided at initial levels with hairs to further initiate turbulence. During exercise or talking, humans shift to "mouth breathing," thus bypassing the nasal passages, and the inhaled air and its dust component go directly through the mouth to the trachea. There are some 32 branches of the conducting airways in the normal adult lung before reaching the distal acinus.[1]

These anatomical branching impacts the direction of airflow, which further serves to increase the potential for dust entrapment. This is because any deviation in the direction of airflow, particularly when it creates "whirlpools" or changes in velocity of flow, increases the chances of sedimentation to occur among the suspended dust particles. These currents can induce perpendicular flow to the walls of the airways, which results in the dust being brought into physical contact with the surfaces. The result of this anatomical design combined with the fact that most surfaces of the conducting airways are lined with "sticky" substances results in highly efficient entrapment of many inhaled particles in the upper airways. The entrapment of larger particles on the mucosa (lining) of the major bronchi is especially prominent where both the direction of flow and the air velocity change abruptly.[1] Lippmann et al.[2] reviewed this process and noted the result of decreasing airway sizes distally, combined with the increasing number of tubes in total cross section, results in decreases in air velocity. The impact of these physical events is that the larger particles get deposited by impaction. At the level of the smallest airways where there are the lowest velocities, the particle entrapment is via sedimentation and diffusion.[2]

The importance of entrapment of inhaled dusts in the conducting airways is critical in preventing it from reaching the lower respiratory tract and potentially compromising the functional respiratory units of the lung. The lung is particularly vulnerable to the toxic gases and dusts in the environment as it represents the largest surface within the body exposed to the external environment.[3] The lungs are responsible for providing oxygen to all cells in the body and for elimination of carbon dioxide produced by these cells. The critical impact of the lungs on the well-being of all parts of the body is emphasized by Witschi[3] in that it is the "only organ in the body in man to receive within 1 minute from one to five times the circulating blood volume." To achieve this objective, the normal lung "filters about 12,000 liters of air per day to 'extract' the fuel needed for survival"[4] and is perfused with more than 6000 L of blood per day to permit normal gas exchange critical for the function of the cells that make up the body.

DOI: 10.1201/9781003431909-3

The functional unit that makes up the majority of the lung parenchyma is the terminal and respiratory units (as shown in Figure 3.1), which when viewed by the eye results in the lung having a "sponge like" appearance. Ochs et al.[5] reported that the average number of alveoli in six adult lungs was 480 million. Weibel[6] equated this very large internal surface as being nearly that of a tennis court. The morphological composition of air sacs and associated lung parenchyma is illustrated in Figure 3.1. The three-dimensional morphology includes the alveoli, the smaller airways, and the associated circulatory components resulting in the lung appearing to be composed of small sack-like structures. The thin lining surrounding the lung tissue is the visceral pleura, which is made up of flattened mesothelium, whereas the predominate cell types of the alveoli are type I and type II pneumocytes (Figure 3.2). Type II pneumocytes are secretory cells that contribute the surfactant lining material necessary to maintain inflation of the air sacks. Type I pneumocytes are cells that form a thin lining over the surface of the air sack and are designed to permit gases (oxygen and carbon dioxide) to be exchanged across the air-blood barrier with the circulating blood that perfuses throughout the numerous small blood capillaries that traverse the regions between the alveoli and the small airways. The surface of the alveoli is designed to be relatively sterile, and inhaled materials are prevented from reaching this level only if the previously described entrapments at the upper airways remove the inhaled particulates from the incoming air. When the alveoli and the surface of small airways are compromised by the presence of inhaled particulates, defense cells from the interstitium are mobilized as a defensive response. Turino[7] appropriately described the lung parenchyma as a "dynamic matrix" that is composed predominantly of collagen, elastin, glycosaminoglycans, and fibronectin. The appropriate balance of these components combined with the proper functional capabilities of the cells that make up the lung parenchyma are critical for a healthy lung. Response to inhaled dusts can acutely or chronically alter the balance and result in reduced lung function and, if sufficiently vigorous and widespread, result in permanent loss of normal respiratory functions in the reactive areas of the lung.

3.2 DUST ELIMINATION FROM THE LUNG

The potential for dust entrapment in the larger airways has been discussed. The effectiveness of the upper airway defense/filtration mechanisms is that the majority of dust particles larger than 3μm in diameter never reach the lower respiratory system or alveolar surfaces.[8] Gross and Detreville[8] projected the defense mechanisms of the lung function at a level of 98–99% efficiency for trapping or removing inhaled particulates. The inefficiency for the removal of 1–2% of inhaled dusts under such assumptions would account for the resultant development of pneumoconiosis (dust diseases). The defense mechanisms of the lung are divided between levels of anatomical divisions. The conducting airways are lined with a sticky blanket of mucus. Columnar lining cells making up a part of the surface lining of the larger conducting airways have specialized hairlike extensions from their surfaces called *cilia*. There are several hundreds of these per cell, and their role is to expedite the movement of the mucous layer and entrapped particulates from the level of deposit to the next higher levels toward the pharynx for elimination as a component of sputa. The cilia beat approximately 1000 times per minute in a coordinated scheme to assure rapid upward movement of the surface layer and any entrapped materials.[9] The combined function of entrapment of particulates in the mucus and the effective transport of the entrapped dusts and mucus with the assistance of the "beating" underlying cilia form a critical clearance mechanism from the lung often referred to as the mucociliary escalator.

The lowest level of the respiratory tract consists of the alveoli that comprise the majority of the lung parenchyma. These fragile-appearing air sacs consist of thin-walled structures formed by the close apposition of a cytoplasmic extension of an epithelial cell on the airway side, an area of basement membrane, and the thin wall of the smallest circulatory blood vessel in the body—the capillary. The extremely thin wall of this region gives it a "spiderweb" appearance in sections when viewed by light microscopy. It is specifically designed anatomically to permit the effective exchange of gases from the air-blood–air compartments. The morphological appearance of the delicate nature of the wall of this structural unit at the light microscopy level led some to consider it initially to be acellular. In reality, the components of the two cell types which populate the air–blood barrier (Figures 3.3 and 3.4) form a total thickness ranging from 0.2 to 0.5 μm, which is up to 20–50 times thinner than a sheet of airmail paper.[4, 6] For proper gas exchange to occur, these sacs must remain open, with minimal congestion and with maintenance of normal wall integrity to assure flexibility for contraction and expansion of the lower lung parenchyma. The surfaces of normal alveoli are protected from foreign material by the previously described defense filtrations that occur in the conducting airways. The alveolar surfaces are ideally maintained in a sterile state. In normal tissue, secreted glycolipoprotein (surfactant) from type II alveolar cells assists in assuring a low surface tension on the surface of the alveoli and helps prevent them from collapsing at low lung volumes.[10] In contrast with the micrograph shown in Figure 3.3, the air-blood barrier in the section from an experimental animal model (Figure 3.4) shows the leakage of horseradish peroxidase (arrow) through the barrier onto the surface of the alveolar sac as an acute response of exposure to asbestos.[11] If congestion occurs in the air sacs as a result of an inflammatory response of defense cells to inhaled particulates or if the walls of the sacks become thickened so that gas exchange is difficult, their functional state as the major respiratory units responsible for proper lung function in the lung is compromised. Particulates that reach this lowest level of the respiratory system (Figure 3.5) represent a population of the smallest structures in the inhaled dusts. These have successfully bypassed the upper-level defense mechanisms and reached a respiratory level where clearance is less effective.

The primary response to dust particles that reach the alveoli is a "call up" of macrophages. These defense cells migrate from the interstitium onto the surface of alveoli. The cells convert to a cellular form capable of functioning in an aerobic environment and display chemotaxis features (Figure 3.6) that permit them to move along the alveolar surface to deposited particulates. Macrophages are the major defense mechanisms of the lower respiratory tract and function by attempting to clear the alveoli of infectious, toxic, and allergic particulates that have evaded the mechanical defenses of the nasal passages, glottis, and mucociliary transport system.[12] Pulmonary macrophages attempt to ingest and isolate foreign particulates and contain internal chemical packages that work to denature or "digest" some ingested microorganisms (Figure 3.7). Werb[13] states "like a chameleon, the macrophage senses alterations in its environment-changes in oxygen tension, the presence of different cells such as lymphocytes, foreign materials, microorganisms or changes in plasma proteins and hormones. Not only is it adaptive to its own environment, but the changes in the structure and functional properties of the macrophage, in general, are reversible. Considering that the macrophage is long lived, with its half-life estimated to be on the order of weeks or months, this cycle of phenotypic response may repeat many times. Macrophages respond to a call for chemotaxis when the fortifications that defend us against an onslaught of microorganisms and other foreign materials have been breached."

A population of macrophages is capable by some yet to be understood mechanisms of relocating to the surface of the more proximal levels of the airways where the more rapid clearance of macrophages and their phagocytized dust particles occur via the mucociliary escalator. Camner et al.[14] studied the efficiency of clearance for various sized particles and found that the deeper the particulates were inhaled, the longer the time was required to clear them from the lung. The average retention after 24 h was around 100% for particles deposited in generations 13–16 (ciliated bronchioles) and around 20% in generations 0–12 (both large and small ciliated airways). It should be recognized that clearance is an ongoing event; thus, periods of elevated dust accumulation may not be totally represented by tissue burden at the time of sampling, particularly if the period from last exposure has covered an appreciable period of months or years.

The impact of smoking and asbestos as combined causal agents of disease in man is discussed in appreciable detail in the section on clinical issues. However, it is appropriate to note that exposure to tobacco smoke alters the cellular composition of the upper airways (resulting in squamous cell metaplasia and goblet cell hyperplasia) and negatively impacts on the effectiveness of the mucociliary escalator to properly function.[15–17] Lippmann et al.[2] noted "cigarette smoking and bronchitis produce a proximal shift in the deposition pattern" and "if the particles penetrate the epithelium, either bare or within macrophages, they may be sequestered within cells or enter the lymphatic circulation and be carried to pleural, hilar, and more distant lymph nodes." Animal studies conducted to assess the effect of smoking and clearance were conducted by the research group led by Dr Andrew Churg. In a study using a guinea pig model,[15] it was determined that "cigarette smoking impedes asbestos clearance, largely by increasing retention of short fibers." They further concluded "increased pulmonary fiber burden may be important in the increased disease rate seen in asbestos workers who smoke." In a companion work,[16] the observations "implied that failure of macrophages clearance and subsequent rerelease of fibers into the medium may at least partially explain the changes in fiber sizes and eventually increases in tissue fiber concentrations in smoke-exposed animals." Thus, clearance in a smoker of all types of dust including asbestosis less efficient than in a nonsmoker.[2, 17–19] Churg and Stevens[20] found that in the case of asbestos-exposed individuals, asbestos recovered from the airway mucosa or parenchyma of smokers was shorter than that in nonsmokers. They concluded that smoking led to enhanced retention of short fibers. The other observation was that many more short fibers were cleared over time in individuals who did not have compromised clearance.

3.3 DUST OVERLOADING AND THE IMPACT ON THE RESPIRATORY TRACT

The process as described for clearance from the lung represents the ideal response to dust inhalation and its rapid elimination from the lung. In many instances, exposure to dust can result in periods of "dust overloading" of the defense mechanisms.[21–24] This phenomenon is due to alterations in the capabilities of macrophages to respond to dust burden partly because of overwhelming the phagocytic component and the number of macrophages stimulated to meet the elevated burden of inhaled dust. This results in "macrophage congestion," including congestion at the level of the alveoli and small airways. This results in some macrophages not being able to leave the congested area. These phagocytic cells eventually die and release the ingested particulates, which in turn trigger an influx of more phagocytic cells in response to the freed dust. Oberdorster[21] suggested impaired alveolar macrophage-mediated lung clearance and the accumulation of high levels of pulmonary dust can result in adverse chronic effects, including inflammation, fibrosis, and tumors. For example, it has been shown that poorly soluble, nonfibrous particles (carbon black, coal dust, diesel soot, nonasbestiform talc, and titanium dioxide) elicit tumors in rats when deposition overwhelms the clearance mechanisms of the lung creating the condition of overloading.[25] The impact of elevated dust burden and the risk of developing permanent pathological changes in the respiratory system lie in part with the level of inherent toxicity associated with the accumulated dust. There is increasing appreciation that the same macrophages that provide front line defense in the lower respiratory system carry a liability for inducing injury to lung tissue. The impact of compound exposures of asbestos has been shown in an animal model where Coin et al.[26] found that after three consecutive inhalation exposures to chrysotile, there were asbestos fibers retained at the 6-month evaluation of the tissue. The "three exposures to chrysotile caused a large increase in DNA synthesis in the epithelium of the terminal bronchioles and more proximal airways. When compared with a single exposure, the triple exposure caused an enhanced inflammatory response and a prolonged period of increased DNA synthesis in the proximal alveolar region. Hyperplastic, fibrotic lesions subsequently developed in the same region and persisted for at least 6 months after exposure." Compound exposures to amosite in an animal model likewise resulted in a newer area of responsiveness involving appreciable neutrophil component, while reactive areas to the earlier exposure were typified as being represented by a majority of cells being macrophages.[27]

Pinkerton et al.[28] evaluated the tissue response after chronic exposures using Fisher 344 rats. They concluded "that during exposure to asbestos fibers, macrophages and alveolar epithelial cells contain statistically significant amounts of asbestos and are associated with histological changes indicating marked epithelial injury. Increased amounts of fibers are also localized in the lung interstitium with continued exposure to asbestos and are associated with progressive interstitial fibrotic reaction. After cessation of exposure, macrophages and epithelial cells are cleared of fibers and resolve toward normal proportions. However, significant clearance of fibers from the lung interstitium does not occur after cessation of exposure, and there is a continuing process of fibrogenesis."

Data from such studies emphasize the need to separate assumptions on the basis of findings from one exposure in animal models from the responses after actual compound exposures that occur in occupationally exposed humans. It is through animal models that many concepts of asbestos-induced pathogenicity have been described. Differences in chrysotile and amphibole risks for induction of disease are described in the chapter involving molecular biological interactions. There are several unique features that suggest that amphiboles may carry more of a risk for inducing malignancy, not the least of which is the potential for inhalation of longer fibers when compared with chrysotile (see section on asbestos characteristics). Indeed, some animal models have been interpreted as indicating chrysotile is less pathogenically active, whereas other studies have shown it to be an appreciably active form of asbestos. For example, Reeves et al.[29] found variations in tumorigenicity between fiber types after exposure, stating that "Two pulmonary cancers were produced in rats exposed to inhalation of crocidolite. Local injection into the pleural or peritoneal cavities caused 5 mesotheliomas in rats after chrysotile treatment and 6 mesotheliomas in rats and rabbits after crocidolite treatment. Guinea pigs and hamsters developed no tumors in this experiment, and with the dose used, there were no tumors in any species in the amosite group." Kimizuka et al.[30] found that "chrysotile induced more prominent cell (leukocyte or macrophages) necrosis and alveolar wall thickening. These findings indicate chrysotile asbestos induces stronger cell reactions in the alveolar wall and is more noxious than amosite."

Hesterberg et al.[31]tested the effects of chronic inhalation in rats of X607 (a rapidly dissolving synthetic vitreous fiber) with those previously reported for RCF1 (a refractory ceramic synthetic vitreous fiber) and chrysotile fiber. As will be discussed in detail within the section on fiber length and pathogenicity, a reference point for the potential pathogenicity of a fiber is its durability/biopersistence in tissue. The study reported that RCF1 and chrysotile asbestos "induced pulmonary fibrosis and thoracic neoplasms (chrysotile induced 32% more pulmonary neoplasms than RCF1). Lung deposition and fiber lengths did not explain the toxicological differences between the three fibers." The authors stated that from their data, "chrysotile dissolution was negligible." Rodelsperger[32] pointed out a reasonable concern when attempting to extrapolate data from rat models (and potential all rodent models) to human experiences regarding the carcinogenic potency of fibers in that "the life span of rats is too low to measure the elimination rate of bio-persistent fibers sufficiently." It is also true that animals have a more rapid clearance rate than humans and obviously smaller airways for more efficient filtration of dusts than occurs in the larger passageways of humans.

The macrophage is a cell type characterized by Brody[33] as being on the "one hand a potential defender of the alveolar environment and on the other hand as a central mediator of lung disease." Simplistically, the surfaces of alveolar sacs in the ideal state are devoid of cells and debris, and when inhaled dust such as asbestos stimulates the call up of macrophages and neutrophils,[34, 35] the balance of the alveolar environment changes, potentially resulting in long-term or permanent pathological alterations. The anatomical area that normally consists of open spaces for gas exchange becomes filled with defense cells and fluid. As the macrophages interact with the inhaled dust, the potential exists for there to be a release of oxidants,[35–37] chemoattractants for other inflammatory cells,[38, 39]proteases,[40, 41] and growth factors that stimulate fibroblasts to replicate from these cells[42–44]and to secrete collagen.[45] The latter two events are pivotal in the induction of fibroproliferative disorders in the lung such as intra-alveolar/interstitial fibrosis[42] or in the case of asbestos-induced fibrosis (asbestosis). Bowden[45, 46] reported that these combinations of deleterious events associated with macrophages in the lung are direct contributors to the development of emphysema and interstitial fibrosis.

Secretions from macrophages occur in the normal process of phagocytosis of bacteria, virus, or dust particles. However, if the dust particulates are particularly toxic, the macrophage may be killed, and the release of internal chemicals occurs immediately. If dust overloading occurs, the macrophages may not be able to escape from the airway because of lack of clearance. When the macrophages reach the end of their life expectancy, they release the dust, which triggers the call up of more macrophages, enzymes, and other chemicals that negatively interact with the cell wall and adjacent cells. Such a scenario would be expected to occur with generation after generation of newly attracted macrophages and thus result in a constant reinforcement of the negative events as described earlier. In part, this concept should be considered as a factor in the continuing development of fibrosis in an asbestotic lung, which can progress long after the individual's contact with asbestos has ceased. Thus, as summarized by brain,[47] "though the macrophages serve as the first line of defense for the alveolar surface, they may also be capable of injuring the host while exercising their defensive role."

3.4 RELOCATION OF PARTICLES FROM THE LUNG VIA THE LYMPHATICS

The most efficient mechanism for dust clearance from the lung follows a pathway that backs up the same route as it entered the airways by the mechanisms described. However, there is another route for clearance or relocation of particulates from the lung, and that is by lymphatic drainage into lymph nodes via lymphatic channels.[2,48–54] The drainage of lymphatics from the lung have long been appreciated as indicated by the evidence of silicotic nodules forming in lymph nodes of silica-exposed individuals[54, 55] as well as observations from numerous animal models as described in detail in a recent publication from our laboratory.[56] In one interesting animal study, Oberdorster et al.[57] studied the transfer of amosite fibers from the lower respiratory system in a dog model. The project incorporated both neutron activated amosite fibers as well as detection of the fibers by scanning electron microscopy at a period of 24 h after exposure. The assessment included both thoracic lymph nodes and postnodal lung lymph. The authors concluded that there was "a fast translocation of fibers from the airspaces of the lung to the lymph nodes and even into postnodal lymph." The findings indicated that the "structures of the peripheral lung and lymph node itself act like size selective filters, permitting only the fine fibre-fraction to penetrate." This conclusion is consistent with our findings of the actual fiber burden in the lung and lymph nodes from exposed humans.[56] Oberdorster et al.[57] further concluded that "fibres below about 9 μm in length and below about 0.5 μm in diameter can be cleared into the postnodal lymph and thus can reach any organ of the body."

The awareness of the communication routes between the lung and the lymphatics is well appreciated as typified by the use of the Naruke lymph node map used by the American Joint Commission for staging the spread of primary carcinomas of the lung.[58]

Furthermore, the characterization as to which level of the lung is drained by the various anatomically located nodes in the chest cavity is described by Netter[59] in his illustrated anatomical text. It is ironic that, previously, only theoretical concepts have been offered regarding asbestos relocation from the lung to the lymph nodes and thus as potential routes to extrapulmonary sites. However, a study[56] from our laboratory provides quantitative data regarding fiber burden and characterization of the fibers found in the lymph nodes as compared with that in lung tissue. The observations are described in applicable sections under topics regarding asbestos in extrapulmonary sites and the relevance of short fibers in assessing accurate tissue burdens.

Dust overload of the usual clearance mechanisms previously described results in the translocation of a portion of the dust to extrapulmonary sites via the lymphatics and lymph nodes as discussed by Cullen et al.[60] The logic of this explanation is that usual clearance route via the mucociliary escalator of dust from the deeper lung is impaired/overwhelmed. Relocation of dust from the lung to the lymph node and the lymphatic drainage has resulted in these sites becoming "reservoirs of retained material" or, in the case of the nodes, as "repositories for dust."[8, 60] With sufficient dust accumulation the lymph nodes become "densely mineralized and stony hard."[8] If dust accumulated in the nodes has appreciable cytotoxicity, pathological changes can occur, including the formation of nodules.[54] This same route through the lymphatic system has been suggested as the mechanism by which asbestos fibers relocate to extrapulmonary sites,[61–63] a concept for which we have now offered quantitative validation.[56]

Another interesting issue regarding relocation of fibrous dust from the lung to lymph nodes and other extrapulmonary sites involves the influence of mixed dust on the process. Davis et al.[64] evaluated the influence of nonfibrous dusts on translocation of respirable size asbestos. The scientists studied translocation and clearance in a rat model after 1 year of exposure and 2 years of follow-up. They acknowledged that rat pleural lining differs from humans in thickness and morphological complexity. Thus, mechanisms of translocation through the visceral pleura may be appreciably different between rats and humans. However, when combining the exposure of chrysotile or amosite with titanium dioxide or quartz, they observed differing levels of reactions and end points (tumor formation). Quartz "greatly increased fibrosis above that produced by the asbestos types alone." The occurrence of pulmonary tumors and mesothelioma in animals receiving asbestos and other dusts was increased. The authors observed the "presence of particulate dusts made little difference in the amounts of amosite fibre retained in the lung tissue, but, with chrysotile, titanium dioxide appeared to increase retention while quartz reduced it."

An evaluation by Pintos et al.[65] from two case–control studies assessed the risk of mesothelioma and occupational exposure to asbestos and man-made vitreous fibers. Not surprisingly, the findings revealed "in workers with exposure levels lower than historical cohort studies and across a wide range of industries, a strong association was found between asbestos, especially when it was amphibole, and mesothelioma." The investigators determined that "subjects exposed to both asbestos and MMVF had particularly high risks, an unexpected result."

The subject of reactions in mixed exposures to nonfibrous and/or mixed fibrous dusts is beyond the focus of this chapter; however, it is useful to remember that most exposures in humans are to mixed dusts. It is also useful to recognize that although the molecular mechanisms discussed in the various sections may emphasize characteristics of fibrous dusts, many of the same mechanisms may have applicability to respired dusts that are of the same elemental composition but not in a fibrous form. A potential synergistic effect between various fibrous and nonfibrous dusts cannot be ruled out as a mechanism resulting in increased risk for development of disease.

3.5 MORPHOLOGICAL FEATURES OF ASBESTOS/ELONGATED MINERAL PARTICLES THAT DETERMINE THE POTENTIAL FOR INHALATION

Asbestos minerals have been used by intent in more than 3000 commercial applications.[66] Asbestos is sometimes a component of minerals mined for many different products that are considered as not containing asbestos or having less than a "regulated percent of content 1%," which trigger the regulatory definition of asbestos-containing material. Thus, millions of individuals are exposed to asbestos-containing products in the workplace or through secondary or bystander exposures from occupational settings. The widespread use of asbestos results from their unique properties including high tensile strength, flexibility, insulating properties, fire resistance, and resistance to strong chemicals—both alkaline and acidic.[66] These attributes in the past made asbestos an important commercial contributor to the economic development of industrialized societies.[67] The problem arises that when asbestos is disturbed, it results in fibers breaking down into respirable-sized dust particles. This fibrous dust is easily inhaled and can cause pathological damage to the lung (e.g., asbestosis, lung cancer, mesothelioma) and extrapulmonary sites.[68]

The term *asbestos* refers to a group of six different fibrous forms of minerals and is generally used in society as a generic nomenclature. The mineral name and the name given to the asbestos and non-asbestos forms of anthophyllite, actinolite, and tremolite are the same. The most widely used form of asbestos in commercial applications (90–95%) is chrysotile, which is a serpentine form of mineral.[69–72] The other five forms of asbestos (amosite, crocidolite, actinolite, tremolite, and anthophyllite) are the asbestiform habits of the amphibole family of mineral groups. The nonfibrous form of these minerals can break along cleavage planes and create elongated cleavage fragments[73] that are sometimes confused with the fibrous form in that they are morphologically similar in appearance, particularly by light microscopy. Although an in-depth discussion of the differentiation between the cleavage fragment and the asbestiform habit is outside the scope of this chapter, suffice it to say that the former is not considered "asbestos" under the definition of regulated fibers. This is not to imply that cleavage fragments of these minerals may not carry their own risk to health if sufficient numbers are inhaled, as will be emphasized later in this chapter.

Amosite and crocidolite were used in commercial applications in the USA while the use of anthophyllite was very limited. In the past, actinolite, tremolite, and anthophyllite have been considered "noncommercial asbestos types." However, their presence in products containing minerals such as vermiculite and talc provides a vehicle for their widespread exposure, even if the exposures are often less intense than those occurring in occupational exposures to commercial forms of asbestos. Compounding the issue of exposure to noncommercial amphiboles is that often the individual has had no idea a product contained asbestiform structures. Tremolite asbestos is considered as a mineral component (often referred to as a contaminant) of Canadian chrysotile. Tremolite asbestos within chrysotile asbestos mined from Canada[66] is suggested by some investigators to be an important factor in diseases associated with exposures to Canadian chrysotile.[74] All types of asbestos have a silicon tetroxide (SiO4) tetrahedral as backbone of the crystal lattice. The X-ray energy dispersive spectra of the types of fibrous mineral entities defined as "asbestos" are illustrated in Chapter 2 of this volume. Chrysotile is a magnesium silicate that is assembled in nature with the layers of linked silica tetrahedral alternating with the layers of magnesium oxide–hydroxide octahedral (brucite). The double layering in this type of structure rolls up onto itself to form hollow tubes or scrolls that are morphologically characteristic of chrysotile. The impact of this internal organization as reflected in the physical features of the fiber is that the longer the fiber becomes, the more likely it is to coil or curl (Figures 3.8, 3.9). Thus, the fiber when seen in cross section displays a true diameter at any one point, which is thinner than the functional diameter of the fiber in an air stream. This greater functional diameter because of morphological curvature of a fiber within an airstream results in less potential for the inhalation of longer, more curved fibers than comparable length straight fibers. The amphiboles, on the other hand, contain aggregates of cations (calcium, sodium, iron, and magnesium) between the strips of linked silica tetrahedral in the form of parallel chains. The variations of the percentage and types of cations determine the type of amphibole asbestos (see illustrations in Chapter 2 this edition). All amphiboles, because of the repeating crystalline units, tend to be straight even as the fiber (crystal) increases in length. Thus, the functional diameter tends to be similar to the actual diameter in an air stream. It is therefore easier to inhale longer fibers of amphiboles than fibers of chrysotile of the same length. This difference alone favors the retention of amphiboles in the lung as short or small entities having a greater potential to be more rapidly cleared.[75] The other side of this issue is that greater numbers of smaller entities may be inhaled over a shorter period of time and lead to dust overloading as previously described. The smaller entities are (as will be extensively described in later sections) the dust particles that are more likely to reach extrapulmonary sites. A final point regarding the smaller entities is that their combined surface area/reactive surface may well exceed that contributed by the larger (in the case of asbestos, longer) structures.[76] A chronic inhalation study by Hesterberg et al.[31] compared the biologic effects in rats of a rapidly dissolving synthetic vitreous fiber with a refractory ceramic synthetic vitreous fiber and chrysotile (Jeffrey Mine, Canada). At the selected end point, the rapidly dissolving synthetic vitreous fiber group did not show fibrosis or tumors, whereas the refractory ceramic synthetic vitreous fiber group and the chrysotile-exposed group showed pulmonary fibrosis and tumors with chrysotile inducing "32% more pulmonary neoplasms than RCF1"—the refractory ceramic fibers. The issue of interpreting chrysotile biopersistence in animal models should be reviewed with the concerns offered by Pezerat[77] that "aggressive pre-treatment of fibers, inducing many faults and fragility in the fibers' structure, may lead to rapid hydration and breaking of long fibers in the lungs." A review of alterations that some procedures may induce in the process of isolating ferruginous bodies/fibers from lung and other samples will be discussed in the section of this chapter on tissue preparation.

There are important differences in surface charges associated with differences in composition of various types of asbestos as has been discussed by Hamilton,[78] Valerio et al.,[79] and Xu et al.[80] Likewise, there are differences in surface cations among the amphibole forms, which result in potential for chemical reactions to occur. Some reactions can produce harmful by-products, including the formation of reactive radicals. A recent study by MacCorkle et al.[81] evaluated the response of cultured human fibroblasts after exposure to amphiboles and several types of chrysotile. They observed that the individual fibers were engulfed into the cytoplasm where they "induced significant mitotic aberrations leading to chromosomal instability and aneuploidy." The observation indicated that the "intracellular asbestos fibers induced aneuploidy and chromosome instability by binding to a subset of proteins that include regulators of the cell cycle, cytoskeleton, and mitotic process." The precoating of fibers with protein complexes blocked the measurable asbestos-induced changes associated with surface reactions without affecting the uptake by the cells. The mechanisms that resulted in the damaging interactions in this study involved surface reactions that did not appear to be dependent on the type of asbestos, which is in contrast with the Fenton–iron-driven reactions that have been emphasized as important in amphibole generation of damaging free radicals because of iron content, particularly with crocidolite and amosite.

These features are discussed in greater detail in the chapter on molecular mechanisms of asbestos interactions with cells and the lung milieu. The significance of asbestos to become a respirable dust is inherent in that the fibers and bundles can dissociate into shorter or thinner units during traumatic disturbance, which can occur in airflow or exerted physical pressure. The upper limits of respirability in humans has been given for a rounded structure as 10 μm in diameter[82, 83]and for a fibrous particulate as 3.5 μm in diameter.[82] The potential for inhaling fibrils (the thinnest unit structure) is evident when recognizing that from our experience the measurements for such structures by analytical transmission electron microscopy (ATEM) for the most commonly used commercial types of asbestos are 0.02–0.08 μm for chrysotile, 0.06–0.35 μm for amosite, and 0.04–0.15 μm for crocidolite.[56, 67] It is evident that bundles or fibers composed of multiple fibrils are well within the respirable range for fibrous dust (Figure 3.10). It should be recognized that the filtration and entrapment processes as described earlier result in many fibrous particulates being trapped higher up the respiratory system and rapidly eliminated. However, the potential for inhalation is a relative issue on the basis of the overall numbers common in many exposures to fibrous dust as the distributions in sizes (diameters) that can comprise the aerosolized dust in the individual's breathing zone are often mixed. Smaller diameter and shorter fibrous particulates are more readily inhaled to a greater depth in the respiratory system and may be inhaled in far greater numbers than the larger counterparts.[83, 84] The issue of fiber size and the potential for inducing irreversible changes in human and/or animal models have been discussed regarding respirability and the inherent physical potential for being more readily cleared/translocated in portions of this section and in subsequent sections of this chapter. However, the impact of surface area as a factor in determination of the potential for inducing molecular/biochemical reactions has received limited attention. One study evaluating the impact of fiber type and surface area was conducted by Timbrell et al.[85] The study involved tissue specimens obtained from postmortem lungs of individuals who had amphibole exposure at mining sites, including Paakkila (Finland—anthophyllite), Wittenoom (Australia—crocidolite), North Western Cape Province (NW Cape, South Africa—crocidolite), and Transvaal (South Africa—amosite and crocidolite). The authors observed that when "mass was used as a parameter of fiber quantity, the fiber concentrations in specimens showing a given degree of fibrosis increased progressively: Wittenoom < NWCape < Transvaal < Paakkila. Significantly, however, when surface area was used as the parameter, the fiber concentrations in specimens showing a given degree of fibrosis were approximately equal: Wittenoom = NW Cape = Transvaal = Paakkila. But when the number was used as the parameter, the fiber concentrations in specimens showing a given degree of fibrosis decreased progressively: Wittenoom » NW Cape » Transvaal » Paakkila. These trends in the concentrations of retained fiber required to produce the same degree of fibrosis are the consequence of large differences in fiber size between the four locations, rather than the differences in type of amphibole. Long-resident chrysotile fibres exhibited roughly the same fibrogenicity per unit of surface area as amphibole fibres, and this was also true for quartz grains."

As discussed in the sections involving macrophagic/clearance response, the repetitious exposures to such dusts may trigger an ongoing inflammatory response resulting in pathological changes in the tissue.

3.6 FERRUGINOUS BODIES IN TISSUE

The term ferruginous body means "iron-rich" body. These structures when found in lung tissue are indicators that the defense cells of the lung—the alveolar macrophages—have interacted with a particulate and deposited an iron-rich coating on its surface. The tissues in some individuals are efficient in coating inhaled fibrous and nonfibrous particulates while some individuals are ineffective in coating of inhaled dusts. If these structures are created on asbestos fibers, they are appropriately called "asbestos bodies." The first reports of these golden-brown structures in lung tissue were by Marchand[86] in 1906. These structures were first recognized by Cooke[87] in 1929, who used the name "curious bodies." In 1931, Gloyne[88] proved that the cores of these structures were asbestos fibers by exposing guinea pigs to asbestos dust. After 6 months, Gloyne[89] found varying degrees of maturing ferruginous bodies in their lung tissue. He also reported a ferruginous body in the lung tissue of a gray rat caught on an asbestos factory premises. Gloyne[89] warned of the complexity of identifying a ferruginous body formed in tissue sections by noting "there is difficulty previously mentioned that an elongated structure such as an asbestosis body rarely lies entirely in one plane." This is a point well remembered before tending to call anything that stains positively with an iron stain a ferruginous body (implying it is consistent with an asbestos body as seen by light microscopy).

There is universal agreement that the coating that forms on asbestos fibers is deposited through interactions with macrophages (Figure 3.11 and Figure 3.12) and appears to preferentially involve deposition on the longer fibers that do not become internalized within the phagocyte. The shorter fibers that can be phagocytized within the macrophages are often found in "iron-rich" organelles as indicated by the Perls-positive nature of the regions. However, the shorter fibers do not morphologically exhibit coatings when isolated from the tissue. In 1970, Davis[90] reported in animal models that the "first coating material of the asbestos bodies seems to be some form of acid mucopolysaccharide, but this coating soon becomes impregnated with ferritin or hemosiderin to form the well-known Perls-positive bodies." In 1972, Governa and Rosanda[91] suggested that mucopolysaccharides might act as a matrix for iron deposition on the coating. Not all animal species readily form asbestos bodies, if at all,[92] and the formation of such bodies in man also varies between individuals.[93–95]

The common link in stimulating the formation of asbestos bodies in tissue is the presence of asbestos fibers longer than 8 μm (with most being over 20 μm in length), with the majority of asbestos fibers in lung being much shorter and uncoated.[92–95] It is evident that diameters and surface irregularities may play a role in the selection process as suggested by the appearance of fibrous cores where the ferruginous coating had been removed[95] and because asbestos bodies represent only a portion of the longer fiber burden within the tissue at a given time.[92–95] It should be noted that other fibrous and nonfibrous inhaled structures stimulate formation of ferruginous bodies. Gross et al. [96] introduced the term "pseudo-asbestos bodies" or "unusual ferruginous bodies" to designate these structures. Fibrous aluminum silicate, silicon carbide whiskers, cosmetic talc, and glass fibers can stimulate ferruginous body formation in animals.[96, 97] Holmes et al.[98]used sized fiberglass to stimulate "pseudo-asbestos body" formation in hamster lung. In human tissue, Churg and Warnock[99] reported ferruginous bodies on cores of sheet silicates (talc, mica, or kaolinite) and carbon. Dodson et al.[100–102] demonstrated ferruginous bodies from human material could form on iron-rich fibers, carbon filaments, elongated talc particles (Figures 3.13, 3.14, 3.15, 3.16), and various sheet silicates (Figure 3.17). Initially, it may seem that the previously mentioned types of ferruginous bodies would make it difficult to differentiate an asbestos body by light microscopy. Churg[94] correctly observed that when a ferruginous body seen by light microscopy as a beaded structure formed on a clear, elongated, transparent, usually straight core, that structure is with a high degree of certainty an asbestos body. In fact, a trained reader can easily distinguish the vast majority of non-asbestos ferruginous bodies by use of the light microscope.[101] Asbestos bodies have been found in tissues outside of the lung.[102–105] The most common location for such observations has been the lymph nodes.[105–107]The question was raised if asbestos bodies could form in extrapulmonary sites on uncoated asbestos fibers relocated from the lung, or was it necessary that they be relocated as mature bodies? In a study from our laboratory, a guinea pig model was used to compare the coating efficiency of fibers introduced into the lung tissue as compared with reactions to fibers from the same preparation injected into the spleen and liver in other groups of animals.[108] The liver and the spleen were found to independently exhibit the inherent capability to form ferruginous bodies, but at a much less efficient rate than within the lung tissue.

The presence of asbestos bodies in sections from lung tissue offers an important indicator of past asbestos exposure. The Pneumoconiosis Council of the College of American Pathologists and the National Institute for Occupational Safety and Health stated that the "minimal criteria that permitted the diagnosis of asbestosis in tissue were demonstration of discrete foci of fibrosis in the walls of respiratory bronchioles associated with the accumulations of asbestos bodies."[109] Crouch and Churg,[110] in recognizing the relative insensitivity of tissue sections for detection of ferruginous bodies, stated that "the demonstration of a single asbestos body on casual inspection of several lung sections implies asbestos exposure many times above background." Compounding the issue of using tissue sections for the identification of asbestos bodies is that the plane of section may only strike one level of the body and not permit visualization of the core material or if the structure is formed on an elongated core.

3.7 DESTRUCTIVE TESTING METHODS USED IN SAMPLING TISSUE AND FLUIDS FOR ASBESTOS BODIES AND UNCOATED ASBESTOS FIBERS AND OTHER ELONGATED PARTICLES

Although light microscopic evaluation of tissue sections in determination of the pathological processes is important, histologic evaluation of tissue sections offers a relatively insensitive method for determining asbestos body and fiber concentrations. Thus, a method that provides an expansion of the amount of tissue sampled involves destruction of relatively large amounts of tissue and collection of the particulates from that tissue on a flat surface for analysis. Some techniques used for tissue sampling include sample filtration,[111] low-temperature ashing,[112] and high-temperature ashing.[113] Additional options for tissue destruction include digestion with ozone,[114, 115] strong bases,[116, 117] sodium hypochlorite, and/or hydrogen peroxide.[118–120] It is important that any tissue preparation where the tissue is destroyed avoids inducing sufficient trauma to cause ferruginous bodies to fragment or asbestos bundles to dissociate into smaller units resulting in a falsely elevated asbestos tissue burden.[121–123]

Ashcroft and Heppleston[116] compared the effects on longer and uncoated fibers induced by drying the tissue before maceration. Their conclusions were: "this effect (of fractures) is evident microscopically on comparing suspension prepared from dried and wet portions of the same lung and it may exaggerate the fibre count. The numbers of fibres from wet and dried asbestotic lung tissue were compared in five cases, a sample of tissue from each being divided into two approximately equal-sized portions showing uniform pathological features." "All five specimens show higher coated fibre counts after drying, and in three specimens the uncoated fibre count is also increased."[116] The concern for breakage of the ferruginous bodies and uncoated asbestos fibers was further expressed by the European Respiratory Society Task Force.[124] The ERS Task Force Report[124] cautions that the potential not only exists for creation of artifacts in fiber/ferruginous body content of tissue due to drying of the tissue before low-temperature ashing, but the "uncontrolled use of ultrasound to disperse the residue may break the fibres, resulting in higher counts and smaller sizes. Fibres may be lost during repeated centrifugation."

Dement et al.[125] concluded the following regarding fiber analysis: "The use of indirect sample transfer for transmission electron microscopy (TEM) of asbestos has been shown to break up the airborne fibers into smaller units. Depending upon the treatment, the observed concentration of fibers and their size distribution change drastically. There is no biological justification for such a violent treatment, and the measured entity is not a biologically justifiable measured quantity. Therefore, the use of indirect sample transfer method for asbestos sampling should be discouraged, and the more gentle direct transfer method should be used."

To safeguard against this occurrence, it has been recommended that two separate samples are taken from each site (when adequate tissue permits). One sample is completely dried and the other samples pooled and used for the digestion procedure.[122] This approach permits determination of wet to dry ratio as used in determining ferruginous bodies or uncoated asbestos fiber per gram of wet or dry tissue. If there is not enough adequate tissue for two comparative samples (dry/wet), then it is advisable the individual sample is maintained/processed in a wet state, and data are given as fibers per gram of wet tissue or deparaffinized wet tissue (if tissue is extracted from paraffin blocks), unless there will be concern for induced changes in the characteristics of the tissue burden as per the previous discussions. Clarification of the sampling scheme and tissue status is critical if comparisons are to be made with the findings of others. When adequate tissue exists, multiple sites should be sampled. The wet samples are weighed and pooled for digestion. It is preferable to use multiple tissue samples to compensate for variations of ferruginous body/fiber burden within various areas of the tissue. The larger number of samples compensates for random sampling issues, although often single or several small tissue samples may be all that are available. Under such conditions, the use of digestion techniques and the screening of digested material for ferruginous bodies by light microscopy and for uncoated asbestos fibers by electron microscopy offer the best evidence concerning past exposure.[125] If a small sample contains asbestos bodies or fibers, it is reasonable that similar "hot" areas are present in the lung. If a small sample is negative, then the concern is that random sampling error has resulted in the tissue not being representative of the general lung/tissue burden. The method for digesting tissue[126] in our laboratory incorporates a modification of the Smith and Naylor[127] bleach digestion technique. The procedure permits the maximum disruption of tissue but with minimal trauma to particulates obtained from the tissue through the application of the most "direct" mode of sample preparation. This is in contrast with "indirect methods" of preparations that often involve additional manipulations of the sample. These may include the filter being ashed to remove more organic debris and the redispersion of the material collected from the ashed preparation as a suspension into an additional liquid for redispersion. In the direct method, the tissue is digested with the material collected on the filter remaining in place throughout the additional treatment, thus avoiding additional manipulations and possible loss or disruption of asbestos bodies or fibers. This is critical because data on the basis of laboratory suspensions of pure chrysotile asbestos indicate fiber size distribution may be greatly affected by indirect preparation procedures with the greatest impact being an increased number of short fibers below 2.5 μm.[67] These would not be included in a count of fibers longer than 5 μm, although they may have been this length or longer in the tissue before the traumatic influence of the preparative procedures. Thus, the indirect method is suspect of splitting and fragmenting chrysotile fibers or bundles and, potentially, ferruginous bodies.

The original bleach digestion procedure[127] works well for some tissues, but the development of the modified version was deemed necessary to digest tissue with considerable mucus content, thus reducing the amount of residual tissue material trapped on the surface of the filter. This procedure also allows digestion of sputum and lavage material to the degree that ferruginous bodies and uncoated asbestos fibers can be quantified.[125, 128, 129] The use of a digested aliquot permits sampling of tissue with the least inherent variation in procedures that could contribute to sampling errors.

The procedure used in our facility is to sample a portion of the aliquot for ferruginous body content of the tissue by collecting a measured amount of the solution on a mixed cellulose ester (MCE) filter. This membrane filter is easily cleared by acetone vapor resulting in a transparent film being left on the surface of a glass slide. This preparation can then be screened by light microscopy for identification of ferruginous bodies. It is critical that the core material of the ferruginous bodies be easily seen to distinguish asbestos bodies from non-asbestos ferruginous bodies. The data from this preparation provide the information used for determining ferruginous body numbers per gram of digested tissue. Such information can be compared with data from a given laboratory for tissue burden per gram wet or dry for tissue from the general population with findings from lung samples from individuals with defined asbestos exposures.

In the technique used in our laboratory, a second sample of the aliquot is passed through a smooth surfaced polycarbonate filter (0.2 µm pored). The material is prepared for evaluation by analytical transmission electron microscopy (ATEM). The pore size chosen for the collection of material is critical if one desires to include the thinner and shorter fibers in a count because considerable numbers of short and long, thin fibers in an aqueous solution can pass through a pore size as small as 0.4 µm in diameter.[130] The counterpoint is that if the digestion procedure selected has not dissolved the majority of the tissue components, the membrane will rapidly occlude even with a 0.4-µm pored filter. This is of concern when the objective of the preparation is to determine uncoated asbestos fiber burden in the tissue as the residue can easily obscure smaller, thinner fibers. This issue is of much less concern when the collection of material to be assessed is for asbestos body content because asbestos bodies are large and easily seen when compared with uncoated asbestos fibers. Selected filters from each polycarbonate lot should be screened for inherent contamination by TEM. These data are used as part of the basis for establishment of laboratory background levels for asbestos in a laboratory. Each solution used in the preparation of the tissue should be prefiltered before use to further protect against introduction of asbestos from non-tissue sources. The use of a polycarbonate filter which has a smooth surface with defined pores as opposed to an irregular surfaced MCE filter for collecting digestate material has recently been further supported by findings in the study of Webber et al.[131] Their study evaluated the performance of membrane filters used for TEM analysis of asbestos. They concluded that "unless substantial care is used in the collapsing of MCE filters with an acetone hot block, grid preparations can suffer and fiber recoveries can be compromised." They further observed that in some phases of etching, the surface of the MCE as part of the preparation for TEM sampling can lead to the loss of short fibers. The comparison of the MCE and the polycarbonate filters for TEM preparations resulted in their conclusion that the latter were favored because of advantages of "straightforward preparation, improved solvents, and reduced contamination" of the PC filters.

3.8 INSTRUMENTATION USE IN TISSUE ANALYSIS FOR ASBESTOS/ELONGATED MINERAL PARTICLES

A discussion regarding the use of the light microscope in determining asbestos burden in tissue requires description of several applications. First, sections cut from paraffin blocks can be mounted on glass slides and screened for ferruginous bodies in H&E or iron-stained preparations. This is an insensitive method, and the evaluation of digested material by light microscopy for asbestos bodies on a filter is more sensitive because the content of much more tissue is evaluated. The use of light microscopy for determination of uncoated asbestos fibers collected from tissue is of limited to no value. Most inhaled fibers are below the level of resolution of the light microscope, and those seen can only be categorized as fibers because distinction between fiber types (asbestos and non-asbestos) cannot be made.[84] The more definitive instruments for asbestos fiber identification are the analytical scanning electron microscope (SEM) and the ATEM.

As pointed out in the Health Effects Institute report on Asbestos in Public and Commercial Buildings,[67] "the scanning electron microscope appears at first review to be a suitable instrument for analysis of fibers collected on a filter (in this case from air samples). SEMs are less costly than analytical transmission electron microscopes, specimen preparations are relatively simple, and they can be equipped with an X-ray energy dispersive analyzer for determination of elemental compositions of particles. They have an acceptable level of resolution to permit identification of the asbestos particles." It is not possible to provide a better description as to the limits of the SEM than provided in the Health Effects Institute report as quoted in the following: "Detection of a small asbestos fiber on the surface of an air filter, using any type of microscope, requires that both resolution and contrast be sufficient. When the SEM is operated at high magnification, a compromise must be made between image resolution and the signal presented to the image-forming system. This compromise leads to a routine detectability for small diameter fibers on the viewing screen that is often only slightly better than that achieved in the PCOM (i.e., approximately 0.2 μm).[132–136] The full resolution of the instrument can be achieved; permitting the detection of the smallest asbestos fibers, but only if each field of view is photographed using a time exposure of about 1 min or more. To produce real-time images at the magnification required, the beam current must be increased, and at the required high-beam currents, the resolution is degraded.[137] Real-time operation is required because each fiber must be identified. The image quality can be improved by using heavy metals, such as gold, to coat the surface of the filter, but this coating compromises the interpretation of the X-ray spectra on which fiber identification is based and may even obscure objects on the filter. Energy dispersive X-ray analysis (EDXA) is the only technique available in the SEM by which fibers can be identified. Identification of fibers by this technique alone has some serious limitations. The approximate chemical composition, derived from an EDXA spectrum, is frequently not sufficient to discriminate between asbestos varieties and some other relatively common minerals.[138] In addition, when attempts are made to identify a fiber by the use of EDXA, contributions to the EDXA spectrum may be made by other particulates close to the fiber under examination. The composite EDXA spectrum thus obtained can lead to ambiguities in identification. Definitive identification of asbestos fibers can often be achieved only by a combination of chemical and electron diffraction data, and this combination of identification techniques is available only in the analytical TEM."[67]

The most accurate instrument for detecting and analyzing asbestos fiber types in a sample and appropriately providing their dimensions is the ATEM. The data derived from fibers collected on a membrane filter from an air sample or from a tissue preparation require the same levels of resolution and analytical interpretation provided only by the ATEM. The Asbestos Hazard Emergency Response Act (Title II of the Toxic Substance Control Act 15, U.S.C. Sections 2641–2654) defines ATEM as the "state-of-the-art" instrument and required the use of ATEM for final clearance in many abatement projects in schools. As of August 1, 1990, laboratories performing analysis for abatement clearance in U.S. schools were required to be accredited by the National Voluntary Laboratory Accreditation Program. This accreditation includes assurance that analysis by ATEM is done consistently and that other laboratories likewise use the same magnification for analysis, including the same dimension fibers in any count scheme, analyzing the fibers in the same way, and reporting the data in the same way. Another important part of the National Voluntary Laboratory Accreditation Program is that of quality assurance. Steps were described earlier as to how our laboratory carries out quality assurance to ensure analysis of the tissue is not altered because of contamination within the laboratory or from other sources. Once particulates to be analyzed, including asbestos fibers, are collected on a filter, it is irrelevant as to whether they are from air, water, or tissue. The only major difference is that considerable numbers of fibers can be lost (as per the concern of the indirect method of tissue preparation) or obscured on the filter surface by debris, thus preventing the analyst from detecting smaller particulates. The count scheme under the Asbestos Hazard Emergency Response Act includes structures (fibers) that are greater than or equal to 0.5 μm in length, have an aspect ratio of at least 5:1, and have parallel sides (in the case of fibers) for most of their length. The analysis includes defining the morphology, the elemental composition (EDXA), and the crystalline characteristics (selected area diffraction). This contrasts with the light microscope counting scheme where fibers counted are 5 μm or longer, have parallel sides for most of their length, and where there is no differentiation as to the type of fiber counted. The power of the ATEM to provide the most accurate information as to uncoated asbestos fiber burden in tissue is only as useful as the quality of the preparation permits and the utilization of the instrument at a sufficient magnification to permit detection of short and long, thin asbestos fibers. The analytical scheme of counting should include fibers below 5 μm, the population of fibers that make up the majority of fibers in human lung and extrapulmonary sites,[56, 84, 139] if the overall representation of fiber burden is to be achieved. To ignore fibers less than 5 μm in a count scheme provides a biased base of information that starts with a decision to exclude most chrysotile in air or tissue samples.

3.9 USEFULNESS OF SPUTUM AND LAVAGE FOR DETERMINATION OF PAST EXPOSURE TO ASBESTOS/ELONGATED MINERAL PARTICLES

Sputum is collected as phlegm produced as a normal process of clearance from the respiratory system. A marker of sputum as being from the deeper regions of the lung is the presence of pulmonary macrophages. As described in the section on clearance mechanisms, macrophages are capable of reaching the mucociliary escalator and bring associated (in the case of asbestos bodies) or ingested dust particles (smaller fibers) to the back of the throat for elimination via swallowing or expectoration. Sputum can be collected via spontaneous or induced methods. In the latter, a mist of salt water triggers a cough reflex to clear more sputum. Smokers produce more sputum, whereas nonsmokers are poor sputum producers. Asbestos bodies formed in the lung can be found in the mucus or macrophage-laden material in the sputum of occupationally exposed individuals. Greenberg et al.[140] evaluated asbestos body production in a group of former amosite workers for approximately a year. Sputa was screened cytologically. One-third of sputa samples from workers contained asbestos bodies that were most numerous in induced sputum samples. Bignon et al.[141] reported an absence of asbestos bodies in sputum when the asbestos body concentration in lung parenchyma was under 1000/cm^3. McLarty et al.,[142] in a further review of the amosite-exposed cohort, concluded that the presence of asbestos bodies in sputa was related to radiographic findings of interstitial fibrosis (asbestosis) and pleural fibrosis and to spirometric findings of restrictive lung disease. Age and cigarette smoking were also related to the number of asbestos bodies found in sputum samples. Modin et al.[143] reviewed the findings of asbestos bodies in sputa and bronchial washings obtained as screening in a general hospital/clinic setting and concluded that finding ferruginous bodies in either sample was a highly specific marker for past asbestos exposure and reflected the presence of a significant asbestos load within the lung. Paris et al.[144] reviewed three consecutive sputum samples collected from 270 retired workers in a textile and friction materials factory. In this study, 53% of samples were positive for ferruginous bodies. The authors concluded that the prevalence of asbestos bodies in sputa was not related to sex, smoking status, or latency.

Sebastien et al.[145] evaluated sputa samples from a cohort of vermiculite miners and millers who were exposed to ore that contained the amphibole tremolite as well as other fibrous amphiboles. Two sputa samples were collected from all but three of the 173 workers. Chest radiographs were scored according to the 1980 ILO classification. They reported that 75% of the workers had from "one to nearly 4000 asbestos bodies in their sputum, and their concentration in sputum and cumulative exposure (intensity × duration) were significantly related." The authors stated "the finding that the radiographic changes were better explained by the sputum index than by cumulative exposure."

Dodson et al.[146] determined asbestos body and uncoated asbestos fiber content in 12 randomly selected sputa samples from former amosite asbestos workers and 12 individuals from the general population with no history of asbestos exposure. The sputa were digested by the procedure previously described by Williams et al.,[126] after which samples were screened by light microscopy and TEM for asbestos bodies/fibers. The inconsistency of finding asbestos bodies in sputa, even from occupationally exposed individuals, was reflected in that none of the 12 sputa samples from former amosite workers contained asbestos bodies, nor were any asbestos bodies found in samples from the general population. However, 10 of 12 samples from the amosite group contained uncoated amosite fibers as detected by electron microscopic evaluation. One short chrysotile fiber was found in our sputum samples from the general population group. The finding of uncoated fibers and no asbestos bodies in sputa from exposed individuals was not surprising because asbestos bodies are larger and less easily brought upward by macrophages than uncoated fibers that are more easily carried upward in mucus or are moved upward within macrophages that have ingested the fibers. Screening for uncoated fibers by electron microscopy increased the sensitivity of sputa analysis for identifying past occupational exposure to asbestos.

The techniques for assessing the various content (including dust particles) in bronchoalveolar lavage (BAL) fluid were developed after the creation of the fiber-optic bronchoscope in the late 1960s. The technique by definition is "a procedure that recovers cellular and noncellular components from the epithelial surface of the lower respiratory tract and differs from bronchial washings that typically refer to aspiration of secretions or small amounts of instilled saline from the large airways."[147] The BAL technique provides clinicians a new mechanism by which they can sample the lung milieu and the free cells that populate the lower respiratory tract. Begin[148] reviewed the array of diseases about which additional information could be learned via application of the BAL technique, including those categorized as inflammatory and interstitial in nature. One particular application is the sampling of lower airway contents for dust particles.

De Vuyst et al.[149–153] provided much of our data concerning the usefulness of lavage assessment in asbestos-exposed individuals. A comparison of the asbestos body content of lavage material was made with content of lung samples from the same individuals, most of whom were undergoing thoracotomy procedures for lung cancer.[151] Their findings were the absence of or low asbestos body (AB) counts (<1 AB/mL BAL fluid) corresponded in about 70% of cases to concentrations of less than 1000 AB/g of dry lung tissue and in 100% of the cases to tissue concentrations of less than 10,000 AB/g. In subjects with BAL containing greater than 1 AB/mL of BAL, it was found that 85% of cases contained more than 1000 AB/g of dry lung tissue. Those individuals with greater than 10 AB/mL of BAL fluid were all found to contain lung burdens of greater than 10,000 AB/g of dry lung tissue. In an earlier companion study, the sensitivity of BAL fluid analysis for indicating past exposure to asbestos was supported; in the study, 28 of 28 individuals with obvious exposures were found to have ABs in lavage material.[150] Among 40 controls, only five were found to have ABs in BAL fluid, and the burden was reported to be 1 AB/mL of BAL fluid. De Vuyst et al.,[149] in another study that included assessment of BAL fluid from white-collar workers, blue-collar workers, and subjects with definite exposure to asbestos, found that ABs were a marker of exposure to asbestos and not an asbestos-induced disease. Asbestos bodies were more likely to be found in BAL fluid from "patients presenting with asbestos-related diseases but in whom exposure is not confirmed by the occupational history (65 of 78 cases)." Sebastien et al.[154] studied BAL fluid from 69 patients with suspected asbestos-related diseases who subsequently underwent lung biopsy or autopsy. They concluded that when the BAL fluid "exceeds 1 AB/mL, it can be quite confidently predicted, however, that the parenchymal concentration is in excess of 1000 AB/g (dry weight) and that the patient has experienced a nontrivial asbestos exposure."

Schwartz et al.[155] concluded that asbestos bodies found in lavage fluid are a reproducible assay for exposure but have little utility in most clinical settings to predict disease presence. Similarly, Oriowski et al.[156] found that the extent of pleural plaques correlated neither with frequency or duration of exposure nor to the number of asbestos bodies in BAL fluid in subjects free of lung parenchymal abnormalities determined by high-resolution computerized tomography. One must remember when reviewing the correlation of asbestos bodies in BAL fluid that they represent only a population of longer fibers (>8 μm) in the lung and tell nothing about the overall burden of longer, uncoated, or shorter asbestos fibers. Furthermore, asbestos-related diseases often occur long after first exposure and not infrequently a considerable time from last exposure. Thus, asbestos bodies in BAL fluid may confirm a level of past exposure to longer fibers but not offer insight to the quantity of the overall fiber burden in the past. Because asbestos bodies form months to years after exposure, their presence can be detected in BAL fluid long before the latency period required for the development of asbestos-induced diseases, for example, often 15–50 years. Asbestos bodies in BAL fluid through representation of a higher percentage of longer fibers in the lung indicates an increased likelihood of occupational exposure to asbestos because asbestos fibers found in general populations are usually short and uncoated.[153, 154, 157, 158]

The information discussed to this point regarding past levels of asbestos exposure as determined from BAL fluid is based on asbestos body content determined by light microscopy. Additional information regarding past exposure can be obtained from BAL samples analyzed by electron microscopy just as the sensitivity of sputum samples is expanded when uncoated fiber composition is included in an analysis. Gellert et al.[159] compared findings by light and electron microscopy of BAL fluid from 15 subjects with exposure to asbestos, 3 of whom had clinical and radiological evidence of asbestosis compared with asbestos BAL fluid concentrations findings in 13 urban-dwelling control subjects. Asbestos fibers were confirmed in BAL fluid from 11 of 15 exposed persons ranging between 133 and 3700 fibers per milliliter of lavage fluid, with the range of asbestos bodies per milliliter of lavage fluid being 0–333. Five exposed subjects with no asbestos bodies detected by light microscopy were found to have uncoated asbestos fibers by electron microscopy (range = 133–2711 fibers/mL of lavage fluid). Only one sample from the control group was found to have a "few" asbestos fibers in the BAL fluid.

The use of BAL fluid has been shown to be of value for assessment of exposures to particular fiber types, including exposures in secondary settings.[153, 160] These include lavage material analyzed from a woman (household contact) with bilateral pleural and diaphragmatic plaques whose only source of exposure was while washing the clothing of her husband who had been an asbestos sprayer. The second individual had been a coal miner for much of his adult life. The presence of crocidolite fibers in the lavage material was attributed to the individual's daily use of personal protection masks during work in the coal mine. These masks were reported to have been used from 1920 to 1970 and contained crocidolite. The third case was of a mason who for 44 years lived in a region of Turkey where exposure to tremolite, as found in his lavage material, was known to occur as a result of environmental exposures. The final case consisted of an individual who had "all of the possible asbestos-related diseases except lung cancer." These were attributed to a short but intense exposure that had occurred 47–51 years before the diagnosis of the specific diseases. Dodson et al.[101] found ferruginous bodies formed on a variety of particulates inhaled by foundry workers. These included fibrous and nonfibrous structures. The most common non-asbestos cores of elongated ferruginous bodies consisted of sheet silicates, graphite (carbon), and iron-rich fibers. Dodson et al.[160] reported that the greatest specificity is obtained for correlating past exposures to asbestos by using a combination of light microscopic quantitation of asbestos bodies correlated with the uncoated asbestos fiber burden as determined by ATEM evaluation of BAL fluid samples.

The high incidence of malignant mesothelioma in villages in Turkey (Tuzkoy/Cappadocia) has been considered a result of environmental exposure to erionite, which is found as a fibrous mineral in the local soil.[161] Dumortier et al.[162] evaluated BAL fluid from 16 subjects originating from Tuzkoy. The authors found ferruginous bodies in 12 subjects. Erionite was the central fiber of 95.7% of the ferruginous bodies while erionite fibers were found in the bronchoalveolar lavage fluid in all subjects. They concluded that the mean concentration of erionite fibers in lavage fluid was similar to that of tremolite fibers in Turks with environmental exposure to tremolite. These exposures illustrate an example of a non-asbestos, naturally occurring fibrous mineral that is considered as a causal agent for mesothelioma in man.

De Vuyst et al.[163] evaluated BAL from six talc workers with pneumoconiosis. Two were defined as mainly exposed to American and Australian talc, and the other four were defined as exposed to French talc (Luzenac). The authors stated: "Talc particles and talc bodies were abundant, sometimes many years after the end of exposure. A qualitative difference was the presence of tremolite asbestos fibres in the two patients exposed to American and Australian talc and its absence in the four French talc workers. The presence of tremolite in lavage is attributed to a geological association of this mineral with the inhaled talc." The authors concluded that lavage "can confirm exposure to talc and provide information about the heterogeneity of inhaled dust."

In another study, the lavaged individuals worked in a cement manufacturing facility that used chrysotile and crocidolite as reflected in the content and type of uncoated asbestos fiber burden in their BAL fluid. A unique observation was obtained when analysis of lavage material was carried out by light and electron microscopic assessment from 15 brake lining workers considered to be only exposed to chrysotile and 44 asbestos cement workers exposed extensively to amphiboles.[164]

As indicated by the authors, the literature is replete with references that chrysotile does not readily stimulate the formation of asbestos bodies unless there is a rare exposure that includes a population of longer chrysotile fibers (Figure 3.18).[164, 165] However, analysis of BAL fluid indicated that an exposure to asbestos among brake lining factory workers occurred for longer fibers of chrysotile because 95.6% of the cores of asbestos bodies were chrysotile. This contrasted with 93.1% of cores of asbestos bodies that were formed on amphiboles analyzed from BAL fluid from asbestos cement workers. A similar observation of chrysotile-cored ferruginous bodies in BAL fluid and lung tissue was found in our laboratory. Lung tissue evaluation from an individual with a unique asbestos exposure during work as a clutch rebuilder indicated the presence of longer fibers of chrysotile and the majority of asbestos bodies found in the lung tissue sample (77.2%) being formed on chrysotile asbestos cores.[165]

Additional publications[166–169] emphasized that brake dust contained predominantly short chrysotile fibers, with most fibers being less than 5 μm. This suggests that exposure to brake dust would not be expected to result in asbestos body formation because, as previously stated, asbestos bodies form on longer fibers usually greater than 8 μm. However, disturbance of friction products during some activities can result in inhalation of longer fibers as verified by the presence of chrysotile-cored ferruginous bodies in lavage materials[164] and in tissue.[165]

The status of existing data regarding evaluation of BAL samples for the presence of asbestos provides the basis of the synopsis offered by Sartorelli et al.,[170] who stated that "fiber concentration in BALF can be considered as a reliable biomarker of past asbestos exposure, even many years after the end of exposure."

3.10 ASBESTOS (FERRUGINOUS) BODY BURDEN IN EXPOSED AND GENERAL POPULATIONS

The asbestos body as a marker of past exposure to asbestos has been discussed in the context of its presence in tissue sections. A more sensitive method of assessing tissue samples for asbestos bodies is by sampling larger amounts of tissue via digestion techniques. The digested material is collected on a thin membrane (filter) and after being made transparent, as previously described, can be subjected to screening by light microscopy. The numbers of asbestos bodies found can be extrapolated to the numbers per gram of wet or dry tissue. Some earlier works combining light and electron microscopy for determining the numbers of asbestos bodies per gram of tissue and core identification were carried out by Churg and Warnock.[99, 118, 171–173] Their observations in tissues from individuals considered as representing the general population from larger cities led them to "arbitrarily consider 100 bodies to be the division between 'environmental' and 'occupational' exposure."[173] If one chooses to use a multiplier of 10 to approximate asbestos bodies per gram of dry weight, then the number would be 1000 per gram dry weight for nonoccupational exposures. These two numbers have been referenced as a "break point" that separates occupational from nonoccupational levels of exposure to asbestos as defined by tissue burdens.[173, 174] The report by the ERS Working Group[124] appropriately notes, "the dry to wet weight ratio varies from 5–20% and should be measured for each sample. The use of a mean conversion factor of 10 for the wet/dry ratio should be avoided." Data from our own experience indicate that the number of asbestos bodies in the nonoccupationally exposed general population per gram of wet tissue is 0–20 asbestos bodies,[157, 175] which is more in keeping with reference levels in general populations as reported by Breedin and Buss[176] and by Roggli et al.[177]

Churg and Warnock[171] analyzed core material of ferruginous bodies by ATEM in 23 autopsy and surgical patients, none of whom had occupational asbestos exposure. Of the 328 bodies examined, 264 (80%) had diffraction patterns consistent with amphibole asbestos whereas only 6 had chrysotile cores. In a separate study of 144 asbestos bodies isolated from 29 persons with fewer than 100 asbestos bodies per gram of wet lung tissue (below occupational levels)[173] analyzed by electron diffraction, 143 were found to be formed on amphiboles whereas only 1 was formed on a chrysotile core. Chemical analysis by XEDA was used to further define the types of amphiboles. Twenty-one were determined to be formed on amosite or crocidolite cores, 13 on anthophyllite asbestos cores, and 1 on a tremolite asbestos core. Commercial amphiboles were the dominant cores of asbestos bodies in men (86%), whereas 57% of the asbestos bodies analyzed from women were formed on anthophyllite or tremolite cores. Cosmetic talc was suggested as the source of these "noncommercial" types of asbestos fibers in the women within the studies.[99, 172]

Roggli et al.[177] studied asbestos body concentrations as related to types of asbestos-induced diseases. The highest numbers of asbestos bodies per gram of tissue were in individuals with asbestosis (≥2000 AB/g wet tissue). Intermediate levels were found in individuals with malignant mesothelioma and the lowest in patients with pleural plaques. As in other studies, the majority of the cores of asbestos bodies were on amphiboles. The explanation of why amphibole cores were most common is that amphiboles, being straight fibers, tend to be more readily inhaled in a longer form than chrysotile. However, when longer fibers of chrysotile are readily available and inhaled, chrysotile cores of asbestos bodies are not uncommon. As stated previously, appreciable numbers of chrysotile-cored asbestos bodies were reported in BAL fluid from brake lining workers[164] and in tissue from a clutch refrabricator.[165]

Moulin et al.[178] analyzed cores of ferruginous bodies in 19 asbestos-exposed individuals and 25 nonexposed urban dwellers from the Belgium urban population. Of the 319 ferruginous bodies analyzed, 315 were formed on asbestos. The non-asbestos cores were on talc and crystalline silica. Eighty-two percent of the asbestos cores were commercial amphiboles (amosite/crocidolite) and 7% were formed on chrysotile cores. The remaining 3.8% were formed on noncommercial amphiboles (anthophyllite/tremolite). In each study, some ferruginous bodies were totally coated and not capable of being analyzed by XEDA or selected area diffraction.

Holden and Churg[179] examined ferruginous body content from lungs of chrysotile miners and found that 64% of the cores were formed on chrysotile and 29% formed on amphiboles, although the amphiboles (tremolite and actinolite) constituted the majority of uncoated fibers in these cases. Levin et al.[180] reported a case of a clutch refabricator where 72% of the ferruginous bodies were formed on chrysotile asbestos cores (Figure 3.18).

An ideal model for determining tissue burden of asbestos fibers would be to develop a multiplier of the number of more easily seen ferruginous bodies (as determined by light microscopy) and extrapolate the concentration of uncoated asbestos fibers from this number. Such an effort is an exercise in futility as the ratio varies widely as does the efficiency for ferruginous body formation between individuals.[93, 107, 181, 182]

For example, Srebro et al.[183] evaluated the tissue content of ferruginous bodies in 18 cases of mesothelioma compared with 19 "control" cases. The data, when combining uncoated asbestos burden, indicated that six mesothelioma cases might be asbestos-related despite asbestos body counts similar to those in the samples from the general population. A prudent recommendation was offered that "electron microscopic analysis of pulmonary mineral fibers may be required to differentiate asbestos-related mesotheliomas from non-asbestos-related cases when asbestos body counts are within the range of background values."

However, asbestos body burden is elevated in many occupationally exposed individuals, given that longer fibers reach the lower airways and thus provide a stimulus for coating as per the described data from our laboratory. In a group of 55 occupationally exposed asbestos individuals with mesothelioma, 46 had concentrations of asbestos bodies above 1000/g dry weight of lung tissue.[181] Of 841 ferruginous bodies analyzed, 781 (92.9%) were formed on amosite, 24 (2.9%) on crocidolite, 8 (1%) on tremolite, 3 (0.4%) on anthophyllite, 3 (0.4%) on actinolite, and 1 (0.1%) on chrysotile cores. Eleven (1.3%) of the ferruginous bodies were formed on non-asbestos cores and 10 (1.2%) were totally coated or successful analysis of the core material could not be achieved. Seven of 15 cases of women with mesotheliomas evaluated in another study had over 1000 asbestos bodies per gram.

Ferruginous body quantitation was carried out in 19 cases of individuals with a prior history of occupational asbestos exposure and lung cancer. The ferruginous body content in 11 cases was found to be over 1000 asbestos bodies per gram of dry tissue.[184] Three individuals lung tissue did not contain asbestos bodies (within limits of detectability of the study), and two were found to have concentrations at general population levels. One individual did not have detectable levels of asbestos fibers, although lung tissue from the remaining four contained asbestos fibers.

As mentioned earlier, asbestos bodies are not readily formed in some individuals although their lung tissue contains elevated numbers of longer asbestos fibers[182, 184, 185] suitable for iron-protein coating. The absence of detectable levels of ferruginous bodies implies little regarding the presence of chrysotile in the majority of samples. This suggests that the number of uncoated asbestos fibers found in tissue is independently important as an indicator of exposure/causation of asbestos-induced disease.[186]

Asbestos bodies have also been reported in colonic tissue from an insulation worker with asbestosis[187]; however, the question exists as to whether the fibers reached the area by ingestion of sputa, which contained the ferruginous bodies/asbestos fibers originally deposited within the lungs, or were relocated via some other route to the site of the tumor.

An excellent study was published that focused on the determination of the epigenetic profiles that distinguish pleural mesothelioma from normal pleura and predict lung asbestos burden and clinical outcome.[188] The authors conducted an elaborate investigation but took liberty to use their findings of asbestos bodies per gram as interchangeable with the overall asbestos burden. Although the increased numbers of ferruginous bodies may indeed be a predictor of mesothelioma, their presence only represents one small component of the overall asbestos burden in tissue. Asbestos bodies represent a selective population of the longer fibers (if the individual coats fibers) and tell us nothing regarding the number of shorter fibers (including most chrysotile in lung) and uncoated longer/thinner fibers that are less likely to coat. It thus remains for the uncoated asbestos burden to be defined before the story is complete.

3.11 UNCOATED ASBESTOS FIBERS/ELONGATED PARTICLES IN OCCUPATIONALLY EXPOSED INDIVIDUALS AND IN LUNG TISSUE FROM THE GENERAL POPULATION

In order evaluate uncoated asbestos fiber concentrations in tissue, it is imperative there is a clear understanding of what techniques were used to obtain asbestos concentration data. The resolution of the light microscope coupled with its lack of ability to distinguish fiber types greatly limits it usefulness in assessing fiber concentration in tissue. Even in the most ideal settings where tissue has been destroyed and there is minimal obstruction of fibers from view, only a small percent is detectable by light microscopic examination. Morgan and Holmes[189] reported that approximately one-half of uncoated fibers would have been detected by light microscopy. Ashcroft and Heppleston[116] reported that only 12–30% of uncoated asbestos fibers from tissue samples in their study were visible by light microscopy. Rood and Streeter[190] compared the detection capabilities of light microscopy versus those of scanning and TEM for chrysotile fibers collected on a filter. All fibers (100%) would have been counted and analyzed by the transmission electron microscope, 60% by SEM, and only 25% of fibers greater than 5 μm long would have been identified with the light microscope (Figures 3.19

and 3.20). The data from our publications[104, 181, 182, 184] generally agrees with the range for optically detectable fibers reported by Ashcroft and Heppleston[116] and by Rood and Streeter,[190] except when the population of asbestos fibers in a tissue sample is predominantly short and/or long, thin fibers.[56, 107, 139, 191] In such cases when the fiber burden is represented by chrysotile and crocidolite, the number of fibers detected by light microscopy is often 0%. Pooley and Ranson[192] correctly stated: "It is possible, using the electron microscope, to predict the asbestos fibre count that would be obtained by light microscopy, the reverse prediction cannot be made: it is impossible to determine the proportion of the various asbestos minerals types using the light microscope." A referral to our laboratory[193] further emphasizes the need to recognize what one "sees" with a given technique and at a given magnification with a specific instrument. A portion of a block of tissue was evaluated by SEM at relatively low magnification and the referring individual wanted to determine the findings via a high magnification evaluation by ATEM. The earlier assessment had evaluated fiber burden at 1000× and included only those fibers <5 μm in the count scheme. The individual had been reported to have had a work history that would have been expected to have specifically included chrysotile dust. One fiber that was considered to be chrysotile was found by SEM. The sheer numbers of short chrysotile fibers (>0.5 μm) and a count scheme at high magnification by ATEM that permitted their detection necessitated a modified count scheme consisting of a reduced count area from the total area we would usually review. Three very small chrysotile-cored ferruginous bodies were also found. Only three of the individual chrysotile fibers <5 μm were not in the form of fibrils. Only 7% of all lengths of chrysotile fibers were not fibrils (0.02–0.05 μm in diameter); thus, length is not the only determinate for detection of a fiber. This illustrates the importance of clearly understanding what is being used to evaluate a sample of fibers from tissue, air, or water and what is being included in a count as well as what is potentially there but not "seen" or included in the count scheme.[194]

In discussing uncoated fiber burden in tissue, it seems reasonable, on the basis of the aforementioned reasons, to compare data obtained by TEM to that generated via similar techniques. It is important to compare data generated at sufficient magnification and with a count scheme that includes "short" and long/thin asbestos fibers, as this population makes up the vast majority of asbestos fibers in lung tissue and extrapulmonary sites.[56, 107, 192–194]

Some of the earliest contributions using ATEM for analysis of tissue digestion from "control populations" were contributed from the research by Churg et al. In a study of individuals from the San Francisco area, Churg and Warnock[118] reported that "80% of uncoated fibers were chrysotile (mean: 130×10^3) with a range of 12×10^3 to 680×10^3 fibers per gram wet lung and 90% of chrysotile fibers less than 5 μm long." Total amphiboles had a mean of 25×10^3 and ranged from 1.3×10^3 to 75×10^3 fibers per gram wet lung tissue. Ninety-five percent were noncommercial amphiboles and two-thirds were less than 5 μm long. Approximately 20% of amosite, crocidolite, and anthophyllite fibers identified were longer than 10 μm. They concluded the following: (1) substantial amounts of asbestos, mainly chrysotile and noncommercial amphiboles, are present in the average lung in an urban environment; (2) most of these fibers are too small to form asbestos bodies or to be visible by light microscopy; (3) asbestos bodies may serve as some indication of exposure to long amphiboles but offer no information about the bulk of fibers present; and (4) it is probable that most of these fibers reflect general environmental contamination.

In a subsequent tissue study of individuals residing in Vancouver, British Columbia, Churg and Wiggs[17] reported the mean chrysotile burden to be "only" 0.2×10^6 g of dry lung when compared with approximately 1.0×10^6 g of dry lung in San Francisco. A possible difference was explained by known outcrops containing chrysotile asbestos in the San Francisco Bay area that might contribute to environmental exposures. However, the conclusion offered was that the majority of fiber types are "more or less the same in both cities."

Langer et al.,[195] in a study involving 28 individuals who resided in New York City, found chrysotile to be present in 24 cases with the other four being considered potentially "positive" by occurrence of background fibril contamination. Langer concluded that unaltered chrysotile is uncommonly found as the core in asbestos bodies removed from lung samples from general populations. The authors correctly stated that the vast majority of chrysotile structures in the lungs of the general population are "fibrillar units" and require ATEM for detection. The same is true from our experience for chrysotile structures isolated from lungs and extrapulmonary tissue from occupationally exposed individuals. In another study, Langer and Nolan[196] evaluated lung burden by ATEM of 126 autopsy cases of persons who died in New York City from 1966 through 1968. They considered 107 of the 126 cases to "probably" be nonoccupationally exposed. Their important observations were that "virtually all the chrysotile in nonoccupationally exposed persons was composed of short fibrils, most equal to or less than 1 μm in length, with the modal class between 0.2 and 0.5 μm." They further concluded that "analysis of selected fibers showed preservation of both chemistry and structure. It would appear, therefore, that in occupational exposure to chrysotile not only are doses higher, but the proportion of longer fibers is greater than in the chrysotile to which the general population is exposed."

Data from our own laboratory tend in many ways to agree with the early studies of Churg and Warnock.[118]The definition of a member of the general population used in our laboratory is that the individual has not been involved in a known asbestos-related work activity, has no disease conditions which may have been caused by asbestos, and has 20 or less (our general population number) asbestos bodies per gram of wet lung tissue. In a study by Dodson et al.,[157] 35% of uncoated asbestos fibers from 33 individuals considered as from the general population were chrysotile and 86% were <5 μm long. Also, 83% of amphiboles in this study were noncommercial amphiboles and 73% of these were <5 μm long. The most commonly found asbestos fiber was chrysotile, which was observed in 14 cases, with anthophyllite being found in 12 cases. Of the 33 cases, 26 cases had no ferruginous bodies detected by light microscopy. Of the 33 individuals, 10 were not found to have asbestos fibers in their lung tissue (within the limit of detection in the procedure). The geometric mean of fiber length for each asbestos type found was less than 3 μm. An additional study of lung samples from 15 individuals considered as representing the general population[158] confirmed the findings from the earlier study. Only four individuals were found to contain asbestos bodies, and only two individuals' lung tissue contained an asbestos fiber in their lung digest (within limits of detection used in the study). In conclusion, our findings indicate that lung tissue from the general population contains low numbers of asbestos fibers. If detected, these fibers will likely be short chrysotile or noncommercial amphibole fibers. When commercial amphiboles are found, the fibers are short (<5 μm) and few in numbers. When a lung tissue sample contains appreciable numbers of asbestos fibers, long fibers, and/or commercial amphiboles (amosite or crocidolite), the suggestion is that the individual had an occupational or paraoccupational/bystander exposure to asbestos.

Additional data exist regarding asbestos burden in tissue from occupationally exposed individuals. As mentioned earlier, the chrysotile form of asbestos constituted 90–95% of asbestos used in commercial applications in the USA. However, chrysotile veins have been reported to be "contaminated" with amphiboles, particularly actinolite, anthophyllite, tremolite, and more recently crocidolite.[197] Quebec chrysotile, which constituted the majority of chrysotile used in the USA, has been stated to have between 1% and 6.9% amphibole asbestos.[196–199] Tremolite has been suggested by McDonald et al.[200] as a "valid marker" for exposure to chrysotile asbestos. This same suggestion was made in a study by Churg et al.[201] of nine chrysotile miners with "asbestos airway disease" (the so-called early asbestosis)[201] but with no evidence of classic asbestosis (interstitial fibrosis) on pathological examination. The findings indicated a strong correlation between the amount of chrysotile and amphibole, suggesting that the amphibole (tremolite) component was a good measure of original (but no longer) chrysotile burden because of the more rapid clearance of the latter. In 1988, Churg[74] reviewed the literature on chrysotile, tremolite, and mesothelioma in man. Dr Churg opined "induction of mesothelioma by chrysotile requires, on average, as great a lung fiber burden as induction of asbestosis by chrysotile, whereas amphibole (amosite or crocidolite)-induced mesotheliomas appear at several hundred-fold smaller lung burden." In an additional study, Churg et al.[202, 203] found that high tremolite fiber concentration was strongly associated with mesothelioma, airway fibrosis, and asbestosis in a study involving chrysotile miners and millers from Thetford

Mines in Quebec. Pleural plaques and carcinoma of the lung were reported to show no relationship to tremolite burden.

Churg et al.[203] measured tissue burden by ATEM from 20 shipyard and insulation workers. The findings in this study indicated "amosite concentration, like chrysotile and tremolite concentration, is closely and directly related to fibrosis at the local lung level." The authors raised an important issue often ignored by those using counting schemes where only longer fibers (>5 μm) are counted, in the "possibility that short fibers may be more important than is commonly believed in the genesis of fibrosis in man." They also expressed their belief that an amosite fiber was more fibrogenic than a chrysotile or tremolite fiber and that tremolite was more fibrogenic than chrysotile.

McDonald et al.[204] concluded "that amphibole fibers could explain most mesothelioma cases in Canada and other inorganic fibers, including chrysotile, very few. Fibrous tremolite, contaminant of many industrial minerals including chrysotile, probably explained most cases in the Quebec (mesothelioma) mining and perhaps 20% elsewhere."

A study consisting of tissue evaluation of "young adults with mesothelioma" was reported by McDonald et al.[205] The project consisted of evaluating tissue from British mesothelioma cases where, because of the age group, "it was thought that most, but not all, work-related exposures would have been since 1970, when the importation of crocidolite, but not amosite, was virtually eliminated." The concentrations in the lung of "crocidolite and amosite fibers, which together could account for 80–90% of the cases, did not differ between occupational categories; those for amosite were appreciably higher than for crocidolite. Tremolite fibers were rarely found." "Contrary to expectation, however, some 90% of cases were in men who had started work before 1970."

Dufresne et al.[206] evaluated lung parenchymal samples by light microscopy and ATEM from 50 workers seeking compensation from the Workers' Compensation Board of Quebec for pleural or peritoneal mesothelioma. The group consisted of 12 from Asbestos township, 11 from Thetford Mines (mining and milling activities), and 27 from other types of industry (including asbestos factory, shipyard, and others). Data were compared with that obtained from a reference population. The fiber types in the three groups were different: "The lungs of workers from the Thetford Mines containing only chrysotile and tremolite; those from Asbestos township containing chrysotile, tremolite, amosite, and crocidolite; and those from other industries containing largely amosite and crocidolite." They concluded that the "fiber types responsible for the tumors are probably different in the three different groups" and that "fiber analysis confirmed occupational asbestos exposure in every case."

An additional study from Churg's laboratory involved a cohort consisting of 144 shipyard workers and insulators from the Pacific Northwest. The major residual fiber type in the lungs from these individuals was amosite, and the lung tissue in most cases contained tremolite and chrysotile fibers.[207] Interestingly, the authors reported that "crocidolite fibers were found in only a very few cases, usually in quite small numbers, and have been excluded from all analysis." This indicates that the exposure to the second most commonly used form of "commercial amphibole," crocidolite, was minimal as reflected in the tissue burden of shipyard workers and insulators. The conclusion from the study was that mesothelioma occurred at much lower lung tissue amosite concentration than did asbestosis, which was in contrast to their conclusion for chrysotile-induced mesothelioma.

A study of lung tissue from former asbestos miners and millers from Thetford Mines and Asbestos regions was carried out by Nayebzadeh et al.[208] There were higher concentrations of tremolite asbestos in lung tissues from the Thetford Mines workers compared with workers from the Asbestos region. Fiber burden was categorized in three sizes: (1) those less than 5 μm long, (2) those greater than 5 μm and less than 10 μm long, and (3) those greater than 10 μm long. The conclusion from review of data was that "no consistent and biologically important difference was found for fiber dimension; therefore, fiber dimension does not seem to be a factor that accounts for the difference in incidence of respiratory diseases between the two groups." "The greater incidence of respiratory diseases among workers of Thetford Mines can be explained by the fact that they had greater exposure to fibers than did workers at the Asbestos region. Among the mineral fibers studied, retention of tremolite fibers was most apparent."

Langer and Nolan[209] reviewed lung tissue from 53 asbestos-exposed workers and one person with secondary exposure. They concluded that amosite was the most prevalent fiber, occurring in 74% of the specimens, with amosite always being found in the lungs of insulators and chrysotile found in only 50% of this group. Crocidolite was found in 24% of this group and increased to 40% of the workers with shipyard exposure. Langer and McCaughey[210] reported that the lung tissue from an individual with pleural mesothelioma and a work history of brake repair was found to contain chrysotile structures. Fibrils less than 1 μm and others longer than 5 μm were present. They noted that the findings were consistent with those of Pooley et al.[211] in that long fibrils have been frequently encountered in lung tissues from occupationally exposed workers[210] but not in persons with only environmental exposure. Ten percent of the fibrils were longer than 10 μm.

One early study from our laboratory emphasized the importance in some cases of assessing not only the asbestos body burden when defining past levels of asbestos exposure but also the uncoated asbestos fiber burden.[185] Analysis of lung tissue from 12 former amosite workers showed 10 with over 1000 ferruginous bodies per gram of dry tissue, whereas no ferruginous bodies were detected in the digest of the other two samples. This was an unexpected finding in that amosite can be readily inhaled in a longer form and is often found as the core of asbestos bodies in occupationally exposed individuals. The initial explanation was that individuals had relatively short exposure (0.5 and 3.3 months), although that exposure was known to be in very dusty occupations. Two samples from the individuals' tissue when analyzed by electron microscopy showed 1.2 and 2.1 million fibers per gram of tissue, respectively. Thus, even with the proper length (>8 μm) and considerable numbers of fibers being present in the lung, the individuals' lungs were apparently not efficient in coating the fibers. The importance of combining data for asbestos body content and uncoated asbestos fibers is further supported in the evaluation of an individual from a group of shipyard workers[107] who was not found to have chrysotile in his lung tissue. When tissue from his lymph node and pleural plaque was analyzed by ATEM, there were 21,000,000 chrysotile fibers per gram of dry tissue in the pleural plaque and 5,500,000 chrysotile fibers per gram of dry tissue in the lymph node. This finding suggests the efficiency of chrysotile clearance from lung tissue.

Amosite asbestos was found in lung tissue from 53 of 55 persons with mesothelioma whose tissue was evaluated by ATEM[181], with 39 patients having greater than 200,000 amosite fibers per gram dry weight of tissue. The geometric mean length of the amosite fibers was 13 μm, which contrasted with that found in lung tissue samples from the general population where amosite fibers are usually less than 5 μm. Forty-three percent of patients' lung tissue contained chrysotile asbestos and 40% contained crocidolite asbestos. Tremolite was the most commonly found of the "noncommercial" amphiboles (33 cases), whereas actinolite and anthophyllite were each found in 21 cases. There was no evidence chrysotile was the source of tremolite in that 11 of the patients had both, but 13 persons whose lungs contained tremolite had no detectable chrysotile. These findings contrast with the suggestion of Srebro and Roggli[212] that tremolite is "nearly ubiquitous and represents the most common amphibole fiber in the lungs of urbanites." The link, statistically, could be more easily made for chrysotile accounting for the amosite compared with the relationship of chrysotile to tremolite. Only a small percent of each type of asbestos would have been detected by light microscopy even of longer fibers of asbestos (based on diameter). In our mesothelioma study,[181] 26 of 5 patients did not have pathologic asbestosis, although most had appreciable ferruginous bodies and uncoated fiber burden.

Tissue from another group of mesothelioma cases from various regions in the USA was evaluated for the presence and numbers of ferruginous bodies and uncoated asbestos fibers.[213] The information generated was compared with that in the earlier 55 case study[181] that predominantly consisted of individuals who had either worked in shipyards, related industries, or lived in adjacent areas to shipyard centers. There were 26 cases in this study that had over 1000 ferruginous bodies per gram of dry tissue. The most common form of asbestos found in this group (as in the 55 group study) was amosite (74%), which was less than the 94% positives in the earlier study. The second and third most common forms of asbestos were anthophyllite (61%) and tremolite (52%), whereas the other commercial forms of asbestos—crocidolite and chrysotile—were found in 43% and 50%, respectively.

There are reports that the presence of tremolite in the lungs of miners and millers "probably" reflects high burden in these cohorts[214] and that the tremolite component has been suggested to be an important contributor to the development of asbestos-related diseases in the mining region of Quebec.[200, 215] Thus, much has been made as to the role tremolite has in inducing diseases among miners and millers in Canada.

A consideration of the impact of tremolite as a "contaminate" of chrysotile has been considered by Finkelstein[216]in an evaluation of data regarding chrysotile/amphibole burden in the lung tissue of brake mechanics as reported by Butnor et al.[166] The findings by Butnor et al.[166] essentially reported an appreciable amphibole (commercial amphibole in some cases) component in the lungs from these individuals whose work history was as brake mechanics (with friction products usually being manufactured with a chrysotile component). The assessment by Finkelstein[216] led him to conclude that the levels of tremolite in the lung tissue of brake mechanics could be explained from exposure to "dusts from friction products manufactured from Canadian chrysotile," which as previously noted contains appreciable tremolite (as per the studies of the lungs of chrysotile miners and millers).

Various agencies grapple with the definition of a "cleavage fragment" versus a fibrous form of the same mineral based, in part, on defining a "regulated fiber" under the asbestos regulations. The variations in the definition of a "fiber" is covered in Chapter 2 of this edition. Obviously, a structure may be considered a fiber by one definition and not by the definition of another definition. There are clearly political, legal, and economic issues driving this discussion as clearly described in an article reviewing the chrysotile/tremolite relationship as written by a Canadian researcher, Dr Bruce Case.[217, 218] Ultimately, the question from a health effect perspective becomes not what is regulated but whether it causes disease in man when inhaled. The Canadian experience would strongly argue that the answer regarding tremolite is "yes." In fact, Dr Case[217] stated that the relationship of chrysotile and tremolite in Canadian chrysotile products caused him at one point to favor a compound phrase "chrysotile/tremolite" to describe mined material and the products containing Canadian chrysotile. Dr Case clearly defines the fact that the issue of tremolite fiber versus tremolite "cleavage fragment" is a distinction often defined by the mineralogists or regulators. The implication for all of those without a locked fixation on length, aspect ratio, and diameter of a structure being the predictor for risk of inducing disease overlooks the obvious question posed by Dr Case if the reaction within a cell or a biosystem discriminates that the mineral form is a "cleavage fragment" from reactions with a fiber of the same general dimensions. His point is well taken in questioning if "potentially affected cells can distinguish between *asbestiform* and *nonasbestiform* fibres having equivalent dimensions."[218] In fact, the discussion in the USA has resulted in numerous industries sponsored "studies" or publications over the last several years focusing on the definition of an elongated "nonasbestiform" entity and emphasizing it is not regulated as such under the Asbestos Standard as a "regulated fiber." In addition, an argument is often offered that exposures of cohorts to these "nonregulated" structures are not available for assessment of elevated occurrence of diseases. Realistically, exposure in the USA and in other parts of the world to "cleavage fragments" of minerals and the fibrous forms of the same minerals may occur simultaneously as well as exposures to other mixed dusts in the work place/environment. However, there does seem to be a concurrence in Canada among several researchers that tremolite is a major concern for causation of disease in chrysotile miners and millers, as previously discussed. The emphasis of a study by Williams-Jones et al.[219] described the relationship of chrysotile veins with other fibrous minerals, including tremolite, in the mining areas. They conducted evaluations of the Jeffrey Mine in Asbestos, Quebec, and found the presence of amphibole group minerals: anthophyllite, cummingtonite, hornblende, and tremolite-actinolite. "The bulk of the amphibole, however, was in the form of tremolite and actinolite, and was found mainly in serpentinite adjacent to or included within felsic dykes. Appreciable quantities of amphibole also are present in pyroxenite (tremolite) and slate (actinolite) in contact with serpentinite distal to the ore zones. Significantly, the chrysotile ores are essentially amphibole free. Most of the amphibole is fibrous, but a small proportion is asbestiform according to criteria established by the U.S. Occupational Safety and Health Administration." A study was conducted of elongated mineral particles within chrysotile ore from another Canadian mine (Bell mine-Thetford, Quebec) by Langer and Nolan.[220] The concluded that "tremolite was detected at very low concentrations, by transmission electron microscopy. The morphology of the particles found, and selected area electron diffraction characterization, showed that they were cleavage fragments, not asbestos fibres. If tremolite asbestos is present in the ore, its concentration must be below the detection level." It is not in debate that elongated minerals in the form of cleavage fragments (occasionally in the morphology identical to a given definition of a fiber) can be respirable-sized dust. Therefore, if the exposure to tremolite is attributable to causing some/most/all the diseases in Canadian miners and millers, by this definition the tremolitic respirable dust would be considered by many as mineralogically definable as a nonasbestiform structure or "cleavage fragment." Additionally elongated particles occur in many minerals where they may be defined as a fiber or cleavage fragment based on the definition used in a count/identification scheme. Given that concern, the French Agency for Food, Environmental and Occupational Health and Safety (ANSES)[221] was charged with review of the "Health Effects and Identification of cleavage fragments of amphiboles from quarried minerals." The following conclusions were offered as their assessments:

"In the light of the epidemiological studies, it is not possible to rule out a risk to health linked to exposure to cleavage fragments from the non-asbestiform species of the five regulated amphiboles;

A relationship between the occurrence of cancers and the exposure of populations to some calcic or sodic-calcic amphiboles present in the form of a mixture of different facies, such as fluoro-edenite, winchite or richterite, has been established in recent assessments;

There are currently no validated scientific toxicological data to confirm that cleavage fragments with the dimensional criteria laid down by the WHO for 'fibre' (L>5 μm; D<3 μm and L:D>3:1 are less toxic than their asbestiform counterparts."

We are aware of the presence of tremolite in Canadian chrysotile in our studies simply on the basis of the previously mentioned concept of chrysotile being "contaminated" with tremolite within the mined product and contained as the minerals are processed during the mining/milling activity. However, in a study of 54 cases of mesothelioma from our laboratory,[213] there is more likelihood of tremolite occurring with anthophyllite (20 cases) than with chrysotile. There were 13 cases with both and 14 cases with chrysotile and no detectable tremolite. This is a common finding in all of our studies in that relationships between the finding of chrysotile in tissue with the expectation of finding tremolite do not occur. The common findings in observations within our reported mesothelioma studies[181, 182, 213] are the presence of various amounts of asbestos in most cases and with a composition often of mixed types of asbestos (commercial and noncommercial). Furthermore, there are some cases in these groups with lower levels of tissue burden.

Mesothelioma is a very rare tumor that occurs in men more than women. This has historically (and logically) been attributable to the higher potential for men to work in areas where occupational exposures to asbestos may occur. However, we evaluated tissue samples from a series of mesothelioma cases that occurred in women.[182] Some individuals were exposed to asbestos by secondary exposure via dust being brought home on the clothing of family members. The most commonly found asbestos in tissue from this series of 15 mesothelioma cases in women was amosite, and the second most commonly found fiber type was tremolite.[182] However, with the exception of the upper third of the study group, the tissue burden was much less than that found in the predominantly male study groups. It should be noted that some tissue burdens in the lower group would not in any way be considered as reflective of past definitions for levels of occupationally exposed individuals. The common link in these cases with the larger study groups made up predominantly of men[181, 213] was that the fiber burden was often of mixed types of asbestos. The majority of fibers in all our mesothelioma publications were less than 5 μm in length, but a population of uncoated fibers within the lung samples were longer than 5 μm. The differences in the lung fiber characteristics (fiber type, concentration, and/or populations of longer fibers) in these mesothelioma cases offer a contrast with those same features reported from tissue analysis conducted on samples of tissue from the general population.

It would be helpful if a specific concentration of asbestos tissue burden could be linked to a specific disease. Some individuals have attempted to develop such a "threshold" concept for induction of disease such as mesothelioma. This usually begins with extracting data from a selected cohort, which may or may not equate with expected findings in another cohort. As pointed out by Warnock and Isenberg[222]: "Because large burdens of asbestos do not always cause pulmonary fibrosis, asbestosis may be a poor marker of fiber-related lung cancer." Indeed, in one of our studies, only 29 mesothelioma cases[181] out of 55 showed pathologic asbestosis. Compounding the issue further is that most reasonable people consider that mesothelioma is often a longer latency, lower dose-induced disease. The result historically is that many heavy dose-exposed individuals simply die from another asbestos-induced disease before living long enough after first exposure to develop mesothelioma. Another issue is that no one can define the vulnerability of an individual to a given asbestos exposure. Finally, mesothelioma can occur outside the lung, and little knowledge exists as to the relevance of the populations of fibers left in the lung over time with those that reach the extrapulmonary sites except as a confirmation of past exposure. As will be described in detail in the section on asbestos in extrapulmonary sites, it is evident that unique populations of asbestos fibers reach these sites.[107, 223]

Further compounding the issue of extrapolating the meaning of fiber burden in the lung with events that induce mesothelioma is that at the time a lung sample is obtained, it is reflective of the dust concentration in the tissue at that time and does not indicate the number of fibers, particularly short fibers, that may have been in the lung and cleared via the mucociliary escalator and/or relocated to other sites within the body.[107] The question is why should these cleared fibers not have played a role in tissue response as well as creating the setting for permanent pathological changes to occur before their departure from the lung? This is particularly important relative to chrysotile or amphiboles, where repeated exposures would be expected to stimulate continued inflammatory responses and potential changes that could lead to pathological responses, including neoplasia, even if the clearance of chrysotile (more preferentially inhaled as shorter structures) is considered to occur more rapidly from the lung than do amphiboles.[75] Although smaller asbestos fibers would logically be more readily cleared from the lung, it is sometimes not adequately appreciated as to the effectiveness of the lung clearance for larger structures, including asbestos bodies as found in samples of sputa.[128, 140, 144] These clearly are very large particulates formed on a population of longer inhaled asbestos fibers. However, the question remains whether most chrysotile (or shorter amphiboles which also reach the lower airways in appreciable numbers) could be eliminated from lung tissue over time since first exposure until a lung sample is collected and yet still be present in appreciable numbers in extrapulmonary sites where they had been relocated from the lung and the clearance process is appreciably slower.[56, 107, 223]

3.12 EXPOSURE FROM ASBESTOS/ELONGATED MINERAL PARTICLES AS COMPONENTS OF OTHER MINERALS

There is potential asbestos exposure from products that are made from minerals that contain asbestos. This is often referred to as *contamination*, although contamination may not be the proper word to describe naturally occurring types of asbestos that occurs as a component of these minerals. Although many products are presented/assumed to not contain asbestos, the reality is that miners/millers and consumers have potential asbestos exposures from their use. Vermiculite, mined in Libby, Montana, is an example. This mineral has been distributed to numerous processing facilities in the USA and used in products ranging from garden products (e.g., potting soil components, packing material) to insulation products. As early as 1986, McDonald et al.[224] stated that tremolite in vermiculite could cause asbestos-related diseases. The elemental chemical analysis of individual fibers by energy dispersive spectrometry reportedly yielded "unsuspected and complicated results." They further clarified that the chemistry of "many fibres was compatible with minerals of the tremolite-actinolite series, the sodium content of some was too high to meet the criteria for tremolite according to the classification of the International Mineralogical Association." Wright et al.[225] reported lung burdens of tremolite asbestos from exposure to asbestos-containing vermiculite of over 8,000,000 asbestos fibers per gram of dry lung in a person with brief exposure in a vermiculite expansion plant during a summer job 50 years prior. Sixty-eight percent of the fibers were tremolite asbestos. Compounding the issue further is that there are nonregulated fibrous amphiboles in the vermiculite vein, and debate rages on as to the implications of the role these nonregulated structures have as contributors in inducing disease.

Later mineralogical clarification of the fibrous component of the mined vermiculite indicated only a minor tremolite component (regulated asbestos) with the majority of the fibrous minerals being of the winchite/richerite series (occurring in asbestiform/fibrous habit but not defined presently as one of the six types of fibrous forms of minerals included in the generic term "asbestos."[226] This mixture of fiber types explains the confusion regarding the elemental analysis in the paper by McDonald[224] although the title attributes "tremolite" as the causative agent inducing disease in miners.

In reality, as discussed in the following case report,[227] the predominant fiber type found in tissues from a miner, was not tremolite. The lung sample was submitted to Dr Dodson's a lab from a Libby Vermiculite Miner who was diagnosed with lung cancer.[227] The tissue digest contained very large numbers of ferruginous bodies (150,830 ferruginous bodies/gram deparaffinized wet weight of tissue) (Figure 3.21), with the abundance of "Libby Amphiboles" present that a "stop count limit" of 100 fiber was easily reached. The 100 "Libby amphiboles" were equivalent to 5,377,090 fibers/gram deparaffinized wet weight of tissue. Exposure to the fibrous materials in the "Libby" vermiculite (often defined as "Libby amphibole") induce all of the types of asbestos-related diseases defined as risks following exposure to asbestos.[228]

Another widely used mineral that can contain asbestos is talc. Kanack[229] provides a useful overview of the definition of talc. He noted that there are two general categories of commonly utilized forms of talc. Cosmetic talc is mined from talc deposits targeted due to the desire of providing the "highest" quality of talc based on "purity, smoothness, particle size" and from sources with lower amounts of accessory minerals. Industrial talc was mined with less stringent characteristics than cosmetic talc. This of course does not mean that cosmetic talc mines do not also sell talc for industrial usage. We have had several cases referred to our laboratory where tissue analysis was requested for tissue where two individuals were occupationally exposed industrial talc in the workplace.[230] The referrals advised that the individuals had worked in a ceramic tile manufacturing facility for various length of time and that talc was utilized in the manufacturing process. Examination of the digested tissue revealed the presence of elongated talc fibers/ribbons as well as elevated numbers of noncommercial amphiboles (anthophyllite and tremolite) as well as an occasional transitional fiber (showing features of talc and anthophyllite).

Kleinfeld et al.[231] and Rohl et al.[232] reported that certain talc formations contained tremolite and anthophyllite asbestos. Thus, these asbestos fibers can occur in consumer talc products. Asbestos bodies and fibers have been reported in lung tissue from workers with asbestos-related diseases who worked in New York State talc mines.[233]The fibers in the lungs consisted of fibrous talc, tremolite, and related mineral series. A considerable burden of asbestos fibers and bodies were identified by Scancarello et al.[234] in individuals with respiratory diseases and bilateral pleural plaques after talc inhalation and as found in BAL fluid and tissue samples. These are a few examples where determining asbestos burden in tissue samples can offer potentially important information in settings where exposures occurred to products not thought to contain asbestos.

Roggli et al.[235] examined lung tissue from 312 mesothelioma cases for fiber burden. The majority of cases were reported to have exposure to dust from products containing asbestos. They concluded that "tremolite in lung tissue samples from mesothelioma victims derives from both talc and chrysotile and that tremolite accounts for a considerable fraction of the excess fiber burden in end-users of asbestos products."

Ghio and Roggli[236] expressed concern about risk of utilization of talc (and therefore associated accessory/elongated mineral particles) in pleurodesis. They noted "even is product is 'asbestos-free', the mechanism of cancer induction by asbestos (i.e., metal-catalyzed radical generation) is similarly pertinent to talc and the occurrence of fibrous forms of the sheet silicate itself." They further indicated "simply stating that talc is 'asbestos-free' should not release us from a responsibility to the patient when safe alternatives are available."

Another issue of concern regarding talc is that some deposits of talc contain fibrous talc. A point of confusion arose regarding the classification of talc containing fibrous talc as a carcinogen. IARC (International Agency for Research in Cancer has issued a clarification on that point. [237, 238] "The review of talc in Supplement 7 led to evaluations for two agents: talc containing asbestiform fibres and talc not containing asbestiform fibres. The term 'asbestiform fibre' has been mistaken as a synonym for 'asbestos fibre' when it should be understood to mean any mineral, including talc, when it grows in an asbestiform habit. To avoid confusion over the term 'asbestiform fibre', the present Working Group decided that it is scientifically more precise to call the agent 'talc not containing asbestos or asbestiform fibres', and this evaluation supersedes the earlier review of talc not containing asbestiform fibres. The present Working Group also decided to expand the name of the Group-1 agent from 'talc containing asbestiform fibres' to 'talc containing asbestos or other asbestiform fibres'. The present Working Group reviewed the earlier Monograph on talc containing asbestiform fibres and determined that the expanded name is consistent with what had been evaluated in Supplement 7. No update was undertaken for this Group-1 agent."

The fact is that talc may contain asbestiform structures (asbestos and/or talc fibers). Kelse and associates[239] reviewed the issue of asbestiform structures as part of an assessment of pneumoconiosis in an industrial talc mining population. In the context of elongated mineral content of the talc. They stated that "the more common pure talc fiber often visually resembles asbestos and is therefore correctly described as asbestiform in appearance." They further referenced that "talc fibers exhibit fiber bundling and dimensions closer to those of amphibole asbestos." Little is often available from clinical histories of mesothelioma/cancer patients (particularly females suffering from mesothelioma or ovarian cancer) if there had been use of cosmetic talc or in some situations had past exposure to industrial talc. The author within the last year asked several outstanding asbestos researchers and/or epidemiologists if cohorts within their studies and presumed exposed to asbestos, were asked if they had used and/or knew if they had been exposed to talc. None of these experts nor the author of this chapter had asked about that potential exposure to talc in the past. We are not aware of tissue burden analysis in the past where ATEM had been used to define the presence of talc in tissue from individuals with "asbestos-related diseases." Our previous study of lung samples from the general population of East Texas evaluated the fiber burden as to type and numbers of uncoated fibers.[157] In that study 6.9% of the non-asbestos fibrous component were MgSi (the elemental composition of talc) and thus having the elemental potential to be talc fibers. This study did not include the composition of the nonfibrous particulates (talc is predominantly found in a platy form). While it offers nothing quantitative data, an attempt was made several years ago to review some of the raw data for the paper and it was found that the limited numbers of talc fibers were present in individuals with the highest levels of anthophyllite and/or tremolite.

Fibrous zeolites (erionite) known to cause mesothelioma in Turkey[161] occur in certain regions of the USA; however, these are mostly in areas with low population density. Recently, Kliment et al.[240] reported a mesothelioma case with appreciable erionite content in the lung tissue. The work history in the case indicated an approximate 2-year history of possible exposure to dust from floor tiles while working in "janitorial and maintenance services." The individual lived for 20–25 years in Mexico. There were no specific erionite exposures defined, although the implication is that the individual's exposure may have been from environmental sources in previous residencies, including in Mexico where erionite had been reported to be part of the environment. There were no specific exposures to erionite originally defined. The findings in this case included plaques and abundance of ferruginous bodies within lung tissue. The digested material contained elevated levels of ferruginous bodies and uncoated erionite structures. There were no "commercial or noncommercial" asbestos fibers reportedly found in the tissue. A case was referred to our laboratory for tissue burden analysis in which his history included working as a welder and with friction products. As with the report by Kliment et al.[240], subsequent assessment of background revealed he had raised in Mexico on a family farm until he left at approximately 18 years of age. The area in Mexico was defined as having erionite present in the environment. Our evaluation indicated the predominate fiber present in the tissue sample was erionite (Figure 3.22), however, we also found a commercial amphibole and all three of the types of noncommercial amphiboles (tremolite, actinolite, anthophyllite) in the tissue digestate.

3.13 ASBESTOS/ELONGATED MINERAL PARTICLES IN EXTRAPULMONARY SITES

The majority of the world's literature regarding asbestos in extrapulmonary sites is based on observations of a few asbestos bodies seen by light microscopy. These sites include the stomach,[241]the liver,[242] the kidney,[103, 242] the spleen,[103, 106, 242] the lymph nodes,[54, 103, 104] and the pleural plaques.[243] The limited occurrence of such observations in pleural samples was noted in 1988 by Churg.[244] His conclusions were that "as a rule asbestos bodies are not seen in pleural plaques, although Rosen et al.[243] claim to have extracted a few bodies in some cases. As mentioned earlier, the asbestos content of plaques and pleurae appears to be quite different from that of the lung, and these sites are not useful for mineral analysis."[244] With respect to asbestos bodies, Dr Churg and our laboratory are in agreement in that we are yet to find an asbestos body in digests of pleural plaques or parietal pleural (fibrotic) tissue. However, the presence of uncoated asbestos fibers in extrapulmonary sites, including pleura, is an important indicator of asbestos translocating from other sites. One cancer of greatest concern from exposure to asbestos is mesothelioma. This is a rare cancer of the serosal membranes of the body and is considered a marker of asbestos disease. Knudson[245] stated that "in the absence of asbestos, mesothelioma is so rare that it might never be studied."

Inhalation of asbestos can result in the occurrence of pathological responses in sites considerably removed from the lung (the original site of deposition).[109] Particulates can relocate through the lymphatic system to hilar lymph nodes and to more distant lymph nodes.[2] Schlesinger[61] described lymph nodes as "reservoirs of retained material." Gross and Detreville[8] stated that lymph nodes were "repositories for dust," and in heavy dust, exposures over time become "densely mineralized and stony hard." In cases of more toxic dust such as silica, lymph nodes may show necrosis, fibrosis, and calcification.[55] For those familiar with anatomy texts, a visit to Netter's[59] illustrated version of the respiratory system provides a refresher of not only the anatomy of the lymphatic drainage system in the chest cavity but also the designation as to which node drains what level of the lung. As proposed by Becklake[62]and Hillerdal,[63] the lymphatic route offers a mechanism for relocation of asbestos from the lung to other parts of the body. Knudson[245] stated that the "transport of the fibers to these surfaces (pleural and peritoneal) can lead to mesothelial proliferation, and after many years, to malignant mesotheliomas." Confirmation of relocation to extrapulmonary sites requires the application of the ATEM for identification of the type and size of asbestos fibers that reach extrapulmonary tissues.

A study in our laboratory was conducted to determine the content of lung and peritracheal lymph node tissue in 21 individuals who also conformed to the definition of general population.[246] Two lymph nodes were positive for at least one ferruginous body. There were no asbestos fibers detected in lymph nodes from eight cases. Five cases with asbestos fibers in lung tissue were not determined to have asbestos in lymph nodes. Nine cases had detectable levels of asbestos in lung and lymph nodes. The most common type of asbestos found in the lymph nodes was anthophyllite (nine cases), with the second most common type being tremolite (six cases). The composition of the asbestos burden (when present) from lymph nodes when compared with findings from samples of lung parenchyma from the general population is the predominance reflective of past exposures to short fibers (<5 µm) of noncommercial amphiboles or chrysotile (if asbestos fibers are detected at all).

Another publication from our laboratory further defines the analytical characterization of the asbestos burden in lung tissue versus the levels of lymph nodes that drain the lung.[56] The individuals had documented exposures to asbestos and died from various asbestos-related diseases. The article reviews the data regarding lymph drainage from the lung as well as experimental studies in animal models that have assessed particulate relocation. For purposes of brevity, only a few significant points will be made from the findings. The lymph nodes have some population of ferruginous bodies but not as elevated as in lung tissue. This is similar to findings in our earlier comparative study of lung burden with composition of lymph node and pleural plaques.[107] The asbestos types found in lymph nodes are consistent with types found in the lung; however, as in the study,[107] the fiber size found in lymph nodes is appreciably shorter than those found in lung. Most fibers found in lymph nodes are a mixture of commercial and noncommercial amphiboles just as in lung tissue. The attempt to quantify the fiber numbers by light microscopy would be worthless because the vast majority would not be "seen" or counted in phase-contrast microscopy. The vast majority of fibers in all sites were <5 µm in length. ATEM is required to both detect and correctly analyze fiber burden in this study.

One of the first quantitative studies evaluating fiber burden in extrapulmonary sites and using ATEM was carried out by Sebastien et al.[223] He and his associates analyzed fiber content of lung samples and parietal pleural tissue from 29 cases sent to them for confirmation of diagnosis. The majority of patients had histories of asbestos exposure. In the study, 16 of 29 samples of parietal pleural tissue contained asbestos (within the detection limit of the study) and 27 lung tissue samples were positive. The pleural samples identified to have asbestos in them contained "almost all chrysotile." The reason light microscopic evaluation of extrapulmonary sites for asbestos is usually negative is evident by fiber size as reported by Sebastien et al.[223] The mean length of fiber in the lung was µm, whereas the average length in the pleura was 2.3 µm. These asbestos fibers were not long enough to trigger asbestos body formation. Likewise, an assessment by light microscopy would not detect short or longer/thinner asbestos fibers from these tissues.

In the study carried out by Dodson et al.[107] on samples of lung tissue, lymph nodes, and pleural plaques obtained from eight former shipyard workers from Italy, no asbestos bodies were found in the pleural plaques, whereas all but one sample of lymph node contained asbestos bodies. This suggests a relocation of mature bodies from the lungs to the lymph nodes, a selective segregation on the basis of the size of fibers that reach the two sites (a predictor of asbestos body formation), or differences in coating efficiency between these extrapulmonary sites. However, the population of longer fibers suitable for stimulation of coating in the lymph nodes constitutes a fraction of the total population when compared with the percent of longer fibers in total burden in lung tissue.

Amphiboles and chrysotile fibers were found at various concentrations in different sites with total concentrations often ranging into the millions of fibers per gram of dry tissue. The average length of chrysotile and amphibole asbestos fibers found in the lung was longer than lengths for the same type of fibers found in the lymph node and pleural plaques. Fibers in all three sites were represented by a majority that were less than 5 µm long with only 4% of the chrysotile in the lung being <10 µm and no chrysotile fiber >10 µm being detected in pleural plaques and lymph nodes. The amphibole content consisted of 80% being less than 10 µm in the lung with only 8% of the fibers in the pleural plaques and 2.5% in the lymph nodes being >10 µm. The importance of including short fibers in a count scheme is illustrated in one individual. The lung tissue from this individual was not determined to have chrysotile (within the limits of detectability). Thus, if this parameter alone was used, one could extrapolate this to mean no or low exposure. However, the pleural plaque tissue contained 21,000,000 fibers of chrysotile per gram of dry tissue and lymph node contained 5,500,000 fibers of chrysotile per gram of dry tissue. If only fibers longer than 5 μm were counted, only 3.1% of the total chrysotile from the plaques of this individual and none in the lymph nodes would have been counted (given sufficient magnification had been used to "see" the thin fibers). These findings indicated a past exposure to chrysotile and emphasized the lung's capability to clear short fibers after cessation of exposure, whereas extrapulmonary sites have less efficient mechanisms to rid their tissue of asbestos.

Suzuki and Yuen[247–248] and Suzuki,Yuen and Ashley [249]analyzed asbestos content in lung and mesothelial tissue from individuals with mesothelioma. Using ATEM, Suzuki and Yuen[247–249] found that the majority of fibers in the lung and the mesothelial tumor tissue were less than 5 μm in length. They also found that the majority of short fibers were chrysotile. Only 4% of fibers fit the Stanton model for a more "pathogenically active" population of fiber (>8 μm long and thinner than 0.25 μm in diameter).[247] They concluded that the majority of fibers in both lung and mesothelial tissues were <5 μm. A comparison made between the average length of asbestos fibers found in pleural tissue in studies by Sebastien et al.[223]and Dodson et al.[107] with those reported by Suzuki and Yuen [247–249] shows a striking similarity in that the fibers are very short. Suzuki et al. [249] evaluated lung and mesothelial tissues from 168 cases of human malignant mesothelioma. Their conclusions were as follows: "(1) long, thin asbestos fibers consistent with the Stanton hypothesis comprised only 2.3% of total fibers (247/10,575) in these tissues; (2) the majority (89.4%) of the fibers in the tissues examined were shorter than or equal to 5 μm in length (9,454 of 10,575), and generally (92.7%) smaller than or equal to 0.25 μm in width (9,808 of 10,575); and (3) among the asbestos types detected in the lung and mesothelial tissues, chrysotile was the most common asbestos type to be categorized as short, thin asbestos fibers." They concluded that "contrary to the Stanton hypothesis, short, thin, asbestos fibers appear to contribute to the causation of human malignant mesothelioma."

The finding of short fibers as the primary component of lymph nodes that drain the lung and in pleural tissue does not bode well for the arguments supporting the "amphibole hypothesis"[250] for explaining most asbestos-induced diseases in extrapulmonary sites. The "amphibole hypothesis" is based, in part, on longer fibers being more pathogenically active (see discussion in section on fiber length and disease), and this, of course, skews risk for causation of cancer toward amphibole fibers, in part, because they are inhaled as longer fibers in the lung (because they tend to be straight) and thus are less readily cleared compared with the shorter chrysotile component that is found in lung tissue. There are some reasonable explanations that seem to support a greater potential for molecular interactions within tissue from interactions with amphiboles than chrysotile fibers. However, there are other models that indicate chrysotile is more reactive.[251] This subject will be covered in detail in the section on molecular biology-induced reactions with asbestos fibers.

It is obvious that the findings of predominantly shorter asbestos in extrapulmonary sites leaves the "chrysophiles"[250] scrambling to explain how the predominate numbers of shorter asbestos fibers in extrapulmonary sites are noncontributors to carcinogenicity or to development of other asbestos-related changes in these sites.

It appeared initially that an excellent study by Boutin et al.[252] had uniquely linked the presence of amphiboles with concentrations of such fibers in areas within the parietal pleura in individuals apparently exposed to aerosols likely containing fossil fuel soot (coal dust). Apparently, the concept of finding black spots in the parietal pleura is rare in the USA (personal communication of Samuel Hammar, MD, who has been involved with thousands of autopsies). In such cases, areas within the parietal pleura contain parietal anthracosis described within "lymphatic vessels of the parietal pleura" and in this study are dubbed "black spots." The authors devised a study in which they looked at fiber burden content in lung and pleural tissue in 14 individuals. Eight individuals had defined asbestos exposure, and six were without defined asbestos exposure. In most subjects exposed to asbestos, "fiber concentrations in the lung and anthracotic pleural samples were $>1 \times 10^6$ fiber per gram, whereas there were practically no fibers in nonanthracotic pleural samples. In 5 of 11 patients, including all three mesothelioma patients, the concentration of fibers was even higher in black spots than in lung samples."

The conclusions from the study included the following: (1) fiber distribution is heterogeneous in the parietal pleura, (2) the fibers concentrate in black spots in high concentrations, and (3) this could explain why parietal pleura is the target organ for mesothelioma and plaques. The following is offered in able to better appreciate the findings that led to each of the conclusions and the issues to consider regarding their findings:

1. If asbestos is relocated from the lung tissue via the lymphatic drainage—which we have analytically confirmed,[56, 107] then it is reasonable that the dust particles, including asbestos particles, could concentrate in the lymphatic-rich areas of the pleura.
2. The concentration of asbestos fibers in plaque areas has been previously shown[107, 223, 252253254] however, most of the fibers in these studies have found chrysotile to often be the prevalent asbestos type, which is in contrast with the findings of amphiboles only as in the study by Boutin et al.[252]

There are several interesting points regarding the study of Boutin et al.[252] that are sometimes over-interpreted as to significance. The first is that the study showed long amphiboles reached the parietal pleural where mesotheliomas develop. This observation is not unique and should be reviewed on the basis of two important findings in the report. First, 99% of the asbestos fibers in the lung were amphiboles, 95% were amphiboles in pleural black spots, and 61% were in non-anthracotic pleura. Thus, if one essentially has only amphiboles in the lung, then that constitutes the asbestos that is available to be translocated to extrapulmonary sites. Second, the issue of fiber length with the emphasis occasionally placed that "longer fibers of amphiboles reach the pleura" can be correct. However, what they said in detail was that in the "black spots" 22.5% of the fibers were 5 μm or longer and 10% were 8 μm or longer. These observations compare with LeBouffant's[253] report, where 7% of the amosite and 5% of the chrysotile in the parietal pleura were 5 μm or longer. Sebastien et al.[223] reported that 24% of the amphibole fibers and 14% of the chrysotile in the parietal pleura exceeded 4 μm in length. In our own study,[107] 10% of the amphiboles and 3.1% of the chrysotile were >5 μm. Thus, the findings in the study by Boutin et al.[252] appear to have shown the same as the previously stated studies in that the vast majority (in their study 77.5%) of the asbestos fibers (in their case amphiboles) in the pleura and in their cases within pleural "black spots" are <5 μm. The authors also offered a sound scientific explanation as to a potential reason that chrysotile was not detected stating: "from a technical point of view, short and thin chrysotile fibers could be less easily detected among a 'background' of particulates in anthracotic samples." For a review of this issue, the reader is referred to the section on tissue preparation and instrument selection previously discussed in this chapter.

3. The question of the anatomical concentration of asbestos in the "black spots" as defining regions with the potential for the development of mesothelioma and pleural plaques has been the subject of several additional European studies. Müller et al.[255] conducted a morphological evaluation of 12 "black spots" (four surgical and eight autopsy specimens) located in the parietal pleura. They concluded that "there were hints for an increased proliferation of mesothelial cells in some areas with black spots," but "our findings do not support the classification of black spots as an obligate early lesion in the development of malignant mesothelioma." They further stated, "our results do not support the hypothesis whereby mesotheliomas develop 'preferentially' in the regions of preexisting black spots. In our collective of former miners of the Ruhr area we do not find asbestos fibers especially amphibole fibers directly located in black spots. But we found silicates, quartz and silicone as well as aluminum-rich minerals such as muscovite. There were no hints that black spots play a possible role in the development of mesotheliomas."

Mitchev et al.[256] evaluated the macroscopic appearance of "black spots" and possible relationships with pleural plaques in 150 consecutive necropsies of urban dwellers. Black spots were observed in 92.7% of cases and were noted mainly in the lower costal and diaphragmatic zones. They reported "there was no relationship between the predominant locations of black spots and hyaline pleural plaques."

In summation, samples of the parietal pleura (specifically plaques) have been reported to contain asbestos fibers in occupationally exposed individuals. A majority of these fibers are less than 5 μm in length and in most cases can only be detected at higher magnification by ATEM. Data derived from any other technical assessment of these tissues should be viewed with caution.

A theoretical review as to how fibers reach the extrapulmonary sites from the lung (site of original deposition) has been offered by Miserocchi et al.[257] Their discussion involves the mechanisms that permit inhaled fibers to pass the alveolar barrier. The proposed concepts include a "paracellular route down a mass water flow due to combined osmotic (active Na+ absorption) and hydraulic (interstitial pressure is subatmospheric) pressure gradient. Fibers can be dragged from the lung interstitium by pulmonary lymph flow (primary translocation) wherefrom they can reach the bloodstream and subsequently distribute to the whole body (secondary translocation)." Their conclusions regarding fiber size and as related to the likelihood for fiber relocation from the lung to extrapulmonary sites creates problems for the "longer fibers cause mesothelioma" concept. They do, however, reflect favorably on the actual findings regarding fiber size and relocation to extrapulmonary sites as previously described. Their specific point is that "ultrafine fibers (length <5 μm, diameter <0.25 μm) can travel larger distances due to low steric hindrance (in mesothelioma about 90% of fibers are ultrafine)."

Approximately 10–15% of mesotheliomas occur in the peritoneal cavity. Recent investigations by Hasanoglu et al.[258]studied the effects of orally ingested asbestos in the lungs and pleura in a rat model. "Histopathological evaluation of lungs and pleura of rats after 6 months revealed significant mesothelial proliferation and asbestos bodies." They further suggested that the ingested asbestos traveled from the gastrointestinal system to the lungs, "likely via a lymphohematological route, leading to mesothelioma proliferation, which may lead to malignancies." Although this is an animal study, the observation is of importance in that the serosal tissues that give rise to peritoneal mesothelioma may receive fibers from the lymphatic drainage from the lungs to lymph system and/or be subjected to delivery of fibers that relocate from inside the gastrointestinal tract. Little is known about what population of asbestos fibers reach the parietal pleura and less regarding the composition of the fiber burden reaching the components of the peritoneal cavity.

Dodson et al.[104] conducted an analytical analysis of lung tissue, omentum, and mesentery (fatty lining tissue in the peritoneal cavity) from 20 mesothelioma cases. Asbestos bodies were found in lung tissue of 18 individuals and in five mesentery and two omentum samples. Uncoated asbestos fibers were found in lung tissue of 19 individuals with 17 individuals having fibers in at least one extrapulmonary site. Ten individuals had over 1.4 million asbestos fibers per gram of dry lung. Fourteen individuals had uncoated asbestos fibers in mesentery and omentum samples. The most common type of asbestos fiber found in omentum and mesentery was amosite, which was also the most prevalent asbestos fiber type found in lung tissue. The second most commonly found form of asbestos in the two sample sites was chrysotile. The fiber type and the concentration in the lung tissue were similar to that found in 55 mesothelioma cases reported in 1997[181] with regard to there being a mixture of asbestos types. Different asbestos fiber types were seen in omentum/mesentery in several individuals. The most common was amosite (consistent with the lung tissue); however, chrysotile was the second most common. Predictors from lung data for fiber presence in omentum and mesentery statistically included asbestos body concentration, amphibole concentration, fiber length, and aspect ratio. Obviously, this study showed asbestos fibers reached the peritoneal cavity in humans where peritoneal mesotheliomas develop.

A comparative study[158] of lung, mesentery, and omental tissue was conducted in tissue from 15 individuals who conformed to the definition of members of the general population (as used in our laboratory)[157] Four lung samples contained asbestos bodies, and two lung samples contained at least one asbestos fiber. The only asbestos fiber found in extrapulmonary sites consisted of one short chrysotile fiber (<3 μm) and one short tremolite fiber (<4 μm) in two samples of omentum.[158]

Monchaux et al.[259]found that translocation of fibers including UICC chrysotile A, UICC crocidolite, and JM 104 glass fibers occurred to various sites after intrapleural injection into rats. Ninety-day postexposure fibers were found in mediastinal lymph nodes, lung parenchyma, spleen, liver, kidneys, and brain. The concentration of fibers per gram of tissue was reported to be in the same range for all sites except in the thoracic lymph nodes where the concentration was reported as 10 to 100× greater. Interestingly, the findings included the observation that the "mean length of fibres observed in lung parenchyma increased with time." "After 210 days, the mean length of all three types of fibres was higher than the initial length; and after 380 days, the mean length of the fibres, and especially chrysotile fibres, was considerably higher than that of the injected fibres." The question was raised from the data as to whether the "hypothesis formulated by Lauweryns and Baert[260] that particles are removed from the pulmonary interstitium via the blood capillaries and the pulmonary lymphatics is correct, (thus) it can be assumed that only short fibres are cleared in this way, whereas long fibres are entrapped within the alveolar walls." Obviously, the findings from our studies support the concept that shorter fibers are the form that are most likely to reach extrapulmonary sites (see section on fiber burden in lymph nodes as well as section on fiber length and pathogenicity).

Uibu et al.[261] evaluated the asbestos fiber burden in para-aortic and mesenteric lymph nodes with that in lung tissue from 22 persons who underwent medicolegal autopsy. The individuals were suspected of having an asbestos-related cause of death. The findings indicated that some fibers >20 μm were found in lymph nodes, which they interpreted to mean that "macrophage migration is not the main transport mechanism for long asbestos fibers." They added "that asbestos fibers reach the parietal pleura with the fluid absorbed from the pleural space and pass along the lymph vessels into the subdiaphragmatic region. Depending on anatomical variations, some fibers accumulate in the PA (para-aortic lymph nodes) and other subdiaphragmatic lymph nodes and some are drained into the thoracic duct and venous systemic circulation." This would imply that macrophage "transport" requires the fiber be phagocytized within the macrophage. However, anyone who has evaluated samples of sputa would appreciate that multiple macrophages are associated with most ferruginous bodies cleared via the mucociliary route. Therefore, these structures are not within a macrophage but are being cleared with attached macrophages. If this association enhances clearance rate at least via the mucociliary escalatory or not remains an open question, but the fact that a directional flow occurs without the bodies being "internalized" within macrophages is factually correct. The authors further concluded that "even low-level occupational exposure results in the presence of crocidolite, amosite, anthophyllite, tremolite, or chrysotile in these abdominal lymph nodes. Our results support the hypothesis of lymph drainage as an important translocation mechanism for asbestos in the human body."

3.14 FIBER LENGTHS AND THE RELATIONSHIP TO PATHOGENICITY

The discussion regarding fiber lengths and their relationships to pathogenicity have evolved into scientific discussions involving differences in opinions on one hand and polarized camps suggestive of representing vested interests on the other. The issue has evolved based in large part on the issue of fiber length versus pathogenicity. To be more specific, the focus of the discussion is often stimulated by economic/legal issues involving chrysotile. This is not a trivial issue because chrysotile was used in over 90+ percent of commercial asbestos products in the USA. The facts already described include the likelihood of chrysotile being aerosolized as a short and/or thin fiber that is not detectable by light microscopy (as acknowledged in the federal regulations), and furthermore, these are the exact size of chrysotile fibers that are found in human tissue. The often intense legal/political arena on the subject has varying levels of positioning. One approach is to simply disavow that chrysotile is harmful. Because most national and international health agencies take a different position, this is not usually a successful approach. Another approach is to simply use the phase-contrast optical microscope (PCOM) to evaluate air samples with the full knowledge that chrysotile fibrils cannot be detected by phase-contrast microscopy,[67] so if the fibers cannot be seen, that portion of the aerosol certainly cannot be used to assess exposure levels.[84] The other strategy is to use an electron microscope with a count scheme (low magnification) that excludes short fibers (<5 μm) or long, thin fibers that are too thin to see at low magnification. In either case, the result is a conclusion that if the chrysotile is not seen it cannot be there. The other extreme is one in which a concept is offered that one fiber can cause cancer. This one is a total nonwinner for both sides. The issues used by the various players—defense and plaintiffs in the legal field—have been discussed in detail by Tweedle and McCullock.[250] The purpose of the following section will be to simply provide the reader with facts concerning what is known about fibers on the basis of their length as it influences counting schemes and as they interact with tissue. With this information, the reader is encouraged to formulate their own opinions as they read future articles. Thus, the intent is to provide the reader with the tools to ask the right questions in an attempt to determine the validity/completeness of the reported observations.

Aerosolized asbestos fibers assessed in the workplace are often counted via reproducible counting schemes by use of phase-contrast light microscopy. This system is based on the definition of a "regulated fiber," which physically is sufficiently thick to be observed by light microscopy under the designated magnification. The count scheme includes fibers that are 5 μm or longer and the instrument cannot distinguish fiber type. This selection criterion was established to permit reproducibility between analysts and provides an inexpensive mode for determining the numbers of fibers in air sampled over a period of time and a certain volume of air. This formed the basis of the terms "action level," "permissible exposure limits," and "excursion levels," which have been used to establish levels of exposure for workers in asbestos-containing environments as defined by OSHA and/or EPA work practices. It is recommended that the reader review the discussion in OSHA regulations regarding the evolving reduction of the PEL over time. The objective of reducing the PEL was an attempt (which when compliance is met in the workplace) to reduce the potential occurrence of asbestosis (a heavy dose, exposure disease). As Langer et al.[73] noted, the light microscopy counting guidelines define the physical definition of a fiber to be included in a count, the aspect ratio for fibers to be included, and the definition of asbestos bundles and other structures as applicable to the count scheme. These selection criteria were based on "practicality and theoretical considerations" rather than having a target of a "more toxic" population of fibers. As already stated from our studies, it is evident that the predominance of asbestos fibers in tissue consist of short or longer/thin fibers that cannot be readily detected with the light microscope, just as in air samples.[65] These shorter fibers can be phagocytized within a cell such as shown in Figure 3.23 and/or can relocate to extrapulmonary sites.

What therefore is the scientific basis that long fibers are more likely to cause disease than short fibers? Simple logic indicates inhalation of longer fibers would result in less likelihood of rapid elimination via lung clearance mechanisms than an equivalent number of inhaled shorter fibers. However, it is unlikely that only long fibers are in the breathing zone; thus, there is a mixture of fiber sizes. There are unique occupational settings where the short fiber grades/types of chrysotile are used, and in these there are few fibers greater than 5 μm.

Many of the most important experimental studies regarding the inherent pathogenicity of fibrous particles on the basis of their morphology were conducted by Stanton et al.[262, 263] in the USA and by Professor Fredrick Pott et al.[264–267] in Germany. The Stanton team used pleural implants of gelatin containing the fibers of interest, whereas the Pott team concentrated most of their studies using intraperitoneal exposures. Both the Stanton group and the Pott group chose models where the dust of interest could be placed directly into the target zone for determination of the level of response. Either technique permitted appreciable fibrous dusts to be given in the models. These animal exposures bypass the physiological route of fiber entry into these sites within the body because the lung and thus the previously described primary body defense systems in the respiratory system are a non-factor. It is evident from our studies and others that a shorter population of fibers reach the extrapulmonary sites as compared with the burden in the lung. Thus, the concern for disease induction in the lung that has excellent clearance mechanisms may have variables for induction of asbestos-related changes that are somewhat different on the basis of fiber characterizations than those for induction of changes in extrapulmonary sites.

However, the concept of fiber length and potential for causation of disease is often referenced in the USA on the basis of the innovative studies by Stanton et al.[262, 263] The conclusions from his work using pleural implants in rats was that "the carcinogenicity of fibers depend on dimension and durability rather than on physicochemical properties."[263] As is evident from the chapter on the molecular mechanisms of asbestos-induced disease, the concept of physically based explanation of the pathogenicity of a fiber is only one factor that can induce pathogenic responses. The quote often attributed to Stanton's[263] observation is "the probability of pleural sarcoma correlated best with numbers of fibers that measured 0.25 µm or less in diameter and more than 8 µm in length." An advocacy that only long fibers induce cancer selects these dimensions as "Stanton Fibers." However, the sentence actually continued with the statement "but relative high correlations were noted with fibers in other size categories having diameters up to 1.5 µm and lengths greater than 4 µm."

Occasionally, the comparison of the population of fibers conforming to a "Stanton Fiber" is given for a particular analysis of tissue (for reference, the defined dimension of a "Stanton Fiber" is often included). In our own papers, the comparison is made with the full appreciation that the Stanton et al.[262, 263] measurements were far from absolute as typified by the following quote taken from Stanton's article: "Of special interest are the data on the amphibole asbestoses: amosite, tremolite, and crocidolite, although estimates of the dimensions of the asbestoses are especially liable to error."[263]

A dimension of a "Stanton Fiber" would seem to have particular importance in a discussion of the reduced relative potential of a chrysotile fiber to induce disease because most fibers of this type found in tissue are shorter than 8 µm. The "Stanton Fiber" is therefore freely used in discussions regarding the potential of this type of asbestos as a "lesser" causal agent of cancer when compared with amphiboles. However, specific data supporting a position that there is a lack of carcinogenicity of chrysotile are lacking when the argument is based on the specifics of the study by Stanton et al.[260, 261] in that they did not use chrysotile as one of the tested fibers. The exact statement is[263] "chrysotile, although as carcinogenic as amphiboles at comparable dimensions, could not be included since it has proved difficult to be measured with any degree of precision." Obviously, this statement is not a good reference if one desires to present an argument that chrysotile is less carcinogenic than amphiboles.

The second series of studies on fiber length as related to pathogenicity was carried out by Pott et al.[264–267] Various sizes of fibrous dusts were injected intraperitoneally into rats to assess their tumorigenicity. Pott reported that asbestos fibers shorter than 10 µm in length could produce tumors.[267] In one experiment, milled "chrysotile A" consisting of 99.8% of fibers being less than 5 µm (few longer than 10 µm) produced tumors in 30% of the animals. They further noted that there were "few fibers less than 10µm in length" in the preparation and that they "did not believe that carcinogenic effect can be limited to fibers with a diameter less than 0.5µm."[267]

Aust and colleagues[268] presented an overview of various aspects by which elongated particulates can induce pathological changes in tissue. A more recent publication from one of the authors[76] reviewed the toxicity potency for a model using elongated particulates and compared the data with the so-called "Stanton Fibers"[262, 263] and determined a more important factor for pathogenicity was total surface area not exclusively a factor based on length of a tested population of fiber.

Fraire et al.[269] conducted a study to assess the cytopathological changes, if any, induced by the injection of short fiberglass (mean length of 2.2 µm and width of 0.15 µm) intrapleurally into rats. The histological changes, as graded by several pulmonary pathologists, included chronic inflammation, fibrosis, foreign body reaction, and more advanced proliferative/neoplastic changes of mesothelial hyperplasia and dysplasia. Surprisingly, the short fiber preparation resulted in mature mesotheliomas in three of 25 rats.

Goodglick and Kane[270]assessed the reactivity of long and short crocidolite asbestos fibers in an in vitro and in vivo experimental model. They found "both long and short crocidolite asbestos fibers were toxic to elicited macrophages in vitro. Similar to native crocidolite asbestos, long and short fibers stimulated the release of reactive oxygen metabolites from elicited macrophages in vitro." "In vivo, a single i.p. injection of long crocidolite fibers stimulates an intense inflammatory reaction, release of reactive oxygen metabolites near sites of fiber deposition, and cell death. In contrast, these events were minimal after a single injection of short fibers due to the removal of fibers from the peritoneal cavity. After five daily injections of short fibers, however, fibers were present on the surface of the mesothelium and provoked an inflammatory response. Cell death was observed on the surface of the mesothelium. Reactive oxygen metabolites were also produced near accumulations of short fibers." Their conclusions suggested "that both long and short crocidolite asbestos fibers are toxic to macrophages in vitro via an oxidant and iron-dependent mechanism. In vivo, short fibers are cytotoxic when the clearance of these fibers is prevented." This study illustrates the significance of considering the impact of cumulative exposures, which are the exposure scenarios that occur with most humans. Likewise, these determinations of intensity of the response are not simply defined by the physical features of a fiber.

Attempts have been made to extrapolate from tissue burden and animal studies the risk for developing specific asbestos-related diseases in humans. Lippmann[271]concluded that asbestosis was most correlated with the number of fibers longer than 2 μm and thicker than 0.15 μm, mesothelioma to the number of fibers longer than "about" 5 μm and thinner than "about" 0.1 μm, and lung cancer to the number of fibers longer than "about" 10 μm and thicker than "about" 0.15 μm. Churg and Vedal[207] concluded from tissue analysis of individuals heavily exposed to amosite and chrysotile that "except for pleural plaques, the association of fiber size and disease remains uncertain." They further concluded that "mesotheliomas are not associated with long fibers and in fact are probably associated with lower-aspect-ratio fibers than found in subjects without asbestos-related disease."

McDonald et al.[205] conducted fiber burden analysis in a series of individuals with mesothelioma who were 50 years or younger at time of diagnosis. They concluded that "shorter fibers were more abundant than longer fibers, and high concentrations of all fiber lengths tended to occur together." "Short, medium, and long fibers (of amphiboles) were all associated with mesothelioma risk: those longer than 10 μm had the greatest increment in risk per fiber, followed by medium [6–10 μm] and then by short [<6 μm]." Nayebzadeh et al.[208] observed that respiratory disease in a group of former Quebec chrysotile miners and millers was not related to fiber dimension but to the fiber burden in the tissue, a conclusion that we believe is more universally correct and has general applicability.

Some asbestos-induced changes in humans may be similar to changes induced by other causes. However, the disease that is specifically considered as a unique "asbestos marker disease" is mesothelioma. This tumor often occurs after a longer latency period from first exposure than other asbestos-induced diseases and can occur in individuals with lower level of exposures (such as secondary). The development of mesothelioma as related to asbestos exposure is best summarized in the following statement from Robinson et al.:[272] "Mesothelioma owes its entire existence as a disease entity to its relation with asbestos." Chen et al.[273] noted that "mesothelioma is a rare fatal neoplasm that originates from cells lining the serosal cavities." They indicate that 90–95% arise in the pleural cavity and 5–10% in the peritoneal cavity. They stated that Hammar[274] noted that the tumor has been reported rarely in the pericardium and tunica vaginalis. Mark and Yokoi[275] reviewed "background level of diffuse malignant mesothelioma" by retrospectively analyzing "the autopsy files of the Massachusetts General Hospital as well as the early literature on thoracic neoplasms." Their conclusions were "that the background level of diffuse malignant mesothelioma in Europe and in the USA prior to 1930 was extremely low. No case was detected at the Massachusetts General Hospital until 1946."

Nishikawa et al.[276] evaluated mortality from pleural mesothelioma from the perspective of a global assessment as correlated with patterns of asbestos use and international bans. They concluded that "observed disparities in global mesothelioma trends likely relate to country-to-country disparities in asbestos use trends."

The risks for the development of mesothelioma following occupational levels of exposure to asbestos are appreciated. The disease has the longest latency among asbestos-related diseases for occurrence from first exposure and occurs in lower dose settings. Thus, it has been the focus of several studies involving risks associated with nonoccupational exposures.

Magnani et al.[277] conducted a population-based case–control study in six areas from Italy, Spain, and Switzerland. Among the risk areas of concern were "cleaning asbestos-contaminated clothes, handling asbestos material and presence of asbestos material susceptible to damage. The estimated OR for high probability of environmental exposure (living within 2000 m of asbestos mines, asbestos cement plants, asbestos textiles, shipyards, or brake factories) was 11.5 (95% CI 3.5–38.2). Living between 2000 and 5000 m from asbestos industries or within 500 m of industries using asbestos could also be associated with an increased risk (of mesothelioma). A dose–response pattern appeared with intensity of both sources of exposure. It is suggested that low-dose exposure to asbestos at home or in the general environment carries a measurable risk of malignant pleural mesothelioma."

Kurumatani and Kumagal[278]assessed the impact of neighborhood exposures in a group of individuals who resided around a former large asbestos cement pipe plant in Amagasaki City, Japan. The time of potential exposure was between 1957 and 1975 when the plant used crocidolite and chrysotile asbestos. They identified 73 mesothelioma deaths (35 men and 38 women) among individuals with no occupational exposure to asbestos. "The regions with significantly elevated standardized mortality ratio reached 2200 m from the plant in the same direction in which the wind predominately blew." The authors concluded that "neighborhood exposure to asbestos can pose a serious risk to residents across a wide area."

Goldberg and Luce[279] evaluated epidemiological data to assess the risk for development of mesothelioma, lung cancer, and other respiratory diseases associated with nonoccupational exposure to asbestos. They concluded studies concerning exposure to naturally occurring asbestos "that begins at birth does not seem to affect the duration of the latency period, but the studies do not show whether early exposure increases susceptibility; they do not suggest that susceptibility differs according to sex. Solid evidence shows an increased risk of mesothelioma among people whose exposure comes from a paraoccupational or domestic source. The risk of mesothelioma associated with exposure as result of living near an industrial asbestos source (mines, mills, asbestos processing plants) is clearly confirmed." The authors further concluded that "nonoccupational exposures to asbestos may explain approximately 20% of the mesotheliomas in industrial countries."

Regulation of asbestos in occupational and bystander settings would be much simpler if only the longer/thicker fibers visible by light microscopy and scanning electron microscopy were the causative agent of all asbestos-related diseases. The accurate counting of fiber burdens would not require the more expensive, extensive preparative processes, and time-consuming use of ATEM. There would be great liability relief provided to those who manufacture products whose dust consists of fibers that predominantly can only be detected by ATEM. In reality, the majority of asbestos dust that makes up the predominate tissue burden found in the lung and extrapulmonary sites is represented by fibers shorter than 5 μm long and/or longer thin fibers not visible by light microscopy. In fact, the same can be said for many preparations and magnifications reported as used in studies involving scanning electron microscopy. The short fibers are the ones most readily cleared from the lung but are also the ones more readily translocated out of the lung to extrapulmonary sites. These are often misrepresented in some analyses of tissue samples by concluding that their absence or lack of detection means they had never been there, thus excluding them from possible participation in pathological mechanisms in the lung and other tissues. The importance of recognizing the presence of short fibers in tissue and/or as potential components of an exposure is shown by the findings of

Professor Carbone and associates. [280] A comprehensive study by SEM and ATEM of the physical dimensions of Turkish (from the area of the "cancer villages") and North Dakota erionite revealed the average length of 3.57 µm in the former and 2.20 µm in the latter. An evaluation of potential exposures to either samples would exclude a major population of the fibers when measuring those only longer than 5 µm.

This ability for short asbestos fibers and especially chrysotile to be cleared over time from the lung lead to the suggestion that occupational histories in some instances may be a better indicator of risk of lung cancer than fiber burden.[281]

An editorial in *Lancet*[282] correctly stated that "asbestos has been linked with diseases such as asbestosis, mesothelioma, and lung cancer" and that "all forms of asbestos are carcinogenic." The authors note "that unlike carcinogens such as tobacco, the risk of developing mesothelioma increases over time, even after exposure to asbestos has been stopped." Furthermore, they noted, "Canada is the only high-income country that still mines asbestos (in the form of chrysotile) (at the time of the article), and it is the second largest exporter of the toxin in the world (after Russia). Despite the country's claims that chrysotile poses a lower health risk than other types of asbestos, it acknowledges that chrysotile is a carcinogen and as such protects its own citizens by limiting its use within Canada; 98% of Canadian asbestos is exported to developing countries including India and Thailand." They conclude "the only way to eliminate asbestos-related illness is to stop the use of all types of asbestos, all over the world." This is a noble statement, but even if the utilization of asbestos is stopped in all countries, there will be years of exposure to degenerating asbestos in place and from demolition and abatement of the materials, particularly if incorrectly done, that will result in release of fibers in the workplace and environment.

3.15 CONCLUSION

The primary conclusions from the data presented in this chapter are that inhaled asbestos fibers cause asbestos-related diseases. The assumption that risks from asbestos exposure in the USA and induction of disease are going away in the near future are put in perspective by two recent articles. Attfield et al.[283] defined the trends in pneumoconiosis mortality and morbidity for the United States from 1968 to 2005 as related to indicators of the extent of exposure. They concluded that "asbestosis deaths from 1968–2005 closely followed the historical trend in asbestos consumption, and appear to be declining in most age groups." However, they noted "given appropriate exposure control, asbestosis could be eliminated by 2050." Obviously, prevention of occupational exposure is critical if this "heavy dose" related disease is to essentially disappear. A CDC/MMWR report[284] in April 2009 reviewed the status and projections for cases of mesothelioma in the USA. The fundamental basis for concern is that this disease has an appreciable latency period from first exposure (often 30–40+ years). The best-case scenario would project the disease to peak in 2010. However, the "annual number of mesothelioma deaths is still increasing, and future cases will continue to reflect the extensive past use of asbestos. New cases also might result through occupational and environmental exposure to asbestos during remediation and demolition of existing asbestos in buildings if controls are insufficient to protect workers and the surrounding community." A newer CDC/MMWR report[285] offers updated review of the status of mesothelioma cases in the USA. A particular area of interest was the reported occurrence of mesothelioma. They noted "the annual number of mesothelioma deaths among women increased significantly, from 489 in 1999 to 614 in 2020; however, the age-adjusted death rate per 1 million women declined significantly, from 4.83 in 1999 to 3.15 in 2020. The largest number of deaths was associated with the health care and social assistance industry (89; 15.7) and homemaker occupation (129; 22.8%)." "Mesothelioma deaths were classified as mesothelioma of the pleura (7.9%), peritoneum (9.2), pericardium (0.3%) and other sites (11.3%)."

A news released from the office of a previous Surgeon General[286] offers a useful overview of asbestos exposure issues by stating: "In recent decades, because of concern about asbestos' health effects, production and use has declined substantially. Most individuals exposed to asbestos, whether in a home, in the workplace, or out-of-doors will not develop disease-but there is no level of asbestos exposure that is known to be safe and minimizing your exposure will minimize your risk of developing asbestos-related diseases."

The tissue burden in individuals with asbestos-induced diseases consists most frequently of mixtures of asbestos types and sizes reflecting the features of many occupational exposures. Data from any tissue analysis for asbestos must be judged on what is included in the observations and what is realistically or potentially excluded by virtue of the limits of the methodologies used in the assessment. This requires an understanding of the impact of preparative techniques, the capabilities/magnification of the selected instrument used in obtaining the information, and the parameters/definition of structures defined in the count scheme used in a given study of a sample. This information is often critical in supplementation of clinical history. For example, few clinical histories have included any mention of past exposure to talc, which has been increasingly of concern due to fibrous materials being a component of both industrial talc and to a lesser extent cosmetic talc. Several cases have been referred to our laboratory for tissue burden analysis where no indication in the history explained the source of past exposure to "vermiculite containing asbestiform amphiboles" as found in the tissue. Further recollection as to past exposure to elongated mineral particles is often flawed or the individuals were not aware of asbestos/elongate mineral particles even being in a particular setting/product. A perfect example of the additional value of tissue burden assessment is a study of malignant mesothelioma in Australia from 1945 to 2000.[287] The data accumulated for this rare tumor indicated from 1945 to 2000 there were 6329 documented cases. The authors presented the data defined by age, sex and potential of occupational/paraoccupational and/or environmental exposures. The initial data also had "no history of exposure" as a category. When a more intensive review of actual history was conducted, they found that 57 of 203 "so classified" as "no history" actually had a history of some exposures identified. Thus, they noted only 19% had "no known history." When actual fiber burden of tissue was conducted the authors concluded that in the "no know history" group that "81% had fiber counts >200,000 fibers/gm dry lung detected," and "30% had more than 10^6 fibers/gm >2 μm including 'long' (>10 μm) fibers" interpreted as suggesting that "nearly all cases have been exposed."

REFERENCES

1. Robertson, B., Basic morphology of the pulmonary defense system, *Eur. J. Respir. Dis. Suppl.*, 61, 21–40, 1980.
2. Lippmann, M., Yeates, D.B., and Albert, R.E., Deposition, retention, and clearance of inhaled particles, *Br. J. Ind. Med.*, 37(4), 337–362, 1980.
3. Witschi, H., Proliferation of type II alveolar cells: A review of common responses in toxic lung injury, *Toxicology*, 5(3), 267–277, 1976.
4. Burri, P.H., Morphology and respiratory function of the alveolar unit, *Int. Arch. Aller. Appl. Immunol.*, 76, 2–12, 1985.
5. Ochs, M., Nyengaard, J.R., Jung, A., et al., The number of alveoli in the human lung, *Am. J. Respir. Crit. Care Med.*, 169(1), 120–124, 2004.
6. Weibel, E.R., How does lung structure affect gas exchange?, *Chest*, 83(4), 657–665, 1983.
7. Turino, G.M., The lung parenchyma — A dynamic matrix, *Am. Rev. Respir. Dis.*, 132(6), 1324–1334, 1985.
8. Gross, P., and Detreville, R.T., The lung as an embattled domain against inanimate pollutants, *Am. Rev. Respir. Dis.*, 106(5), 684–691, 1972.
9. Breeze, R., and Turk, M., Cellular structure, function and organization in the lower respiratory tract, *Environ. Health Perspect.*, 55, 3–24, 1984.
10. Mason, R.J., Dobbs, L.G., Greenleaf, R.D., and Williams, M.C., Alveolar type II cells, *Fed. Proc.*, 36(13), 2697–2702, 1977.
11. Ford, J.O., Dodson, R.F., and Williams, M.G., An ultrastructual study of the blood/air barrier in the guinea pig, *Tissue Cell*, 16(1), 53–63, 1984.
12. Rubins, J.B., Alveolar macrophages: Wielding the double-edged sword of inflammation, *Am. J. Respir. Crit. Care Med.*, 167(2), 103–104, 2003.

13. Werb, Z., How the macrophage regulates its extracellular environment, *Am. J. Anat.*, 166(3), 237–256, 1983.
14. Camner, P., Anderson, M., Philipson, K., et al., Human bronchiolar deposition and retention of 6-, 8-, and 10-mm particles, *Exp. Lung Res.*, 23(6), 517–535, 1997.
15. McFadden, D., Wright, J.L., Wiggs, B., and Churg, A., Smoking inhibits asbestos clearance, *Am. Rev. Respir. Dis.*, 133(3), 372–374, 1986.
16. Churg, A., Thon, V., and Wright, J.L., Effects of cigarette smoke exposure on retention of asbestos fibers in various morphological compartments of the guinea pig lung, *Am. J. Pathol.*, 129(2), 385–393, 1987.
17. Churg, A., and Wiggs, B., Mineral particles, mineral fibers, and lung cancer, *Environ. Res.*, 37(2), 364–372, 1985.
18. Churg, A., Wright, J.L., Hobson, J., and Stevens, B., Effects of cigarette smoke on the clearance of short asbestos fibers from the lung and a comparison with the clearance of long asbestos fibres, *Int. J. Exp. Pathol.*, 73(3), 287–297, 1992.
19. Albin, M., Pooley, F.D., Stromberg, U., et al., Retention patterns of asbestos fibres in lung tissue among asbestos cement workers, *Occup. Environ. Med.*, 51(3), 205–211, 1994.
20. Churg, A., and Stevens, B., Enhanced retention of asbestos fibers in the Airways of human smokers, *Am. J. Respir. Crit. Care Med.*, 151(5), 1409–1413, 1995.
21. Oberdorster, G., Lung particle overload: Implications for occupational exposures to particles, Regulat, *Toxicol. Pharmacol.*, 27, 123–135, 1995.
22. Morrow, P.E., Possible mechanisms to explain dust overloading of the lungs, *Fundam. Appl. Toxicol.*, 10(3), 369–384, 1988.
23. Pritchard, J.N., Dust overloading causes impairment of pulmonary clearance: Evidence from rats and humans, *Exp. Pathol.*, 37(1–4), 39–42, 1989.
24. Stober, W., Morrow, P.E., and Hoover, M.D., Compartment modeling of the Long-term retention of insoluble particles deposited in the alveolar region of the lung, *Fundam. Appl. Toxicol.*, 13(4), 823–842, 1989.
25. Castranova, V., Driscoll, K., Harkema, J., et al., The relevance of the rat lung response to particle overload for human risk assessment: A workshop consensus report, *Inhal. Toxicol.*, 12(1–2), 1–17, 2000.
26. Coin, P.G., Osornio-Vargas, A.R., Roggli, V.L., and Brody, A.R., Pulmonary Fiberogenesis after three consecutive inhalation exposures to chrysotile asbestos, *Am. J. Respir. Crit. Care Med.*, 154(5), 1511–1519, 1996.
27. Dodson, R.F., and Ford, J.O., Tissue reaction following a second exposure to amosite asbestos, *Cytobios*, 68(272), 53–62, 1991.
28. Pinkerton, K.E., Pratt, P.C., Brody, A.R., and Crapo, J.D., Fiber localication and its relationship to lung reaction in rats after chronic inhalation of chrysotile asbestos, *Am. J. Pathol.*, 117(3), 484–498, 1984.
29. Reeves, A.L., Puro, H.E., Smith, R.G., and Vorwald, A.J., Experimental asbestos carcinogenesis, *Environ. Res.*, 4(6), 496–511, 1971.
30. Kimizuka, G., and Shinozaki, H.Y., Comparison of the pulmonary responses to chrysotile and amosite asbestos administrated intratracheally, *Acta Pathol. Jpn.*, 42(10), 707–711, 1992.
31. Hesterberg, T.W., Hart, G.A., Chevalier, J., Miiller, W.C., Hamilton, R.D., Bauer, J., and Thevenaz, P., The importance of fiber biopersistence and lung dose in determining the chronic inhalation effects of X607, RCF1, and chrysotile asbestos in rats, *Toxicol. Appl. Pharmacol.*, 153(1), 68–82.1998.
32. Rodelsperger, K., Extrapolation of the carcinogenic potential of fibers from rats to humans, *Inhal. Toxicol.*, 16(11–12), 801–807, 2004.
33. Brody, A.R., Whither goes the alveolar macrophage? Another small chapter is written on the localized response of this crucial cell, *J. Lab. Clin. Med.*, 131(5), 391–392, 1998.
34. Dodson, R.F., Williams, M.G., and Hurst, G.A., Acute lung response to amosite asbestos: A morphological study, *Environ. Res.*, 32(1), 80–90, 1983.
35. Hasselbacher, P., Binding of immunoglobulin and activation of complement by asbestos fibers, *J. Aller Clin. Immunol.*, 64(4), 294–298, 1979.
36. Johnson, R.B. Jr., Godzik, C.A., and Cohn, Z.A., Increased superoxide anion production by immunologically activated and chemically elicited macrophages, *J. Exp. Med.*, 148, 127, 1978.
37. Hoidal, J.R., Beall, G.D., and Repine, J.E., Production of hydroxyl radical by human alveolar macrophages, *Infect. Immun.*, 26(3), 1088–1094, 1979.
38. Hunninghake, G.W., Gadek, J.E., Fales, H.M., and Crystal, R.G., Human alveolar macrophage-derived chemotactic factor for neutrophils, *J. Clin. Invest.*, 66(3), 473–483, 1980.
39. Rennard, S.I., Hunninghake, G.W., Bitterman, P.B., and Crystal, R.G., Production of fibronectin by the human alveolar macrophage: Mechanism for recruitment of fibroblasts to sites of tissue injury in interstitial lung diseases, *Proc. Natl Acad. Sci. USA*, 78(11), 7147–7151, 1981.

40. Werb, Z., and Gordon, S., Secretion of a specific collagenase by stimulated macrophages, *J. Exp. Med.*, 142(2), 346–360, 1975.
41. Werb, Z., and Gordon, S., Elastase secretion by stimulated macrophages, *J. Exp. Med.*, 142(2), 361–377, 1975.
42. Henke, C., Marineili, W., Jessurun, J., et al., Macrophage production of basic fibroblast growth factor in the fibroproliferative disorder of alveoli fibrosis after lung injury, *Am. J. Pathol.*, 143(4), 1189–1199, 1993.
43. Bitterman, P.B., Rennard, S.I., Hunninghake, G.W., and Crystal, R.G., Human alveolar macrophage growth factor for fibroblasts: Regulation and partial characterization, *J. Clin. Invest.*, 70(4), 806–822, 1982.
44. Bitterman, P.B., Rennard, S.I., Adelberg, S., and Crystal, R.G., Role of fibronectin as a growth factor for fibroblasts, *J. Cell Biol.*, 97(6), 1925–1932, 1983.
45. Bowden, D.H., Macrophages, dust, and pulmonary diseases, *Exp. Lung Res.*, 12(2), 89–107, 1987.
46. Bowden, D.H., The alveolar macrophage, *Environ. Health Perspect.*, 55, 327–341, 1984.
47. Brain, J.D., Macrophage damage in relation to the pathogenesis of lung diseases, *Environ. Health Perspect.*, 35, 21–28, 1980.
48. Corry, D., Kulkarni, P., and Lipscomb, M.F., The migration of bronchoalveolar macrophages into hilar lymph nodes, *Am. J. Pathol.*, 225(3), 321–328, 1984.
49. Snipes, M.B., Long-term retention and clearance of particles inhaled by mammalian species, *Crit. Rev. Toxicol.*, 20(3), 175–211, 1989.
50. Ferin, J., and Feldstein, M.L., Pulmonary clearance and hilar lymph node content in rats after particle exposure, *Environ. Res.*, 16(1–3), 342–352, 1978.
51. Lauweryns, J.M., The juxta-alveolar lymphatics in the human adult lung histologic studies in 15 cases of drowning, *Am. Rev. Respir. Dis.*, 102(6), 877–885, 1970.
52. Lauweryns, J.M., and Baert, J.H., The role of the pulmonary lymphatics in the defenses of the distal lung: Morphological and experimental studies of the transport mechanisms of intratracheally instillated particles, *Ann. N. Y. Acad. Sci.*, 221, 244–275, 1974.
53. Camner, P., Alveolar clearance, *Eur. J. Respir. Dis.*, 61, 59–72, 1980.
54. Tosi, P., Franzinelli, A., Miracco, C., et al, Silicotic lymph node lesions in non-occupationally exposed lung carcinoma patients, *Eur. J. Respir. Dis.*, 68(5), 362–369, 1988.
55. Craighead, J.E., Kleinerman, J., Abraham, J.L., et al, Diseases associated with exposure to silica and nonfibrous silicate minerals, *Arch. Pathol. Lab. Med.*,112. 673–720, 1988.
56. Dodson, R.F., Shepherd, S., Levin, J., and Hammar, S.P., Characteristics of the asbestos concentration in various levels of lymph nodes that collect drainage from the lung, *Ultrastruct. Pathol.*, 31(2), 95–153, 2007.
57. Oberdorster, G., Morrow, P.E., and Spurny, K., Size dependent lymphatic short-term clearance of amosite fibres in the lung, *Ann. Occup. Hyg.*, 32 (Supplement 1), 149–156, 1988.
58. Hammar, S.P., Common neoplasms, in Dail, D.H., and Hammar, S.P., eds. *Pulmonary Pathology*, Springer-Verlag, New York, pp. 1123–1278, 1994..
59. Netter, F.H., Respiratory system, in Divertie, M.B., and Brass, A., eds. *The Ciba Collection of Medical Illustrations*, Ciba Pharmaceutical, CIBA-Summit, NJ, pp. 32–33, 1979.
60. Cullen, R.T., Tran, C.L., Buchanan, D., Davis, J.M.G., Searl, A., and Jones, A.D., Inhalation of poorly soluble particles. I. Differences in inflammatory response and clearance during exposure, *Inhal. Toxicol.*, 12(12), 1089–1111, 2000.
61. Schlesinger, R.B., Clearance from the respiratory tract, *Fundam. Appl. Toxicol.*, 5(3), 435–450, 1985.
62. Becklake, M.R., Asbestos-related diseases of the lung and other organs: Their epidemiology and implications for clinical practice, *Am. Rev. Respir. Dis.*, 114(1), 187–227, 1976.
63. Hillerdal, G., The pathogenesis of pleural plaques and pulmonary asbestosis: Possibilities and impossibilities, *Eur. J. Respir. Dis.*, 61(3), 129–138, 1980.
64. Davis, J.M.G., Jones, A.D., and Miller, B.G., Experimental studies in rats on the effects of asbestos inhalation coupled with the inhalation of titanium dioxide or quartz, *Int. J. Exp. Pathol.*, 72(5), 501–525, 1991.
65. Pintos, J., Parent, M.-E., Case, B.W., Rousseau, M.-C., and Siemiatycki, J., Risk of mesothelioma and exposure to asbestos and man-made vitreous fibers: Evidence from two case-control studies in Montreal, Canada, *JOEM*, 51, 1177–1184, 2009.
66. Craighead, J.E., and Mossman, B.T., The pathogenesis of asbestos-associated diseases, *N. Engl. J. Med.*, 306(24), 1446–1455, 1982.
67. Upton, A.C., Barrett, J.C., Becklake, M.R., et al., *Health Effects Institute-Asbestos Research: Asbestos in Public and Commercial Buildings. A Literature Review and Synthesis of Current Knowledge*, Health Effects Institute, Cambridge, 1991.

68. Bowles, O., *Asbestos: The Silk of the Mineral Kingdom*, The Ruberoid Co., New York, 1946.
69. Kaplan, J. P., *Syracuse Research Corporation Under Contract No.205-1999-00024, Toxicological Profile for Asbestos (Update)*, Agency for Toxic Substances and Disease Registry, Atlanta, GA, p. 1, 2001.
70. Hendry, N.W., The geology occurrences and major user of asbestos, in Boland, B., ed. *Annals of the New York Academy of Sciences*, The New York Academy of Sciences, New York, p. 12, 1965.
71. Clifton, R.A., *Asbestos, in Bureau of Mines Minerals Yearbook*, Bureau of Mines United States Department of the Interior, Washington, DC, pp. 1–5, 1973.
72. Bignon, J., Peto, J., and Saracci, R., (eds.), *Non-occupational Exposure to Mineral Fibres*. IARC Scientific Publication No. 90, World Health Organization International Agency for Research on Cancer, Oxford University Press , New York, p. 330, 1989.
73. Langer, A.M., Nolan, R.P., and Addison, J., Distinguishing between amphibole asbestos fibers and elongate cleavage fragments of their non-asbestos analogues, in Brown, R.C., et al., eds. *Mechanisms in Fibre Carcinogenisis*, Plenum Press, New York, pp. 253–267, 1991.
74. Churg, A., Chrysotile, tremolite, and malignant mesothelioma in man, *Chest*, 93(3), 621–628, 1988.
75. Bernstein, D.M., Chevlier, J., and Smith, P., Comparison of calidria chrysotile asbestos to pure tremolite: Inhalation biopersistence and histopathology following short-term exposure, *Inhal. Toxicol.*, 15(14), 1387–1419, 2003.
76. Cook, P.M., Swinek, J., Dawson, T.D., Chapman, D., Etterson, M.A., and Hoff, D., Quantitative structure-mesothelioma potency model optimization for complex mixtures of elongated particles in rat pleura: A retrospective study, *J. Tox. Env. Health Part B. Spec. Ed.*, 19, 5–6, 266–288, 2016.
77. Pezerat, H., Chrysotile biopersistence, *Int. J. Occup. Environ. Health*, 15(1), 102–106, 2009.
78. Hamilton, J.A., Asbestos fibers, plasma and inflammation, *Environ. Health Perspect.*, 51, 281–285, 1983.
79. Valerio, F., Balducci, D., and Lazzarotto, A., Adsorption of proteins by chrysotile and crocidolite: Role of molecular weight and charge density, *Environ. Res.*, 44(2), 312–320, 1987.
80. Xu, A., Zhou, H., Yu, D., and Hei, T., Mechanisms of the genotoxicity of crocidolite asbestos in mammalian cells: Implication from mutation patterns induced by reactive oxygen species, *Environ. Health Perspect.*, 110(10), 1003–1008, 2002.
81. MacCorkle, R.A., Slattery, S.D., Nash, D.R., and Brinkley, B.R., Intracellular protein binding to asbestos induces aneuploidy in human lung fibroblasts, *Cell Motil. Cytoskeleton*, 63(10), 646–657, 2006.
82. Lee, K.P., Lung response to particulates with emphasis on asbestos and other fibrous dusts, *CRC Crit. Rev. Toxicol.*, 14(1), 33–86, 1985.
83. Anonymous, Task group on lung dynamics: Deposition and retention models for internal dosimetry of the human respiratory tract, *Health Phys.*, 12, 173–207, 1966.
84. Dodson, R.F., Atkinson, M.A.L., and Levin, J.L., Asbestos fiber length as related to potential pathogenicity: A critical review, *Am. J. Ind. Med.*, 44(3), 291–297, 2003.
85. Timbrell, V., Ashcroft, T., Goldstein, B., Heyworth, F., Meurman, L.O., Rendall, R.E.G., Reynolds, J.A., Shilkin, K.B., and Whitaker, D., Relationships between retained amphiboles fibres and fibrosis in human lung tissue specimens, *Ann. Occup. Hyg., Supplement*, 1(32), 323–340, 1988.
86. Marchand, F., Uber eigentumliche pigmentkristalle in den Lungen, *Verh. Deut Ges. Pathol.*, 17, 223–228, 1906.
87. Cooke, W.E., Asbestos dust and the curious bodies found in pulmonary asbestosis, *Br. Med. J.*, 2(3586), 578–580, 1929.
88. Gloyne, S.R., The formation of the asbestos body in the lung, *Tubercle*, 12(9), 399–401, 1931.
89. Gloyne, S.R., The morbid anatomy and histology of asbestosis, *Tubercle*, 14(12), 550–558, 1933.
90. Davis, J.M.G., Further observations on the ultrastructure and chemistry of the formation of asbestos bodies, *Exp. Mol. Pathol.*, 13(3), 346–358, 1970.
91. Governa, M., and Rosanda, C., A histochemical study of the asbestos body coating, *Br. J. Ind. Med.*, 29(2), 154–159, 1972.
92. Dodson, R.F., O'Sullivan, M.F., Williams, M.G., and Hurst, G.A., Analysis of cores of ferruginous bodies from former asbestos workers, *Environ. Res.*, 28(1), 171–178, 1982.
93. Dodson, R.F., O'Sullivan, M., and Corn, C.J., Relationships between ferruginous bodies and uncoated asbestos fibers in lung tissue, *Arch. Environ. Health*, 16, 637–647, 1996.
94. Churg, A., The diagnosis of asbestosis, *Hum. Pathol.*, 20(2), 97–99, 1989.
95. Dodson, R.F., Williams, M.G., and Hurst, G.A., Method for removing the ferruginous coating from asbestos bodies, *J. Toxicol. Environ. Health*, 11(4–6), 959–966, 1983.

96. Gross, P., Tuma, J., and deTreville, R.T.P., Unusual ferruginous bodies, *Arch. Environ. Health*, 22(5), 534–537, 1971.
97. Gross, P., deTreville, R.T.P., Cralley, L.J., and Davis, J.M.G., Pulmonary ferruginous bodies, *Arch. Pathol.*, 85(5), 539–546, 1968.
98. Holmes, A., Morgan, A., and Davison, W., Formation of pseudo-asbestos bodies on sized glass fibres in the hamster lung, *Ann. Occup. Hyg.*, 27(3), 301–313, 1983.
99. Churg, A., and Warnock, M.L., Asbestos and other ferruginous bodies, *Am. J. Pathol.*, 102(3), 447–456, 1981.
100. Dodson, R.F., O'Sullivan, M.F., Corn, C., Williams, M.G., and Hurst, G.A., Ferruginous body formation on a nonasbestos mineral, *Arch. Pathol. Lab. Med.*, 109(9), 849–852, 1985.
101. Dodson, R.F., O'Sullivan, M., Corn, C.J., Garcia, J.G.N., Stocks, J.M., and Griffith, D.E., Analysis of ferruginous bodies in bronchoalveolar lavage from foundry workers, *Br. J. Ind. Med.*, 50(11), 1032–1038, 1993.
102. Dodson, R.F., O'Sullivan, M.F., Corn, C.J., and Hammar, S.P., Quantitative comparison of asbestos and talc bodies in an individual with mixed exposure, *Am. J. Ind. Med.*, 27(2), 207–215, 1995.
103. Auerbach, O., Conston, A.S., Garfinkel, L., Parks, V.R., Kaslow, H.D., and Hammond, E.C., Presence of asbestos bodies in organs other than the lung, *Chest*, 77(2), 133–137, 1980.
104. Dodson, R.F., O'Sullivan, M., Huang, J., Holiday, D.B., and Hammar, S.P., Asbestos in extrapulmonary sites omentum and mesentery, *Chest*, 117(2), 486–493, 2000.
105. Roggli, V.L., and Benning, T.L., Asbestos bodies in pulmonary hilar lymph nodes, *Mod. Pathol.*, 3(4), 513–517, 1990.
106. Godwin, M.C., and Jagatic, J.J., Asbestos and mesotheliomas, *Environ. Res.*, 3, 391–416, 1970.
107. Dodson, R.F., Williams, M.G., Corn, C.J., Brollo, A., and Bianchi, C., Asbestos content of lung tissue, lymph nodes and pleural plaques from former shipyard workers, *Am. Rev. Respir. Dis.*, 142(4), 843–847, 1990.
108. Williams, M.G., Dodson, R.F., Dickson, E.W., and Fraire, A.E., An assessment of asbestos body formation in extrapulmonary sites, liver and spleen, *Toxicol. Ind. Health*, 17(1), 1–6, 2001.
109. Craighead, J.E., Abraham, J.L., Churg, A., et al., The pathology of asbestos-associated diseases of the lungs and pleural cavities: Diagnostic criteria and proposed grading schema, *Arch. Pathol. Lab. Med.*, 106(11), 544–596, 1982.
110. Crouch, E., and Churg, A., Ferruginous bodies and the histological evaluation of dust exposure, *Am. J. Surg. Pathol.*, 8(2), 109–116, 1984.
111. Millette, J.R., Twyman, J.D., Hansen, E.C., Clark, P.J., and Pansing, M.F., Chrysotile, palygorskite, and halloysite in drinking water, *Scan. Electron Microsc.*, 1, 579–586, 1979.
112. Berkley, C., Churg, J., Selikoff, I.J., and Smith, W.E., The detection and localization of mineral fibers in tissue, in Boland, B., Hitchcock, J., and Kates, S., eds. *Biological Effects of Asbestos*, The New York Academy of Sciences, New York, pp. 48–63, 1965.
113. Carter, R.E., and Taylor, W.F., Identification of particular amphibole asbestos fiber in tissue of persons exposed to a high oral intake of the mineral, *Environ. Res.*, 21(1), 85–93, 1980.
114. Chatfield, E.J., Preparation and analysis of particulate samples by electron microscopy, with special reference to asbestos, *Scan. Electron Microsc.*, 1, 563–578, 1979.
115. Chatfield, E.J., and Dillon, M.J., Some aspects of specimen preparation and limitations of precision in particulate analysis by SEM and TEM, *Scan. Electron Microsc.*, 1, 487–496, 1978.
116. Ashcroft, T., and Heppleston, A.G., The optical and electron microscopic determination of pulmonary asbestos fiber concentration and its relation to the human pathological reaction, *J. Clin. Pathol.*, 26(3), 224–234, 1973.
117. Langer, A.M., Rubin, I.B., and Selikoff, I.J., Chemical characterization of asbestos body cores by electron microprobe analysis, *J. Histochem. Cytochem.*, 20(9), 723–734, 1972.
118. Churg, A., and Warnock, M.L., Asbestos fibers in the general population, *Am. Rev. Respir. Dis.*, 122(5), 669–678, 1980.
119. Stasny, J.T., Husach, C., Albright, F.R., Schumacher, D.V., Sweigart, D.W., and Boyer, K., Development of methods to isolate asbestos from spiked beverages and foods for SEM characterization, *Scan. Electron Microsc.*, 1, 587–595, 1979.
120. Sundius, N., and Bygden, A., Isolation of the mineral dust in lungs and sputum, *J. Ind. Hyg. Toxicol.*, 20, 351–359, 1938.
121. Vallyathan, V., and Green, F.H.Y., The role of analytical techniques in the Diagnosis of asbestos-associated disease, *CRC Crit. Rev. Clin. Lab. Sci.*, 22(1), 1–42, 1985.

122. Gylseth, B., Baunan, R.H., and Bruun, R., Analysis of inorganic fibre Concentrations in biological samples by scanning electron microscopy, *Scand. J. Work Environ. Health*, 7(2), 101–108, 1981.
123. Gylseth, B., and Baunan, R.H., Topographic and size distribution of asbestos Bodies in exposed human lungs, *Scand. J. Work Environ. Health*, 7(3), 190–195, 1981.
124. DeVuyst, P., Karjalainen, A., Dumortier, P., Pairon, J-C., Monso, E., Brochardi, P., Teschler, H., Tossavainen, A., and Gibbs, A., Guidelines for mineral fibre analysis in biological samples: Report of the ERS working group, *Eur. Respir. J.*, 11(6), 1416–1426, 1998.
125. Dement, J.M., Overview on fiber toxicology research needs, Environmetal, *Health Perspect.*, 88(117), 261–268, 1990.
126. Williams, M.G., Dodson, R.F., Corn, C., and Hurst, G.A., A procedure for the isolation of amosite asbestos and ferruginous bodies from lung tissue and sputum, *J. Toxicol. Environ. Health*, 10(4–5), 627–638, 1982.
127. Smith, M.J., and Naylor, B., A method of extracting ferruginous bodies from sputum and pulmonary tissue, *Am. J. Clin. Pathol.*, 58(3), 250–254, 1972.
128. Dodson, R.F., Williams, M.G., McLarty, J.W., and Hurst, G.A., Asbestos bodies and particulate matter in sputum from former asbestos workers, *Acta Cytol.*, 27(6), 635–640, 1983.
129. Dodson, R.F., Garcia, J.G.N., O'Sullivan, M., et al., The usefulness of bronchoalveolar lavage in identifying past occupational exposure to asbestos, A light and electron microscopy study, *Am. J. Ind. Med.*, 19(5), 619–628, 1991.
130. O'Sullivan, M.F., Corn, C.J., and Dodson, R.F., Comparative efficiency of Nuclepore filters of various pore sizes as used in digestion studies of tissue, *Environ. Res.*, 43(1), 97–103, 1987.
131. Webber, J.S., Czuhanich, A.G., and Carhart, L.J., Performance of membrane filters used for TEM analysis of asbestos, *J. Occup. Environ. Hyg.*, 4(10), 780–789, 2007.
132. Middleton, A.P., and Jackson, E.A., A procedure for the estimation of asbestos collected on membrane filters using transmission electron microscopy (TEM), *Ann. Occup. Hyg.*, 25(4), 381–391, 1982.
133. Middleton, A.P., Visibility of fine fibres of asbestos during routine electron microscopical analysis, *Ann. Occup. Hyg.*, 25(1), 53–62, 1982.
134. Small, J.A., *Proceeding of the Asbestos Fibers Measurements in Building Atmospheres*, Ontario Research Foundation, Mississauga, ON, p. 69, 1982.
135. Teichert, U., *Proceedings of the Fourth International Colloquium on Dust Measuring Techniques and Strategies*, Asbestos International Association, Edinburgh, Scotland and London, p. 130, September 20–23, 1982.
136. Small, J.A., Newbury, D.E., and Myklebust, R.L., *Proceedings of the 18th Annual Conference of the Microbeam Analysis Society*, San Francisco Press, San Francisco, CA, 1983.
137. Lee, R.J., *Basic Concepts of Electron Diffraction and Asbestos Identification Using Selected Area Diffraction*, SEM, O'Hare, IL, 1978.
138. Ruud, C.D., Russell, P.A., and Clark, R.L., Selected area electron diffraction and energy dispersive X-ray analysis for the identification of asbestos fibers, a comparison, *Micron*, 7, 115–132, 1976.
139. Dodson, R.F., O'Sullivan, M.F., and Corn, C.J., Technique dependent variations in asbestos burden as illustrated in a case of nonoccupational exposed mesothelioma, *Am. J. Ind. Med.*, 24(2), 235–240, 1993.
140. Greenberg, S.D., Hurst, G.A., Matlage, W.T., Christianson, C., Hurst, I.J., and Mabry, L.C., Sputum cytopathological findings in former asbestos workers, *Tex. Med.*, 72(1), 39–43, 1976.
141. Bignon, J., Sebastien, P., Jaurand, M.C., and Hem, H., Microfiltration method for quantitative study of fibrous particles in biological specimens, *Environ. Health Perspect.*, 9, 155–160, 1974.
142. McLarty, J.W., Greenberg, S.D., Hurst, G.A., et al., The clinical significance of ferruginous bodies in sputa, *J. Occup. Med.*, 22(2), 92–96, 1980.
143. Modin, B.E., Greenberg, S.D., Buffler, P.A., Lockhart, J.A., Seitzman, L.H., and Awe, R.J., Asbestos bodies in a general Hospital/Clinic population, *Acta Cytol.*, 26(5), 667–670, 1982.
144. Paris, C., Galateau-Salle, F., Creveuil, C., et al., Asbestos bodies in sputum of asbestos workers: Correlation with occupational exposure, *Eur. Respir. J.*, 20(5), 1167–1173, 2002.
145. Sebastien, P., Armstrong, B., Case, B.W., Barwick, H., Keskula, H., and McDonald, J.C., Estimation of amphibole exposure from asbestos body and macrophage counts in sputum: A survey in vermiculite miners, *Ann. Occup. Hyg.*, 32 (Supplement 1), 195–201, 1988.
146. Dodson, R.F., Williams, M.G., Corn, C.J., Idell, S., and McLarty, J.W., Usefulness of combined light and electron microscopy evaluation of sputum samples for asbestos to determine past occupational exposure, *Mod. Pathol.*, 2(4), 320–322, 1989.
147. Goldstein, R.A., Rohatgi, P.K., Bergofsky, E.H., Block, E.R., Daniele, R.P., Dantzker, D.R., Davis, G.S., Hunninghake, G.W., King, T.E., Metzger, W.J., Rankin, J.A., Reynolds, H.Y., and Turino, G.M., Clinical

role of bronchoalveolar lavage in adults with pulmonary disease, *Am. Rev. Respir. Dis.*, 142(2), 481–486, 1990.
148. Begin, R.O., Bronchoalveolar lavage in the pneumoconioses, *Chest*, 94(3), 454, 1988.
149. de Vuyst, P., Dumortier, P., Moulin, E., Yourassowsky, N., and Yernault, J.C., Diagnostic value of asbestos bodies in bronchoalveolar lavage fluid, *Am. Rev. Respir. Dis.*, 136(5), 1219–1224, 1987.
150. de Vuyst, P., Jedwab, J., Dumortier, P., Vandermoten, G., Vande Weyer, R., and Yernault, J.C., Asbestos bodies in bronchoalveolar lavage, *Am. Rev. Respir. Dis.*, 126(6), 972–976, 1982.
151. de Vuyst, P., Dumortier, P., Moulin, E., et al., Asbestos bodies in bronchoalveolar lavage reflect lung asbestos body concentration, *Eur. Respir. J.*, 1(4), 362–367, 1988.
152. Dumortier, P., Coplu, L., de Maertelaer, V., Emri, S., Baris, Y.I., and deVuyst, P., Assessment of environmental asbestos exposure in Turkey by bronchoalveolar lavage, *Am. J. Respir. Crit. Care Med.*, 158(6), 1815–1824, 1998.
153. de Vuyst, P., Dumortier, P., and Gevenois, P.A., Analysis of asbestos bodies in BAL from subjects with particular exposures, *Am. J. Ind. Med.*, 31(6), 699–704, 1997.
154. Sebastien, P., Armstrong, B., Monchaux, G., and Bignon, J., Asbestos bodies in bronchoalveolar lavage fluid and in lung parenchyma, *Am. Rev. Respir. Dis.*, 137(1), 75–78, 1988.
155. Schwartz, D.A., Galvin, J.R., Burmeister, L.F., Merchant, R.K., Dayton, C.S., Merchant, J.A., and Hunninghake, G.W., The clinical utility and reliability of asbestos bodies in bronchoalveolar fluid, *Am. Rev. Respir. Dis.*, 144, 684–688, 1991.
156. Oriowski, E., Pairon, J.C., Ameille, J., et al., Pleural plaques, asbestos exposure, and asbestos bodies in bronchoalveolar lavage fluid, *Am. J. Ind. Med.*, 26(3), 349–358, 1994.
157. Dodson, R.F., Williams, G., Huang, J., and Bruce, J.R., Tissue burden of asbestos in nonoccupationally exposed individuals from East Texas, *Am. J. Ind. Med.*, 35(3), 281–286, 1999.
158. Dodson, R.F., O'Sullivan, M., Brooks, D.R., and Bruce, J.R., Asbestos content of omentum and mesentery in nonoccupationally exposed individuals, *Toxicol. Ind. Health*, 17(4), 138–143, 2001.
159. Gellert, A.R., Kitajewska, J.Y., Uthayakumar, S., Kirkham, J.B., and Rudd, R.M., Asbestos fibres in bronchoalveolar lavage fluid from asbestos workers: Examination by electron microscopy, *Br. J. Ind. Med.*, 43(3), 170–176, 1986.
160. Dodson, R.F., O'Sullivan, M., Brooks, D.R., and Levin, J.L., The sensitivity of lavage analysis by light and analytical electron microscopy in correlating the types of asbestos from a known exposure setting, *Inhal. Toxicol.*, 15(5), 461–471, 2003.
161. Artivinli, M., and Baris, Y.I., Environmental fiber-induced pleuro-pulmonary diseases in an Antolian Village: An epidemiology study, *Arch. Environ. Health*, 37(3), 177–181, 1982.
162. Dumortier, P., Coplu, L., Broucke, I., Emir, S, Selcuk, T, Maertelaer, V, De Vuyst, P, and Baris, I., Erionite bodies and fibres in bronchoalveolar lavage fluid (BALF) of residents from Tuzkoy, Cappadocia, Turkey, *Occup. Environ. Med.*, 58(4), 261–266, 2001.
163. de Vuyst, P., Dumortier, P., Leophonte, P., Vande Weyer, R., and Yernault, J.C., Mineralogical analysis of bronchoalveolar lavage in talc pneumoconiosis, *Eur. J. Respir. Dis.*, 70(3), 150–156, 1987.
164. Dumortier, P., de Vuyst, P., Strauss, P., and Yernault, J.C., Asbestos bodies in bronchoalveolar lavage fluids of brake lining and asbestos cement workers, *Br. J. Ind. Med.*, 47(2), 91–98, 1990.
165. Levin, J.L., O'Sullivan, M.F., Corn, C.J., and Dodson, R.F., An individual with a majority of ferruginous bodies formed on chrysotile cores, *Arch. Environ. Health*, 50(6), 462–465, 1995.
166. Butnor, K., Sporn, T., and Roggli, V.L., Exposure to brake dust and malignant mesothelioma: A study of 10 cases with mineral fiber analysis, *Ann. Occup. Hyg.*, 47(4), 325–330, 2003.
167. Paustenbach, D., Richter, R., Finley, B., and Sheehan, P., An evaluation of the historical exposures of mechanics to asbestos in brake dust, *Appl. Occup. Environ. Hyg.*, 18(10), 786–804, 2003.
168. Weir, F., and Meraz, L., Morphological characteristics of asbestos fibers released during grinding and drilling of friction products, *Appl. Occup. Environ. Hyg.*, 16(12), 1147–1149, 2001.
169. Weir, F., Tolar, G., and Meraz, L., Characterization of vehicular brake service personnel exposure to airborne asbestos and particulate, *Appl. Occup. Environ. Hyg.*, 16(12), 1139–1146, 2001.
170. Sartorelli, P., Scancarello, G., Romeo, R., et al., Asbestos exposure assessment by mineralogical analysis of bronchoalveolar lavage fluid, *J. Occup. Environ. Med.*, 43(10), 872–881, 2001.
171. Churg, A., and Warnock, M.L., Analysis of the cores of ferruginous (asbestos) bodies from the general population. I. Patients with and without lung cancer, *Lab. Investig.*, 37(3), 280–286, 1977.
172. Churg, A., and Warnock, M.L., Analysis of the cores of ferruginous (asbestos) bodies from the general population. III. Patients with environmental exposure, *Lab. Investig.*, 40(5), 622–626, 1979.
173. Churg, A., and Warnock, M.L., Correlation of quantitative asbestos body counts and Occupation in urban patients, *Arch. Pathol. Lab. Med.*, 101(12), 629–634, 1977.

174. Mollo, F., Magnani, C., Bo, P., Burlo, P., and Cravello, M., The attribution of lung cancers to asbestos exposure: A pathological study of 924 unselected cases, Anatom, *Pathologe*, 117, 90–95, 2002.
175. Dodson, R.F., Greenberg, S.D., Williams, M.G., Corn, C.J., O'Sullivan, M.F., and Hurst, G.A., Asbestos content in lungs of occupationally and nonoccupationally exposed individuals, *J. Am. Med. Assoc.*, 252(1), 68–71, 1984.
176. Breedin, P.H., and Buss, D.H., Ferruginous (asbestos) bodies in the lungs of rural dwellers, urban dwellers and patients with pulmonary neoplasms, *South. Med. J.*, 69(4), 401–404, 1976.
177. Roggli, V.L., Pratt, P.C., and Brody, A.R., Asbestos content of lung tissue in asbestos associated diseases: A study of 110 cases, *Br. J. Ind. Med.*, 43(1), 18–28, 1986.
178. Moulin, E., Yourassowsky, N., Dumortier, P., de Vuyst, P., and Yernault, J.C., Electron microscopic analysis of asbestos body cores from the Belgian urban population, *Eur. Respir. J.*, 1(9), 818–822, 1988.
179. Holden, J., and Churg, A., Asbestos bodies and the diagnosis of asbestosis in chrysotile workers, *Environ. Res.*, 39(1), 232–236, 1986.
180. Levin, J., O'Sullivan, M., Corn, C., Williams, M.G., and Dodson, R.F., Asbestosis and small cell lung cancer in a clutch refabricator, *Occup. Environ. Med.*, 56(9), 602–605, 1999.
181. Dodson, R.F., O'Sullivan, M., Corn, C., McLarty, J.W., and Hammar, S.P., Analysis of asbestos fiber burden in lung tissue from mesothelioma patients, *Ultrastruct. Pathol.*, 21(4), 321–336, 1997.
182. Dodson, R.F., O'Sullivan, M., Brooks, D.R., and Hammar, S.P., Quantitative analysis of asbestos burden in women with mesothelioma, *Am. J. Ind. Med.*, 43(2), 188–195, 2002.
183. Srebro, S.H., Roggli, V.L., and Samsa, G.P., Malignant mesothelioma associated with low pulmonary tissue asbestos burdens: A light and scanning electron microscopic analysis of 18 cases, *Mordern Pathol.*, 8(6), 614–621, 1995.
184. Dodson, R.F., Brooks, D.R., and O'Sullivan, M., Quantitative analysis of asbestos burden in a series of individuals with lung cancer and a history of exposure to asbestos, *Inhal. Toxicol.*, 16(9), 637–647, 2004.
185. Dodson, R.F., Williams, M.G., O'Sullivan, M.F., Corn, C.J., Greenberg, S.D., and Hurst, G.A., A comparison of the ferruginous body and uncoated fiber content in the lungs of former asbestos workers, *Am. Rev. Respir. Dis.*, 132(1), 143–147, 1985.
186. Warnock, M.L., and Wolery, G., Asbestos bodies or fibers and the diagnosis of asbestosis, *Environ. Res.*, 44(1), 29–44, 1987.
187. Ehrlich, A., Rohl, A.N., and Holstein, E.C., Asbestos bodies in carcinoma of colon in an insulation worker with asbestosis. *JAMA*, 254(20), 2932–2933, November 22/29, 1985.
188. Christensen, B.C., Houseman, E.A., Godleski, J.J., Marsit, C.J., Longacker, J.L., Roelofs, C.R., Karagas, M.R., Wrensch, M.R.Y.R.F., Nelson, H.H., Wiemels, J.L., Zheng, S., Wiencke, J.K., Bueno, R., Sugabarker, D.J., and Kelsey, K.T., Epigentic profiles distinguish pleural mesothelioma form normal pleura and predict lung asbestos burden and clinical outcome, *Cancer Res.*, 69: 227–233. 2009.
189. Morgan, A., and Holmes, A., The distribution and characteristics of asbestos fibers in the lungs of Finnish anthophyllite mine-workers, *Environ. Res.*, 33(1), 62–75, 1984.
190. Rood, A.P., and Streeter, R.R., Size distributions of occupational airborne asbestos textile fibres as determined by transmission electron microscopy, *Ann. Occup. Hyg.*, 28(3), 333–395, 1984.
191. Dodson, R.F., Williams, M.G., and Satterley, J.D., Asbestos burden in two cases of mesothelioma where the work history included manufacturing of cigarette filters, *J. Toxicol. Environ. Health A*, 65(16), 1109–1120, 2002.
192. Pooley, F.D., and Ranson, D.L., Comparison of the results of asbestos fibre dust counts in lung tissue obtained by analytical electron microscopy and light microscopy, *J. Clin. Pathol.*, 39(3), 313–317, 1986.
193. Dodson, R.F., Hammar, S.P., and Poye, L.W., A technical comparison of evaluating asbestos concentration by phase-contrast microscopy (PCM), Scanning Electron Microscopy (SEM), and Analytical Transmission Electron Microscopy (ATEM) as illustrated from data generated from a case report, *Inhal. Toxicol.*, 20(7), 723–732, 2008.
194. Dodson, R.F., and Atkinson, M.A.L., Measurements of asbestos burden in tissues, *Ann. N. Y. Acad. Sci.*, 1076, 281–291, 2006.
195. Langer, A.M., Chrysotile asbestos in the lungs of persons in New York City, *Arch. Environ. Health*, 22(3), 348–361, 1971.
196. Langer, A.M., and Nolan, R.P., Chrysotile biopersistence in the lungs of persons in the general population and exposed workers, *Environ. Health Perspect.*, 102 (Supplement 5), 235–239, 1994.
197. Egilman, D., Fehnel, C., and Bohme, S., Exposing the "myth" of ABC, "anything but chrysotile: A critique of the Canadian asbestos mining industry and McGill University chrysotile studies", *Am. J. Ind. Med.*, 44(5), 540–557, 2003.
198. Lindell, F.D.K., Magic, menace, myth and malice, *Ann. Occup. Hyg.*, 41(1), 3–12, 1997.

199. Addison, J., and Davies, L.S.T., Analysis of amphibole asbestos in chrysotile and other minerals, *Ann. Occup. Hyg.*, 34(2), 159–175, 1990.
200. McDonald, J.C., Armstrong, B.G., Edwards, C.W., et al., Case referent survey of young adults with mesothelioma: I. Lung fibre analysis, *Ann. Occup. Hyg.*, 45(7), 513–518, 2001.
201. Churg, A., Asbestos fiber content of the lungs in patients with and without asbestos airways disease, *Am. Rev. Respir. Dis.*, 127(4), 470–473, 1983.
202. Churg, A., Wright, J.L., and Vedal, S., Fiber burden and patterns of asbestos-related disease in chrysotile miners and millers, *Am. Rev. Respir. Dis.*, 148(1), 25–31, 1993.
203. Churg, A., Wright, J., Wiggs, B., and Depaoli, L., Mineralogic parameters related to amosite asbestos-induced fibrosis in humans, *Am. Rev. Respir. Dis.*, 142(6 Pt 1), 1331–1336, 1990.
204. McDonald, J.C., Armstrong, B., Case, B., Doell, D., McCaughey, W.T.E., McDonald, A.D., and Sebastien, P., Mesothelioma and asbestos fiber type-Evidence from lung tissue analysis, *Cancer*, 63(8), 1544–1547, 1989.
205. McDonald, J.C., Edwards, C.W., Gibbs, A.R., Lloyd, H.M., Pooley, F.D., Ross, D.J., and Rudd, R.M., Case-referent survey of young adults with mesothelioma: II occupational analysis, *Ann. Occup. Hyg.*, 45(7), 519–523, 2001.
206. Dufresne, A., Begin, R., Chrug, A., and Masse, S., Mineral fiber content of lungs in patients with mesothelioma seeking compensation in Quebec, *Am. J. Respir. Crit. Care Med.*, 153(2), 711–718, 1996.
207. Churg, A., and Vedal, S., Fiber burden and patterns of asbestos-related disease in workers with heavy mixed amosite and chrysotile exposure, *Am. J. Respir. Crit. Care Med.*, 150(3), 663–669, 1994.
208. Nayebzadeh, A., Dufresne, A., Case, C., et al., Lung mineral fibers of former miners and millers from Thetford-mines and asbestos regions: A comparative study of fiber concentration and dimension, *Arch. Environ. Health*, 56, 65–76, 2001.
209. Langer, A.M., and Nolan, R.P., Non-occupational exposure to mineral fibres, fibre type and burden in parenchymal tissues of workers occupationally exposed to asbestos in the United States, *IARC Sci. Pub.*, 90, 330–335, 1989.
210. Langer, A.M., and McCaughey, W.T.E., Mesothelioma in a brake repair worker, *The Lancet*, November 13, 1101–1103, 1982.
211. Pooley, F.D., Oldham, F.D., Chang-Hyum, U.M., and Wagner, J.C., The detection of asbestos in tissues, in Shirpio, H.A., ed. *Pnuemonoconiosis: Proceeding of 2nd International Conference (Johannesburg)*, Oxford University Press, London, pp. 108–116, 1970.
212. Srebro, S.H., and Roggli, V.L., Asbestos-related disease associated with exposure to asbestiform tremolite, *Am. J. Ind. Med.*, 26(6), 809–819, 1994.
213. Dodson, R.F., Graef, R., Shepherd, S., O'Sullivan, M., and Levin, J.L., Asbestos burden in cases of mesothelioma from individuals from various regions of the United States, *Ultrast Path*, 29, 415–433, 2005.
214. Churg, A., Wright, J.L., and Vedal, S., Fiber burden and patterns of asbestos-related disease in chrysotile miners and millers, *Am. Rev. Respir. Dis.*, 148(1), 25–31, 1993.
215. McDonald, J.C., and McDonald, A.D., Chrysotile, tremolite and mesothelioma: Letter published, *Science*, 267, 775–776, 1995.
216. Finkelstein, M.M., Asbestos fibre concentrations in the lungs of brake workers: Another look, *Ann. Occup. Hyg.*, 52(6), 455–461, 2008.
217. Case, B.W., Health effects of tremolite. The third wave of asbestos disease: Exposure to asbestos in place-public health control, *Ann. N. Y. Acad. Sci.*, 643, 491–504, 1991.
218. Case, B.W., On talc, tremolite, and tergiversation, *Br. J. Ind. Med.*, 48(5), 357–360, 1991.
219. Williams-Jones, A.E., Normand, C., Clark, J.R., Vali, H., Martin, R.F., Dufresne, A., and Nayebzadeh, A., Controls of amphibole formation in chrysotile deposits; evidence from the Jeffrey mine, asbestos, Quebec; The health effects of chrysotile asbestos: Contribution of science to risk-management decisions, *Can. Mineral. Spec Pub.*, 5, 89–194, 2001.
220. Langer, A.M., and Nolan, R.P., Chrysotile: Its occurrence and properties as variables controlling biological effects, *Ann. Occup. Hyg.*, 18(4), 427–431.
221. French Agency for Food, Opinion of the French agency for food, environmental and occupational health and safety on health effects and the identification of cleavage fragments of amphiboles from quarried minerals, in *Environmental and Occupational Health & Safety*. ANSES opinion, request No. 2014_SA_0196; Maison-alfort, pp. 1–14, December 4, 2015.
222. Warnock, M.L., and Isenberg, W., Asbestos burden and the pathology of lung cancer, *Chest*, 89(1), 20–26, 1986.

223. Sebastien, P., Jason, X., Gaudichet, A., Hirsch, A., and Bingnon, J., Asbestos retention in human respiratory tissues: Comparative measurements in lung parenchyma and in parietal pleura, in Wagner, J.C., ed. *Biological Effects of Mineral Fibers*, IARC, Lyon, pp. 237–246, 1980.
224. McDonald, J.C., McDonald, A.D., Armstrong, B., and Sebastien, P., Cohort study of mortality of vermiculite miners exposed to tremolite, *Br. J. Ind. Med.*, 43(7), 436–444, 1986.
225. Wright, R.S., Abraham, J.L., Harber, P., Burnett, B.R., Morris, P., and West, P., Fatal asbestosis 50 years after brief high intensity exposure in a vermiculite expansion plant, *Am. J. Respir. Crit. Care Med.*, 165(8), 1145–1149, 2002.
226. Meeker, G.P., Bern, A.M., Brownfield, I.K., Lowers, H.A., Sutley, S.J., Hoefen, T.M., and Vance, J.S., The composition and morphology of amphiboles from the rainy creek complex, near Libby, Montana, *Am. Mineral.*, 88(11–12), 1955–1969, 2003.
227. Black, B., Dodson, R.F., Bruce, J.R., Poye, L.W., and Henschke, C., Loewen; A clinical assessment and lung tissue burden from an individual who worked as a Libby vermiculite miner, *Inhal. Toxicol.*, 29(9), 404–413, 2017.
228. Antao, V.C., Larson, T.C., and Horton, D.K., Libby vermiculite exposure and risk Developing asbestos-related lung and pleural diseases, *Curr. Opin. Pulm. Med.*, 18(2), 161–167, 2012.
229. Kanark, M.S., and Liegel, J.C.O., Asbestos in talc and mesothelioma: Review of causality using epidemiology, *Med, Res.Arch.*, 8, 1–13, 2020.
230. Dodson, R.F., and Poye, L.W., Tissue burden evaluation of elongated mineral particles in two individuals with mesothelioma and whose work history included manufacturing tile, *Ultrastruct. Pathol.*, 44(1), 17–31, 2020.
231. Kleinfeld, M., Messite, J., and Langer, M., A study of workers exposed to asbestiform minerals in commercial talc manufacture, *Environ. Res.*, 6(2), 132–143, 1973.
232. Rohl, A.N., Langer, A.M., Selikoff, I., et al., Consumer talcums and powders: Mineral and chemical characterization, *J. Toxicol. Environ. Health*, 2(2), 255–284, 1976.
233. Hull, M.J., Abraham, J.L., and Case, B.W., Mesothelioma among workers in asbestos fiber-bearing mines in New York State, *Ann. Occup. Hyg.*, 1, 132–135, 2002.
234. Scancarello, G., Romeo, R., and Sartorelli, E., Respiratory disease as a result of talc inhalation, *J. Occup. Environ. Med.*, 38(6), 610–614, 1996.
235. Roggli, V.L., Vollmer, R.T., Butnor, K.J., and Sporn, T.A., Tremolite and mesothelioma, *Ann. Occup. Hyg.*, 46, 447–453, 2002.
236. Ghio, A.J., and Roggli, V., Talc should not be used for pleurodesis in patients with nonmalignant pleural effusions, *Am. J. Respir. Crit. Care Med.*, 164(9), 174–173, 2001.
237. IARC (International Agency for Research on Cancer), IARC monograph on the evaluation of the carcinogenic risk of chemicals to humans, *Carbon Black Titanium Talc*, 93, 278, 2006.
238. IARC, *Report of the Advisory Group to Review the Amended Preamble to the IARC Monographs*, International Agency for Research on Cancer, Lyon, 2006 Internal Report No.06/001.monographstest.iarc.fr/ENG/Preamble/Preamble-IntReport.pdf.
239. Kelse, J.W., Gamble, J.F., and Boehlecke, B.A., The occurrence of pneumoconiosis in a talc mining population exposed to non-asbestos elongated mineral particle, *J Epid, Prev. Med.*, 3(2), 128, 2017.
240. Kliment, C.R., Clemens, K., and Ory, T.D., North American erionite-associated mesothelioma with pleural plaques and pleural fibrosis: A case report, *Int. J. Clin. Exp. Pathol.*, 2(4), 407–410, 2009.
241. Telischi, M., and Rubenstone, A.I., Pulmonary asbestosis, *Arch. Pathol.*, 72, 116–125, 1961.
242. Langer, A.M., Inorganic particles in human tissues and their association with neoplastic disease, *Environ. Health Perspect.*, 9, 229–233, 1974.
243. Rosen, P., Gordon, P., Savino, A., and Melamed, M., Ferruginous bodies in benign fibrous pleural plaques, *Am. J. Clin. Pathol.*, 60(5), 608–617, 1980.
244. Churg, A., and Green, F.H.Y., Quantitative assessment of asbestos bodies from lung tissue, in Churg, A., and Green, F.H.Y., eds. *Pathology of Occupational Lung Disease*, Igaku-Shoin, New York, pp. 385–386, 1988.
245. Knudson, A., Asbestos and mesothelioma: Genetic lessons from a tragedy, *Proc. Natl Acad. Sci. USA.*, 92(24), 10819–10820, 1995.
246. Dodson, R.F., Huang, J., and Bruce, J.R., Asbestos content in the lymph nodes of nonoccupationally exposed individuals, *Am. J. Ind. Med.*, 37(2), 169–174, 2000.
247. Suzuki, Y., and Yuen, S.R., Asbestos tissue burden study on human malignant mesothelioma, *Ind. Health*, 39(2), 150–160, 2001.
248. Suzuki, Y., and Yuen, S.R., Asbestos fibers contributing to the induction of human malignant mesothelioma, *Ann. N. Y. Acad. Sci.*, 1, 1–14, 2002.

249. Suzuki, Y., Yuen, S.R., and Short, A.R., Thin asbestos fibers contribute to the development of human malignant mesothelioma: pathological evidence, *Int. J. Hyg. Environ. Health*, 208(3), 201–210, 2005.
250. Tweedale, G., and McCulloch, J., Chrysotile versus Chrysophobes-the white asbestos controversy, 1950-2004 Isis overview of Chrysophiles versus Chrysophobes, *The Hist. Sci. Soc.*, 95, 239–259, 2004.
251. Kamp, D.W., and Weitzman, S.A., The molecular basis of asbestos induced lung injury, *Thorax*, 54(7), 638–652, 1999.
252. Boutin, C., Dumortier, R.F., Viallat, J.R., and De Vuyst, P., Black spots concentrate oncogenic asbestos fibers in the parietal pleural-Thoracospic and mineral study, *Am. J. Respir. Crit. Care Med.*, 153, 444–449, 1996.
253. LeBouffant, L., Physics and chemistry of asbestos dust, in Wagner, J.C., ed. *Biological Effects of Mineral Fibres*, IARC Scientific Publications, Lyon, France, pp. 15–33, 1980.
254. Kohyama, N., and Suzuki, Y., Analysis of asbestos fibes in lung parenchyma, pleural plaques, and mesothelioma tissues of North American insulation workers, *Ann. N. Y. Acad. Sci.*, 643(1), 27–52, 1991.
255. Muller, K-M., Schmitz, I., and Konstantinidis, K., Black spots of the parietal pleura: Morphology and formal pathogenesis, *Respiration*, 69, 261–267, 2002.
256. Mitchev, K., Dumortier, P., and DeVuyst, P., "Black Spots" and hyaline pleural plaques on the parietal pleura of 150 urban necropsy cases, *Am. J. Surg. Pathol.*, 25(9), 1198–1206, 2002.
257. Miserocchi, G., Sancini, G., Mantegazza, F., and Chiappino, G., Translocation pathways for inhaled asbestos fibers-A. Review, *Environ. Health*, 7(1), 2008.
258. Hasanoglu, H.C., Bayram, E., Hasanoglu, A., and Demirag, F., Orally ingested chrysotile asbestos affects rat lungs and pleura, *Arch. Env. Occ Health*, 63(2), 71–75, 2008.
259. Monchaux, G., Bignon, J., Hirsch, A., and Sebastien, P., Translocation of mineral fibres through the respiratory system after injection into the pleural cavity of rats, *Ann. Occup. Hyg.*, 26(1–4), 309–318, 1982.
260. Lauweryns, J.M., and Baert, J.H., State of the art. Alveolar clearance and the role of the pulmonary lymphatics, *Am. Rev. Respir. Dis.*, 115(4), 625–683, 1977.
261. Uibu, T., Vanhala, E., Sajantila, A., Lunetta, P., Makela-Bengs, P., Goebeler, S., Jantti, M., and Tossavainen, A., Asbestos fibers in para-aortic and mesenteric lymph nodes, *Am. J. Ind. Med.*, 52(6), 464–470, 2009.
262. Stanton, M.F., and Wrench, C., Mechanisms of mesothelioma induction with asbestos and fibrous glass, *J. Natl Cancer Inst.*, 48(3), 797–821, 1972.
263. Stanton, M.F., Layard, M., Tegeris, E., et al., Relation of particle dimension to carcinogenicity in amphibole asbestoses and other fibrous minerals, *J. Natl Cancer Inst.*, 67(5), 965, 1981.
264. Pott, F., Problems in defining carcinogenic fibres, *Ann. Occup. Hyg.*, 31(4B), 799–802, 1987.
265. Pott, F., Ziem, U., Reiffer, F.J., Huth, F., Ernst, H., and Mohr, U., Carcinogenicity studies on fibres, metal compounds, and some other dusts in rats, *Exp. Pathol.*, 32(3), 129–152, 1987.
266. Pott, F., Roller, M., Ziem, U., et al., Carcinogenicity studies on natural and man-made fibres with the intraperitoneal test in rats, Symposium on Mineral. Fibres in the Non-occupational Environment, Lyon, September 8–10, 1987, Lyon, 1–4(90), 1988.
267. Pott, F., Huth, F., and Friedrichs, K.H., Tumorigenic effect of fibrous dusts in experimental animals, *Environ. Health Perspect.*, 9, 313–315, 1974.
268. Aust, A.E., Cook, P.M., and Dodson, R.F., Morphological and chemical mechanisms of elongated mineral particle toxicities, *J. Toxicol. Environ. Health Part B Crit. Rev.*, 14(1–4), 40–75, 2011.
269. Fraire, A.E., Greenberg, S.D., Spjut, H.J., et al., Effect of fibrous glass on rat pleural mesothelium, *Am. J. Respir. Crit. Care Med.*, 1509, 521–527, 1994.
270. Goodglick, L.A., and Kane, A.B., Cytotoxicity of long and short crocidolite sbestos fibers in vitro and in vivo, *Cancer Res.*, 50(16), 5153–5163, 1990.
271. Lippmann, M., Review: Asbestos exposure indices, *Environ. Res.*, 46(1), 86–106, 1988.
272. Robinson, B.W.S., Musk, A.W., and Lake, R.A., Seminar-Malignant Mesothelioma, *The Lancet* 366(9483), 397–408, July 30, 2005.
273. Chen, H.C., Tsai, K.B., Wang, C.S., Hsieh, T.J., and Hsu, J.S., Duodenal Metastasis of malignant Pleural mesothelioma, *J. Formos. Med. Assoc.*, 107(12), 961–964, 2008.
274. Hammar,S.P., Macroscopic, histological, histochemical, immunohistochemical, and ultrastructual features of mesothelioma, *Ultrastruct. Pathol.*, 30(1), 3–17, 2006.
275. Mark, E.J., and Yokoi, T., *Absence of Evidence for a Significant Background Incidence of Diffuse Malignant Mesothelioma Apart from Asbestos Exposure. Part 8. The Neoplasms of Asbestos Exposure; the Third Wave of Asbestos Diseases: Exposure to Asbestos in Place-Public Health Control*, The New York Academy of Sciences, New York, NY, vol. 643, pp. 196–204, 1991.

276. Nishikawa, K., Takahashi, K., Karjalainen, A., Wen, C-P., Furuya, S., Hoshuyama, T., Todoroki, M., Kiyomoto, Y., Wilson, D., Higashi, T., Ohtaki, M., Pan, G., and Wagner, G., Recent mortality from pleural mesothelioma, historical patterns of asbestos use, and adoption of bans: A global assessment, *Environ. Health Prespect.*, 116, 1675–1680, 2008.
277. Magnani, C., Agudo, A., Gonzalez, C.A., Andrion, A., Calleja, A., Chellini, E., Dalmasso, P., Escolar, A., Hernandez, S., Ivaldi, C., Mirabelli, D. Ramirez, J., Turuguet, D., Usei, M., and Terracini, B., Multicentric study on malignant pleural mesothelioma and non-occupational exposure to asbestos, 83(1), 104–111, 2000.
278. Kurumatani, N., and Kumagal, S., Mapping the risk of mesothelioma due to neighborhood asbestos exposure, *Am. J. Respir. Crit. Care Med.*, 178(6), 624–629, 2008.
279. Goldberg, M., and Luce, D., The health impact of nonoccupational exposure to asbestos: What do we know?, *Eur. J. Cancer Prev.*, 18(6), 489–503, 2009.
280. Carbone, M., Baris, Y.I., Bertino, P., Brass, B., Comertpay, S., Dogan, A.U., Gaudino, G., Jube, S., Kanodia, S., Partridge, C.R., Pass, H.I., Rivera, Z.S., Steele, I., Tuncer, M., Way, S., Yang, H., and Miller, A., Erionite exposure in North Dakota and Turkish villages with mesothelioma, *PNAS*, 108(33), 13618–13623, 2011.
281. Henderson, D., Rantanen, J., Barhart, S, Dement, J.M., DeVuyst, P., Hillerdal, G., Huuskonen, M.S., Kivisaari, L., Kusaka, Y., Lahdensuo, A., Langard, S., Mowe, G., Okubo, T., Parker, J.E., Roggli, V.L., Rodelsperger, K., Rosler, J., Tossavainen, A., and Woitowitz, J., Asbestos, asbestosis, and cancer: The Helsinki criteria for diagnosis and attribution, *Scand. J. Work Environ. Health*, 23(4), 311–316, 1997.
282. Editorial, Lancet, *Asbestos-Relat. Dis. Preventable Burden*, 371, 2009, 1927.
283. Attfield, M.D., Bang, K.M., Petsonk, E.L., Schleiff, P.L., and Mazurek, J.M., Trends in pneumoconiosis mortality and morbidity for the United States, 1968–2005, and relationship with indicators of extent of exposure, Inhaled Particulates X, *J. Phys. Conf. S.*, 151, 2009.
284. Anonymous, *Morbidity and Mortality Weekly Report*, Centers for Disease Control, No. 15, Malignant Mesothelioma Mortality, pp. 1990–2005, April 24, 2009.
285. Mazurek, J.M., Blackley, D.J., and Weissman, D.N., Morbidity and mortality Weekley report, 71(19), 645–649, May 13, 2022.
286. Galson, S.K., *Statement from Acting Surgeon General Steven K. Galson about National Asbestos Week*, Office of the Surgeon General, April 1, 2009.
287. Leigh, J., Davidson, P., Hendrie, L., and Berry, D., Malignant mesothelioma in Australia, 1945–2000, *Am. J. Ind. Med.*, 41(3), 188–201, 2002.

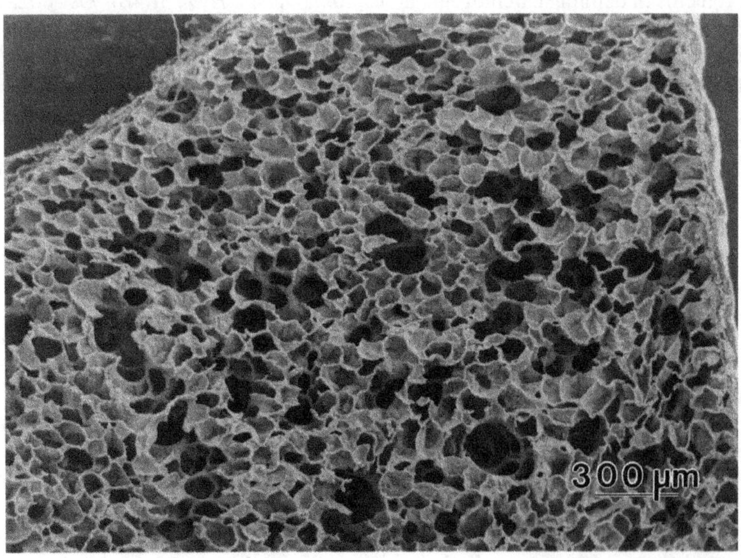

FIGURE 3.1 The lung parenchyma as seen in this lower magnification scanning electron micrograph shows the three-dimensional morphology of the alveoli, smaller airways, and associated circulatory components that result in the lung appearing to be comprised of small sac-like structures.

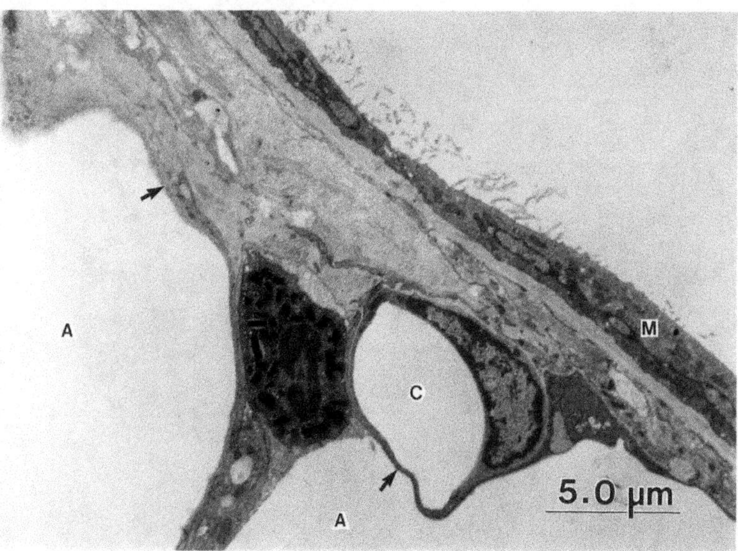

FIGURE 3.2 This low-magnification transmission electron micrograph shows the thin visceral pleura surface consisting of a layer of mesothelial cells (M). The alveoli (A) are lined by type I (arrow) and type II pneumocytes. A cross section through an interstitial capillary (C) shows the close association between the vascular space and the alveolar spaces.

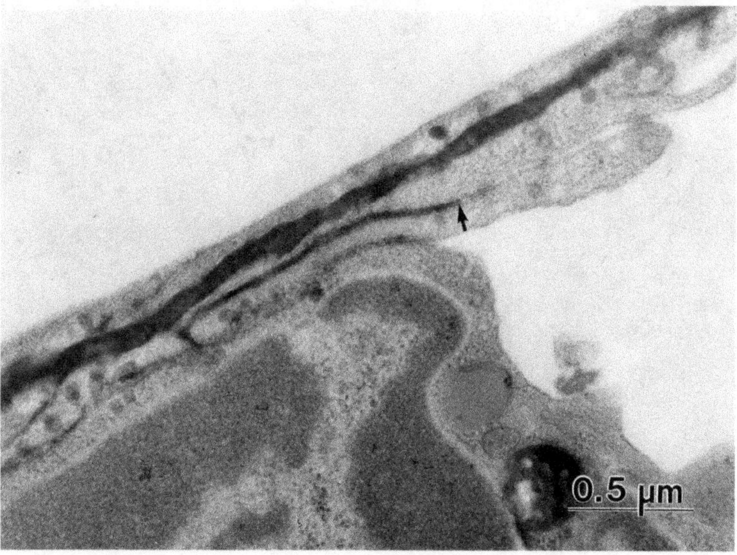

FIGURE 3.3 This transmission electron micrograph shows the boundaries of the alveolar-air/blood barrier. The dark material illustrates the penetration of the tracer horseradish peroxidase to the level of the junctions between the alveolar cells (arrow) that prevents its leakage into the airway.

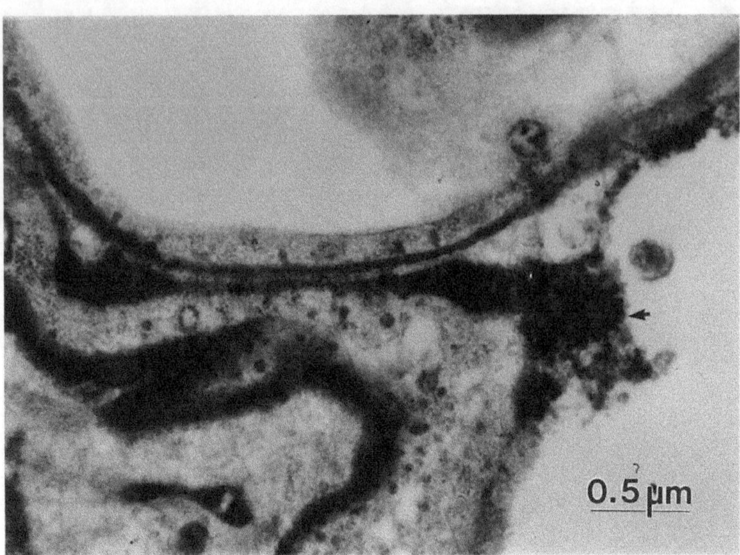

FIGURE 3.4 In contrast with the micrograph shown in Figure 3.3, the air-blood barrier in this section from an experimental animal model shows the leakage of horseradish peroxidase (arrow) through the barrier onto the surface of the alveolar sac. The change was induced as an early response to asbestos exposure.

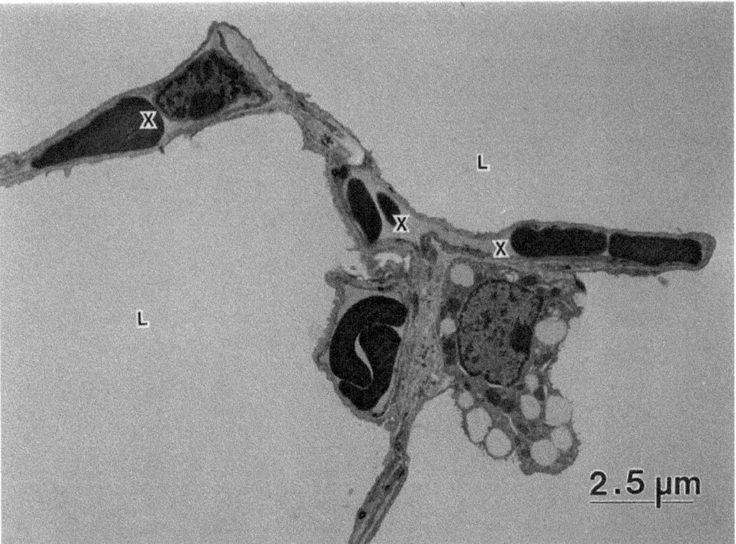

FIGURE 3.5 The delicate architecture of the alveolar level is shown in this transmission electron micrograph. The thin cellular separation between the blood compartment-capillary (X) and the air compartment of the alveoli (L) is shown in this micrograph.

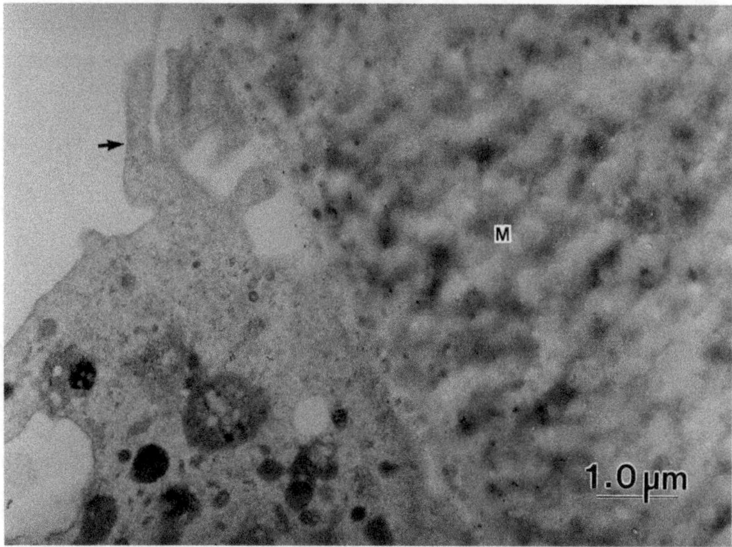

FIGURE 3.6 This micrograph illustrates the cross-section of an activated macrophage that has been cultured on medium (M). The stimulated macrophage shows surface projections (arrow) that extend from the cell surface and provide the mechanism by which the cells move toward a stimulus either on culture medium or in tissue.

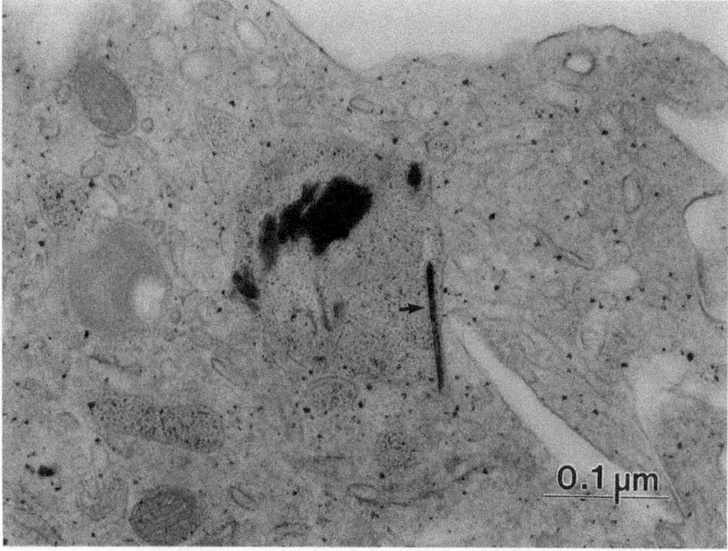

FIGURE 3.7 This small amosite fiber (arrow) in this transmission electron micrograph is being isolated within a sidersome of a macrophage.

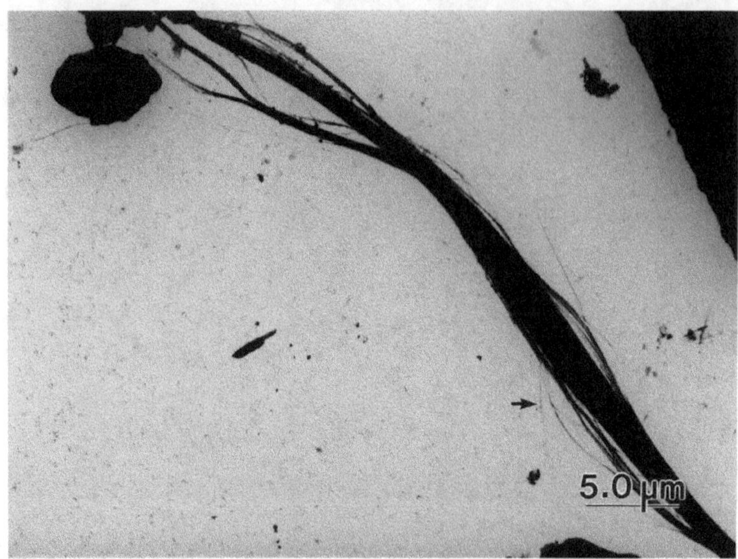

FIGURE 3.8 The large bundle of chrysotile fibers was obtained from digested lung tissue of a chrysotile miner. The curved morphology of the chrysotile is evident even in this large bundle. There are number of areas on the bundle which show the fraying characteristic that can result in separation into smaller/thinner units including separation to the fibrillar level . (Tissue provided courtesy of Dr. Andrew Churg).

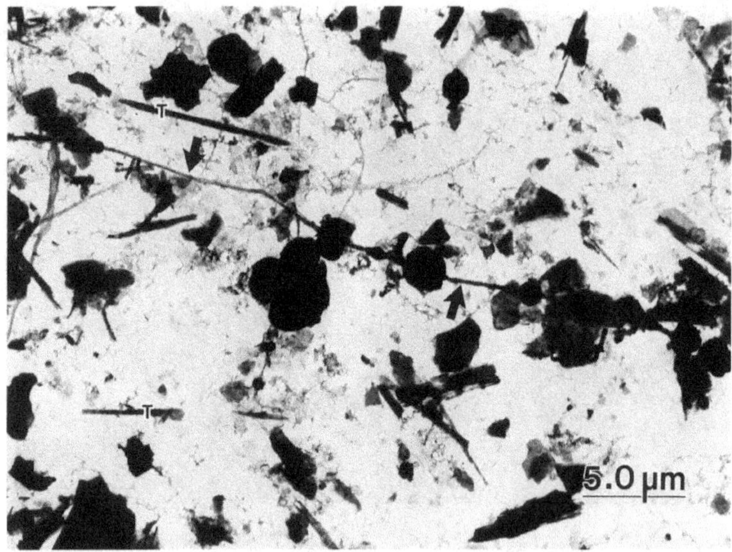

FIGURE 3.9 The long chrysotile cored asbestos body shown in the center of the photograph (arrow) illustrates tendencies in several areas for a curvature to occur in the fiber. This contrasts with the straight fibers seen as uncoated tremolite asbestos (T) within the field. This tissue sample was from an individual who had been a chrysotile asbestos miner exposed to both chrysotile and tremolite in their work environment. (Material courtesy of Dr. Andrew Churg).

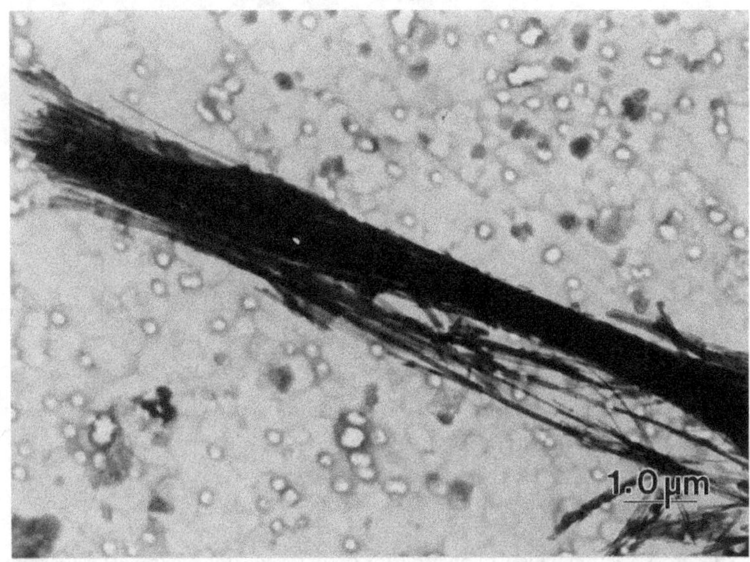

FIGURE 3.10 This bundle of chrysotile asbestos was isolated by digestion techniques from an occupationally exposed individual. The disassociation of the bundle into smaller units including fibrils is evident in the micrograph.

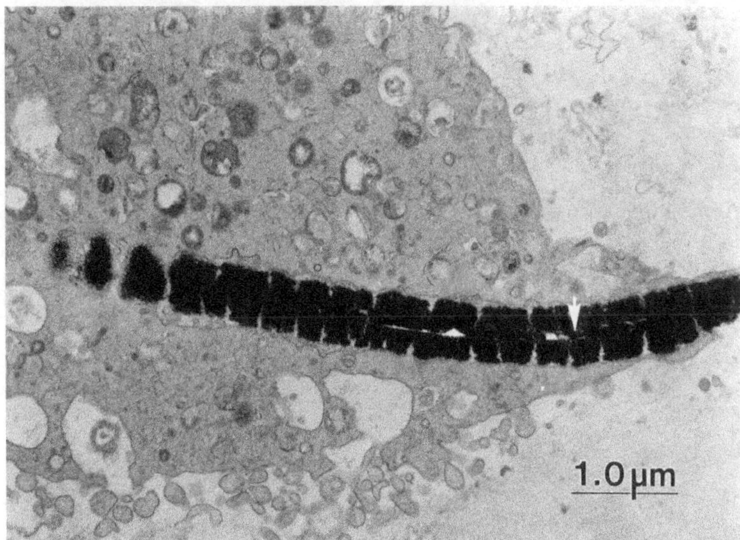

FIGURE 3.11 The section of the asbestos body seen in this field is surrounded by a macrophage. The asbestos fiber is in the center of the asbestos body (arrow) is surrounded by the iron-protein coat deposited through surface interactions with reactive macrophages.

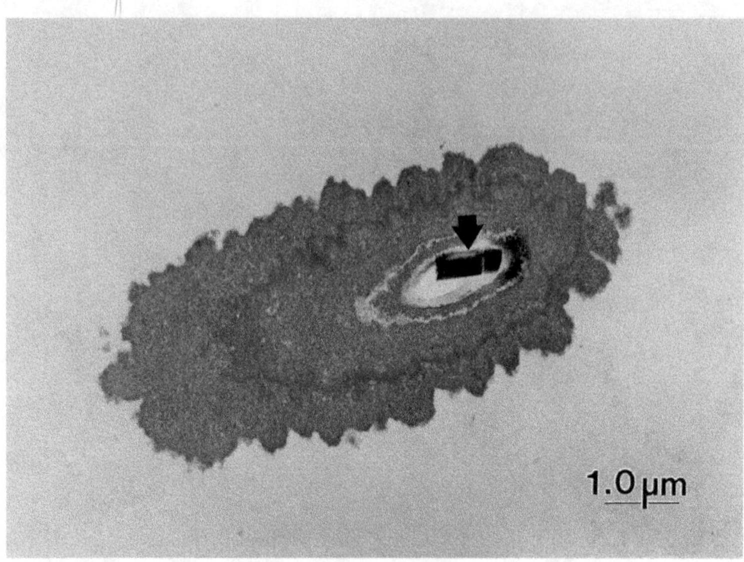

FIGURE 3.12 This cross-sectional view of an asbestos body reveals the central asbestos core (arrow) as surrounded by layers of iron-rich coating.

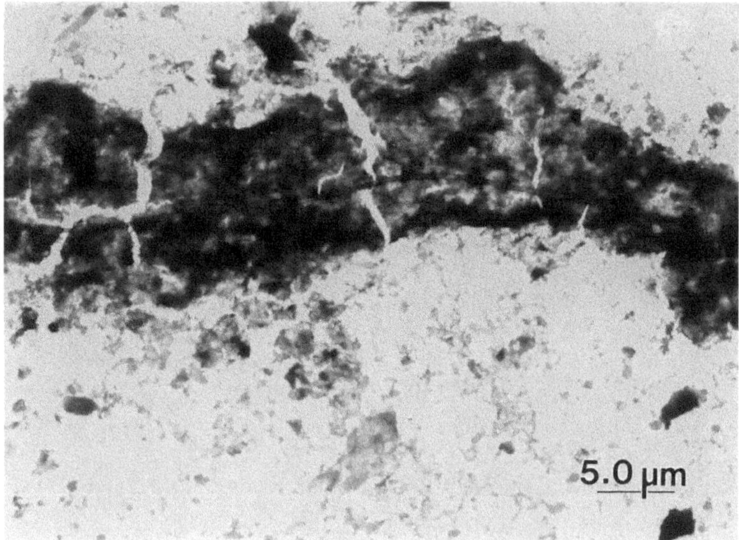

FIGURE 3.13 The ferruginous body seen in this field is formed on an iron-rich fiber as shown as a black rod in center of the structure.

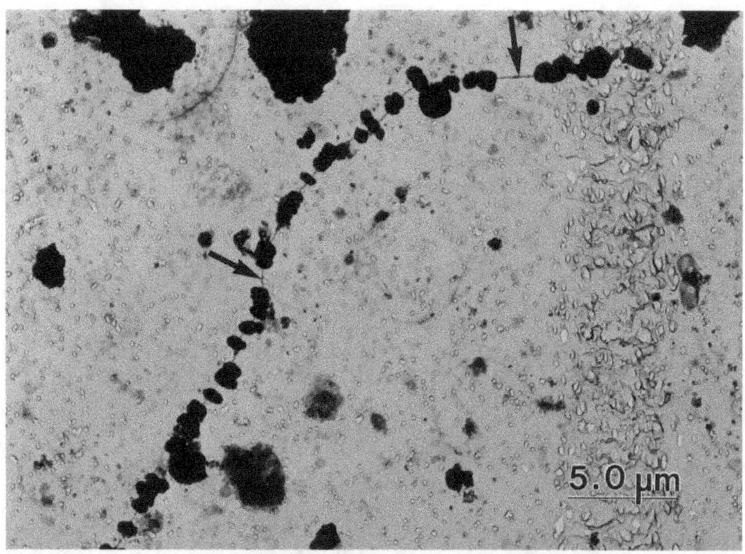

FIGURE 3.14 The core of this ferruginous body is formed on a graphite (organic) filament (arrow).

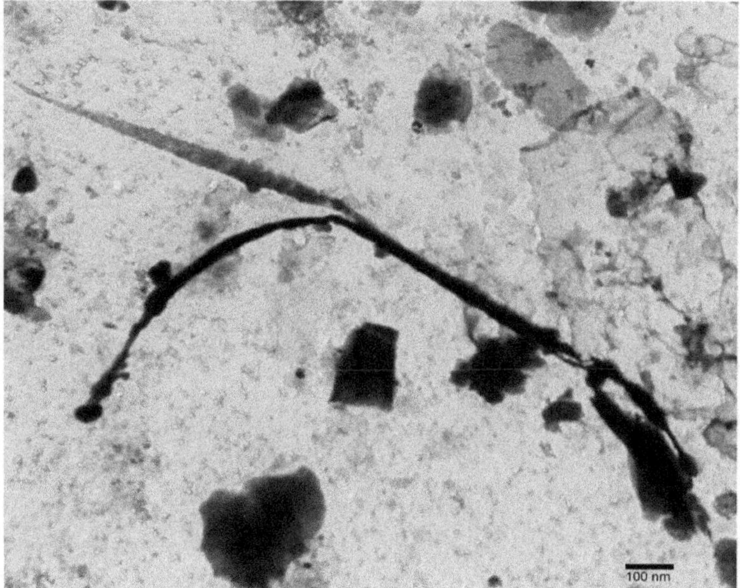

FIGURE 3.15 The core of this ferruginous body is a talc ribbon. Small deposits of coating material are evident at several areas along the central core.

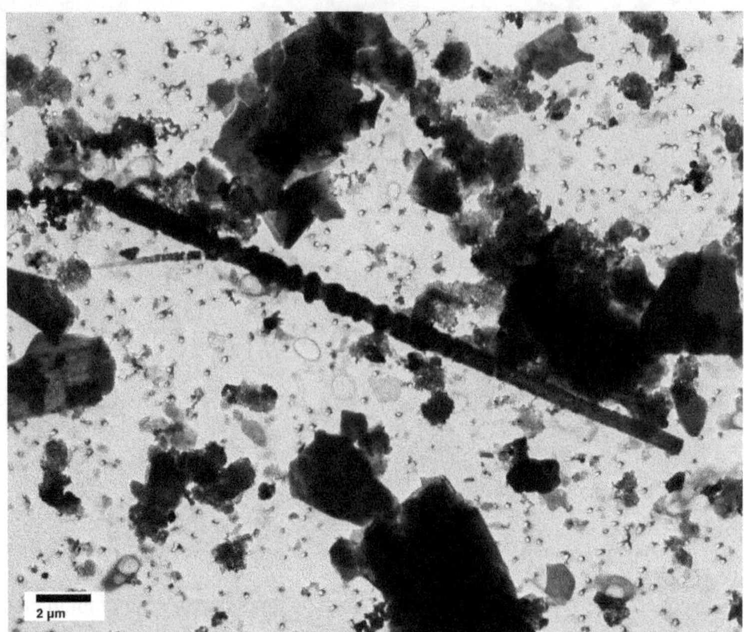

FIGURE 3.16 This ferruginous body was formed on a talc "transitional" fiber. This designation denotes those areas of the fiber display features consistent with anthophyllite asbestos and others with features of talc.

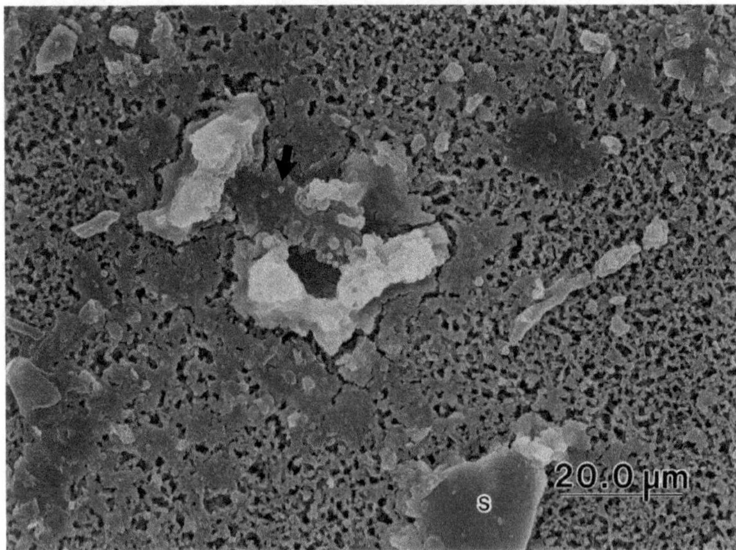

FIGURE 3.17 The ferruginous bodies seen in this scanning electron micrograph indicate that ferruginous coatings can occur on nonfibrous dusts. One of the bodies was formed on a central core of a thick rectangular dust particle at the top center of the micrograph, while the second ferruginous body was formed on a "plate-like" silicate (S) particle.

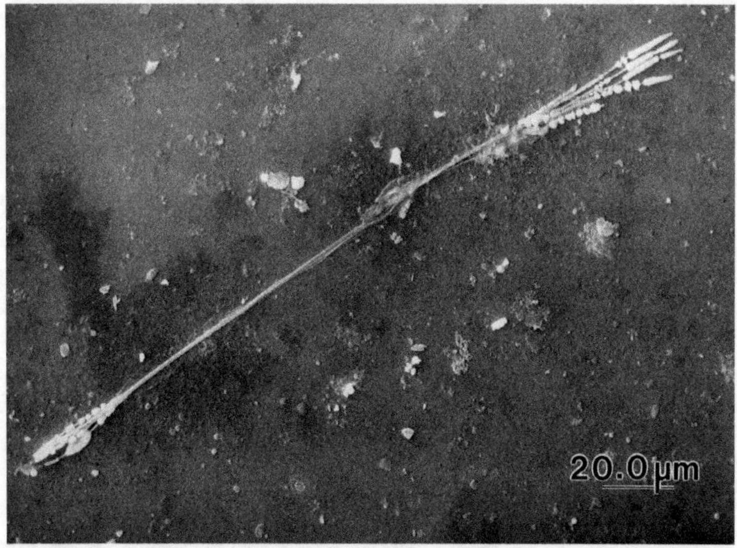

FIGURE 3.18 Although chrysotile-cored ferruginous bodies are less common than those formed on amphibole cores, when longer fibers of chrysotile are inhaled the formation on such cores can occur as indicated in this micrograph. The beaded material representing the ferruginous coating is primarily located on the frayed ends of the fibers.

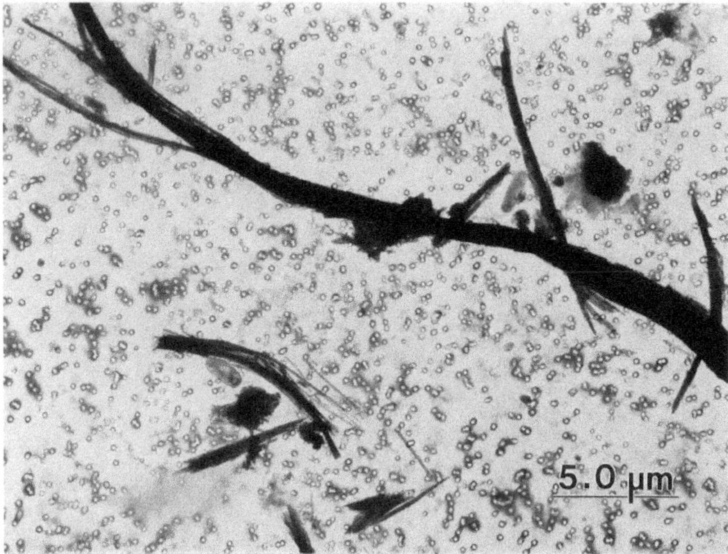

FIGURE 3.19 Bundles of chrysotile asbestos obtained from new brake components are shown in this field. The tendency is evident for the bundles to disassociate into smaller and smaller units, which indicate the potential that many of these units would be below the level of detection in the light microscope analysis of air samples.

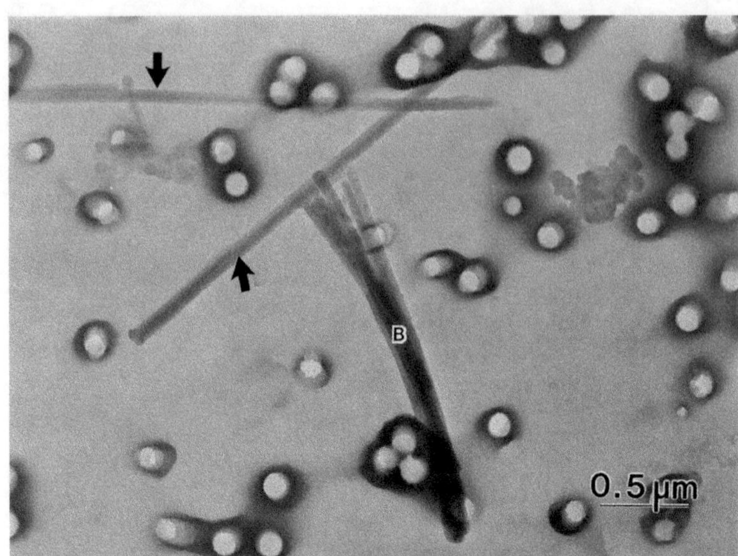

FIGURE 3.20 Neither the fibrils (arrows) of chrysotile asbestos nor the bundle (B) of chrysotile isolated from tissue would have been counted in a typical phase-contrast light microscope counting scheme. The former due to the fact that the fibrils are too thin to be detected in the light microscope and the latter in that the bundle is shorter than the 5 μm length included in 7400 count scheme of "fibers." This provides an example of the problems of interpreting environmental exposures or tissue burdens when large populations of fibers are excluded due to the limits of the count scheme or the magnification/resolution of the instrument of choice.

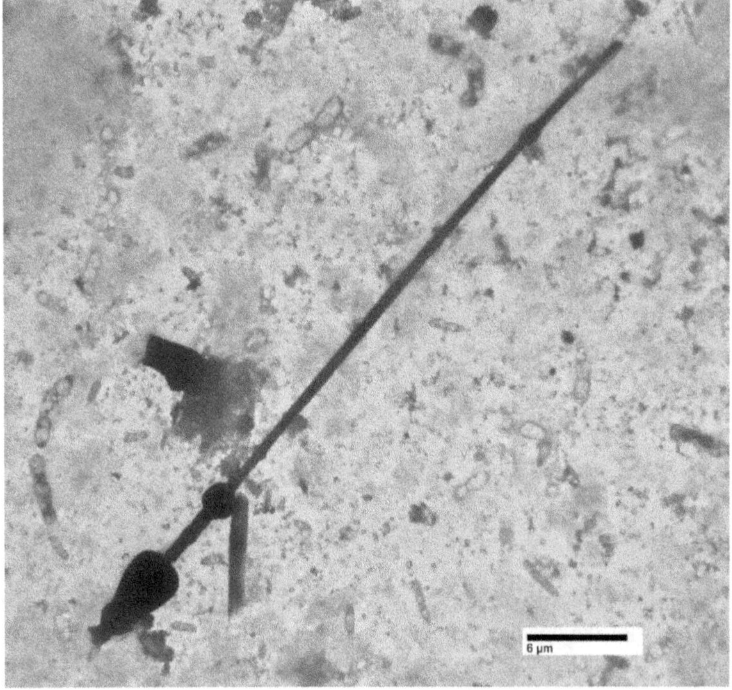

FIGURE 3.21 The core of this ferruginous body is a "Libby amphibole." The fibrous component of this vermiculite consists of winchite/richterite which are sodium-calcium amphiboles reported to comprise up to 80% of the elongated minerals within the vermiculite. The structure is consistent with asbestos cored ferruginous bodies, but this type of fiber is not presently listed as one of the six regulated fibrous forms of minerals in the USA despite being asbestiform in habit and inducing asbestos-related disease once inhaled.

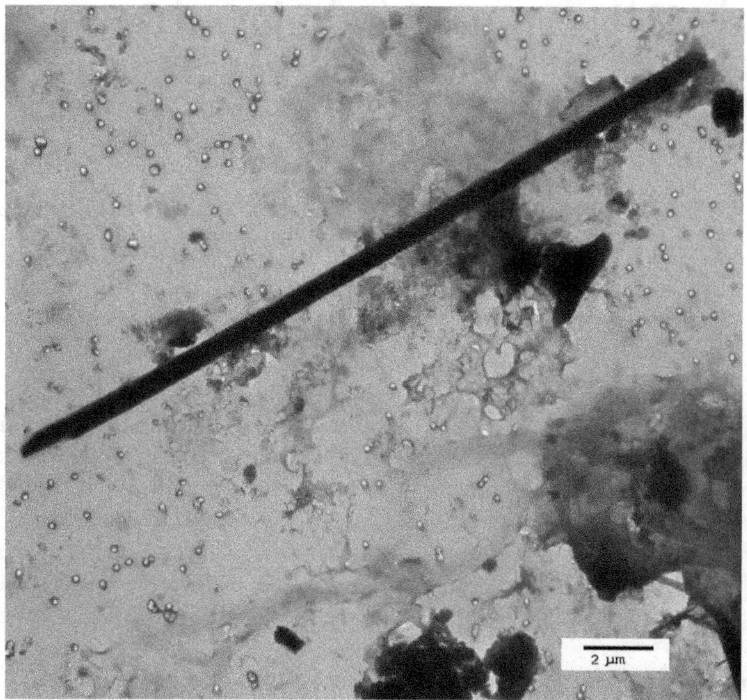

FIGURE 3.22 The erionite fiber found in this micrograph was collected from the digestate of lung tissue from an individual who grew up where erionite was a component of the environment.

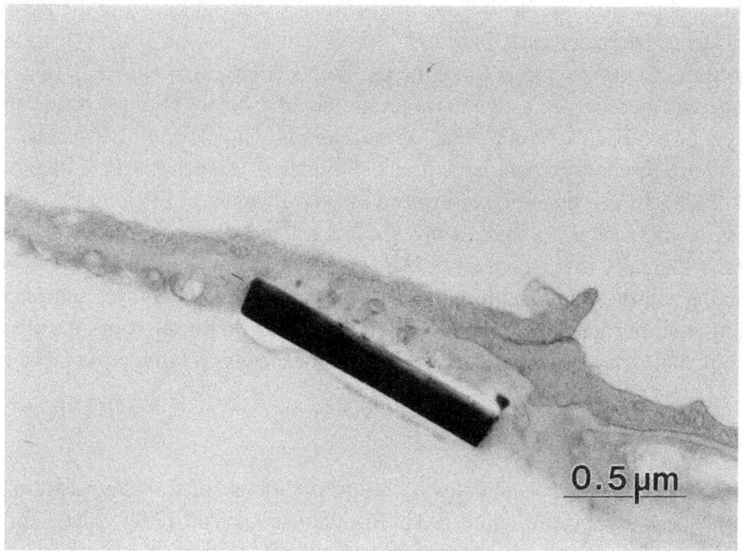

FIGURE 3.23 The short amosite fiber shown in this field is within the cytoplasm of a lining cell. Such "short" fibers in dividing cells create a physical challenge to proper cell division.

4 Evaluation of Asbestos Exposure

Silvia Damiana Visonà, Barbara Bertoglio, Cristina Favaron, Silvana Capella, Elena Belluso, Chandra Bortolotto, Alessandra Marrocco, and Claudio Colosio

Although malignant mesothelioma (MM) is well known to be associated with asbestos, not all cases of MM are attributable to a previous asbestos exposure. Other causes such as exposure to other mineral fibers, radiation, and chronic inflammation have been recently reviewed (Attanoos et al. 2018; Jasani and Gibbs 2012). Moreover, in some genetically predisposed individuals MM can occur as a consequence of asbestos exposures below background (Carbone et al. 2019). Due to the current restrictions or ban of asbestos use in most developed countries, and the decreasing of occupationally exposed individuals, the percentage of MM not related to asbestos has been reported to be increasing (Roggli et al. 2023). In this context, the causal attribution of MM is becoming more difficult.

Causal attribution of other asbestos-related diseases, such as lung cancer and lung fibrosis, is even more complicated, as in most cases they are not asbestos-related and many other factors are known to contribute in causing them, such as exposure to other dusts and cigarette smoking.

In the evaluation of single cases, rather than populations or cohorts, histories of exposure are of limited value, as patients may not know about past exposures or have forgotten them, for example in case of short occupational exposures or non-occupational ones related to leisure activities. On the other hand, some people might refer to exposure to "dust," without knowing the asbestos content of that particular dust (Carbone et al. 2023).

Pleural plaques (PP), lung fibrosis ferruginous bodies (FBs), and, above all, asbestos burden in lung tissue are generally regarded as the main predictors of asbestos etiology of the abovementioned diseases (Roggli et al. 2023). About 90% of individuals who develop MM and whose asbestos lung burden is above the background have medical evidence of such markers of asbestos exposure (Carbone et al. 2023). In this chapter, we explore the significance of PP, lung fibrosis, and FBs, and their usefulness in the causal attribution of asbestos-related diseases to past asbestos exposures, which is crucial, especially in the context of litigations for compensation purposes. We are going to focus, in particular, on the relationship between the presence of the abovementioned markers and the asbestos lung fiber burden determined by analytical electron microscopy. We also deepen imaging and pathological diagnostic issues that are crucial for the correct diagnosis of PP and asbestosis.

4.1 PLEURAL PLAQUES

The term "**pleural plaque**" (PP) indicates a benign pathology of the pleural lining known to be associated with asbestos exposure since 1933 (Roodhouse Gloyne 1933), when, for the first time, hyaline formations were observed at autopsy in patients affected from asbestosis. PP are a marker of previous exposure (Clarke et al. 2006), retention and biological response to asbestos or erionite fibers (Broaddus et al. 2011). PP are believed to be the most common non-malignant asbestos-related conditions (Maxim, Niebo, and Utell 2015; Van Cleemput et al. 2001). They occur typically more than 20 years after the beginning of asbestos exposure (Norbet et al. 2015; Broaddus et al. 2011; Myers 2012). There is no consensus in literature about the exact latency period of PP, that

 DOI: 10.1201/9781003431909-4

has been reported to be between 15 and 40 years (Maxim, Niebo, and Utell 2015), even though some authors reported a latency as short as 8.6 years for PP occurred as a consequence of Libby amphibole inhalation (Larson et al. 2010). However, Libby amphibole, compared to other kinds of asbestos, is known to be highly toxic for pleural tissue (Broaddus et al. 2011).

From a clinical point of view, traditionally they are not associated with any functional impairment (Clarke et al. 2006); recent evidence suggests, instead, that PP, if of remarkable dimensions, can cause restrictive lung functional alterations, such as a decrease of total lung capacity, of forced expiratory volume in 1 sec and forced vital capacity (Clin et al. 2011).

PP must be distinguished from the other asbestos-related pleural benign conditions, especially pleural effusion and diffuse pleural thickening.

Pleural effusions are inflammatory manifestations characterized by a mixed cellularity (they are usually exudative, often hemorrhagic and eosinophilic) (Norbet et al. 2015). They can occur early (in the first 10–20 years) after asbestos exposure and may represent the first manifestation of a malignant mesothelioma (Norbet et al. 2015). The pleural effusion is not specifically related to asbestos exposure, but it can be due to pneumonia, tuberculosis, connective tissue diseases, and many other conditions. Asbestos pleuritis and benign asbestos pleural effusion (BAPE) can be recognized at imaging by the presence of pleural effusion associated with exposure to asbestos and exclusion of other causes (e.g., cardiopulmonary). It tends to have a chronic course and it can be recognized both by X-ray and computed tomography/high-resolution computed tomography (CT/HRCT). CT/HRCT also allows the definition of the density of the effusion, which can be fluid or sovrafluid. Some authors state that benign pleural effusion from asbestos pleuritis may be part of the pathogenic pathway of the diffuse pleural thickening after the reabsorption of the fluid (al Jarad et al. 1991).

Diffuse pleural thickening, also called diffuse pleural fibrosis, is a relatively common condition that can occur as a consequence of asbestos exposure, although less commonly than PP. Microscopically it is similar to a plaque, but it is more extended (usually more than four rib spaces) and typically begins in the visceral pleura (Figure 4.1).

As a consequence of progressive fibrosis, both visceral and parietal pleura can be involved (Schwartz 1991), in that case the adhesion between the two layers of the pleura can cause functional restrictive impairment (Norbet et al. 2015; Schwartz 1991; Myers 2012). Unlike PP, it rarely calcifies. It is believed that diffuse pleural thickening is related to the amount of asbestos exposure, but it is less specific than PP, as can be observed in multiple other conditions, such as fibrothorax, empyema, mesothelioma, and metastatic disease (Norbet et al. 2015). Diffuse pleural thickening, unlike PP, commonly extends into the costophrenic angle, and is usually unilateral. The pathogenesis of this manifestation is poorly understood and it was proposed that it represents an extension of lung fibrosis to pleural cavity (Schwartz 1991). From a radiological point of view, pleural thickening is generally regarded as a thickening of at least 3 mm which makes costophrenic angles more round/blunt. The ILO classification identifies with numbers (Mazzei et al. 2017; Aberle et al. 1988; Gamsu, Aberle, and Lynch 1989; Elshazley et al. 2011) the extent of the involvement on the lateral aspect of the lung on a chest X-ray and with letters (A, B, C) the thickness of the diffuse pleural thickening (International Labour Organization 2022).

4.1.1 Pathology

PP are located in the parietal pleura, usually bilaterally (Clarke et al. 2006; Norbet et al. 2015). They are described macroscopically as discrete, raised, irregularly shaped, smooth or finely nodular areas of grayish-white to ivory white color, most frequently located in the posterior or lower half of the thorax. They can be easily stripped away from the costal wall, while they are adherent to the diaphragm. They are often calcified (Figure 4.2).

Histologically, they are characterized by dense bands of avascular collagen and pseudoelastic tissue (the latter stained black as for elastic tissue in Verhoeff-van Gieson). The plaques are mostly acellular and only occasional fibroblasts were found (Roberts 1971). In PP abundant asbestos fibers have been found, but no FBs (Roberts 1971; Norbet et al. 2015).

4.1.2 Pathogenesis

It has been proposed that the pathogenesis of PP may be related to the abrasive action of the point of asbestos fibers, anchored in visceral pleural tissue and protruding in the pleural space, that produces continuous scratching and consequent inflammation, fibrinous exudation and then fibrosis and calcification due to the poor vascularization of the PP (Roberts 1971). This theory, not supported by pathological data, never gained wide consensus (Schwartz 1991; Hillerdal 1980).

On the basis of the existing literature, it seems that the translocation of asbestos fibers from airways to the pleural space is crucial to explain both the benign pleural manifestations and the mesothelial carcinogenesis induced by asbestos, as well as the exceptionally long latency between the exposure and the onset of the diseases. After the inhalation of long and thin asbestos fibers, macrophages in the alveoli try to phagocyte them in order to digest the fibers or to bring them to the lymph nodes for disposal. As most asbestos fibers are too long and needle-like (especially amphiboles[1]), macrophages' membranes are disrupted and cells are killed. Moreover, the "frustrated phagocytosis" stimulates the production of reactive oxygen species and inflammatory cytokines. This process is repeated many times until asbestos reaches the pleural cavity due to the lymphatic flow according to the negative pressure in the pleural cavity (Toyokuni 2019). Due to the negative pressure in the pleural cavity, the lymphatic direction goes from the lung to the pleural cavity, whereas the direction is opposite in the peritoneal cavity, going from the periphery to the thoracic duct (Toyokuni 2019). This is the reason why the MM originates from parietal pleura and from visceral peritoneum and PP involves parietal pleura. Finally, asbestos reaches the pleural cavity; since mesothelial cells are phagocytic, they phagocyte asbestos fibers, which exert their fibrogenic effect (leading to PP formation) and carcinogenic action (provoking MM in susceptible individuals). Also an alternative, coexisting route, through the costal vascular system, has been proposed to explain the translocation of asbestos to pleural space (Schwartz 1991). This process might require different periods of time according to the physical characteristics of the fibers, being different between chrysotile and amphiboles, the latter having more penetration force; however, very few data are present in literature about pleural asbestos content, and the determination of asbestos fibers in the pleural tissues, unlike the analysis of lung content, is not performed routinely for diagnostic purposes. In a 1975 study about lung and pleural asbestos distribution in exposed individuals, the authors observed the accumulation of asbestos, especially of chrysotile type, in peripheral areas of lungs (especially lower lobes) (Sebastien et al. 1975; Hillerdal 1980). Chrysotile has been detected also within PP (Churg 1982). Caraballo-Arias et al. recently reviewed 12 studies in which asbestos pleural content has been assessed (Caraballo-Arias et al. 2022): the majority of the 142 examined pleural samples (78%) contained asbestos, and in most cases both chrysotile and amphibole fibers were detected. Broaddus et al. stated that most studies about inorganic fiber burden in lung and pleura of patients with PP report short chrysotile fibers in the pleura and long amphibole fibers in the lung (Broaddus et al. 2011). This is in line with the hypothesis that chrysotile is easily removed from the lung by macrophages, due to its crystalline structure, more friable and fragmentable in the acid lung microenvironment (Bernstein 2014) and it accumulates in pleural space.

Warnock et al. (Warnock, Prescott, and Kuwahara 1982) identified significantly higher median concentrations of amosite and crocidolite in lungs of subjects with PP, but they did not investigate the lung content in PP and pleural tissue.

Overall, it is not known which kind of asbestos is more capable of causing PP. In our recent work (Visonà et al. 2024) we did not find the prevalence of any particular kind of asbestos in lungs of people with PP compared to asbestos-exposed patients without PP.

4.1.3 Imaging

For imaging identification and assessment of PP, HRCT is currently the technology with the highest specificity and sensitivity compared to conventional CT and chest X-ray. From a diagnostic standpoint, chest radiography is the standard method used in most screenings for pneumoconiosis, but it has important limitations in detecting early, subtle pleural plaques, whereas a CT scan allows the diagnosis of thin or tiny non-calcified plaques (Mazzei et al. 2017; Aberle et al. 1988; Gamsu, Aberle, and Lynch 1989; Elshazley et al. 2011; Kim et al. 2015). Size, location, shape, degree of calcification and the technical quality of the radiograph have impacts on the correct evaluation of pleural plaques through chest radiograph. Autopsy studies highlighted a considerable rate of false negatives in radiographic recognition of PP. On the other hand, anatomic variations, such as extrapleural muscle and fat, can lead to false-positive diagnoses with a frequency of up to 20% of cases (Jones, McLoud, and Rockoff 1988; Peacock, Copley, and Hansell 2000; Mizell, Morris, and Carter 2009). Different studies suggested that the use of CT gives a higher degree of sensitivity in detecting pleural disease, with particular effectiveness for the plaques located in the paravertebral and posterior aspects of the costal pleural, which are not optimally visualized in routine radiographs (Aberle et al. 1988; Aberle, Gamsu, and Ray 1988; Lozewicz et al. 1989; Oksa et al. 1994). Al Jarad et al. provided a comparison between chest radiographs: CT allowed to identify distinct PP in 95% of patients, while chest radiography identified them only in 59% of patients (al Jarad et al. 1991). Also Friedman et al. compared HRCT and a four-view radiographic series (posteroanterior, lateral, and two oblique): they found out that the positive predictive value for the detection of pleural disease is greater using HRCT, which also eliminates false positives determined by subpleural fat, found in a range of 10–29% of patients who were supposed to have non-calcified pleural plaques (Friedman et al. 1988). Neri and colleagues demonstrated that HRCT is able to identify PP and early lung involvement even when amosite-exposed workers have no symptoms and chest radiographs are apparently normal (Neri et al. 1994).

HRCT has been considered more accurate than conventional CT in detecting PP due to its higher spatial resolution. According to Aberle et al., PP were detected in 100% of patients using HRCT and in 93% using conventional CT (Aberle et al. 1988). Friedman et al. reported that HRCT has a sensitivity of 97% and a specificity of 100% in the assessment of pleural changes. The authors suggested that HRCT, rather than conventional CT, should be requested when any abnormality other than calcified PP is suspected on radiography, mainly to exclude false-positive results (Friedman et al. 1988).

4.1.3.1 Chest X-rays

The posteroanterior (PA) chest radiography allows to optimize the visualization of PP on the lateral chest wall, because they are viewed tangentially. In this projection they are displayed as focal areas of pleural thickening along the lateral chest walls (between the sixth and ninth ribs) and diaphragm, typically not involving the apices and the costophrenic angles (Kusaka, Hering, and Parker 2005). Over the diaphragm, they may manifest as either curvilinear calcifications or scalloping (Ilsen et al. 2016). Usually bilateral and asymmetric, PP can also be unilateral in the 25% of the case (Benamore, Warakaulle, and Traill 2008). They are typically well defined, with smooth, even contours and can range from several millimeters to many centimeters in length but rarely extend more than four interspaces (Gevenois and de Vuyst 2006). Calcification is reported in 10–15% of cases (Peacock, Copley, and Hansell 2000). Their location, their extent in length and in thickness and the presence of calcification on the PA chest radiograph can be evaluated according to the ILO Classification of Radiographs of Pneumoconioses (International Labour Organization 2022). In the ILO classification, plaques that occur on the lateral chest wall are described as being "in profile." Less commonly, when seen on the anterior or posterior chest wall, they are perpendicular to the X-ray beam and are described as "face on" or "en face" (International Labour Organization 2022). When viewed en face, PP may appear as hazy densities and their recognition could be challenging except when they are large and calcified and are identified as multiple and bilateral nodular, patchy, irregular, leaf-shaped or "geographic" opacities (Ilsen et al. 2016). In addition to the chest wall and the diaphragm, the ILO classification also includes the mediastinal pleura in the para-spinal or para-cardiac location as other sites of plaque occurrence (International Labour Organization 2022). PP nearly always involve the parietal pleura, but can occasionally arise from the visceral pleura in the lower aspects of the interlobar fissures, where they can simulate pulmonary nodules on chest radiographs (Rockoff et al. 1987) (Figure 4.3, 4.4).

On chest radiographs, non-calcified PP can be difficult to distinguish from the normal muscle and fat "companion shadows" of the chest wall. In this regard, HRCT allows for ruling out false-positive diagnoses and to differentiate between pleural plaques and pseudo-plaques, structures that simulate plaques on radiography. One of the most common causes of pseudo-plaques is extrapleural fat prominence. Indeed, about 10–20% of patients diagnosed with pleural plaques on radiographs have prominent extrapleural fat, which is well demonstrated on HRCT (Gefter and Conant 1988). The shadows of the origins of the serratus anterior and external oblique muscles may appear as densities between the intercostal spaces and therefore may be confused with plaques on chest X-rays. The so-called companion shadow, which is parallel to the medial surface of the first three or four ribs and is thought to be a combination of the shadows of the intercostal muscles and fat, may be also mistaken for PP (Clarke et al. 2006). Rib fracture callus and early pleural metastatic disease may also mimic pleural plaques on chest X-ray (Gevenois and de Vuyst 2006). Furthermore, HRCT allows the distinction of face-on PP from pulmonary nodules and confluent PP from diffuse pleural thickening (McLoud 1998) (Figure 4.5, 4.6).

4.1.3.2 High-Resolution Computed Tomography

The International Classification of HRCT for Occupational and Environmental Respiratory Diseases (ICOERD) defines PP as focal, well-circumscribed areas of pleural thickening with soft tissue attenuation values that sometimes include calcifications. PP can have a typical plateau shape or be a flat thickening of the pleura. What defines their parietal nature are their smooth and sharply demarcated edges, well separated from adjacent extrapleural tissue and from adjacent lung parenchyma (Kusaka, Hering, and Parker 2005). A thin layer of fat separates them from the underlying rib and adjacent extrapleural soft tissues (Peacock, Copley, and Hansell 2000). PP typically have edges that are thicker than the central part and can increase in size, extent, and calcification over time (Hallifax et al. 2017; Qureshi and Gleeson 2006) (Figure 4.7).

CT enables to identify their characteristic distribution on the posterolateral chest wall, between the seventh and tenth ribs, on the lateral wall, between the sixth and ninth ribs, on the dome of the diaphragm and on the mediastinal pleura, especially over the pericardium, but also reveals anterior and paravertebral plaques, which are not well visualized on chest radiography (Roach et al. 2002) (Figure 4.8).

In the paravertebral region, intercostal vessels can sometimes mimic pleural thickening, but the presence of thickening on multiple levels, the visibility of extrapleural fat between the pleura and intercostal vessels, or the presence of calcification, may help to establish the pleural origin of the opacity (Kusaka, Hering, and Parker 2005). PP may also have a nodular surface and may slightly impinge on the adjacent lung parenchyma; this can lead to focal hypoventilation, which may result in the occurrence of a pulmonary subpleural curvilinear line adjacent to the plaque (Ilsen et al. 2016). Additionally, a focal stripe of parenchymal ground-glass opacity may sometimes be seen adjacent to thick parietal PP, and this is probably a consequence of focal alveolar dysventilation (Kusaka, Hering, and Parker 2005). PP are usually bilateral and asymmetric, but they occasionally display uncommon attributes of unilateral or single lesions, that require a differential diagnosis due to the pleural thickening or the calcification generated by other factors, such as trauma, surgery, or pulmonary infection (Kim et al. 2015; Cugell and Kamp 2004). Visceral PP are rarer and may be associated with abnormalities in the immediately surrounding lung parenchyma suggesting localized fibrosis, that consists of short interstitial lines (<1 cm) radiating from the plaque, giving rise to the term "hairy plaques" (Roach et al. 2002) (Figure 4.9).

Several studies have been conducted on the detection and quantification of PP on CT. A recent study by Benlala et al. reports the use of the integration of an automated artificial intelligence (AI)-driven and CT scans for the quantification of PP among a population of former workers who were exposed to asbestos (Benlala et al. 2022). AI provides an automated quantification of the volume of PP and their volumetric progression over a period of five years. In this way, the volumetric assessment of PP becomes reproducible and may be useful to further research in order to better understand the relationship between PP, respiratory function and the occurrence of thoracic malignancies (Benlala et al. 2022).

4.1.4 Link with Asbestos Exposure and Dose

The importance of PP is mainly related to their role as hallmarks of previous asbestos exposure. In fact, even though there are other causes of PP formation, there is wide consensus in literature in considering them as markers of asbestos exposure. According to many authors, the evidence of bilateral, scattered calcified PP can be regarded as pathognomonic of asbestos exposure (Norbet et al. 2015), even though not the totality of PP, but the 80–90% of them, are due to previous asbestos exposure (Wolff et al. 2015). Among the other causes, the most represented are exposure to other materials, such as erionite, silicates and manmade fibers (Clarke et al. 2006), tuberculosis, previous rib fractures and calcified hemothorax (Hourihane and McCaughey 1966). Recently, Paris et al. demonstrated an effect of exposure to refractory ceramic fibers (RCFs) or mineral wool fibers (MWFs) on PP formation (Christophe Paris et al. 2023).

Kraynie et al., based on a large series of lung content analyses, stated that the predictive value of PP in indicating an asbestos etiology is 99% (Kraynie et al. 2016).

The main limitation of PP as a marker of asbestos exposure is their lack of statistical sensitivity, as some people with previous asbestos exposure do not develop PP. The occurrence of PP has been estimated between 14% and 62% among occupationally exposed individuals and 2-17% in those with environmental exposure (Boraschi et al. 1999).

In fact, the tendency to PP formation is related to an individual susceptibility, as not in the totality of cases asbestos exposure causes PP; the reason why some subjects present PP as a result of asbestos exposure and others do not is still not known (Broaddus et al. 2011).

A large study conducted in Turin on 898 autopsies concluded that PP are useful indicators of past asbestos exposure in populations, but their reliability in the single case is limited, as individual factors play an important role in the development of PP after asbestos exposure (Mollo et al. 1983) and not all the people exposed to asbestos develop PP.

Kato et al. found that PP were present in 89.4% among 2132 subjects previously exposed to asbestos (Kato et al. 2018), consistently with Barbieri et al., who found them in 89.51% of 124 individuals who died from asbestos-related diseases (Barbieri, Consonni, and Somigliana 2019). In a study conducted on 73 asbestos-cement workers, with a cumulative exposure that ranged from 16.4 to 98.7 fiber-years/mL (mean 26.3 fiber-years/mL) the authors found PP in 70% of them (Van Cleemput et al. 2001). In a work concerning the causal attribution of lung carcinoma to previous asbestos exposure, conducted in Italy on 414 patients, PP were present at autopsy in 82% of the men, and in 54% of women. The authors observed that the presence of PP was a good indicator of previous exposure to asbestos, as using PP the proportion of lung carcinomas attributable to asbestos (around 60%) is the same found applying Helsinki criteria (Bianchi et al. 1999).

In a recent work of our group conducted in a series of 95 exposed individuals who died from MM, PP have been found, at autopsy, in 53.68% of them (Visonà et al. 2024). This is a quite low prevalence compared to other previous studies, especially considering that the subjects have strong exposure histories. In fact, they had occupational, neighborhood or familiar exposure during the activity of a large asbestos-cement plant located in Broni, a small town in Northern Italy. In a recent study, Roggli reported that PP are present in more or less 50% of MM patients investigated in his laboratory (Roggli et al. 2023) and this percentage has remained stable during the last 40 years, with a maximum peak of 61.4% in the 2010s.

PP can be observed also in the general population (people with negative history of asbestos exposure and without any known asbestos-related diseases). In 1991, Schwartz reviewed 16 studies about the prevalence of PP in the general population, reporting that they were present in 12.2% (range = 0.5–39.3%) of the necropsies (Schwartz 1991). Karjalainen et al. found PP in 58% of a series of 288 random consecutive necropsies performed in Finland in 1991-92, one of the highest occurrences of PP in a random autopsy population.

Andrion et al. reported that, among 1019 consecutive autopsies (during which PP were actively searched), performed on adults in Turin, PP were found in 24.5% of males and in less than 1% of females (Andrion et al. 1982). In fact, in the absence of anamnestic evidence of asbestos exposure, especially if the autopsy is ordered for other reasons, unrelated to asbestos litigation, PP may be overlooked, because the pathologist might not examine thoroughly the parietal pleura (Gefter and Conant 1988). Literature about the existence of a dose-response relationship for PP is controversial.

Hefin Roberts in 1971 found PP in 41 cases out of 334 consecutive necropsies (Roberts 1971). The deceased individuals belonged to a heavily industrialized urban population, where many shipbuilding industries were located. Among the 41 subjects with PP, 13 worked in shipyards and other 20 had jobs that implied likely asbestos exposure. In 35 out of 41 cases asbestos bodies (ABs) were found in basal smears. There was a statistically significant difference in the incidence of PP between individuals with and without ABs in the smears. Moreover, they found a relation between the amount of ABs and the incidence of PP.

Warnock et al. compared the lung content in a series of 20 deceased individuals with PP discovered at autopsy with 11 control subjects with less than 100 ABs per gram of wet lung, finding a greater concentration of amosite, crocidolite, and occasionally "tremolite/actinolite/anthophyllite"[2] in subjects with PP than in the control group (Warnock, Prescott, and Kuwahara 1982).

Nevertheless, they observed an overlapping of asbestos concentrations between PP and controls.

Karjalainen et al. studied a series of consecutive necropsy cases who died for causes other than MM and lung cancer, evaluating the link between the asbestos lung burden and PP, finding a dose-response relationship, but also that PP were present in subjects with less than 100 000 ff/gdw (fibers/gram of dry weight) and unlikely previous exposure (Karjalainen et al. 1994). Yet the authors clearly stated that the role of chrysotile could have been underestimated due to the fast clearance of this mineral from lungs.

Van Cleemput et al., studying a series of 73 asbestos-cement workers, did not find any significant correlation between the extent of PP (measured through CT imaging) and cumulative asbestos exposure (estimated through industrial hygiene measurements) (Van Cleemput et al. 2001). Paris et al. pointed out a relationship between PP and both cumulative dose of exposure and time since the first exposure (Paris et al. 2009), though the mathematical model showed that the time since first exposure has a greater effect on PP occurrence than cumulative exposure. In a review written in 1998 by Boffetta, the importance of time since the first exposure in determining the occurrence of PP, greater than cumulative exposure and duration of exposure, had already been stated (Boffetta 1998). Soulat et al. found a link between the presence of PP and both intensity and duration of asbestos exposure (assessed through questionnaires) (Soulat et al. 1999). Another large study conducted on 4 446 workers who reported asbestos exposure found a significant correlation between time since first exposure, duration of exposure and cumulative exposure and the risk to develop PP (Eisenhawer et al. 2014). On the other hand, Mastrangelo et al. found a correlation between PP and time since first exposure and peak exposure, but not with cumulative exposure, in formerly exposed workers (Mastrangelo et al. 2009). However, in these studies the cumulative dose of asbestos exposure was evaluated through occupational hygiene measurements, job-exposure matrix and/or questionnaires, but lung content was not determined (obviously, since the subjects of such studies were alive people). Studies about the link between PP and exposure to Libby amphibole showed that the probability to develop PP increases with cumulative exposure and the duration of exposure (Rohs et al. 2008; Lockey et al. 2015). Moreover, both studies demonstrated that low cumulative exposures (assessed using industrial hygiene measurements) can provoke PP, showing significant ORs for cumulative lifetime exposures ranges of 0.81–1.99 fiber/cc-years and 2.00–19.03 fiber/cc-years.

A strong positive relationship between the presence of PP and asbestos lung burden [determined using scanning electron microscope equipped with energy dispersive spectroscopy (SEM-EDS)] has been described by Barbieri et al., who also found a significant correlation between the extension of PP and asbestos levels in lungs (Barbieri, Consonni, and Somigliana 2019). Instead, they found scarce or no correlation between presence or extension of PP and time since the beginning and the end of exposure, age and duration of exposure.

A few studies investigated the relationship between ABs in digested lung tissue and PP (Kishimoto et al. 1989; Churg 1982; Yusa et al. 2015).

In the most recent of them, the authors observed a significant relationship between PP extent and the concentration of ABs in lungs. Namely, 75% of the patients determined to have extensive plaques had more than 5 000 ABs/gdw (the cut-off value used in Japan for causal attribution of lung cancer to asbestos)(Yusa et al. 2015). However, as stated by the authors, the amount of ABs is not necessarily correlated with asbestos fiber concentration. Moreover, there were some lung cancer patients with extensive plaques but a low level of ABs. On the other hand, many lung cancer patients without extensive plaques had high levels of ABs. Therefore, the conclusions of this study must be interpreted carefully.

In the abovementioned study by our group (Visonà et al. 2024), we compared the asbestos burden (assessed using SEM-EDS) in lungs of exposed subjects with and without PP, without finding any statistically significant difference.

It is important to underline that, even though there is good agreement in literature that the presence of PP correlates with an increased risk to develop both lung cancer and MM after asbestos exposure, they are neither preneoplastic nor an independent risk factor, as it is not demonstrated that two individuals equally exposed to asbestos, one with PP and one without, have different risk to develop MM or lung cancer (Maxim, Niebo, and Utell 2015). The correlation is explained by the fact that both MM (as well as lung cancer) and PP are due to previous asbestos exposure (Myers 2012).

Moreover, the amount of asbestos exposure necessary to develop PP is not known. Some authors stated that it is likely to be elevated (Broaddus et al. 2011), while others believe that PP can occur as a consequence of "low exposures" (Wolff et al. 2015), even though it is rarely specified what is "elevated" and "low." Hourihane and McCaughey suggested that the dose of asbestos necessary to develop PP is intermediate between that necessary to develop MM and asbestosis (Hourihane and McCaughey 1966). It is in line with what stated by Churg and, previously, by the pioneer Selikoff's study: pleural tissue seems to be much more sensitive to the fibrogenic effect of asbestos compared to lung parenchyma (Churg 1982; Selikoff and Lee 1978). In a 1992 study on 386 factory workers previously exposed to high concentrations of amosite, PP have been demonstrated 20 years after intense exposures as short as a month (Ehrlich et al. 1992).

Sichletidis et al. conducted a study on dentists with PP, finding that they had been previously subjected to very low exposures (measured in air using contrast phase microscopy), but repeated daily (Sichletidis et al. 2009). Whitwell found that all people with PP had more than 20 000 ff/gdw (Whitwell, Scott, and Grimshaw 1977), identifying for the first time a "critical dose" of asbestos related to the development of PP.

In a recent work (Visonà et al. 2024) we attempted to identify "optimal" asbestos levels in order to develop PP, performing cut-point analyses by creating Receiver Operating Characteristic (ROC) curves to assess the significance and accuracy of the predictive model. Then we calculated the Youden Index to determine optimal cut-point of asbestos concentration at which both specificity and sensitivity are maximized.

According to our results, the "critical" concentration of asbestos which best predicted the presence of PP was 19 700 ff/gdw (with a sensitivity of 0.6471 and a specificity of 0.6667). This concentration is remarkably low, well below 100 000 ff/gdw, that is the threshold value considered indicative of a previous asbestos exposure (Wolff et al. 2015), and also below the "background exposure" identified by our laboratory (that is below 100 000 ff/gdw). This means that it is theoretically possible to observe PP in people without a significantly increased risk of developing MM. On the other hand, as we observed in the abovementioned work, not all exposed individuals who died from MM developed PP.

In conclusion, the finding of PP can be regarded as "red flag" in clinical context, as a patients with PP at radiological imaging should be subjected to a close follow-up for the risk of MM development (regardless the history of exposure), but when it comes to a forensic evaluation of the causal attribution of MM to previous asbestos exposure, PP alone cannot be used for causal attribution of lung cancer to asbestos exposure, as they can occur as a consequence of low levels of exposure (Wolff et al. 2015). Therefore, in legal contexts they must be used carefully and, if possible, coupled with other markers of exposure, above all lung content analysis.

4.2 ASBESTOSIS

Asbestosis is defined as a bilateral diffuse interstitial fibrosis of lungs caused by the inhalation of asbestos (Lazarus and Philip 2011; Norbet et al. 2015; American Thoracic Society 2004).

The relationship between asbestos inhalation and lung fibrosis had been suspected since at least 1927 (Cooke 1927). The first case reported to the authorities was that of a worker examined by Dr. Murrey in 1899 but then officially reported only in 1906 (Murray 1990). Subsequently, the case of a woman who died at the age of 33 with the clinical and X-ray picture of severe asbestosis after working for 18 years in an asbestos factory was described by Cooke in 1924 (Cooke 1924). In this article the clinical picture of the condition was reported for the first time as characterized by cough, dyspnea and signs of lung fibrosis.

The term "asbestosis" was then used for the first time in 1927 (Cooke 1927) in a report that for the first time described the histopathology of asbestosis, as well as the "foreign bodies" which only subsequently have been called "asbestos bodies." Asbestosis has been a compensable disease in Great Britain since 1930 (Hourihane and McCaughey 1966).

Despite the restrictions of asbestos mining and use introduced in most Western countries in the 1990s, asbestosis still represents a public health concern, especially in countries where asbestos is still largely mined and used. WHO estimated that around 1.3 million people in the USA and 125 million workers worldwide have experienced asbestos exposure due to its varied form of use (Stayner, Welch, and Lemen 2013). Examining the WHO data about mortality in 55 countries, it is estimated that 13 885 individuals died from asbestosis in the period from 1994 to 2010, with 180 000 potential years of life lost (Diandini et al. 2013). The median age at which death occurs is 79 years (Bang et al. 2014). Moreover, it is important to underline that the presence of asbestosis increases the risk of developing lung cancer, as it was demonstrated in a study on a large cohort of North American insulators (Markowitz et al. 2013).

In some South American, Eastern European and Asian countries the production and consumption of asbestos products is still high (Stayner, Welch, and Lemen 2013). In a study on Chinese asbestos factory workers it was observed that out of 586 male workers, 259 died and 39 of these deaths were due to asbestosis (Wang, Courtice, and Lin 2013).

In an Italian work investigating the hospitalization rate due to asbestosis and silicosis between 2001 and 2015, 17 220 hospital admissions for asbestosis have been reported, with an annual average of 1 148; the mean age of the patient was 71.6 years (Ferrante 2019).

We can summarize the pathogenesis of asbestosis as follows. When asbestos fibers are inhaled, they reach the respiratory bronchioles and the alveoli and elicit a foreign body reaction; alveolar macrophages try to phagocyte them, being damaged or activated and release cytotoxic oxidant species and inflammatory cytokines such as tumor necrosis factor alpha (TNF-α), interleukin 1 and arachidonic acid metabolites which recruit additional inflammatory cells to the alveolar epithelial surface and wall, as well as fibroblasts, that deposit connective tissue around the alveoli (Norbet et al. 2015). Also neutrophils and type II pneumocytes play an important role in the development of fibrosis (Robledo and Mossman 1999).

The released TNF-α activates mitogen-activated protein kinase that mediates further release of TNF-α and cellular apoptosis in activated macrophages. If on one hand the induced apoptosis stops the macrophages from releasing additional inflammatory kinases and so limit the inflammatory process, on the other hand its release causes further recruitment of inflammatory cells and cellular damage (Robledo and Mossman 1999).

The described inflammatory process is followed by a reparative phase in which there is the release of growth factors such as fibroblast growth factor, platelet-derived growth factors and insulin-like growth factor by the alveolar macrophages that stimulate the recruitment and the proliferation of fibroblasts and type II pneumocytes and the production of fibronectin and collagen resulting in the development of fibrosis (Fujimura 2000).

Individual susceptibility, maybe on a genetic basis, is an important factor in the development and progression of fibrosis. In a study on pneumoconiosis, polymorphism in the TNF-α gene, especially in case of A-308 genotype, has shown an increased risk for the development of fibrosis (Zhai et al. 1998). Other studies pointed out the role of polymorphisms in genes involved in detoxification of oxygen radicals in the pathogenesis of asbestosis (Franko et al. 2021; Franko et al. 2013).

Discussing extensively the clinical aspects of asbestosis is beyond the scope of this chapter. However, for completeness, we briefly summarize the main clinical features.

The clinical picture of asbestosis depends on the grade and extension of the disease, as patients with grade 1 or 2 asbestosis can have no symptoms nor signs at radiologic imaging (Dodson and Hammar 2011). The clinical presentation of asbestosis do not differ significantly from other kinds of lung fibrosis, but usually asbestosis progresses more slowly and is clinically milder (Oury, Sporn, and Roggli 2014). They consist of gradual and progressive dyspnea, at the beginning manifesting only in condition of exertion, dry cough, chest pain or tightness, fine end-expiratory crackles, especially at the bases, then expanding to the rest of the lung with increasing severity. In cases of very advanced disease, it is also possible to encounter clubbing of fingers and when the pulmonary fibrosis is extensive and severe it can cause a right heart failure with resulting cyanosis, jugular vein distention, hepatojugular reflux and edema (Lazarus and Philip 2011). Lung function tests are indicative of restrictive impairment, showing reduced diffusion capacity, while obstructive alterations are observed in patients with cigarette smoking habits (Caceres and Venkata 2023). Asbestosis can evolve, as it occurs for the other fibrotic pulmonary pathologies, to a restrictive or mixed pattern (restrictive-obstructive) respiratory failure. In severe cases it can evolve in chronic right heart failure and cause death by cardiopulmonary failure (Lazarus and Philip 2011). Asbestosis is often associated with PP: recently, Keskitalo et al. found them in 96% of 116 patients with asbestosis (Keskitalo et al. 2023).

The main criteria for diagnosis of asbestosis, according to the American Thoracic Society, are evidence of pathology at imaging or histology, as well as the presence of exposure markers, such as ABs, asbestos fibers or PP, and the exclusion of other possible causes (American Thoracic Society 2004).

In particular, the diagnosis of asbestosis requires the presence of asbestos fibers in lung tissue or the finding of FBs in association with interstitial lung fibrosis (Musk et al. 2020).

There is still no consensus on the levels of fibers above which the correlation between lung fibrosis and previous asbestos exposure is definitely proved. According to Helsinki criteria, revised in 2015, a level of fibers comparable to those found in other asbestosis cases (according to the parameters identified in each laboratory) is sufficient to proceed with the diagnosis (Wolff et al. 2015).

The Helsinki criteria for identifying subjects with a high probability of previous asbestos exposure require over 0,1 million amphibole fibers (longer than 5 μm) or over 1 million of amphibole fibers (longer than 1 μm) or over 1, 000 ABs/gdw.

In living patients, analysis of bronchoalveolar lavage fluid, sputum or transbronchial biopsies can be useful in diagnosing asbestosis, as the presence of ABs or fibers is highly specific in the differential diagnosis of asbestosis (Dodson and Hammar 2011). In bronchoalveolar lavage the Helsinki criteria recommend more than 1 asbestos body per mL as measured in a qualified laboratory (Wolff et al. 2015).

At imaging (as we are going to illustrate in the next paragraph) the lung fibrosis found in asbestosis is indistinguishable from the idiopathic pulmonary fibrosis (American Thoracic Society 2004). The presence of PP and a confirmed history of exposure can aid in the differentiation and in the diagnosis of asbestosis. Anyway, no clinical, imaging or histological characteristics can serve to differentiate asbestosis from other forms of lung fibrosis without the detection of increased levels of ABs or asbestos fibers in lung tissue.

For this reason a detailed occupational history, with information on working tasks and material used and the presence or use of personal protective devices should be assessed (Gulati and Redlich 2015). It is also important to inquire about the occupation or possible contact with asbestos fibers of relatives that live in close quarters with the patient.

4.2.1 Imaging

Imaging plays a critical role in differentiating other causes of fibrosis from asbestosis including hypersensitivity pneumonitis, nonspecific interstitial pneumonitis (NSIP), and to a lesser extent, idiopathic pulmonary fibrosis (IPF) (Roggli et al. 2010; Akira et al. 2003; Copley et al. 2003).

The imaging techniques used are chest radiography, high-resolution computed tomography (HRCT). Specific imaging methods, such as low-dose CT or Magnetic Resonance MR, are currently taking hold in the asbestosis diagnosis.

The latest update of the Helsinki criteria provides new guidelines for clinical individual evaluation or for research purposes in the exposed population, regarding PP and parenchymal disease (asbestosis). In particular, the use of HRCT is recommended, because conventional computed tomography and HRCT are more sensitive than chest radiography in the diagnosis of both parenchymal and pleural diseases related to asbestos, especially in the mild or early asbestosis (Staples et al. 1989; Gevenois et al. 1994).

CT and specifically HRCT allow direct visualization of the lung tissue, whereas radiographs have some limitations: (i) poorer contrast resolution; (ii) interference from superimposed soft tissue; (iii) more easily influenced by patient positioning and varying degrees of inspiration (Wolff et al. 2015; Paris et al. 2008).

Furthermore, in asbestos-exposed individuals, the diagnostic specificity and sensitivity are low when asbestosis is evaluated only via chest radiograph (Friedman et al. 1988; Spyratos et al. 2012). Previous studies have shown that 10% to 18% of patients with biopsy-proven asbestosis do not have any radiographic abnormalities on chest X-ray (Epler et al. 1978; Kipen et al. 1987). Moreover, Kipen et al. found that there was no correlation between chest radiographic findings and histopathological grade in 80% of patients with biopsy-proven asbestosis (Kipen et al. 1987).

Staples and colleagues found out that among 169 individuals exposed to asbestos with a strong suspicion of asbestosis on CT scans, 57 of them (34%) exhibited regular chest X-ray (Staples et al. 1989). This means that an abnormal chest X-ray does not rule out the possibility of asbestosis in an asbestos-exposed person.

It is estimated that the positive predictive value for an abnormal finding from a chest radiograph alone is approximately 40% and may be lower if the prevalence of asbestosis in the study population is less than 5% (Ross 2003).

On the other hand, Friedman and colleagues additionally noted that among 60 chest radiographs initially identified as indicative of asbestosis, 18 were determined to be false positives (Friedman et al. 1988). Subsequent CT scans revealed that the anomalies in the chest radiographs attributed to asbestosis were actually caused by emphysema, obscuration of the lung by en face extensive plaques, or focal parenchymal scarring from surgery or old infection like tuberculosis (Friedman et al. 1988).

4.2.1.1 Chest X-ray

Despite the acknowledged problems associated with the chest radiograph, it remains the common entry point into the diagnostic imaging algorithm and continues to be used as an epidemiological tool (American Thoracic Society 2004). Chest X-ray is available worldwide and is associated with an accepted classification scheme for the evaluation of pneumoconiosis, the International Labor Organization (ILO) classification of Radiographs of Pneumoconioses, resulting from a collaboration between ILO and the U.S. National Institute for Occupational Safety & Health (NIOSH), revised recently in 2022 (International Labour Organization 2022). The classification provides a tool for the systematic description and recording of chest radiographic abnormalities caused by the inhalation of dusts occurring in all types of pneumoconiosis in a simple and reproducible manner. The guidelines of the ILO classification state that "The Classification neither defines pathological entities nor takes into account working capacity" and underlines the importance of the differential diagnosis of any chest radiographic abnormalities saying that "No radiographic features are pathognomonic of dust exposure. Some radiographic features that are unrelated to inhaled dust may mimic those caused by dust." For the purpose of ILO interpretation, only the posteroanterior (PA) view is used. It consists of a set of standard digitally acquired chest radiographs and the guidelines document to compare the case subject chest radiograph with the standard ones. The set of standard digital radiographs provide different types of parenchymal abnormalities, such as small opacities, classified by shape, size, lobes distribution and concentration (score of "profusion"), and large opacities; it also takes into account alterations in the pleura (such as PP, calcification, obliteration of costophrenic angles, and diffuse thickening of the pleura) as well as other characteristics linked to, or occasionally mistaken for, occupational lung conditions. The findings are then recorded in a structured provided form.

The early radiographic features of asbestosis consist of bilateral small, irregular or reticular opacities, mostly seen in the lower pulmonary lobes, suggesting peribronchiolar and neighboring alveolar interstitial fibrosis (Chong et al. 2006). Over time, the distribution and density/concentration, also known as "profusion," of opacities can extend through the middle and upper region of the lung. Although irregular opacities are most common from asbestos exposure, mixed irregular and rounded opacities are often present. In more advanced cases, honeycombing could be evident on chest radiographs (Kim and Lynch 2002). Furthermore, the presence of pleural thickening or PP might also become evident.

According to the ATS 2004 statement the 1/0 on the profusion score of irregular opacities is a boundary between positive and negative chest radiograph for asbestosis, describing it like "presumptively diagnostic but not unequivocal," and may correlate with an early stage of asbestosis" (American Thoracic Society 2004). On the other hand, the ACCP consensus (2009) states that chest radiographic findings of 1/0 small irregular opacities are a good screening method but lack specificity in definitively diagnosing asbestosis (Banks et al. 2009). In addition, ACCP was in consensus that a chest radiograph showing irregular opacities and profusion score of more than 1/1, coupled with a history of asbestos exposure, are sufficient for a diagnosis of asbestosis (Banks et al. 2009) (Figure 4.10).

4.2.1.2 CT and HRCT

In the most recent revision of the Helsinki Criteria in 2014 (Wolff et al. 2015), it is proposed that incorporating CT imaging into the diagnosis of asbestos-related illnesses could offer value and should be an additional tool to chest X-rays in the specific situations outlined below:

1) A borderline finding of lung fibrosis (ILO grade 0/1–1/0).
2) Divergence between lung function findings indicating restriction and radiographs classified as normal.
3) Extensive pleural alterations that significantly affect the radiographic visualization of lung parenchyma.

CT imaging should be done using state-of-the-art multislice scanner technology and high-resolution reconstruction algorithms. Exposure to ionizing radiation should be kept as low as possible. The use of low-dose CT (LDCT), and even ultralow dose, is becoming more widespread for early diagnosis of lung cancer and some experience demonstrate its suitability in occupationally exposed populations for the evaluation of pleural disease and also for parenchymal disease even in early-stage interstitial lung abnormalities (ILA) (Harris et al. 2021; Brims et al. 2022).

The Helsinki criteria (Wolff et al. 2015) also advise utilizing the International Classification of HRCT for Occupational and Environmental Respiratory Diseases (ICOERD) to assess HRCT findings associated with asbestosis, as previously proposed by other authors (Suganuma et al. 2009). The semi-quantitative ICOERD model, analogous to the ILO classification for standard chest radiograms, aims to standardize and make comparable the reporting of HRCT of occupational lung interstitial diseases. It includes the following as main classificatory elements for lung parenchyma: small nodular or irregular/linear opacities, large opacities, ground glass and honeycombing areas, emphysema and round atelectasis. The profusion of small opacities is stratified into four grades (0–3), to be assigned to each of the three regions of the lung (with a possible range from 0 to 18). Pleural abnormalities are also recorded, distinguishing between parietal and visceral (Kusaka, Hering, and Parker 2005).

According to Helsinki Consensus of 2014, the occurrence of limited lung fibrosis among the general population makes the definition of a threshold value for asbestosis important, and they recommend that fibrosis sufficient for asbestosis according to the ICOERD system could represent the sum grade of ≥2–3 irregular opacities or bilateral honeycombing (sum grade ≥2) (Wolff et al. 2015; Apostoli et al. 2019). Nonetheless, the preface to the ICOERD document states that "The Coding System is to be applied as a strictly descriptive system and is not diagnostic. [...] The purpose of the HRCT Classification is to describe and code parenchymal and pleural manifestation of diffuse non-malignant occupational and environmental respiratory diseases. The Classification gives a semi-quantitative tool for early detection of fibrotic changes induced by occupational and environmental dust exposure. Positive scoring by the HRCT Classification does not always mean the presence of pneumoconiosis" (Tamura et al. 2015).

The need for codified and standardized evaluation of parenchymal features of the asbestos-induced parenchymal disease may benefit in the future from several new tools that are rapidly spreading in the radiology field, such as artificial intelligence applications able to rapidly perform automated, standardized, and cost-effective evaluation of asbestosis patients (Groot Lipman et al. 2023).

The common HRCT findings of early asbestosis include subpleural dot-like or branching opacities, subpleural curvilinear lines, parenchymal bands, and ground-glass opacity; late-stage disease is characterized by thickening of the intralobular lines, irregular thickening of the interlobular septa, signs of parenchymal distortion such as traction bronchiectasis or bronchiolectasis, and honeycombing (Aberle et al. 1988; Akira et al. 1990).

CT abnormalities linked with asbestosis commonly emerge in the lower lung, particularly in the posterior and basal subpleural regions, with a higher impact on centrilobular areas. As the condition advances, irregularities also manifest in the central and upper lung zones, but they frequently spare the apices. These CT findings commonly appear on both sides of the chest and often exhibit a notable symmetry (Akira et al. 2003; Akira et al. 1990, 1991). Given the early involvement of the posterior lung areas in asbestosis, it is crucial to perform scans on individuals with asbestos exposure in the prone position in order to discern between normal dependent atelectasis from early-stage asbestosis in the posterior lung (Aberle et al. 1988; Staples 1992; Aberle, Gamsu, and Ray 1988).

The initial CT changes in asbestosis comprise subpleural dot-like or branching opacities located a few millimeters away from the pleura in the lower lung regions. Some of these opacities manifest as thin branching structures, and some are in connection with the most peripheral branch of the pulmonary artery. Certain nodules may present as faint ground-glass opacity (GGO). From a histopathological perspective, subpleural nodules correlate with the development of peribronchiolar fibrosis (Akira et al. 1990, 1991).

As the number of subpleural dot-like or branching opacities increases, confluence of the dots creates subpleural curvilinear lines. These are defined as linear areas of increased attenuation within 1 cm of the pleura (mostly <0.5 cm) and parallel to the inner chest wall (Cha et al. 2016). The emergence of subpleural curvilinear lines has been linked to peribronchiolar fibrotic thickening along with the flattening and collapse of alveoli due to fibrosis (Akira et al. 1990, 1991). These lines could also suggest the presence of atelectasis, often occurring adjacent to plaques (Cha et al. 2016).

If curvilinear lines are observed at distance of about 1.5–2 cm from the inner chest wall they are more likely due to the thickened secondary lobular septa or plate-like atelectasis in the corticomedullary junction of the lung (Kusaka, Hering, and Parker 2005).

Parenchymal bands are linear densities, from 2 to 5 cm in length and usually contact the pleural surface (Aberle, Gamsu, and Ray 1988). The bands indicate the progression of fibrosis along the bronchovascular bundles or the interlobular septa, resulting in the distortion of lung parenchyma due to the traction force of thickened pleura (Akira et al. 1990). In cases of asbestosis, these bands are frequently seen in proximity to areas of PP and are commonly found in the lower parts of the lungs (Aberle et al. 1988). According to Akira et al, parenchymal bands are significantly more common in patients with diffuse pleural thickening than in others, but they may appear also without asbestosis (Akira et al. 2003). Gevenois et al. (Gevenois et al. 1998) noted the co-occurrence of parenchymal bands and diffuse pleural thickening within the same cluster and this might imply that these bands could reflect fibrosis of the visceral pleural rather than interstitial fibrosis. Because of concomitant pleural abnormalities, infolding collapse of the lung can occur (rounded atelectasis).

Ground glass opacity (GGO) is a feature generally associated with other fibrotic findings (Akira et al. 2003; al-Jarad et al. 1992). In the subpleural location, GGOs are discontinuous and generally do not disappear when the patient is in the prone position. Areas of ground-glass opacity have been shown to be the result of mild alveolar wall and intralobular septal thickening due to fibrosis or edema (Akira et al. 1990).

As parenchymal fibrosis spreads from the peribronchiolar regions into the residual lobules, other characteristic CT findings of pulmonary fibrosis develop (Akira et al. 2003; Aberle et al. 1988; Akira et al. 1990). Interlobular septal thickening is related to interlobular fibrotic or edematous thickening and intralobular interstitial thickening correlates with peribronchiolar fibrosis with subsequent alveolar ducts involvement (Cha et al. 2016). Later, small cystic spaces with thick walls are seen, intermixed with other areas of increased attenuation. Honeycombing refers to the presence of clustered cystic air spaces, commonly of similar size, ranging from 3 to 10 millimeters in diameter, although sometimes they might reach up to 2.5 cm. They are typically located in subpleural areas and have distinct, well-defined walls. If a scan in the end-expiration phase is acquired, lobular areas of low attenuation, representing areas of air trapping, may be seen in the affected lung. In this late stage, there is overlap between the HRCT appearances of asbestosis and usual interstitial pneumonia UIP (Akira et al. 1990; Cha et al. 2016) (Figure 4.11, 4.12).

4.2.1.3 Differential Diagnosis

Differentiating asbestosis from other forms of pulmonary fibrosis at imaging can be challenging, as they may share similar radiological features.

Although it is well known that pleural involvement is more common in asbestosis than in other types of lung fibrosis, Akira et al. investigated the significant differences in CT findings between asbestosis and IPF exclusively on the basis of lung parenchymal findings other than those associated with pleural abnormalities (Akira et al. 2003). They reported that the CT features that stood out as relatively specific indicators of asbestosis, including subpleural dot-like opacities and subpleural curvilinear lines, have been observed in 81% and 69% of cases, compared with 25% and 28% in IPF, respectively. Further specific CT findings included parenchymal band and mosaic perfusion in

48% and 49% of cases, compared with 4% and 11% in IPF. Honeycombing cysts, bronchiolectasis, and traction bronchiectasis were more frequent in patients with IPF while GGO, interlobular septal thickening and emphysema were similar in both groups (Akira et al. 2003). Ultimately, they suggest that the HRCT findings that most effectively discriminate asbestosis from IPF are PP, subpleural lines within 5 mm of the inner thoracic wall, subpleural dots and parenchymal bands. In the late stage of asbestos disease, these opacities are usually observed in the less affected lung portions (Akira and Morinaga 2016).

Copley et al. compare CT features between asbestosis and IPF, testing findings in a subset of histopathologically proven UIP and NSIP. CT showed that the fibrosis in patients with asbestosis was coarser than in those with IPF. Additionally, asbestosis cases exhibited more severe fibrosis than NSIP cases, but comparable to that seen in UIP cases. All subgroups presented with a basal and subpleural distribution of disease, but this was notably more prominent in asbestosis than in UIP or NSIP (Copley et al. 2003).

Arakawa et al. conducted a study on 33 asbestos-exposed patients with confirmed pulmonary fibrosis, out of which 15 had asbestosis and 18 had different types of fibrosis; the sole distinguishing feature between asbestosis and other chronic interstitial pneumonia was the CT finding of subpleural curvilinear lines (Arakawa et al. 2016).

In their research, Ma et al. emphasized the resemblances and distinctions in HRCT discoveries among individuals with asbestosis and FHP (fibrotic hypersensitivity pneumonitis). They noted that pleural irregularities, parenchymal bands, and rounded atelectasis exhibited substantial diagnostic significance for identifying asbestosis (Ma et al. 2022). To some degree, subpleural dots and diaphragmatic pleural abnormalities could differentiate between asbestosis and FHP.

These findings highlight that asbestos-induced pulmonary disease is more easily distinguishable from other pathological entities in early stages than in late stages of interstitial disease, when parenchymal distortion and radiologic signs tends to be less specific. Subpleural dot-like opacities and subpleural curvilinear lines are the most useful features.

4.3 PATHOLOGY

The presence of lung fibrosis, if the diagnostic criteria for asbestosis are fulfilled, can be indicative of causal attribution of MM or lung cancer to asbestos exposure. In addition, asbestosis itself is a compensable disease; therefore, the distinction of this disease from other forms of lung fibrosis is crucial from a medicolegal point of view.

The histologic diagnosis of asbestosis is particularly useful when clinical features and imaging are not sufficient for the diagnosis. In this case, however, the cost-benefit ratio does not justify the choice of performing a lung biopsy, as usually the material obtained by a transbronchial biopsy is too little to be representative for lung asbestos burden (American Thoracic Society 2004) and a more extensive approach is not feasible without therapeutic indications. The histologic diagnosis of asbestosis is achievable at autopsy and when, in a patient with MM or lung cancer, samples of lung parenchyma unaffected by cancer are available in surgical specimens (Roggli et al. 2010).

Histologically, asbestosis is characterized by peribronchiolar fibrosis obliterating surrounding alveoli and extending outward (Hourihane and McCaughey 1966). Although very similar to UIP (usual interstitial pneumonia), some important differences can be observed in lung sections. First, asbestosis begins as fibrosis of alveolar walls next to the respiratory bronchioles and progresses in a centrifugal direction, while UIP starts at the periphery of the secondary lobules and evolves centripetally (Caceres and Venkata 2023).

Moreover, the presence of fibroblastic foci is much more pronounced in UIP, as well as honeycombing changes (the latter being present only in very advanced asbestosis) (Dodson and Hammar 2011; Roggli et al. 2010). According to the 2010 update of the pathologic criteria of asbestosis by the College of American Pathologists and Pulmonary Pathology Society, two more morphologic differences between UIP and asbestosis (other than the presence of asbestos) can be useful: the presence of inflammation, usually absent in asbestosis but more marked in UIP, and the fibrosis of visceral pleura, almost always present in asbestosis but not in UIP (Roggli et al. 2010).

The histologic criteria for the diagnosis of asbestosis have been classified by the College of American Pathologists into four classes depending on the severity of the pathology (Craighead et al. 1982), with the grading based on the most severe areas, not an average (Hammar and Abraham 2015). Starting with the least severe, in grade 1 the pathologic changes affect the wall of at least one bronchiole with or without extension into the adjacent alveolar septa, in grade 2 alveolar ducts or one or two layers of adjacent alveoli are involved; a zone of non-fibrotic alveolar septa are still present between bronchioles. In grade 3 the alveoli of a whole acinus are involved with thickening of the septa and complete obliteration of some alveoli. Grade 4 asbestosis is defined by honeycombing (the formation of new pathologic spaces with diameter up to 1 cm) and diffuse, irregular interstitial fibrosis.

The significance of fibrosis classified as "grade 1" according to the 1986 CAP-NIOSH guidelines (Craighead et al. 1982) in regard to past asbestos exposure is uncertain. Bellis et al., investigating 199 necropsies, concluded that minimal pathological changes compatible with grade 1 asbestosis (small airway lesions) can be an important finding, especially in patients died from MM or lung cancer, and when this histologic pattern occurs together with ABs it is rightly ascribable to grade 1 asbestosis (Bellis et al. 1989).

The Asbestosis Committee of the College of American Pathologists and Pulmonary Pathology Society stated that bronchiolar wall fibrosis should not be referred to as asbestosis and the term "asbestos airways disease" should be used to describe bronchiolar wall fibrosis associated with ABs in the absence of proper alveolar septa fibrosis (Roggli et al. 2010). The decision to remove bronchiolar wall fibrosis as part of the definition of grade 1 asbestosis was hardly criticized by Hammar and Abraham (Hammar and Abraham 2015), who argued that bronchiolar wall fibrosis is the first fibrotic lesion of asbestosis, since asbestos fibers deposits in the respiratory bronchioles.

The pathology of asbestosis has also been classified in three grades according to the extension of the disease: in grade A only occasional bronchioles are involved, in grade B less than a half of bronchioles in a section are involved; in grade C more than half of bronchioles are involved.

As already pointed out in the paragraph about imaging, lung fibrosis might be histologically detectable even if radiological criteria are not fulfilled (Wolff et al. 2015).

According to the 2010 update of the pathologic criteria of asbestosis by the College of American Pathologists and Pulmonary Pathology Society, the microscopic diagnosis of asbestosis "requires an appropriate pattern of interstitial fibrosis plus the finding of ABs. Both components must be present" (Roggli et al. 2010). The Committee recommends that at least 2 ABs/cm^2 of lung, together with an appropriate septal fibrosis, are necessary for a diagnosis of asbestosis. They stated that, as only in rare cases of asbestosis fewer ABs are detected in histologic sections; therefore, fiber analysis using analytical electron microscopy should be considered an adjunctive technique that can be applied, for example, for excluding a diagnosis of asbestosis in individuals with diffuse pulmonary fibrosis and a history of asbestos exposure but without the required number of ABs in histological sections (Roggli et al. 2010).

The requirement of at least two ABs per cm^2 of lung section for asbestosis diagnosis raises some doubts for a number of reasons, which will be deepened in the section about ABs. In short, the relationship between ABs in histologic sections, ABs in digested tissue and, above all, with the real amount of inhaled asbestos fibers is far from certain (Roggli and Pratt 1983; Warnock and Isenberg 1986; Warnock and Wolery 1987). Therefore, the number of ABs that one can observe in 1 cm^2 of lung section could not reflect the amount of asbestos that had been inhaled by the subject. Moreover, there is evidence in literature suggesting that the probability of developing lung fibrosis after asbestos inhalation depends on many factors, such as the amount of asbestos present in lungs, the kind and dimensions of fibers (as explained in the next paragraph) and the individual susceptibility, as in some subjects relatively low asbestos concentrations could be sufficient to develop asbestosis, whereas for other they are not (Dodson et al. 1997; Morgan and Holmes 1985).

4.4 ASBESTOSIS AND ASBESTOS EXPOSURE

Asbestosis typically occurs after around 20 years since the beginning of exposure and requires heavy, continuous exposure (Norbet et al. 2015). A prolonged exposure (usually over 10 to 20 years) is usually associated with asbestosis, even though some individuals with asbestosis (typically shipyard workers) report very intense but short exposures to asbestos, lasting from several months to one year (American Thoracic Society 2004).

Fibrosis of the lungs very similar to those observed in asbestosis can be related to exposure to mineral dusts other than asbestos, such as coal, talc, mica, silica, aluminum oxide, iron oxide (Churg and Wright 1983; Wright et al. 1992). It was suggested that cigarette abuse can lead to lung fibrosis similar to asbestosis (Bledsoe, Christiani, and Kradin 2015). However, asbestos is much more potent in causing lung fibrosis compared to other minerals and cigarette smoking, even though cigarette smoking can worsen the pathologic changes induced by asbestos, possibly increasing the retention of asbestos in lungs by reducing the clearance and suppressing the innate immune system, as suggested by studies on animal models (Churg, Tron, and Wright 1987; Morris et al. 2015).

All types of asbestos can cause asbestosis. However, a dose-response relationship between asbestosis and amphibole asbestos has been reported, but not with chrysotile, that is considered less fibrogenic compared to amphiboles (Roggli et al. 2010). The more marked fibrogenic potency of amphiboles compared to chrysotile is likely to be due to fiber size, aspect ratio and biodurability (Roggli et al. 2010). In fact, it has been shown that longer fibers produce a much greater fibrogenic effect (Ye et al. 1999). In lung microenvironment, chrysotile fibers are known to fragment readily into short fibrils that can be removed by macrophages, resulting in a rapid clearance from lungs: in studies on animal models the removal of most of the inhaled chrysotile from lungs has been observed after 90 days, while amphiboles persist in human lungs for decades (Churg and Wright 1994; Churg and Vedal 1994; Bernstein et al. 2020). Wagner et al. found much higher asbestos fiber burden in asbestosis and lung cancer patients compared to MM. Moreover, they found that in MM, lung cancer and asbestosis the vast majority of asbestos was composed of amphiboles, whereas in controls (people operated for lung cancer without history of asbestos exposure) chrysotile was the most represented type (Wagner et al. 1989). In our recent study (Visonà et al. 2024) deceased patients with lung fibrosis presented higher concentrations of amosite, crocidolite and tremolite/actinolite (assessed using SEM-EDS) compared to exposed MM patients without lung fibrosis. This correlation is in line with previous studies who found a correlation between lung fibrosis and amphibole lung burden (Schneider, Sporn, and Roggli 2010; Roggli 1991; Churg, Wright, and Vedal 1993). We hypothesize that, beside the intrinsic more intense fibrogenicity of amphiboles, this fact is likely to be due to the longer persistence of amphiboles in lungs compared to chrysotile, that leads to their recovery in lung tissue after many years since the exposure has ceased.

An evident dose-response and dose-effect relationship between asbestos exposure and the consequent development of asbestosis has been demonstrated.

This leads to the problem of identifying a minimal cumulative dose that has the ability of causing a clinically relevant asbestosis. This is a particularly critical point, as it is for the other asbestos-related pathologies, that is still under discussion. The 1997 Helsinki criteria suggested a threshold of 25 fibers/mL/year for asbestosis ("Asbestos, Asbestosis, and Cancer: The Helsinki Criteria for Diagnosis and Attribution" 1997).

The various reports about the possible threshold cumulative dose of asbestos necessary for clinical manifestations of asbestosis had been reviewed by Roggli et al. in the 2010 guideline (Roggli et al. 2010). Comprehensively, most studies, conducted between 1984 and 2002, found a threshold cumulative dose for asbestosis development around 20–25 ff/mL/year. However, in a study conducted in 2002 on asbestos-exposed workers extracted from German Mesothelioma Registry, a weak correlation between cumulative dose and asbestos burden in lungs was observed (Fischer, Günther, and Müller 2002). Moreover, in the same study, in 24% of patients with a cumulative dose equal or above 25 fiber-years, no elevated asbestos concentrations were demonstrated in their lung tissues; on the other hand, 42% of patients with asbestos-associated lung fibrosis had a cumulative exposure below 25 fiber-years. Other studies found that asbestosis development is possible also as a consequence of exposures as low as 2–5 ff/mL/year (Burdorf and Swuste 1999; Dement et al. 1983; Sluis-Cremer 1991). However, at such low exposures one should consider the possibility of unknown or forgotten exposures to high doses or asbestos (maybe for shorter periods of time) and, on the other hand, the differential diagnosis of idiopathic fibrosis (Roggli et al. 2010). In particular, Sluis-Cramer et al. found that nearly half of the workers exposed to 20–50 fiber-years/mL developed asbestosis, while at a cumulative exposure exceeding 300 fiber-years/mL and 45 years or more years of residence time, 82% (64/78) of the workers developed asbestosis. For lower cumulative exposures (such as 2–5 fiber-years/mL) only four cases out of 56 (mostly with a very long residency time) developed asbestosis.

Lifetime cumulative exposure, even though not considered reliable in determining the exact amount of inhaled asbestos by some authors (Sluis-Cremer 1991), was found to be positively correlated with asbestos lung burden (Green et al. 1997) in a study conducted on 54 chrysotile workers. By contrast, Fisher et al. found only weak correlation between cumulative lifetime exposures and asbestos burden in lungs in a study on 366 patients from German Mesothelioma Registry (Fischer, Günther, and Müller 2002).

In a recent study, we found a moderate correlation between the retrospective estimate of lifetime cumulative exposure to asbestos and the total asbestos fiber count in the autoptic lung (Visonà et al. 2022). Retrospective exposure assessment was made by a team of expert occupational physicians, based on detailed information on occupational, environmental, and household exposure circumstances. It is worth noting that no chrysotile has been found in lung samples at SEM-EDS investigation; therefore, such conclusions must be limited to amphiboles.

On the whole, the above-summarized findings suggest that the reliability of retrospective estimation of lifetime cumulative exposure to asbestos is not consistent across the various studies and must be used carefully in the causal attribution of asbestos-related diseases only when very detailed and extensive information is available. In fact, such evaluation is based on anamnestic data, that, as suggested by Carbone et al., might be unreliable in case of forgotten or unknown exposures and, on the other hand, in case of exposure to "dust" at the workplace without knowing the nature of the dust (Carbone et al. 2023).

Despite the well-established dose-response relationship for asbestosis, the tendency to develop lung fibrosis as a consequence of asbestos exposure varies according to individual susceptibility. "Heavy" exposures or "excessive amounts" of inhaled asbestos are not always necessary to develop asbestosis. On the other hand, in our and other authors' experience (Dodson et al. 1997; Warnock and Isenberg 1986) some MM patients with very high concentrations of asbestos in lungs do not show lung fibrosis.

Paris et al., in a large HCRT study on 5 545 previously exposed workers, found asbestosis in 6.8%. The analysis demonstrated a clear correlation of asbestosis with the cumulative exposure and with the level of exposure, but not with the time since the first exposure (that was, instead, related to PP) (Paris et al. 2009).

In our recent study (Visonà et al. 2024) we found lung fibrosis in 28.42% of a series of 95 subjects deceased from MM, a prevalence that is in line with a previous study on asbestos-exposed individuals (Kato et al. 2018). Dodson found lung fibrosis in 52.7% cases of MM, in a cohort of 55 cases mainly exposed occupationally (Dodson et al. 1997).

4.5 ASBESTOSIS AND ASBESTOS LUNG BURDEN

In a work conducted by our group, we found higher asbestos concentrations in individuals who died from asbestosis compared to MM (Visonà et al. 2021a). This is in line with previous studies (Wagner et al. 1989; Roggli, Pratt, and Brody 1986; Churg and Vedal 1994). We found no chrysotile in MM nor in asbestosis patients, and this result could be explained by the long period of time elapsed between the end of exposure and death (at least 8 years), that allowed the complete clearance of chrysotile from lungs. This means that, as already pointed out by other authors, the dose of asbestos required for developing asbestosis is much higher compared to MM.

Our results are in line with Roggli et al. (Roggli, Pratt, and Brody 1986), who investigated the lung content in 110 cases of asbestos-related diseases. They found the highest concentrations of both ABs and uncoated fibers in asbestosis patients; all of them had more than 2 000 ABs per gram of wet lung, with a median concentration of 100 000 ABs/g. All patients with more than 100 000 ABs/g had asbestosis and there was no overlap in asbestos concentration between asbestosis and controls (either healthy and with idiopathic lung fibrosis) (Roggli, Pratt, and Brody 1986). They also found a significant correlation between the grade of asbestosis and the lung content (considering both ABs and uncoated fibers), but the best correlation was found between the grade of asbestosis and the total fibers and the uncoated fibers counted by SEM. Also Gibbs et al. found a positive correlation between the grade of fibrosis and the concentration of amosite and ABs (Gibbs et al. 1994), as well as Green et al. (Green et al. 1997)

In our recent study (Visonà et al. 2024) lung fibrosis appeared to be related to significantly higher lung concentrations of asbestos compared to MM patients without lung fibrosis, but not with higher ABs concentrations (counted at SEM), confirming what was previously stated by Roggli and Shelburne (Roggli and Shelburne 1982). Dodson et al. found a higher concentration of both asbestos fibers and ABs in MM patients with asbestosis, even though they pointed out that the dose-response relationship for asbestosis is not constant, given the wide range of asbestos and ABs concentrations reported in asbestosis patients (Dodson et al. 1997). Notably, Bellis et al. found low asbestos fibers in some asbestosis patients (Bellis et al. 1989).

Our results are in line with these data, as the estimation of the critical concentration of asbestos in lung that show the best relationship with lung fibrosis (26 400 ff/gdw) is, indeed, much lower that the value typically observed in patients with asbestosis (several million fibers per gdw) (Roggli 1991). Furthermore, 15 cases with lung fibrosis (always characterized by alveolar septal fibrosis) showed less than 100 000 ff/gdw, and in two cases no asbestos fibers at all; on the other hand, two cases with more than 100,000 ff/gdw had no lung fibrosis.

In previous studies, asbestosis patients without MM showed asbestos concentrations in lungs ranging from 30 321 to 5 689 685 ff/gdw, with a median of 297 895 ff/dgw (IQR 30 321.4–881 567.5) (Visonà et al. 2021a; Visonà et al. 2021b).

Such data confirm the known dose-response relationship for asbestosis, but also the impossibility to predict the onset of this disease based on asbestos lung content, as previously stated by Dodoson et al (Dodson et al. 1997)

4.6 ASBESTOS BODIES

Asbestos bodies (ABs) (Figures 4.13–4.16) are asbestos fibers covered in an iron-protein coat (Figures 4.13–4.16).

The first description of ABs was made in 1906 by Marchand. He defined them as "peculiar pigment crystals" and was able to demonstrate that the pigment surrounding the central fiber was iron. They were then labeled as "curious bodies" by Cooke in 1929 (Cooke 1929) but without proposing a connection to asbestos fibers. It was then Stewart and Haddow that realized that these bodies were caused by inhaled asbestos fibers and as a consequence they called them "asbestosis bodies" (Stewart and Haddow 1929). Only after observing that ABs correlated with the exposure to asbestos and are not necessarily an indicator of disease, the name was changed into "asbestos bodies" (Churg and Warnock 1981). Studies on animal models conducted in the 1960s demonstrated bodies very similar to ABs after inhalation of inorganic fibers other than asbestos, such as aluminum silicate and fiberglass (Gross et al. 1968). At this point Gross suggested to call "ferruginous bodies" all the fibers surrounded by an iron-protein coat and to limit the use of the term "asbestos bodies" for those in which the nature of the central fiber was proved to be asbestos (Gross, Cralley, and DeTreville 1967). To identify the core fiber of ferruginous bodies (FBs) it is necessary to use analytical electron microscopy analyzing an area in which the fiber is not covered with iron, or either more sophisticated techniques, such as X-ray fluorescence and X-ray adsorption spectroscopy (Pascolo et al. 2011; Bardelli et al. 2017). Churg and Warnock suggested that the great majority of FBs characterized by a thin, translucent fibrous core have, indeed, an asbestos core (Churg and Warnock 1977).

In this chapter, we chose to use the term "ferruginous bodies" (FBs) if we refer to those observed at histology, while "asbestos bodies" (ABs) is preferred when they are detected at SEM-EDS. If we refer to other authors' work, we are going to use the original term.

The coating of asbestos fibers with iron and organic matter, mainly ferritin and hemosiderin (Bardelli et al. 2017), has been regarded as a defense mechanism of the lung against the fiber, as ABs are less cytotoxic compared to uncoated asbestos fibers (Ghio, Churg, and Roggli 2004). The iron coating of the fibers is never homogenous and often presents with multiple round "pearls" whose shapes and dimensions are highly variable (Pascolo et al. 2011). In a study on animal models it was shown that at the beginning of its formation the iron coat presents a sheathlike appearance and that it becomes fragment only with time. The entire cycle requires about 40 weeks in experimental models (Botham and Holt 1971).

When inorganic fibers are inhaled and deposited in the lungs, the nearby macrophages try to phagocyte them. This leads to their activation and to the start of the inflammatory cascade. In cases in which the inhaled fiber is longer than 20 μm, a single macrophage is unable to phagocyte the whole fiber. As a consequence, in these macrophages a series of inflammatory mechanisms promote the accumulation of iron in their cytoplasm. These cytoplasmic iron accumulate around the fiber and form ferruginous micelles that together with matrix material, ferritin and hemosiderin form a sort of coating around the fiber (Oury, Sporn, and Roggli 2016). The accumulation of iron in turn causes more inflammation leading to the recruitment of more phagocytes, triggering a vicious cycle.

The iron deposited on the fiber surface is then reduced to Fe^{2+} by reductants present in the lungs. In its reduced form, iron produces oxidative stress.

Taking this into consideration it is possible to say that if FBs are an attempt of the organism to protect itself from inorganic fibers, even though it is also true that their formation leads to an intrinsic cytotoxic effect due to the generation of reactive oxygen species (Ghio et al. 2008; Ghio, Churg, and Roggli 2004). Not all ABs are composed of iron, fibers coated with calcium oxalate crystals or calcium phosphate spherules have been reported (Ghio et al. 2003; de Vuyst et al. 1982).

Although the finding of ABs in histology sections is generally regarded as a pillar in the diagnosis of asbestos-related diseases (Roggli et al. 2010; Kraynie et al. 2016), their significance in relation to previous asbestos exposures is still a much-debated topic.

ABs are present not only in asbestos-exposed individuals but also in the general population. The threshold concentration in digested tissue suggested by Roggli et al. as not indicative of previous asbestos exposure was 0–20 ABs/g of wet lung—which corresponds, more or less, to 0–200 ABs/gdw (Roggli, Pratt, and Brody 1986). Roggli et al. stated that ABs can be found in the lungs of virtually all adults living in industrialized countries (Oury, Sporn, and Roggli 2014). However, this statement is based on a series of studies conducted in the 1970s and 1980s, when asbestos was much more diffused than today in Europe and the USA. A study carried out about 55 individuals from the general population of Milan deceased between 2009 and 2011 revealed typical ABs in 16.4% of them, always in very low concentrations, ranging from 10 to 110 ABs/gdw (Casali et al. 2015).

Recently, we investigated the lung content of 50 individuals from the general population, who died from traumatic causes between 2000 and 2023, without any history of asbestos exposure and/or of lung diseases (Visonà et al. 2023). In 11 of them (22%) we found ABs in digested lung tissue at SEM-EDS, with a maximum value of 30 600 ABs/gdw and an average of 2 013 ABs/gdw. Note that using SEM-EDS instead of light microscopy to count ABs, can lead to underestimation of their actual amounts, as less lung tissue can be examined. Even more so, taking this into account, the ABs concentrations we found in the general population appear to be higher than expected based on other studies (Roggli, Pratt, and Brody 1986; Casali et al. 2015; Churg and Warnock 1981). This implies the possibility of finding FBs in histologic sections of unexposed individuals and therefore of the erroneous attribution of lung diseases to previous asbestos exposures if only this parameter is taken in consideration. Similar conclusions had already been reached in 1969 by Gaensler and Addington (Gaensler and Addington 1969), based on the lack of relationship between the ABs and uncoated fibers, as well as between ABs and the presence and severity of lung fibrosis.

In asbestos-exposed individuals, the relationship between the number of FBs observed in histologic sections, ABs in digested tissue and asbestos is far from certain.

Roggli and Pratt found an excellent correlation between ABs in histological sections and ABs in digested lungs, proposing that an average of two ABs on a 4 cm^2 lung section is equivalent to approximately 200 ABs per gram of wet fixed lung tissue (Roggli and Pratt 1983). However, other studies did not find the same correlation. In the work by Warnock and Isenberg (Warnock and Isenberg 1986) none of seven cases with grossly visible fibrosis, previous asbestos exposure and asbestos concentration in lungs ranging from 10^5 to 10^6 ff/gdw had enough ABs in histologic sections to fulfill the criteria for asbestosis diagnosis proposed by Roggli et al. several years later (at least two ABs for cm^2 of lung section) (Roggli et al. 2010). Moreover, ABs are not evenly distributed within lungs and across different sections, so it is possible that in one section there are no ABs while in the adjacent one they are abundant. In our recent work (Visonà et al. 2024) we investigated the inorganic fibers and FBs lung content using SEM-EDS in 95 individuals with previous documented occupational, familiar or neighborhood exposure to asbestos deceased from MM. At least five sections per case, stained with both H&E and Perls, were examined, without finding any correlation between the asbestos concentration in lungs and the presence of FBs at histological sections. Moreover, in 38 out of 95 subjects who died from MM (and were certainly exposed to asbestos) no FBs have been observed in histologic sections. It is also worth noting that in 5 out of 27 individuals with asbestosis (of any grade) no FBs were observed. It is clear that, in our case series, if FB were used as criteria for causal attribution of MM or lung fibrosis to previous asbestos diseases they would have failed in many cases of our series.

Furthermore, in 11 out of 95 cases, FBs were not observed at histology but were detected at SEM-EDS. Most importantly, in 29 out of 88 cases (33%) no FBs were detected at histological examination but asbestos was observed at SEM-EDS. However, in only two of them the asbestos concentration in lungs was above the threshold that, based on previous investigations on asbestos-exposed individuals and general population, we consider as background exposure in our laboratory (100 000 ff/gdw). Such data corroborated the doubts expressed by Hammar and Abraham about the requirement of at least two ABs in lung sections required for asbestosis diagnosis (Hammar and Abraham 2015).

As rightly pointed out by Hammar and Abraham, the finding of ABs in histologic sections requires the observation of a higher number of high-power fields the lower is the amount of ABs in one particular subject (Hammar and Abraham 2015). As reported by Roggli, for instance, in order to find one AB in the histologic sections of an individual with 100 ABs/g wet lung, one should observe 1 810 fields at a magnification of 400×, while in the case of an individual with 500 ABs, 362 fields are necessary (Oury, Sporn, and Roggli 2014). It is evident that examining such a high number of fields is hardly feasible and, above all, the number of ABs found at histology depends too much on the number of observed fields to be reliable and reproducible.

The correlation between ABs and uncoated asbestos fibers is not consistent across different studies. The efficiency of the coating process depends on several factors, regarding both the kind of fibers and individual characteristics of the subject. In some individuals with grade 4 asbestosis ABs can be very few or absent, while in others with analogous asbestos exposure and histological changes they can be abundant (Dodson and Hammar 2011). On the contrary, Roggli et al. found a good correlation between ABs counted using light microscopy and both coated and uncoated fibers counted by SEM (Roggli, Pratt, and Brody 1986). Also Green et al. found a strong correlation between ABs in histologic sections and both total amphibole and chrysotile fibers counted by analytical transmission electron microscope (TEM-EDS) (Green et al. 1997).

Warnock and Wolery detected fewer than 0.5 histologic ABs/cm^2 in five subjects with a total amphibole concentration that was similar to that in subjects with much more histologic ABs. They concluded that ABs in histologic sections may be scarce or absent in some subjects with over 500 000 total amphibole fibers/gdw (the background threshold identified by the authors) (Warnock and Wolery 1987). Monsò et al. investigated the inorganic fiber burden in lungs of patients diagnosed with idiopathic pulmonary fibrosis using standard criteria (they had no ABs in histologic sections). Some of them showed high amounts of asbestos fibers if the analytical electron microscopy is performed and, on the other hand, patients with diagnosed asbestosis with low counts of both ABs and fibers (Monsó et al. 1991).

In our experience, we found that in most cases (around 89% of those investigated in our previous studies) the concentration of uncoated fibers was higher compared to ABs (both counted by SEM-EDS) (Visonà et al. 2021a). A significant correlation between the amount of asbestos and ABs (counted by SEM-EDS) was detected, but the ratio between asbestos and ABs was extremely variable, ranging from 0.0085 to 157. An extremely wide range of ratios between uncoated asbestos fibers and ABs had been previously reported (Visonà et al. 2021a; Warnock and Isenberg 1986; Dodson et al. 1985). Moreover, we saw subjects with zero asbestos fibers but ABs in their lungs, and vice versa. As pointed out by other authors (e.g., Dodson et al. 1985), who found no ABs in two occupationally exposed individuals with respectively 780 000 and 1.2 million ff/gdw, the tendency to cover asbestos fibers is related to each individual response, and some individuals are "poor coaters" (Dodson et al. 1997). A different coating efficiency has been described even in different areas of the same individual's lung (Morgan and Holmes 1985). In our recent study (Visonà et al. 2024) the "critical" concentration of asbestos in lungs necessary to develop ABs at histology was estimated as 27 371 ff/gdw, a value well below the threshold considered indicative of past exposures to asbestos and currently used for causal attribution of asbestos-related diseases (100 000 ff/gdw) (Wolff et al. 2015). This suggests that it is possible to observe FBs in histologic sections also in individuals with exposure below background. Indeed, as pointed out by Schneider et al., in some isolated cases ("good coaters"), using only FBs counts at light microscopy can lead to a false-positive diagnosis of asbestosis (Schneider, Sporn, and Roggli 2010).

Another problem regarding the reliability of FBs as markers of previous exposure is the different capability of the various kinds of asbestos to form ABs. In particular, it is thought that chrysotile fibers rarely form ABs (Dodson and Hammar 2011); therefore, a person exposed mainly to chrysotile might have no ABs despite having been exposed. Roggli reported that 0.5% of ABs analyzed in his laboratory have a chrysotile core, while 2% of those investigated by other researchers (Oury, Sporn, and Roggli 2014). Dodson et al. found that only one out of 841 FBs had a chrysotile core (Dodson et al. 1997). In a 1979 study by Chrug and Warnock, of 144 bodies examined by electron diffraction, only one contained a chrysotile core (Churg and Warnock 1979). On the contrary, in a study by Holden and Churg on chrysotile miners and millers, in all of the 25 cases ABs were detected in standard H&E sections (Holden and Churg 1986). At electron microscopy, in all of the four cases examined they found ABs. Namely, 46 of 72 bodies (64%) had chrysotile cores, while 21 (29%) had cores of "tremolite" or "actinolite." This can be due to the fact that chrysotile millers are usually exposed to high amounts of long chrysotile fibers, which tend to be coated more than shorter ones.

Instead, the EDS analysis of uncoated fibers showed that the majority of them were amphiboles ("tremolite," "actinolite," that are well known to be part of that specific chrysotile ore). The authors explained such findings suggesting that although uncoated chrysotile fibers had been cleared from these lungs, ABs formed on chrysotile fibers persisted. It means that in case of chrysotile workers the finding of ABs is more reliable in determining past exposure compared to uncoated fibers. However, it must be underlined that this study has been performed only on four cases.

In our case series, 5 out 95 MM patients with documented exposure to asbestos ceased at least 8 years before death had no asbestos fibers at SEM-EDS examination but they have ABs at SEM and in histological sections (Visonà et al. 2023). We know that in their exposure setting (an asbestos-cement factory) chrysotile was used, together with crocidolite and small amounts of amosite (Oddone et al. 2017). We hypothesize that that five subjects were exposed mainly to chrysotile and, as proposed by Holden and Churg, chrysotile fibers had been cleared from lung parenchyma, while ABs formed on chrysotile cores persisted, as they were sequestered in the interstitium and cannot be removed by the immune system.

Another factor that can influence the coating of asbestos is the fiber's length. Morgan and Holmes showed that fibers shorter than 20 μm rarely become ABs, while most fibers longer than 80 μm are coated (Morgan and Holmes 1980). This can be explained by the possible complete phagocytosis of shorter fibers by macrophages. In fact, if a fiber is longer than about 20 μm, a single cell is not able to ingest it entirely, consequently the "frustrated phagocytosis" triggers a series of inflammatory mechanisms that promote the accumulation of iron in the cells (Oury, Sporn, and Roggli 2014). Moreover, thicker fibers are more easily coated compared to thinner ones and this can partly explain the low rate of ABs formation on chrysotile cores (Morgan and Holmes 1985).

Finally, we have to keep in mind that some people exposed to other types of dust show pseudoasbestos bodies (Dodson and Hammar 2011), that are not easy to distinguish from ABs at light microscopy without a specific competence in this field. In fact, even though Churg and Warnock suggested that ABs can be morphologically distinguishable from other FBs based on their transparent core, at light microscope magnifications this distinction might not be easy, and a FBs without asbestos core can be confused with an ABs. This fact further limits the reliability of histological FBs.

Based on all that is reported above, if ABs counted in digested tissue cannot be an accurate indicator of the retention of asbestos in lungs, the finding of FBs in histologic sections appears to be even less reliable. Therefore, even though the presence of FBs is suggestive of previous asbestos exposure, the current evidence suggests that FBs in histological sections, as well as ABs in digested tissue, should not be regarded as a compulsory criterion for causal attribution of a disease to past asbestos exposure, and they cannot provide any reliable quantitative information about the actual asbestos lung content. On the other hand, the low value of asbestos concentration we estimated as "cut-off" for the presence of FBs at histology confirms that FBs can be identified in people with exposure within background (Casali et al. 2015).

4.7 ASBESTOS BURDEN IN LUNG TISSUE

The assessment of inorganic lung content using analytical electron microscopy is considered the most useful and reliable tool in order to evaluate past asbestos exposure, especially in postmortem samples and in medicolegal contexts (Capella, Bellis, and Belluso 2016; Visonà et al. 2022).

Techniques, methods and significance of asbestos in tissue have been extensively discussed by Ronald Dodson in Chapter 3. Here we are going to synthesize the strengths and pitfalls of lung content analysis in the evaluation of past asbestos exposure, taking into account the results obtained by our group and other authors in previous studies.

Analytical electron microscopy [i.e., scanning electron microscope (SEM) or transmission electron microscope (TEM) equipped with energy-dispersive spectroscopy (EDS)] provides morphological, dimensional, and compositional information, allowing quantifying inorganic fibers, and, at the same time, classifying them according to their EDS spectrum. Analytical electron microscopy represents, therefore, an irreplaceable tool for the assessment of asbestos exposure, and despite the costs and the time required (several days for some samples very rich in fibers), it is crucial in the evaluation of past asbestos exposures.

The first disadvantage that hinders the extensive application of electron microscopy is the limited availability of suitable samples. In fact, for the proper implementation of this technique, sufficient amounts of normal lung parenchyma (free from neoplastic invasion) are required. The samples should preferably be still in formalin (not paraffin embedded), even though the analysis of formalin-fixed, paraffin-embedded samples, after paraffin removal, is possible. Yet, in that case, the accurate assessment of the dry weight, essential to normalize the detected fibers to 1 g of dry tissue as indicated by international guidelines (De Vuyst et al. 1998), is hampered. Moreover, for comparison, the sampling site should be consistent across the different cases. The inferior lobe of the right lung, which, for well-known anatomical and gravity reasons (Cooke 1929), is reached by the greatest number of fibers, is considered the best sampling site (Belluso et al. 2006). Performing lung content analysis in living patients is difficult due to the paucity of lung tissue available from biopsies, usually not enough to be representative (Oury, Sporn, and Roggli 2014). The most suitable situation to perform such analysis is the autopsy, where abundant lung tissue is available for both histology and lung content analysis.

One crucial question still to be answered is the existence of a threshold concentration of asbestos in lungs, that allows distinguishing between previous exposures capable of increasing the risk to develop MM and background exposure.

Background exposure can be defined as the asbestos exposure that each person can encounter in life but does not significantly increase the risk to develop MM. In literature, few scientists attempted to identify the concentration of asbestos in lungs that derives from "background exposure." Carbone et al. stated that, even though there is no "magic number" that differentiate between background exposure and exposure that can increase the risk of developing MM, a concentration of asbestos in lungs below 500 000 ff/gdw can be considered within background (Carbone et al. 2012). They decided to lower the threshold previously reported by Berry et al. in the IARC publication regarding the non-occupational exposure (Bignon, Peto, and Saracci 1989), that was 1 million ff/gdw.

Studies investigating inorganic fibers lung content in the general population are useful in order to clarify the concept of background exposure. However, these studies are often limited by the paucity of information available about occupation, residencies and precise history of exposure of the investigated subjects. Case et al. analyzed a series of 65 healthy subjects deceased mostly from traumatic causes, finding chrysotile in 60% of samples, "tremolite" in 20% and commercial amphiboles in only 11% (Case, Sebastien, and McDonald 1988).

More recently, Casali et al. analyzed multiple lung samples taken during autopsies of 55 subjects, deceased in Milan between 2009 and 2011, without any diagnosis of asbestos-related diseases, finding a median concentration of 0.11 million ff/gdw (Casali et al. 2015). They found asbestos in 64% of cases and ABs in only 16%. Interestingly, no correlation between asbestos fibers and ABs has been observed. Non-commercial and commercial amphiboles were equally represented. Previously, Capella et al. performed the SEM-EDS analysis of lung samples taken from people who resided in Torino all their life, without any history of exposure to asbestos, died from causes not related to asbestos exposure. In most of these subjects, a low amount of asbestos, belonging to tremolite/actinolite asbestos and chrysotile/asbestiform antigorite groups, was detected (Capella et al. 2020).

Such data, together with environmental studies conducted in similar urban settings (Chiappino, Sebastien, and Todaro 1991) suggest that the general population is potentially exposed to a low amount of asbestos. Yet, evidently, such "background" exposure is not sufficient, in most cases, by itself, to cause MM.

Studies that compare asbestos lung burden in the general population and in MM patients are rare and the results are difficult to compare due to the different techniques and units of measure.

Wagner and coll. were among the first to undertake this research; in 1982 they studied, on post-mortem samples, the asbestos lung content of former employees of an asbestos textile factory using transmission microscopy (Wagner, Berry, and Pooley 1982) comparing them to controls (patients died from other causes). Interestingly, they found similar concentrations of asbestos, and in particular of crocidolite and chrysotile, in MM and controls, suggesting that MM is not related to any peculiar kind of asbestos.

Churg and Wiggs (Churg and Wiggs 1986) found much higher levels of both chrysotile and "tremolite" in miners and processed ore workers, with a mean concentration of 0.3 million fibers of chrysotile/gdw in controls compared to 11 and 94 in, respectively, processed ore workers and miners, 0.4 million fibers of "tremolite" in controls compared to 3.3 and 221 in processed ore workers and miners. In this setting the raw chrysotile was associated with "tremolite," which allowed the detection of chrysotile exposure even after its clearance. It is worth noting that not all the chrysotile ore presents "tremolite" contamination.

Howel et al., studying lung content in 147 cases of MM and 122 controls, found concentrations of asbestos lower than 0.1 million amphibole fibers/gdw in 46% of controls, between 0.1 and 0.9 in 18% and between 1 and 4.9 in 13%, while only 6 controls had more than 5 million amphibole ff/gdw (Howel et al. 1999). They found much higher chances to have higher amphibole concentrations for MM compared to controls, but it is noteworthy that in a non-negligible number of controls asbestos concentration was suggestive of elevated (certainly above-background) exposures.

One caveat is that most of the previous studies comparing lung content in MM and controls were conducted on subjects who lived between the 1950s and the 1990s, when asbestos-containing materials were extremely diffused and when previous asbestos exposures, even if unknown or forgotten, were very likely.

Barbieri et al. analyzed eight cases of MM and 13 controls, finding a significant difference in asbestos concentration only between MM with occupational exposure and the control group. Notably, in the latter group, asbestos was found in 6 subjects (Barbieri et al. 2012). The concentration of asbestos in environmentally exposed MM and controls were not statistically significant.

In a recent work of our group (Visonà et al. 2023), we compared asbestos lung burden in 95 exposed individuals who died from MM with 50 subjects randomly selected among the general population of similar age (died between 2000 and 2023 from traumatic causes and without any known asbestos exposure nor lung diseases). We observed asbestos in lungs of 28% of controls and in all of them the asbestos concentration in lungs was below 100 000 ff/gdw, suggesting that as a possible current threshold for background exposure, consistently with what proposed by Helsinki criteria for causal attribution (Wolff et al. 2015). The most represented types of asbestos in our controls were tremolite/actinolite asbestos (detected in 24% of them), while chrysotile was observed in 6%, amosite in only one case (2%) and crocidolite in none.

In 2016, Kranye et al. reported the results of asbestos lung content analysis (performed using ATEM) in 546 cases of MM (Kraynie et al. 2016). The authors considered five parameters for causal attribution of MM to previous asbestos exposure: count of ABs at light microscopy, count of ABs at electron microscopy, total commercial amphiboles (amosite + crocidolite), total non-commercial amphiboles ("tremolite" + "actinolite" + "anthophyllite"), total chrysotile. Based on such criteria, they found that 83 out of 546 cases of MM were not attributable to asbestos, as they had all of the five parameters under the background (previously estimated by the authors in a reference population). However, three of them had PP and for two of these patients MM has been confirmed to be not related to asbestos based on lung content analysis (the exposure history is not mentioned). We are wondering if MM in subjects with asbestos lung burden below background can be related to previous chrysotile exposure, that can have been cleared from the lungs and therefore it might not have been detected at electron microscope analysis, even more so considering that authors counted only fibers longer than 5 μm.

From the mineralogical point of view, chrysotile is very different from amphiboles in regard to the chemical composition and structure (Bernstein et al. 2013; Bernstein 2014). It is well known that the retention of chrysotile in human lungs is much lower compared to amphiboles, due to its rapid clearance, rather than a lower rate of deposition (Churg 1994). The mechanism of chrysotile clearance, even though not fully understood, is related to the fragmentation of the fibers (Oberdörster 1994).

In fact, chrysotile, compared to amphiboles, is characterized by chemical instability in the acid lung microenvironment, that leads to the dissociation of magnesium from the crystalline structure. As a consequence, the structure of chrysotile becomes friable and fragments into very short fibrils that can be phagocytized and removed from the alveoli (Bernstein et al. 2013). Experimental studies on rats and baboons confirmed a very rapid clearance of chrysotile from lungs (with very few fibers after 90 days since the end of exposure, compared to high concentration of amphiboles after the same period of time) (Bernstein et al. 2020; Rendall and Du Toit 1994).

However, other studies showed a longer persistence of chrysotile. For instance, a recent paper by Feder et al. showed that chrysotile is stable in human lungs for up to 37 years (Feder et al. 2017), and they observed mostly chrysotile in human lung samples using a high-resolution type of electron microscope, a FEG-SEM. Similarly, previous studies on animals, as well as on humans, pointed out the presence of chrysotile as late as 60 years after exposure (Neumann, Löseke, and Tannapfel 2011).

Churg and De Paoli, in 1988 (Churg and DePaoli 1988), measuring the asbestos fiber burden in lungs of subjects with different time intervals since exposure cessation, concluded that inhaled chrysotile may end up as two populations: one is cleared quickly from the air spaces and the other, composed of fibers which managed to reach the interstitium, remain for longer. Such observations suggested that the degradation of chrysotile in human lungs, leading to its clearance, must occur at a very early time since inhalation and after that the remaining chrysotile, not degraded in a short time, is not significantly cleared in the following years. Also longitudinal splitting of asbestos bundles has been observed (Germine and Puffer 2015).

Until now we investigated, using SEM-EDS, asbestos lung burden in a series of 120 subjects exposed to asbestos during the activity of an important asbestos-cement plant located in Broni, a small town in Northern Italy (Visonà et al. 2021a, Visonà et al. 2023, Visonà et al. 2024). All of them had a compelling history of occupational, household and/or neighborhood exposure (widely documented by the records of a trial), died with asbestos-related diseases and underwent a forensic autopsy. We compared them with a series of healthy controls of similar age and sex distribution selected from the general population.

Overall, we found that it is possible to have asbestos concentrations below SEM-EDS detection limits in exposed individuals, most likely due to the complete degradation and removal of chrysotile. Indeed, we detected no asbestos in 26.3% of exposed subjects. In our case series, the time intervals since the cessation of the exposure (occupational or anthropogenic environmental) were extremely inhomogeneous (range: 8–44 years), but we did not notice any relationship between the time since the end of exposure and chrysotile concentration, suggesting that the clearance of this mineral occurs relatively rapidly, consistently with what was previously known (Churg 1994; Churg and Wright 1994). Moreover, we noticed a significantly higher concentration of chrysotile in women compared to men. This finding, together with the presence of larger fibers in males compared to females, suggests that there might be sex-related differences in the immune response to asbestos, determining a more efficient fragmentation and longitudinal splitting of chrysotile in females (explaining both the higher concentration and the thinner fibers) and, on the other hand, maybe a more efficient sequestration of chrysotile in females (that explains the longer biopersistence).

This can mean that electron microscopy analysis of lung content might not be totally reliable for chrysotile, especially in males.

Lung clearance does not regard only chrysotile, but was experimentally demonstrated for amphiboles by Rendall and Du Toit, who estimated a half-life of about 50 months for crocidolite and 18 months for amosite (Rendall and Du Toit 1994). These results correlate well with observations conducted on humans by the same authors (Rendall 1988). Despite a certain grade of clearance, amphiboles persist for long years in human lungs, as demonstrated by studies conducted on lung content of individuals whose exposure has ceased several decades ago (Visonà et al. 2021b) and amphibole concentration, estimated using electron microscopy, generally correlates well with retrospective assessments made using retrospective methods, such as job-exposure matrix, databases and literature (Visonà et al. 2022). Therefore, we suggest relying on amphibole concentration, rather than chrysotile, in assessing previous asbestos exposure.

In conclusion, asbestos lung content is subjected to deep changes with the passing of time after the end of exposure, especially for what concerns chrysotile. Therefore, SEM-EDS evaluation should be interpreted carefully, especially in a legal context, where the causal attribution of asbestos-related diseases depends on this assessment, as the asbestos lung content at the moment of death, even though considered the most reliable tool for assessing previous exposure, may not exactly reflect the actual amount of asbestos which was inhaled by the subject during life. In particular, we believe that a case of MM with negative asbestos fiber analysis should not automatically be considered as idiopathic, but an accurate evaluation of history of exposure and the presence of other markers of previous exposure (such as PP, lung fibrosis or FBs) should be carried out. Each of these parameters, alone, is not sufficient for causal attribution, but a sensible evaluation of all of the available information and pathological data should be carried out.

Finally, it is worth underlining that asbestos burden assessment is commonly performed in lungs and not in pleural tissue, where it exerts its pathogenicity in relation to MM. Very few studies in literature, reviewed by Caraballo-Arias et al. (Caraballo-Arias et al. 2022), investigated the asbestos content in pleural tissue. The majority of them found asbestos in pleural samples, and in most cases both chrysotile and amphibole fibers were detected. Therefore, chrysotile might be present in pleural tissue but have been cleared from lungs. This mean that, in workers exposed only to chrysotile, lung content analysis might give a negative result, while chrysotile may have been removed from lung parenchyma and partly translocated to pleural cavity, where it was phagocyted by mesothelial cells and give rise to carcinogenesis. More research is necessary to clarify the relationship between asbestos lung content and pleural lung content and the mechanisms involved in asbestos translocation to the pleura.

NOTES

1. As not all amphiboles are asbestos, it is important to underline that in this chapter the term "amphiboles" is used for shortness, but we are referring only to amphiboles classified as asbestos.
2. As the last asbestos nomenclature (2006) recommends that the terms tremolite, actinolite, and anthophyllite are followed by "asbestos," in this chapter, we put between brackets these terms when referring to papers published previously.

REFERENCES

Aberle, D. R., G. Gamsu, and C. S. Ray. 1988. "High-Resolution CT of Benign Asbestos-Related Diseases: Clinical and Radiographic Correlation." *AJR. American Journal of Roentgenology* 151 (5): 883–91.

Aberle, D. R., G. Gamsu, C. S. Ray, and I. M. Feuerstein. 1988. "Asbestos-Related Pleural and Parenchymal Fibrosis: Detection with High-Resolution CT." *Radiology* 166 (3): 729–34.

Akira, Masanori, and Kenji Morinaga. 2016. "The Comparison of High-Resolution Computed Tomography Findings in Asbestosis and Idiopathic Pulmonary Fibrosis." *American Journal of Industrial Medicine* 59 (4): 301–6.

Akira, Masanori, Satoru Yamamoto, Yoshikazu Inoue, and Mitsunori Sakatani. 2003. "High-Resolution CT of Asbestosis and Idiopathic Pulmonary Fibrosis." *AJR. American Journal of Roentgenology* 181 (1): 163–69.

Akira, M., K. Yokoyama, S. Yamamoto, T. Higashihara, K. Morinaga, N. Kita, S. Morimoto, J. Ikezoe, and T. Kozuka. 1991. "Early Asbestosis: Evaluation with High-Resolution CT." *Radiology* 178 (2): 409–16.

Akira, M., S. Yamamoto, K. Yokoyama, N. Kita, K. Morinaga, T. Higashihara, and T. Kozuka. 1990. "Asbestosis: High-Resolution CT-Pathologic Correlation." *Radiology* 176 (2): 389–94.

Al Jarad, N., N. Poulakis, M. C. Pearson, M. B. Rubens, and R. M.Rudd. 1991. "Assessment of Asbestos-Induced Pleural Disease by Computed Tomography–Correlation with Chest Radiograph and Lung Function." *Respiratory Medicine* 85 (3): 203–8.

Al Jarad, N., B. Strickland, M. C. Pearson, M. B. Rubens, and R.M. Rudd. 1992. "High Resolution Computed Tomographic Assessment of Asbestosis and Cryptogenic Fibrosing Alveolitis: A Comparative Study." *Thorax* 47 (8): 645–50.

American Thoracic Society. 2004. "Diagnosis and Initial Management of Nonmalignant Diseases Related to Asbestos." *American Journal of Respiratory and Critical Care Medicine* 170 (6): 691–715.

Andrion, A., A. Colombo, M. Dacorsi, and F. Mollo. 1982. "Pleural Plaques at Autopsy in Turin: A Study on 1,019 Adult Subjects." *European Journal of Respiratory Diseases* 63 (2): 107–12.

Apostoli, Pietro, Paolo Boffetta, Massimo Bovenzi, Pier Luigi Cocco, Dario Consonni, Alfonso Cristaudo, Gianluigi Discalzi, et al. 2019. "Position Paper on Asbestos of the Italian Society of Occupational Medicine." *La Medicina Del Lavoro* 110 (6): 459–85.

Arakawa, Hiroaki, Takumi Kishimoto, Kazuto Ashizawa, Katsuya Kato, Kenzo Okamoto, Koichi Honma, Seiji Hayashi, and Masanori Akira. 2016. "Asbestosis and Other Pulmonary Fibrosis in Asbestos-Exposed Workers: High-Resolution CT Features with Pathological Correlations." *European Radiology* 26 (5): 1485–92.

"Asbestos, Asbestosis, and Cancer: The Helsinki Criteria for Diagnosis and Attribution." 1997. *Scandinavian Journal of Work, Environment & Health* 23 (4): 311–16.

Attanoos, Richard L., Andrew Churg, Francoise Galateau-Salle, Allen R. Gibbs, and Victor L. Roggli. 2018. "Malignant Mesothelioma and Its Non-asbestos Causes." *Archives of Pathology & Laboratory Medicine* 142 (6): 753–60.

Bang, Ki Moon, Jacek M. Mazurek, John M. Wood, and Scott A. Hendricks. 2014. "Diseases Attributable to Asbestos Exposure: Years of Potential Life Lost, United States, 1999–2010." *American Journal of Industrial Medicine* 57 (1): 38–48.

Banks, Daniel E., Runhua Shi, Jerry McLarty, Clayton T. Cowl, Dorsett Smith, Susan M. Tarlo, Feroza Daroowalla, John Balmes, and Michael Baumann. 2009. "American College of Chest Physicians Consensus Statement on the Respiratory Health Effects of Asbestos. Results of a Delphi Study." *Chest* 135 (6): 1619–27.

Barbieri, Pietro Gino, Dario Consonni, and Anna Somigliana. 2019. "Relationship between Pleural Plaques and Biomarkers of Cumulative Asbestos Dose. A Necropsy Study." *La Medicina Del Lavoro* 110 (5): 353–62.

Barbieri, Pietro Gino, Dario Mirabelli, Anna Somigliana, Domenica Cavone, and Enzo Merler. 2012. "Asbestos Fibre Burden in the Lungs of Patients with Mesothelioma Who Lived near Asbestos-Cement Factories." *The Annals of Occupational Hygiene* 56 (6): 660–70.

Bardelli, Fabrizio, Giulia Veronesi, Silvana Capella, Donata Bellis, Laurent Charlet, Alessia Cedola, and Elena Belluso. 2017. "New Insights on the Biomineralisation Process Developing in Human Lungs around Inhaled Asbestos Fibres." *Scientific Reports* 7 (March): 44862.

Bellis, D., A. Andrion, L. Delsedime, and F. Mollo. 1989. "Minimal Pathologic Changes of the Lung and Asbestos Exposure." *Human Pathology* 20 (2): 102–6.

Belluso, Elena, Donata Bellis, Elisa Fornero, Silvana Capella, Giovanni Ferraris, and Sergio Coverlizza. 2006. "Assessment of Inorganic Fibre Burden in Biological Samples by Scanning Electron Microscopy – Energy Dispersive Spectroscopy." *Microchimica Acta* 155 (1): 95–100.

Benamore, R. E., D. R. Warakaulle, and Z. C. Traill. 2008. "Imaging of Pleural Disease." *Bildgebung = Imaging* 20 (4): 236–51.

Benlala, Ilyes, Baudouin Denis De Senneville, Gael Dournes, Morgane Menant, Celine Gramond, Isabelle Thaon, Bénédicte Clin, et al. 2022. "Deep Learning for the Automatic Quantification of Pleural Plaques in Asbestos-Exposed Subjects." *International Journal of Environmental Research and Public Health* 19 (3). https://doi.org/10.3390/ijerph19031417.

Bernstein, David M. 2014. "The Health Risk of Chrysotile Asbestos." *Current Opinion in Pulmonary Medicine* 20 (4): 366–70.

Bernstein, David M., Jacques Dunnigan, Thomas Hesterberg, Robert Brown, Juan Antonio Legaspi Velasco, Raúl Barrera, John Hoskins, and Allen Gibbs. 2013. "Health Risk of Chrysotile Revisited." *Critical Reviews in Toxicology* 43 (2): 154–83.

Bernstein, D. M., B. Toth, R. A. Rogers, D. E. Kling, P. Kunzendorf, J. I. Phillips, and H. Ernst. 2020. "Evaluation of the Exposure, Dose-Response and Fate in the Lung and Pleura of Chrysotile-Containing Brake Dust Compared to TiO2, Chrysotile, Crocidolite or Amosite Asbestos in a 90-Day Quantitative Inhalation Toxicology Study - Interim Results Part 1: Experimental Design, Aerosol Exposure, Lung Burdens and BAL." *Toxicology and Applied Pharmacology* 387 (January): 114856.

Bianchi, C., A. Brollo, L. Ramani, and C. Zuch. 1999. "Asbestos Exposure in Lung Carcinoma: A Necropsy-Based Study of 414 Cases." *American Journal of Industrial Medicine* 36 (3): 360–64.

Bignon, Jean, J. Peto, and Rodolfo Saracci. 1989. *Non-occupational Exposure to Mineral Fibres*. International Agency for Research on Cancer.

Bledsoe, Jacob R., David C. Christiani, and Richard L. Kradin. 2015. "Smoking-Associated Fibrosis and Pulmonary Asbestosis." *International Journal of Chronic Obstructive Pulmonary Disease* 10: 31–7.

Boffetta, P. 1998. "Health Effects of Asbestos Exposure in Humans: A Quantitative Assessment." *La Medicina Del Lavoro* 89 (6): 471–80.

Boraschi, P., S. Neri, G. Braccini, R. Gigoni, B. Leoncini, and G. Perri. 1999. "Magnetic Resonance Appearance of Asbestos-Related Benign and Malignant Pleural Diseases." *Scandinavian Journal of Work, Environment & Health* 25 (1): 18–23.

Botham, S. K., and P. F. Holt. 1971. "Development of Asbestos Bodies on Amosite, Chrysotile and Crocidolite Fibres in Guinea-Pig Lungs." *The Journal of Pathology* 105 (3): 159–67.

Brims, Fraser, Edward Ja Harris, Chellan Kumarasamy, Amie Ringuet, Brendan Adler, Peter Franklin, Nick de Klerk, Bill Musk, and Conor Murray. 2022. "Correlation of Lung Function with Ultra-Low-Dose CT-Detected Lung Parenchymal Abnormalities: A Cohort Study of 1344 Asbestos Exposed Individuals." *BMJ Open Respiratory Research*.

Broaddus, V. Courtney, Jeffrey I. Everitt, Brad Black, and Agnes B. Kane. 2011. "Non-neoplastic and Neoplastic Pleural Endpoints Following Fiber Exposure." *Journal of Toxicology and Environmental Health. Part B, Critical Reviews* 14 (1–4): 153–78.

Burdorf, A., and P. Swuste. 1999. "An Expert System for the Evaluation of Historical Asbestos Exposure as Diagnostic Criterion in Asbestos-Related Diseases." *The Annals of Occupational Hygiene* 43 (1): 57–66.

Caceres, Jose Diego, and Anand N. Venkata. 2023. "Asbestos-Associated Pulmonary Disease." *Current Opinion in Pulmonary Medicine* 29 (2): 76–82.

Capella, Silvana, Donata Bellis, and Elena Belluso. 2016. "Diagnosis of Asbestos-Related Diseases: The Mineralogist and Pathologist's Role in Medicolegal Field." *The American Journal of Forensic Medicine and Pathology* 37 (1): 24–8.

Capella, Silvana, Donata Bellis, Elena Fioretti, Roberto Marinelli, and Elena Belluso. 2020. "Respirable Inorganic Fibers Dispersed in Air and Settled in Human Lung Samples: Assessment of Their Nature, Source, and Concentration in a NW Italy Large City." *Environmental Pollution* 263 (Pt B): 114384.

Caraballo-Arias, Yohama, Paola Caffaro, Paolo Boffetta, and Francesco Saverio Violante. 2022. "Quantitative Assessment of Asbestos Fibers in Normal and Pathological Pleural Tissue-A Scoping Review." *Life* 12 (2): 296.

Carbone, Michele, Prasad S. Adusumilli, H. Richard Alexander Jr, Paul Baas, Fabrizio Bardelli, Angela Bononi, Raphael Bueno, et al. 2019. "Mesothelioma: Scientific Clues for Prevention, Diagnosis, and Therapy." *CA: A Cancer Journal for Clinicians* 69 (5): 402–29.

Carbone, Michele, Bevan H. Ly, Ronald F. Dodson, Ian Pagano, Paul T. Morris, Umran A. Dogan, Adi F. Gazdar, Harvey I. Pass, and Haining Yang. 2012. "Malignant Mesothelioma: Facts, Myths, and Hypotheses." *Journal of Cellular Physiology* 227 (1): 44–58.

Carbone, Michele, Haining Yang, Harvey I. Pass, and Emanuela Taioli. 2023. "Did the Ban on Asbestos Reduce the Incidence of Mesothelioma?" *Journal of Thoracic Oncology: Official Publication of the International Association for the Study of Lung Cancer* 18 (6): 694–97.

Casali, Michelangelo, Michele Carugno, Andrea Cattaneo, Dario Consonni, Carolina Mensi, Umberto Genovese, Domenico Maria Cavallo, Anna Somigliana, and Angela Cecilia Pesatori. 2015. "Asbestos Lung Burden in Necroscopic Samples from the General Population of Milan, Italy." *The Annals of Occupational Hygiene* 59 (7): 909–21.

Case, B. W., P. Sebastien, and J. C. McDonald. 1988. "Lung Fiber Analysis in Accident Victims: A Biological Assessment of General Environmental Exposures." *Archives of Environmental Health* 43 (2): 178–79.

Cha, Yoon Ki, Jeung Sook Kim, Yookyung Kim, and Yoon Kyung Kim. 2016. "Radiologic Diagnosis of Asbestosis in Korea." *Korean Journal of Radiology: Official Journal of the Korean Radiological Society* 17 (5): 674–83.

Chiappino, G., P. Sebastien, and A. Todaro. 1991. "Atmospheric asbestos pollution in the urban environment: Milan, Casale Monferrato, Brescia, Ancona, Bologna and Florence." *La Medicina del lavoro* 82 (5): 424–38.

Chong, Semin, Kyung Soo Lee, Myung Jin Chung, Joungho Han, O. Jung Kwon, and Tae Sung Kim. 2006. "Pneumoconiosis: Comparison of Imaging and Pathologic Findings." *Radiographics: A Review Publication of the Radiological Society of North America, Inc* 26 (1): 59–77.

Churg, A. M. 1982. "Asbestos Fibers and Pleural Plaques in a General Autopsy Population." *The American Journal of Pathology* 109 (1): 88–96.

Churg A. M. 1994. Deposition and Clearance of Chrysotile Asbestos. *Annals of Occupational Hygiene* 38(4) (August): 625–33, 424–5.

Churg, A. M., and L. DePaoli. 1988. "Clearance of Chrysotile Asbestos from Human Lung." *Experimental Lung Research* 14 (5): 567–74.

Churg, A. M., and M. L. Warnock. 1979. "Analysis of the Cores of Ferruginous (Asbestos) Bodies from the General Population. III. Patients with Environmental Exposure." *Laboratory Investigation; a Journal of Technical Methods and Pathology* 40 (5): 622–26.

Churg, A. M., and M. L. Warnock. 1981. "Asbestos and Other Ferruginous Bodies: Their Formation and Clinical Significance." *American Journal of Pathology* 102(3) (March): 447–56.

Churg, A., V. Tron, and J. L. Wright. 1987. "Effects of Cigarette Smoke Exposure on Retention of Asbestos Fibers in Various Morphologic Compartments of the Guinea Pig Lung." *The American Journal of Pathology* 129 (2): 385–93.

Churg, A., and S. Vedal. 1994. "Fiber Burden and Patterns of Asbestos-Related Disease in Workers with Heavy Mixed Amosite and Chrysotile Exposure." *American Journal of Respiratory and Critical Care Medicine* 150 (3): 663–69.

Churg, A., and M. L. Warnock. 1977. "Analysis of the Cores of Ferruginous (Asbestos) Bodies from the General Population. I. Patients with and without Lung Cancer." *Laboratory Investigation; a Journal of Technical Methods and Pathology* 37 (3): 280–86.

Churg, A., and B. Wiggs. 1986. "Fiber Size and Number in Workers Exposed to Processed Chrysotile Asbestos, Chrysotile Miners, and the General Population." *American Journal of Industrial Medicine* 9 (2): 143–52.

Churg, A., and J. L. Wright. 1983. "Small-Airway Lesions in Patients Exposed to Nonasbestos Mineral Dusts." *Human Pathology* 14 (8): 688–93.

Churg, A., and J. L. Wright. 1994. Persistence of Natural Mineral Fibers in Human Lungs: An Overview. *Environmental Health Perspectives* 102(Suppl 5) (October): 229–33.

Churg, A., J. L. Wright, and S. Vedal. 1993. "Fiber Burden and Patterns of Asbestos-Related Disease in Chrysotile Miners and Millers." *The American Review of Respiratory Disease* 148 (1): 25–31.

Clarke, Chester C., Fionna S. Mowat, Michael A. Kelsh, and Mark A. Roberts. 2006. "Pleural Plaques: A Review of Diagnostic Issues and Possible Nonasbestos Factors." *Archives of Environmental & Occupational Health* 61 (4): 183–92.

Clin, Bénédicte, Christophe Paris, Jacques Ameille, Patrick Brochard, Françoise Conso, Antoine Gislard, François Laurent, et al. 2011. "Do Asbestos-Related Pleural Plaques on HRCT Scans Cause Restrictive Impairment in the Absence of Pulmonary Fibrosis?." *Thorax* 66 (11): 985–91.

Cooke, W. E. 1924. "Fibrosis of the Lungs Due To the Inhalation of Asbestos Dust." *British Medical Journal* 2 (3317): 147–140.2.

Cooke, W. E. 1927. "Pulmonary Asbestosis." *British Medical Journal* 2(3491) (December 3): 1024–5.

Cooke, W. E. 1929. "Asbestos Dust and the Curious Bodies Found in Pulmonary Asbestosis." *British Medical Journal* 2(3586) (September 28): 578–80.

Copley, Susan J., Athol U. Wells, Pathanamathan Sivakumaran, Michael B. Rubens, Y. C. Gary Lee, Sujal R. Desai, Sharyn L. S. MacDonald, et al. 2003. "Asbestosis and Idiopathic Pulmonary Fibrosis: Comparison of Thin-Section CT Features." *Radiology* 229 (3): 731–36.

Craighead, J. E., J. L. Abraham, A. Churg, F. H. Green, J. Kleinerman, P. C. Pratt, T. A. Seemayer, V. Vallyathan, and H. Weill. 1982. "The Pathology of Asbestos-Associated Diseases of the Lungs and Pleural Cavities: Diagnostic Criteria and Proposed Grading Schema. Report of the Pneumoconiosis Committee of the College of American Pathologists and the National Institute for Occupational Safety and Health." *Archives of Pathology & Laboratory Medicine* 106 (11): 544–96.

Cugell, David W., and David W. Kamp. 2004. "Asbestos and the Pleura: A Review." *Chest* 125 (3): 1103–17.

Dement, J. M., R. L. Harris Jr, M. J. Symons, and C. M. Shy. 1983. "Exposures and Mortality among Chrysotile Asbestos Workers. Part II: Mortality." *American Journal of Industrial Medicine* 4 (3): 421–33.

De Vuyst, P., A. Karjalainen, P. Dumortier, J. C. Pairon, E. Monsó, P. Brochard, H. Teschler, A. Tossavainen, and A. Gibbs. 1998. "Guidelines for Mineral Fibre Analyses in Biological Samples: Report of the ERS Working Group. European Respiratory Society." *The European Respiratory Journal: Official Journal of the European Society for Clinical Respiratory Physiology* 11 (6): 1416–26.

Diandini, Rachmania, Ken Takahashi, Eun-Kee Park, Ying Jiang, Mehrnoosh Movahed, Giang Vinh Le, Lukas Jyuhn-Hsiarn Lee, Vanya Delgermaa, and Rokho Kim. 2013. "Potential Years of Life Lost (PYLL) Caused by Asbestos-Related Diseases in the World." *American Journal of Industrial Medicine* 56 (9): 993–1000.

Dodson, R. F., and Samuel P. Hammar. 2011. *Asbestos: Risk Assessment, Epidemiology and Health Effects. 6000 Broken Sound Parkway NW, SUite 300.* Boca Raton, FL: CRC Press, Taylor and Francis Group.

Dodson, R. F., M. O'Sullivan, C. J. Corn, J. W. McLarty, and S. P. Hammar. 1997. "Analysis of Asbestos Fiber Burden in Lung Tissue from Mesothelioma Patients." *Ultrastructural Pathology* 21 (4): 321–36.

Dodson, R. F., M. G. Williams Jr, M. F. O'Sullivan, C. J. Corn, S. D. Greenberg, and G. A. Hurst. 1985. "A Comparison of the Ferruginous Body and Uncoated Fiber Content in the Lungs of Former Asbestos Workers." *The American Review of Respiratory Disease* 132 (1): 143–47.

Ehrlich, R., R. Lilis, E. Chan, W. J. Nicholson, and I. J. Selikoff. 1992. "Long Term Radiological Effects of Short Term Exposure to Amosite Asbestos among Factory Workers." *British Journal of Industrial Medicine* 49 (4): 268–75.

Eisenhawer, Christian, Michael K. Felten, Miriam Tamm, Marco Das, and Thomas Kraus. 2014. "Radiological Surveillance of Formerly Asbestos-Exposed Power Industry Workers: Rates and Risk Factors of Benign Changes on Chest X-Ray and MDCT." *Journal of Occupational Medicine and Toxicology* 9 (April): 18.

Elshazley, Momen, Eiji Shibata, Naomi Hisanaga, Gaku Ichihara, Ashraf A. Ewis, Michihiro Kamijima, Sahoko Ichihara, et al. 2011. "Pleural Plaque Profiles on the Chest Radiographs and CT Scans of Asbestos-Exposed Japanese Construction Workers." *Industrial Health* 49 (5): 626–33.

Epler, G. R., T. C. McLoud, E. A. Gaensler, J. P. Mikus, and C. B. Carrington. 1978. "Normal Chest Roentgenograms in Chronic Diffuse Infiltrative Lung Disease." *The New England Journal of Medicine* 298 (17): 934–39.

Feder, Inke Sabine, Iris Tischoff, Anja Theile, Inge Schmitz, Rolf Merget, and Andrea Tannapfel. 2017. "The Asbestos Fibre Burden in Human Lungs: New Insights into the Chrysotile Debate." *The European Respiratory Journal: Official Journal of the European Society for Clinical Respiratory Physiology* 49 (6).

Ferrante, Pierpaolo. 2019. "Asbestosis and Silicosis Hospitalizations in Italy (2001–2015): Results from the National Hospital Discharge Registry." *European Journal of Public Health* 29 (5): 876–82.

Fischer, M., S. Günther, and K. M. Müller. 2002. "Fibre-Years, Pulmonary Asbestos Burden and Asbestosis." *International Journal of Hygiene and Environmental Health* 205 (3): 245–48.

Franko, A., V. Dolžan, N. Arnerić, and M. Dodič-Fikfak. 2013. "The Influence of Gene-Gene and Gene-Environment Interactions on the Risk of Asbestosis." *BioMed Research International* (July): 405743.

Franko, Alenka, Katja Goricar, Metoda Dodic Fikfak, Viljem Kovac, and Vita Dolzan. 2021. "The Role of Polymorphisms in Glutathione-Related Genes in Asbestos-Related Diseases." *Radiology and Oncology* 55 (2): 179–86.

Friedman, A. C., S. B. Fiel, M. S. Fisher, P. D. Radecki, A. S. Lev-Toaff, and D. F. Caroline. 1988. "Asbestos-Related Pleural Disease and Asbestosis: A Comparison of CT and Chest Radiography." *AJR. American Journal of Roentgenology* 150 (2): 269–75.

Fujimura, N. 2000. "Pathology and Pathophysiology of Pneumoconiosis." *Current Opinion in Pulmonary Medicine* 6 (2): 140–44.

Gaensler, E. A., and W. W. Addington. 1969. "Asbestos or Ferruginous Bodies." *The New England Journal of Medicine* 280 (9): 488–92.

Gamsu, G., D. R. Aberle, and D. Lynch. 1989. "Computed Tomography in the Diagnosis of Asbestos-Related Thoracic Disease." *Journal of Thoracic Imaging* 4 (1): 61–7.

Gefter, W. B., and E. F. Conant. 1988. "Issues and Controversies in the Plain-Film Diagnosis of Asbestos-Related Disorders in the Chest." *Journal of Thoracic Imaging* 3 (4): 11–28.

Germine, Mark, and John H. Puffer. 2015. "Analytical Transmission Electron Microscopy of Amphibole Fibers From the Lungs of Quebec Miners." *Archives of Environmental & Occupational Health* 70 (6): 323–31.

Gevenois, P. A., V. de Maertelaer, A. Madani, C. Winant, G. Sergent, and P. De Vuyst. 1998. "Asbestosis, Pleural Plaques and Diffuse Pleural Thickening: Three Distinct Benign Responses to Asbestos Exposure." *The European Respiratory Journal: Official Journal of the European Society for Clinical Respiratory Physiology* 11 (5): 1021–27.

Gevenois, Pierre Alain, and Paul de Vuyst. 2006. *Imaging of Occupational and Environmental Disorders of the Chest.* Springer Science & Business Media.

Gevenois, P. A., P. De Vuyst, S. Dedeire, J. Cosaert, R. Vande Weyer, and J. Struyven. 1994. "Conventional and High-Resolution CT in Asymptomatic Asbestos-Exposed Workers." *Acta Radiologica* 35 (3): 226–29.

Ghio, Andrew J., Andrew Churg, and Victor L. Roggli. 2004. "Ferruginous Bodies: Implications in the Mechanism of Fiber and Particle Toxicity." *Toxicologic Pathology* 32 (6): 643–49.

Ghio, Andrew J., Victor L. Roggli, Judy H. Richards, Kay M. Crissman, Jacqueline D. Stonehuerner, and Claude A. Piantadosi. 2003. "Oxalate Deposition on Asbestos Bodies." *Human Pathology* 34 (8): 737–42.

Ghio, Andrew J., Jacqueline Stonehuerner, Judy Richards, and Robert B. Devlin. 2008. "Iron Homeostasis in the Lung Following Asbestos Exposure." *Antioxidants & Redox Signaling* 10 (2): 371–77.

Gibbs, A. R., M. J. Gardner, F. D. Pooley, D. M. Griffiths, B. Blight, and J. C. Wagner. 1994. "Fiber Levels and Disease in Workers from a Factory Predominantly Using Amosite." *Environmental Health Perspectives* 102 (Suppl 5): 261–63.

Green, F. H., R. Harley, V. Vallyathan, R. Althouse, G. Fick, J. Dement, R. Mitha, and F. Pooley. 1997. "Exposure and Mineralogical Correlates of Pulmonary Fibrosis in Chrysotile Asbestos Workers." *Occupational and Environmental Medicine* 54 (8): 549–59.

Groot Lipman, Kevin B. W., Cornedine J. de Gooijer, Thierry N. Boellaard, Ferdi van der Heijden, Regina G. H. Beets-Tan, Zuhir Bodalal, Stefano Trebeschi, and Jacobus A. Burgers. 2023. "Artificial Intelligence-Based Diagnosis of Asbestosis: Analysis of a Database with Applicants for Asbestosis State Aid." *European Radiology* 33 (5): 3557–65.

Gross, P., L. J. Cralley, and R. T. DeTreville. 1967. "'Asbestos' Bodies: Their Nonspecificity." *American Industrial Hygiene Association Journal* 28 (6): 541–42.

Gross, P., R. T. de Treville, L. J. Cralley, and J. M. Davis. 1968. "Pulmonary Ferruginous Bodies. Development in Response to Filamentous Dusts and a Method of Isolation and Concentration." *Archives of Pathology* 85 (5): 539–46.

Gulati, Mridu, and Carrie A. Redlich. 2015. "Asbestosis and Environmental Causes of Usual Interstitial Pneumonia." *Current Opinion in Pulmonary Medicine* 21 (2): 193–200.

Hallifax, R. J., A. Talwar, J. M. Wrightson, A. Edey, and F. V. Gleeson. 2017. "State-of-the-Art: Radiological Investigation of Pleural Disease." *Respiratory Medicine* 124 (March): 88–99.

Hammar, Samuel P., and Jerrold L. Abraham. 2015. "Commentary on Pathologic Diagnosis of Asbestosis and Critique of the 2010 Asbestosis Committee of the College of American Pathologists (CAP) and Pulmonary Pathology Society's (PPS) Update on the Diagnostic Criteria for Pathologic Asbestosis." *American Journal of Industrial Medicine* 58 (10): 1034–39.

Harris, Edward J. A., Kuan P. Lim, Yuben Moodley, Brendan Adler, Nita Sodhi-Berry, Alison Reid, Conor P. Murray, et al. 2021. "Low Dose CT Detected Interstitial Lung Abnormalities in a Population with Low Asbestos Exposure." *American Journal of Industrial Medicine* 64 (7): 567–75.

Hillerdal, G. 1980. "The Pathogenesis of Pleural Plaques and Pulmonary Asbestosis: Possibilities and Impossibilities." *European Journal of Respiratory Diseases* 61 (3): 129–38.

Holden, J., and A. Churg. 1986. "Asbestos Bodies and the Diagnosis of Asbestosis in Chrysotile Workers." *Environmental Research* 39 (1): 232–36.

Hourihane, D. O., and W. T. McCaughey. 1966. "Pathological Aspects of Asbestosis." *Postgraduate Medical Journal* 42 (492): 613–22.

Howel, D., A. Gibbs, L. Arblaster, L. Swinburne, M. Schweiger, E. Renvoize, P. Hatton, and F. Pooley. 1999. "Mineral Fibre Analysis and Routes of Exposure to Asbestos in the Development of Mesothelioma in an English Region." *Occupational and Environmental Medicine* 56 (1): 51–8.

Ilsen, Bart, Frederik Vandenbroucke, Cathérine Beigelman-Aubry, Carola Brussaard, and Johan de Mey. 2016. "Comparative Interpretation of CT and Standard Radiography of the Pleura." *JBR-BTR: Organe de La Societe Royale Belge de Radiologie* 100 (1): 106.

International Labour Organization. 2022. *Guidelines for the Use of the ILO International Classification of Radiographs of Pneumoconioses*. Revised Edition. Geneva: International Labour Organization.

Jasani, Bharat, and Allen Gibbs. 2012. "Mesothelioma Not Associated with Asbestos Exposure." *Archives of Pathology & Laboratory Medicine* 136 (3): 262–67.

Jones, R. N., T. McLoud, and S. D. Rockoff. 1988. "The Radiographic Pleural Abnormalities in Asbestos Exposure: Relationship to Physiologic Abnormalities." *Journal of Thoracic Imaging* 3 (4): 57–66.

Karjalainen, A., P. J. Karhunen, K. Lalu, A. Penttilä, E. Vanhala, P. Kyyrönen, and A. Tossavainen. 1994. "Pleural Plaques and Exposure to Mineral Fibres in a Male Urban Necropsy Population." *Occupational and Environmental Medicine* 51 (7): 456–60.

Kato, Katsuya, Kenichi Gemba, Kazuto Ashizawa, Hiroaki Arakawa, Satoshi Honda, Naomi Noguchi, Sumihisa Honda, Nobukazu Fujimoto, and Takumi Kishimoto. 2018. "Low-Dose Chest Computed Tomography Screening of Subjects Exposed to Asbestos." *European Journal of Radiology* 101 (April): 124–28.

Keskitalo, Eerika, Johanna Salonen, Hanna Nurmi, Hannu Vähänikkilä, and Riitta Kaarteenaho. 2023. "Comorbidities and Causes of Death of Patients With Asbestosis." *Journal of Occupational and Environmental Medicine. American College of Occupational and Environmental Medicine* 65 (4): 349–53.

Kim, Jeung Sook, and David A. Lynch. 2002. "Imaging of Nonmalignant Occupational Lung Disease." *Journal of Thoracic Imaging* 17 (4): 238–60.

Kim, Yookyung, Jun-Pyo Myong, Jeong Kyong Lee, Jeung Sook Kim, Yoon Kyung Kim, and Soon-Hee Jung. 2015. "CT Characteristics of Pleural Plaques Related to Occupational or Environmental Asbestos Exposure from South Korean Asbestos Mines." *Korean Journal of Radiology: Official Journal of the Korean Radiological Society* 16 (5): 1142–52.

Kipen, H. M., R. Lilis, Y. Suzuki, J. A. Valciukas, and I. J. Selikoff. 1987. "Pulmonary Fibrosis in Asbestos Insulation Workers with Lung Cancer: A Radiological and Histopathological Evaluation." *British Journal of Industrial Medicine* 44 (2): 96–100.

Kishimoto, T., T. Ono, K. Okada, and H. Ito. 1989. "Relationship between Number of Asbestos Bodies in Autopsy Lung and Pleural Plaques on Chest X-Ray Film." *Chest* 95 (3): 549–52.

Kraynie, Alyssa, Gustaaf G. de Ridder, Thomas A. Sporn, Elizabeth N. Pavlisko, and Victor L. Roggli. 2016. "Malignant Mesothelioma Not Related to Asbestos Exposure: Analytical Scanning Electron Microscopic Analysis of 83 Cases and Comparison with 442 Asbestos-Related Cases." *Ultrastructural Pathology* 40 (3): 142–46.

Kusaka, Yukinori, Kurt G. Hering, and John E. Parker, eds. 2005. *International Classification of HRCT for Occupational and Environmental Respiratory Diseases.* PDF. 2005th Edition. Tokyo, Japan: Springer.

Larson, Theodore C., Cristopher A. Meyer, Vikas Kapil, Jud W. Gurney, Robert D. Tarver, Charles B. Black, and James E. Lockey. 2010. "Workers with Libby Amphibole Exposure: Retrospective Identification and Progression of Radiographic Changes." *Radiology* 255 (3): 924–33.

Lazarus, Angeline A., and Andrew Philip. 2011. "Asbestosis." *Disease-a-Month: DM* 57 (1): 14–26.

Lockey, James E., Kari Dunning, Timothy J. Hilbert, Eric Borton, Linda Levin, Carol H. Rice, Roy T. McKay, et al. 2015. "HRCT/CT and Associated Spirometric Effects of Low Libby Amphibole Asbestos Exposure." *Journal of Occupational and Environmental Medicine. American College of Occupational and Environmental Medicine* 57 (1): 6–13.

Lozewicz, S., R. H. Reznek, M. Herdman, J. E. Dacie, A. McLean, and R. J. Davies. 1989. "Role of Computed Tomography in Evaluating Asbestos Related Lung Disease." *British Journal of Industrial Medicine* 46 (11): 777–81.

Markowitz, Steven B., Stephen M. Levin, Albert Miller, and Alfredo Morabia. 2013. "Asbestos, Asbestosis, Smoking, and Lung Cancer. New Findings from the North American Insulator Cohort." *American Journal of Respiratory and Critical Care Medicine* 188 (1): 90–6.

Ma, Ruimin, Shuang Li, Yuanying Wang, Shuqiao Yang, Na Bao, and Ye Qiao. 2022. "High-Resolution Computed Tomography Features of Asbestosis versus Fibrotic Hypersensitivity Pneumonitis: An Observational Study." *BMC Pulmonary Medicine* 22 (1): 207.

Mastrangelo, Giuseppe, Maria N. Ballarin, Ernesto Bellini, Fabio Bicciato, Federica Zannol, Francesco Gioffrè, Antonio Zedde, et al. 2009. "Asbestos Exposure and Benign Asbestos Diseases in 772 Formerly Exposed Workers: Dose-Response Relationships." *American Journal of Industrial Medicine* 52 (8): 596–602.

Maxim, L. Daniel, Ronald Niebo, and Mark J. Utell. 2015. "Are Pleural Plaques an Appropriate Endpoint for Risk Analyses?." *Inhalation Toxicology* 27 (7): 321–34.

Mazzei, Maria Antonietta, Francesco Contorni, Francesco Gentili, Susanna Guerrini, Francesco Giuseppe Mazzei, Antonio Pinto, Nevada Cioffi Squitieri, et al. 2017. "Incidental and Underreported Pleural Plaques at Chest CT: Do Not Miss Them-Asbestos Exposure Still Exists." *BioMed Research International* (June): 6797826.

McLoud, T. C. 1998. "CT and MR in Pleural Disease." *Clinics in Chest Medicine* 19 (2): 261–76.

Mizell, Kelly N., Christopher G. Morris, and J. Elliot Carter. 2009. "Antemortem Diagnosis of Asbestosis by Screening Chest Radiograph Correlated with Postmortem Histologic Features of Asbestosis: A Study of 273 Cases." *Journal of Occupational Medicine and Toxicology* 4 (June): 14.

Mollo, F., A. Andrion, E. Pira, and M. P. Barocelli. 1983. "Indicators of Asbestos Exposure in Autopsy Routine. 2. Pleural Plaques and Occupation." *La Medicina Del Lavoro* 74 (2): 137–42.

Monsó, E., J. M. Tura, J. Pujadas, F. Morell, J. Ruiz, and J. Morera. 1991. "Lung Dust Content in Idiopathic Pulmonary Fibrosis: A Study with Scanning Electron Microscopy and Energy Dispersive X Ray Analysis." *British Journal of Industrial Medicine* 48 (5): 327–31.

Morgan, A., and A. Holmes. 1980. "Concentrations and Dimensions of Coated and Uncoated Asbestos Fibres in the Human Lung." *British Journal of Industrial Medicine* 37 (1): 25–32.

Morgan, A., and A. Holmes. 1985. "The Enigmatic Asbestos Body: Its Formation and Significance in Asbestos-Related Disease." *Environmental Research* 38 (2): 283–92.

Morris, Gilbert F., Svitlana Danchuk, Yu Wang, Beibei Xu, Roy J. Rando, Arnold R. Brody, Bin Shan, and Deborah E. Sullivan. 2015. "Cigarette Smoke Represses the Innate Immune Response to Asbestos." *Physiological Reports* 3 (12). https://doi.org/10.14814/phy2.12652.

Murray, R. 1990. "Asbestos: A Chronology of Its Origins and Health Effects." *British Journal of Industrial Medicine* 47 (6): 361–65.

Musk, A. W., N. de Klerk, A. Reid, J. Hui, P. Franklin, and F. Brims. 2020. "Asbestos-Related Diseases." *The International Journal of Tuberculosis and Lung Disease: The Official Journal of the International Union against Tuberculosis and Lung Disease* 24 (6): 562–67.

Myers, Renelle. 2012. "Asbestos-Related Pleural Disease." *Current Opinion in Pulmonary Medicine* 18 (4): 377–81.

Neri, S., A. Antonelli, F. Falaschi, P. Boraschi, and L. Baschieri. 1994. "Findings from High Resolution Computed Tomography of the Lung and Pleura of Symptom Free Workers Exposed to Amosite Who Had Normal Chest Radiographs and Pulmonary Function Tests." *Occupational and Environmental Medicine* 51 (4): 239–43.

Neumann, Volker, Stefan Löseke, and Andrea Tannapfel. 2011. "Mesothelioma and Analysis of Tissue Fiber Content." *Recent Results in Cancer Research. Fortschritte Der Krebsforschung. Progres Dans Les Recherches Sur Le Cancer* 189: 79–95.

Norbet, Christopher, Amanda Joseph, Santiago S. Rossi, Sanjeev Bhalla, and Fernando R. Gutierrez. 2015. "Asbestos-Related Lung Disease: A Pictorial Review." *Current Problems in Diagnostic Radiology* 44 (4): 371–82.

Oberdörster, G. 1994. "Macrophage-Associated Responses to Chrysotile." *The Annals of Occupational Hygiene* 38 (4): 601–15, 421–22.

Oddone, Enrico, Daniela Ferrante, Sara Tunesi, and Corrado Magnani. 2017. "Mortality in Asbestos Cement Workers in Pavia, Italy: A Cohort Study." *American Journal of Industrial Medicine* 60 (10): 852–66.

Oksa, P., H. Suoranta, H. Koskinen, A. Zitting, and H. Nordman. 1994. "High-Resolution Computed Tomography in the Early Detection of Asbestosis." *International Archives of Occupational and Environmental Health* 65 (5): 299–304.

Oury, T. D., T. A. Sporn, and V. L. Roggli. 2014. *Pathology of Asbestos-Associated Diseases.* Third Edition. Verlag Berlin Heidelberg: Springer.

Oury, Tim D., Thomas A. Sporn, and Victor L. Roggli. 2016. *Pathology of Asbestos-Associated Diseases.* Berlin Heidelberg: Springer.

Paris, Christophe, Aurélie Martin, Marc Letourneux, and Pascal Wild. 2008. "Modelling Prevalence and Incidence of Fibrosis and Pleural Plaques in Asbestos-Exposed Populations for Screening and Follow-up: A Cross-Sectional Study." *Environmental Health: A Global Access Science Source* 7 (June): 30.

Paris, Christophe, Isabelle Thaon, François Laurent, Anastasia Saade, Pascal Andujar, Patrick Brochard, Julia Benoist, et al. 2023. "Pleural Plaques and the Role of Exposure to Mineral Particles in the Asbestos Post-Exposure Survey." *Chest* 164 (1): 149–58.

Paris, C., S. Thierry, P. Brochard, M. Letourneux, E. Schorle, A. Stoufflet, J. Ameille, F. Conso, J. C. Pairon, and National APEXS Members. 2009. "Pleural Plaques and Asbestosis: Dose- and Time-Response Relationships Based on HRCT Data." *The European Respiratory Journal: Official Journal of the European Society for Clinical Respiratory Physiology* 34 (1): 72–9.

Pascolo, Lorella, Alessandra Gianoncelli, Burkhard Kaulich, Clara Rizzardi, Manuela Schneider, Cristina Bottin, Maurizio Polentarutti, Maya Kiskinova, Antonio Longoni, and Mauro Melato. 2011. "Synchrotron Soft X-Ray Imaging and Fluorescence Microscopy Reveal Novel Features of Asbestos Body Morphology and Composition in Human Lung Tissues." *Particle and Fibre Toxicology* 8 (1): 7.

Peacock, C., S. J. Copley, and D. M. Hansell. 2000. "Asbestos-Related Benign Pleural Disease." *Clinical Radiology* 55 (6): 422–32.

Qureshi, Nagmi R., and Fergus V. Gleeson. 2006. "Imaging of Pleural Disease." *Clinics in Chest Medicine* 27 (2): 193–213.

Rendall, R. E. G. 1988. *The Retention and Clearance of Inhaled Glass Fibre and Different Variation of Asbestos by the Lung.* Johannesburg, SA: University of the Witwaterstrand Johannesburg South Africa.

Rendall, R. E. G., and R. S. J. Du Toit. 1994. "The Retention and Clearance of Glass Fibre and Different Varieties of Asbestos by the Lung." *The Annals of Occupational Hygiene* 38 (inhaled_particles_VII): 757–61.

Roach, Huw D., Gareth J. Davies, Richard Attanoos, Michael Crane, Adams Haydn, and Siân Phillips. 2002. "Asbestos: When the Dust Settles an Imaging Review of Asbestos-Related Disease." *Radiographics: A Review Publication of the Radiological Society of North America, Inc* 22 (October): S167–84.

Roberts, G. H. 1971. "The Pathology of Parietal Pleural Plaques." *Journal of Clinical Pathology* 24 (4): 348–53.

Robledo, R., and B. Mossman. 1999. "Cellular and Molecular Mechanisms of Asbestos-Induced Fibrosis." *Journal of Cellular Physiology* 180 (2): 158–66.

Rockoff, S. D., E. Kagan, A. Schwartz, D. Kriebel, W. Hix, and P. Rohatgi. 1987. "Visceral Pleural Thickening in Asbestos Exposure: The Occurrence and Implications of Thickened Interlobar Fissures." *Journal of Thoracic Imaging* 2 (4): 58–66.

Roggli, V. L. 1991. "Scanning Electron Microscopic Analysis of Mineral Fiber Content of Lung Tissue in the Evaluation of Diffuse Pulmonary Fibrosis." *Scanning Microscopy* 5 (1): 71–80; discussion 80–3.

Roggli, Victor L., Allen R. Gibbs, Richard Attanoos, Andrew Churg, Helmut Popper, Philip Cagle, Bryan Corrin, et al. 2010. "Pathology of Asbestosis- An Update of the Diagnostic Criteria: Report of the Asbestosis Committee of the College of American Pathologists and Pulmonary Pathology Society." *Archives of Pathology & Laboratory Medicine* 134 (3): 462–80.

Roggli, Victor L., Cynthia L. Green, Beiyu Liu, John M. Carney, Carolyn H. Glass, and Elizabeth N. Pavlisko. 2023. "Chronological Trends in the Causation of Malignant Mesothelioma: Fiber Burden Analysis of 619 Cases Over Four Decades." *Environmental Research* 230 (August): 114530.

Roggli, V. L., and P. C. Pratt. 1983. "Numbers of Asbestos Bodies on Iron-Stained Tissue Sections in Relation to Asbestos Body Counts in Lung Tissue Digests." *Human Pathology* 14 (4): 355–61.

Roggli, V. L., P. C. Pratt, and A. R. Brody. 1986. "Asbestos Content of Lung Tissue in Asbestos Associated Diseases: A Study of 110 Cases." *British Journal of Industrial Medicine* 43 (1): 18–28.

Roggli, Victor L., and John Shelburne. 1982. "New Concepts in the Diagnosis of Mineral Pneumoconioses." *Seminars in Respiratory and Critical Care Medicine* 4 (02): 138–48.

Rohs, Amy M., James E. Lockey, Kari K. Dunning, Rakesh Shukla, Huihao Fan, Tim Hilbert, Eric Borton, et al. 2008. "Low-Level Fiber-Induced Radiographic Changes Caused by Libby Vermiculite: A 25-Year Follow-Up Study." *American Journal of Respiratory and Critical Care Medicine* 177 (6): 630–37.

Roodhouse Gloyne, S. 1933. "The Morbid Anatomy and Histology of Asbestosis." *Tubercle* 14 (12): 550–58.

Ross, Robert M. 2003. "The Clinical Diagnosis of Asbestosis in This Century Requires More than a Chest Radiograph." *Chest* 124 (3): 1120–28.

Schneider, Frank, Thomas A. Sporn, and Victor L. Roggli. 2010. "Asbestos Fiber Content of Lungs with Diffuse Interstitial Fibrosis: An Analytical Scanning Electron Microscopic Analysis of 249 Cases." *Archives of Pathology & Laboratory Medicine* 134 (3): 457–61.

Schwartz, D. A. 1991. "New Developments in Asbestos-Induced Pleural Disease." *Chest* 99 (1): 191–98.

Sebastien, P., A. Fondimare, J. Bignon, G. Monchaux, J. Desbordes, and G. Bonnaud. 1975. "Topographic Distribution of Asbestos Fibres in Human Lung in Relation to Occupational and Non-occupational Exposure." *Inhaled Particles* 4 (Pt 2) (September): 435–46.

Selikoff, Irving J., and Douglas Harry Kedgwin Lee. 1978. *Asbestos and Disease*. Academic Press.

Sichletidis, L., D. Spyratos, D. Chloros, K. Michailidis, and I. Fourkiotou. 2009. "Pleural Plaques in Dentists from Occupational Asbestos Exposure: A Report of Three Cases." *American Journal of Industrial Medicine* 52 (12): 926–30.

Sluis-Cremer, G. K. 1991. "Asbestos Disease at Low Exposures after Long Residence Times." *Annals of the New York Academy of Sciences* 643 (December): 182–93.

Soulat, J. M., D. Lauque, Y. Esquirol, M. Déprés, J. Giron, R. Claudel, and P. Carles. 1999. "High-Resolution Computed Tomography Abnormalities in Ex-Insulators Annually Exposed to Asbestos Dust." *American Journal of Industrial Medicine* 36 (6): 593–601.

Spyratos, Dionisios, Diamantis Chloros, Bettina Haidich, Loukas Dagdilelis, Stamatia Markou, and Lazaros Sichletidis. 2012. "Chest Imaging and Lung Function Impairment after Long-Term Occupational Exposure to Low Concentrations of Chrysotile." *Archives of Environmental & Occupational Health* 67 (2): 84–90.

Staples, C. A. 1992. "Computed Tomography in the Evaluation of Benign Asbestos-Related Disorders." *Radiologic Clinics of North America* 30 (6): 1191–207.

Staples, C. A., G. Gamsu, C. S. Ray, and W. R. Webb. 1989. "High Resolution Computed Tomography and Lung Function in Asbestos-Exposed Workers with Normal Chest Radiographs." *The American Review of Respiratory Disease* 139 (6): 1502–8.

Stayner, Leslie, Laura S. Welch, and Richard Lemen. 2013. "The Worldwide Pandemic of Asbestos-Related Diseases." *Annual Review of Public Health* 34 (January): 205–16.

Stewart, M. J., and A. C. Haddow. 1929. "Demonstration of the Peculiar Bodies of Pulmonary Asbestosis (Asbestosis Bodies) in Material Obtained by Lung Puncture and in the Sputum." *The Journal of Pathology and Bacteriology* 32: 172.

Suganuma, Narufumi, Yukinori Kusaka, Kurt G. Hering, Tapio Vehmas, Thomas Kraus, Hiroaki Arakawa, John E. Parker, et al. 2009. "Reliability of the Proposed International Classification of High-Resolution Computed Tomography for Occupational and Environmental Respiratory Diseases." *Journal of Occupational Health* 51 (3): 210–22.

Tamura, Taro, Narufumi Suganuma, Kurt G. Hering, Tapio Vehmas, Harumi Itoh, Masanori Akira, Yoshihiro Takashima, Harukazu Hirano, and Yukinori Kusaka. 2015. "Relationships (I) of International Classification of High-Resolution Computed Tomography for Occupational and Environmental Respiratory Diseases with the ILO International Classification of Radiographs of Pneumoconioses for Parenchymal Abnormalities." *Industrial Health* 53 (3): 260–70.

Toyokuni, Shinya. 2019. "Iron Addiction with Ferroptosis-Resistance in Asbestos-Induced Mesothelial Carcinogenesis: Toward the Era of Mesothelioma Prevention." *Free Radical Biology & Medicine* 133 (March): 206–15.

Van Cleemput, J., H. De Raeve, J. A. Verschakelen, J. Rombouts, L. M. Lacquet, and B. Nemery. 2001. "Surface of Localized Pleural Plaques Quantitated by Computed Tomography Scanning: No Relation with Cumulative Asbestos Exposure and No Effect on Lung Function." *American Journal of Respiratory and Critical Care Medicine* 163 (3): 705–10.

Visonà, Silvia Damiana, Silvana Capella, Sofia Bodini, Paola Borrelli, Simona Villani, Eleonora Crespi, Andrea Frontini, Claudio Colosio, and Elena Belluso. 2021a. "Inorganic Fiber Lung Burden in Subjects with Occupational and/or Anthropogenic Environmental Asbestos Exposure in Broni (Pavia, Northern Italy): An SEM-EDS Study on Autoptic Samples." *International Journal of Environmental Research and Public Health* 18 (4). https://doi.org/10.3390/ijerph18042053.

Visonà, Silvia D., Silvana Capella, Sofia Bodini, Paola Borrelli, Simona Villani, Eleonora Crespi, Claudio Colosio, Carlo Previderè, and Elena Belluso. 2021b. "Evaluation of Deposition and Clearance of Asbestos (Detected by SEM-EDS) in Lungs of Deceased Subjects Environmentally and/or Occupationally Exposed in Broni (Pavia, Northern Italy)." *Frontiers in Public Health* 9: 980.

Visonà, S. D., E. Crespi, E. Belluso, S. Capella, S. De Matteis, F. Filippi, M. Lai, et al. 2022. "Reconstructing Historical Exposure to Asbestos: The Validation of 'Educated Guesses.'" *Occupational Medicine* 72 (8): 534–40.

Visonà, S. D., B. Bertoglio, S. Capella, E. Belluso, B. Austoni, C. Colosio, Z. Kurzhunbaeva, T. Ivic-PavlicicE. Taioli. 2024. "Asbestos Burden in Lungs of Mesothelioma Patients with Pleural Plaques, Lung Fibrosis and/or Ferruginous Bodies at Histology: A Postmortem SEM-EDS Study." Carcinogenesis 45 (3): 131–139. doi: 10.1093/carcin/bgad090

Visonà, S. D., B. Bertoglio, C. Favaron, S. Capella, E. Belluso, C. Colosio, S. Villani, T. Ivic-PavlicicE. Taioli. 2023. "A Postmortem Case Control Study of Asbestos Burden in Lungs of Malignant Mesothelioma Cases." *Journal of Translational Medicine* 21 (1): 875. doi: 10.1186/s12967-023-04761-9

Vuyst, P. de, J. Jedwab, Y. Robience, and J. C. Yernault. 1982. "'Oxalate Bodies', Another Reaction of the Human Lung to Asbestos Inhalation?" *European Journal of Respiratory Diseases* 63 (6): 543–49.

Wagner, J. C., G. Berry, and F. D. Pooley. 1982. "Mesotheliomas and Asbestos Type in Asbestos Textile Workers: A Study of Lung Contents." *British Medical Journal* 285 (6342): 603–6.

Wagner, J. C., M. L. Newhouse, B. Corrin, C. E. Rossiter, and D. M. Griffiths. 1989. "Correlation between Lung Fibre Content and Disease in East London Asbestos Factory Workers." *IARC Scientific Publications* 90(90): 444–48.

Wang, Xiaorong, Midori N. Courtice, and Sihao Lin. 2013. "Mortality in Chrysotile Asbestos Workers in China." *Current Opinion in Pulmonary Medicine* 19 (2): 169–73.

Warnock, M. L., and W. Isenberg. 1986. "Asbestos Burden and the Pathology of Lung Cancer." *Chest* 89 (1): 20–6.

Warnock, M. L., B. T. Prescott, and T. J. Kuwahara. 1982. "Numbers and Types of Asbestos Fibers in Subjects with Pleural Plaques." *The American Journal of Pathology* 109 (1): 37–46.

Warnock, M. L., and G. Wolery. 1987. "Asbestos Bodies or Fibers and the Diagnosis of Asbestosis." *Environmental Research* 44 (1): 29–44.

Whitwell, F., J. Scott, and M. Grimshaw. 1977. "Relationship between Occupations and Asbestos-Fibre Content of the Lungs in Patients with Pleural Mesothelioma, Lung Cancer, and Other Diseases." *Thorax* 32 (4): 377–86.

Wolff, Henrik, Tapio Vehmas, Panu Oksa, Jorma Rantanen, and Harri Vainio. 2015. "Asbestos, Asbestosis, and Cancer, the Helsinki Criteria for Diagnosis and Attribution 2014: Recommendations." *Scandinavian Journal of Work, Environment & Health* 41 (1): 5–15.

Wright, J. L., P. Cagle, A. Churg, T. V. Colby, and J. Myers. 1992. "Diseases of the Small Airways." *The American Review of Respiratory Disease* 146 (1): 240–62.

Ye, J., X. Shi, W. Jones, Y. Rojanasakul, N. Cheng, D. Schwegler-Berry, P. Baron, G. J. Deye, C. Li, and V. Castranova. 1999. "Critical Role of Glass Fiber Length in TNF-Alpha Production and Transcription Factor Activation in Macrophages." *The American Journal of Physiology* 276 (3): L426–34.

Yusa, Toshikazu, Kenzo Hiroshima, Fumikazu Sakai, Takumi Kishimoto, Kazuo Ohnishi, Ikuji Usami, Tetsuyuki Morikawa, et al. 2015. "Significant Relationship between the Extent of Pleural Plaques and Pulmonary Asbestos Body Concentration in Lung Cancer Patients with Occupational Asbestos Exposure." *American Journal of Industrial Medicine* 58 (4): 444–55.

Zhai, R., M. Jetten, R. P. Schins, H. Franssen, and P. J. Borm. 1998. "Polymorphisms in the Promoter of the Tumor Necrosis Factor-Alpha Gene in Coal Miners." *American Journal of Industrial Medicine* 34 (4): 318–24.

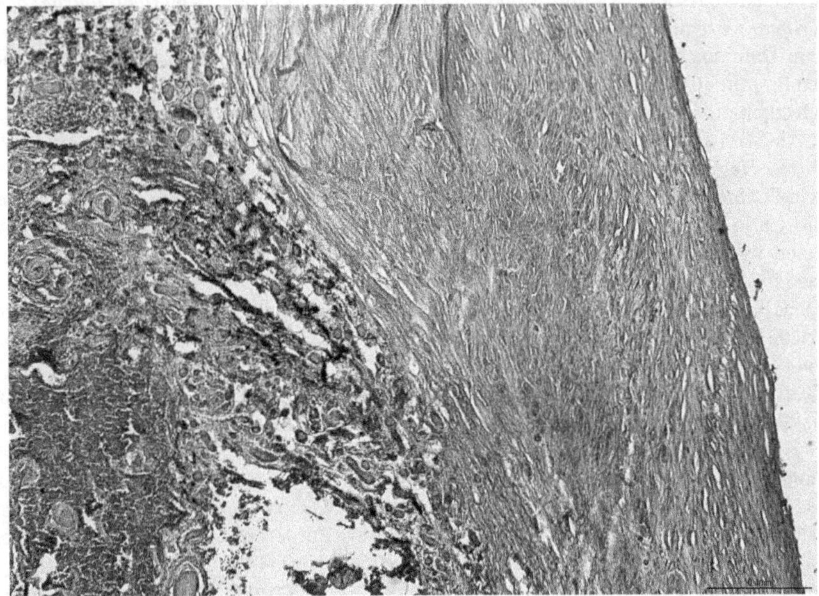

FIGURE 4.1 Low-magnification light microscopy appearance of diffuse pleural thickening, H&E. Note the many subpleural ferruginous bodies.

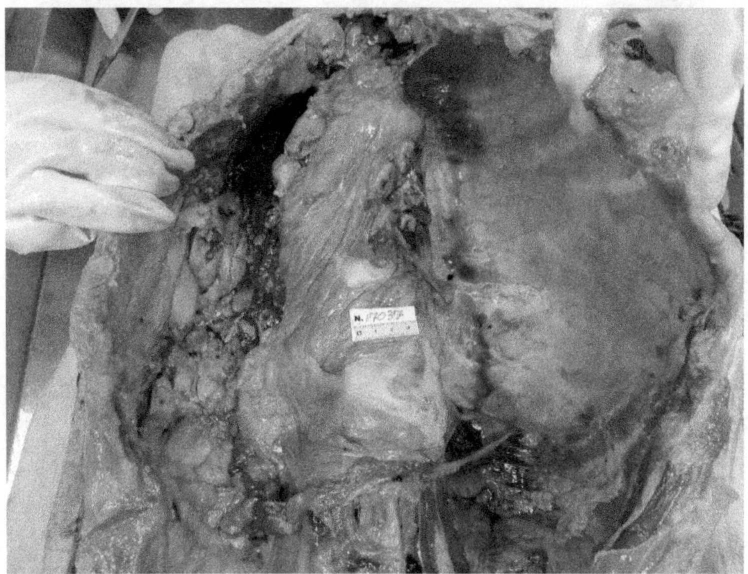

FIGURE 4.2 Macroscopic appearance of pleural plaques at autopsy. After removing the thoracic organs it was possible to observe typical plaques on the pericardial external surface and on the diaphragm.

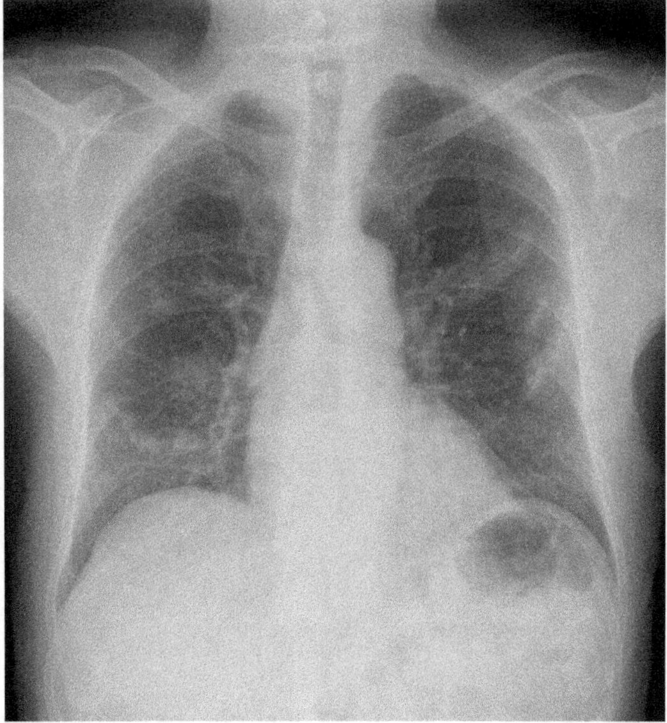

FIGURE 4.3 Pleural plaques on chest X-ray.

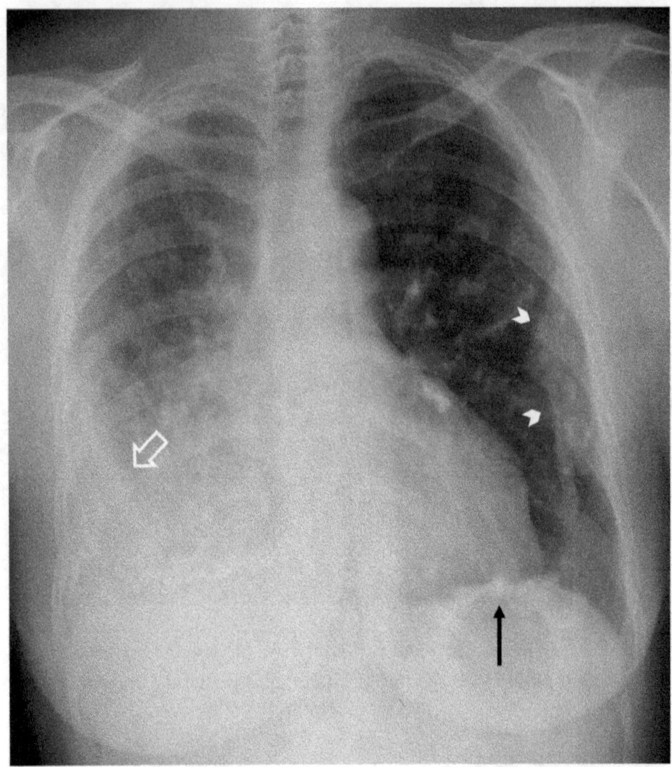

FIGURE 4.4 Chest X-ray. Pleural plaques on lateral chest wall (*arrowheads*) and on diaphragm (*black arrow*); pleural effusion (*white empty arrow*).

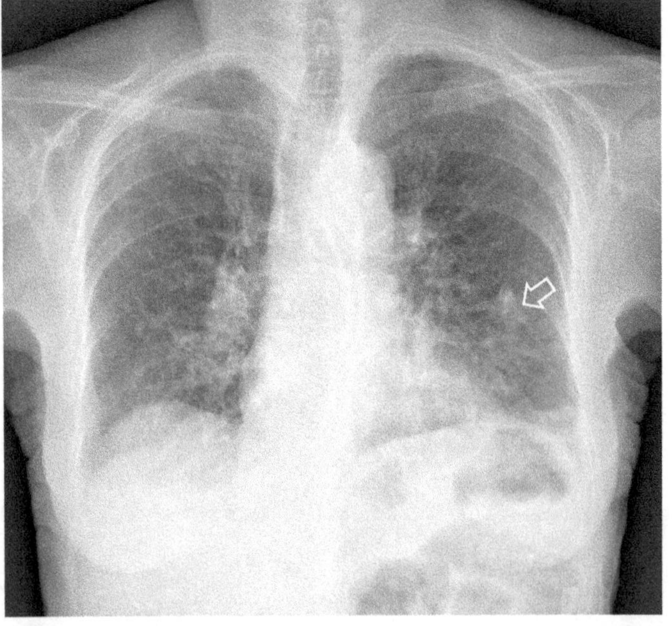

FIGURE 4.5 Pleural plaque "en face" on chest X-ray.

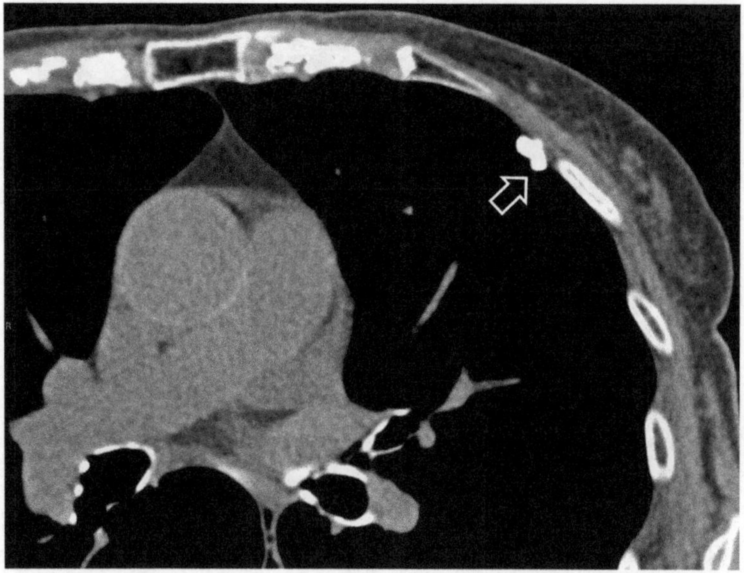

FIGURE 4.6 The same pleural plaque on the anterior chest wall on HRCT.

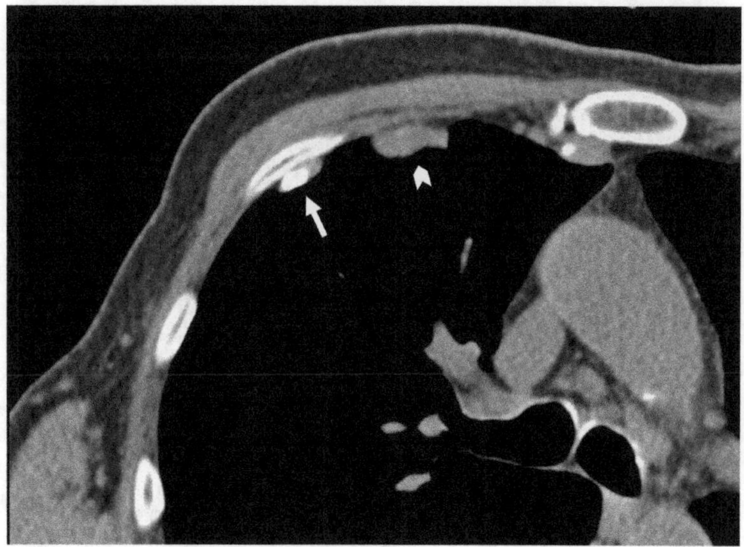

FIGURE 4.7 HRCT. Non-calcified pleural plaque (*arrowhead*) and calcified pleural plaque (*arrow*).

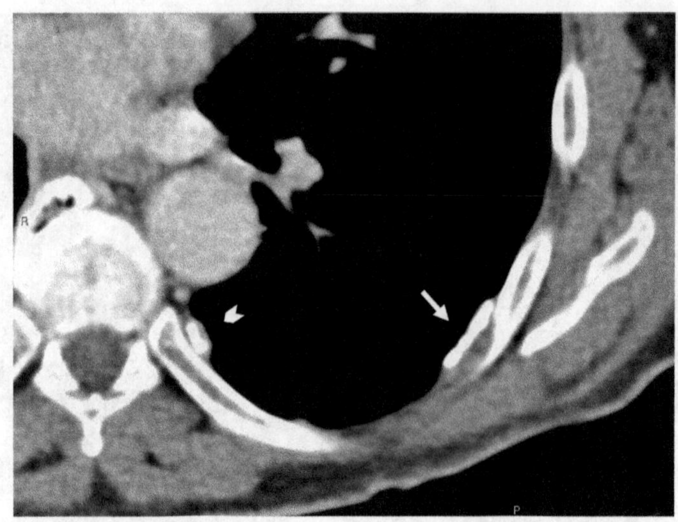

FIGURE 4.8 HRCT. Pleural plaques on the posterolateral chest wall (*arrow*) and in the paravertebral region (*arrowhead*).

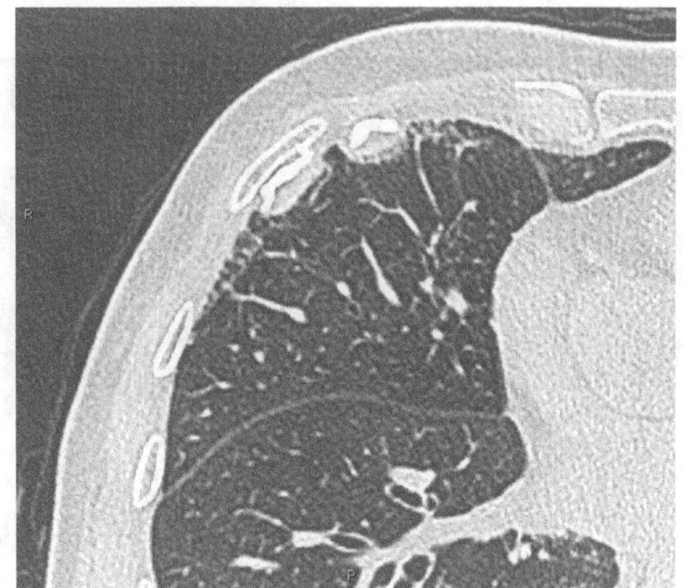

FIGURE 4.9 Pleural plaques with adjacent parenchymal fibrosis (CT).

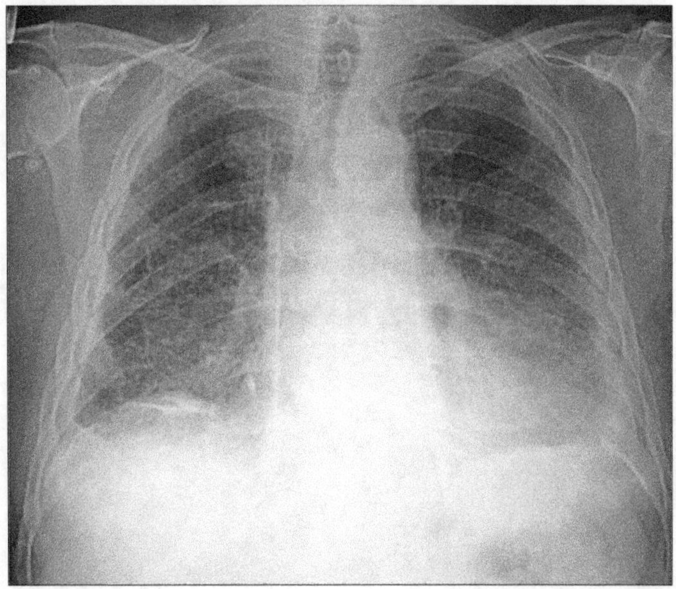

FIGURE 4.10 Asbestosis—interstitial fibrosis in the lower and middle lung zones. Chest X-ray.

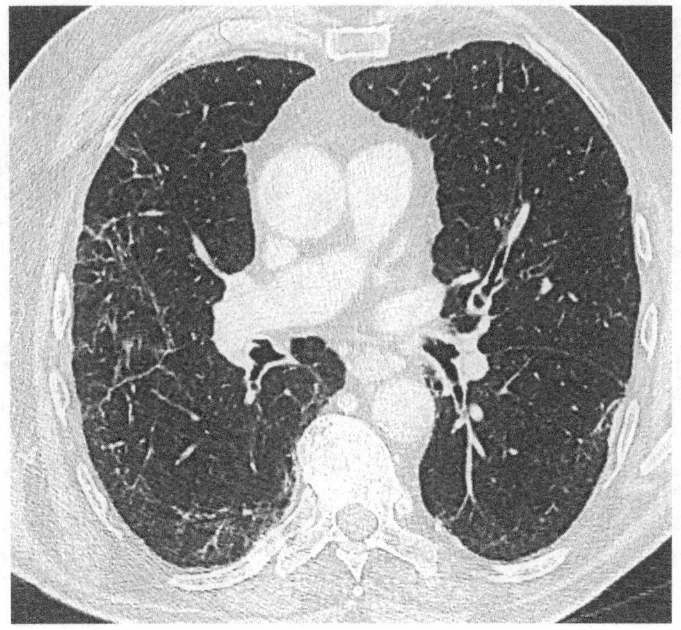

FIGURE 4.11 Asbestosis—subpleural branching opacities (CT).

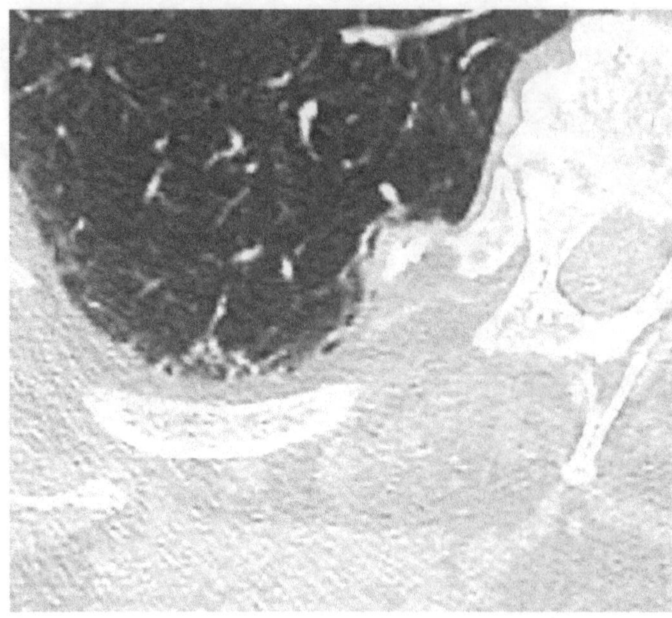

FIGURE 4.12 Asbestosis—parenchymal fibrosis and pleural plaque (a close-up view) (CT).

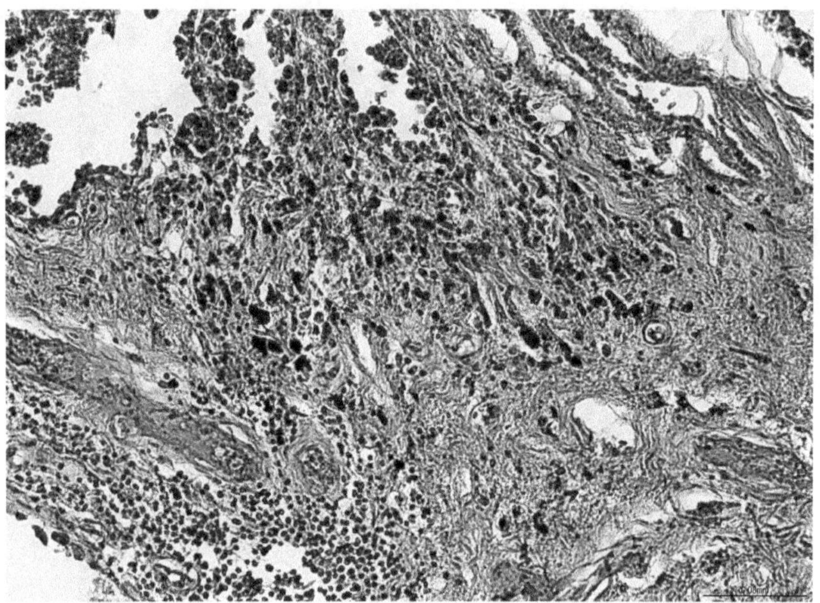

FIGURE 4.13 Medium-magnification image of multiple asbestos bodies in a lung section of an asbestos-exposed MM patient with lung fibrosis (light microscopy, H&E).

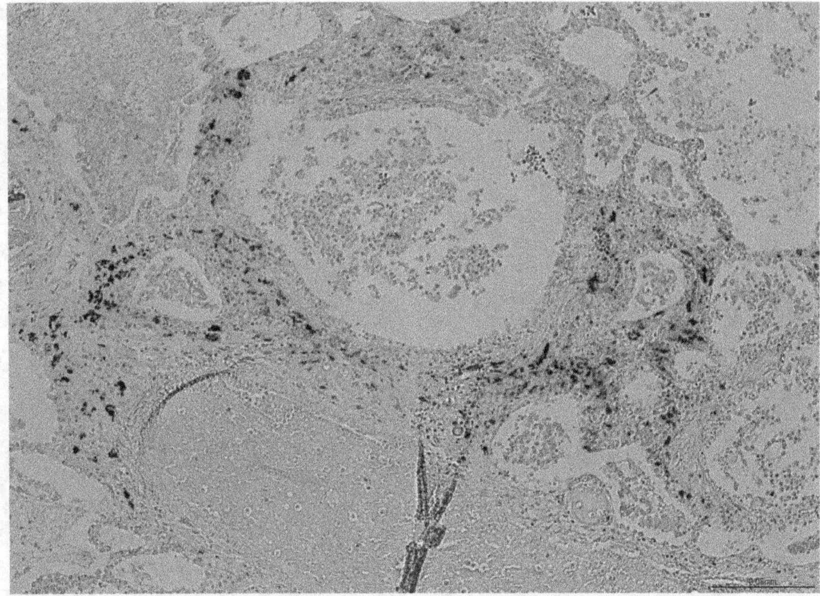

FIGURE 4.14 Low-magnification microscopic image of multiple interstitial asbestos bodies in a lung section of an asbestos-exposed MM patient with lung fibrosis (light microscopy, Perls staining).

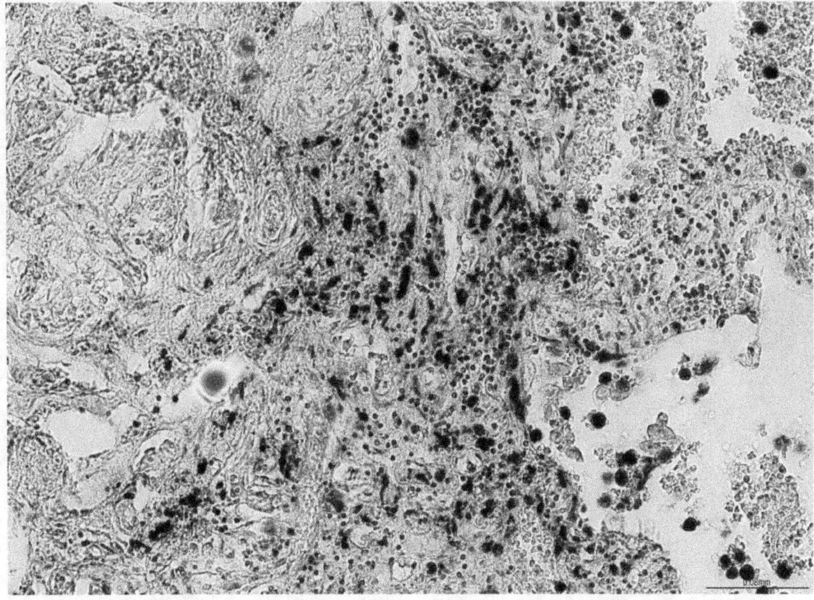

FIGURE 4.15 High-magnification microscopic image of multiple interstitial asbestos bodies in a lung section of an asbestos-exposed MM patient with lung fibrosis (light microscopy, Perls staining).

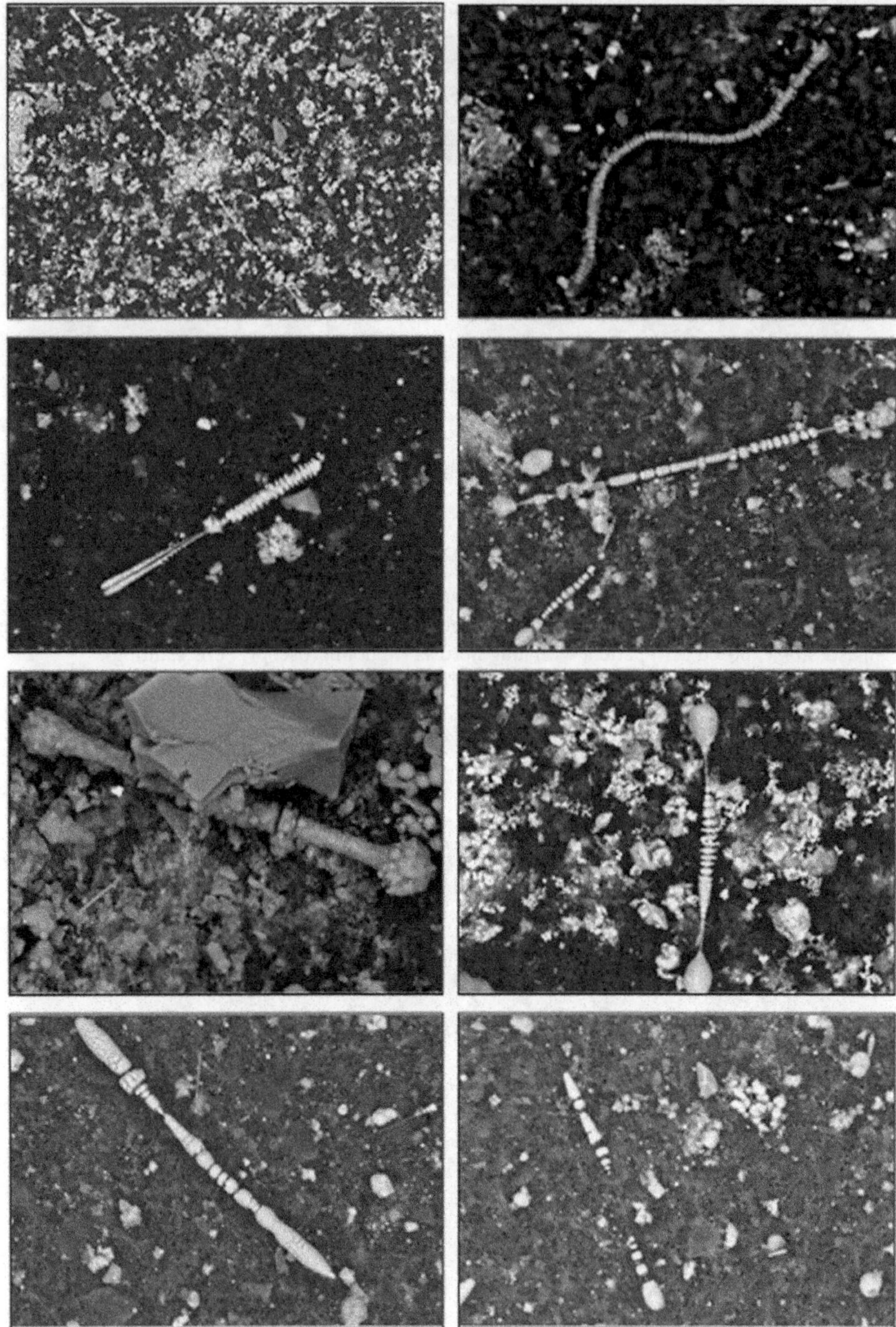

FIGURE 4.16 SEM images of asbestos bodies in digested lung tissue from MM patients.

5 Mechanisms of Asbestos Carcinogenesis

Giovanni Gaudino and Haining Yang

5.1 INTRODUCTION

The term "asbestos" used in national regulatory documents encompasses six commercially exploited minerals, including five amphiboles (crocidolite, actinolite, tremolite, anthophyllite, and amosite) and one serpentine (chrysotile). However, the natural environment contains approximately 400 additional minerals, and many of them have similar physical and chemical properties that have not been regulated and can be used without restrictions (Baumann and Carbone 2016). Some of these minerals have already shown carcinogenic properties and, when dispersed in the air, they can impact local communities. This highlights the inadequacy of the current terminology (Baumann, Ambrosi et al. 2013). For instance, residents of certain Cappadocian villages in Turkey and North Dakota, United States, are exposed to naturally occurring erionite fibers, which are more carcinogenic than regulated asbestos but have been utilized in construction or road paving materials (Carbone, Emri et al. 2007; Carbone, Baris et al. 2011).

Malignant mesothelioma is a cancer that originates from the transformation of mesothelial cells lining various body cavities. The most common site of this tumor is the pleura (thoracic cavity) with the second most common occurrence being the serosal membranes of the peritoneum (abdominal cavity). Occasionally mesothelioma develops from the transformed mesothelial cells of the pericardium or the serosal membranes of tunica vaginalis testis. The development of mesothelioma has been associated with exposure to carcinogenic mineral fibers, primarily asbestos (Carbone and Yang 2017).

The widespread use of asbestos in the mid-20th century, due to its insulating properties and cost-effectiveness, led to a significant increase in the incidence of mesothelioma and related mortality rates in developed countries. Consequently, these countries strictly regulated (United States) or banned (Europe, Australia) the use of asbestos after in vitro toxicology studies and rodent experiments demonstrated its carcinogenic nature (Carbone, Adusumilli et al. 2019).

The mechanisms of asbestos carcinogenesis have remained enigmatic until recently. Human mesothelial cells (HMs), the cells that when transformed give rise to mesothelioma, are uniquely susceptible to asbestos-induced cell death. It should be noted here that rodent mesothelial cells are more resistant to asbestos-induced cell death. When HMs are exposed to asbestos in tissue culture, they die within 1–2 weeks from exposure. How could asbestos, a toxic agent that kills mesothelial cells in tissue culture, cause mesothelioma? Remarkably, other human cell types, for example, human fibroblasts are resistant to asbestos cytotoxicity, yet asbestos does not cause fibrosarcomas. Yang et al. discovered that when human mesothelial cells are exposed to asbestos in the presence of TNF-α, which is either added exogenously to the cells in culture or is produced by macrophages exposed to asbestos in co-culture experiments, some mesothelial cells survive asbestos exposure and form tridimensional foci—i.e., loss of contact inhibition, evidence of in vitro cell transformation (Yang, Bocchetta et al. 2006). It was found that this process was mediated by the release of high mobility group box 1 (HMGB1) by dying mesothelial cells that trigger tumor necrosis factor alpha (TNF-α) release, and the release of other cytokines [interleukin 6 (IL-6), IL-8], as well as

DOI: 10.1201/9781003431909-5

active secretion of HMGB1, etc., by nearby mesothelial cells and macrophages. These cytokines in concert promote HM survival, growth, and transformation (Yang, Rivera et al. 2010), reviewed in Chen, Gaudino et al. (2017). These findings pointed to the chronic inflammatory process caused by the deposition of asbestos in tissues as the key factor that promotes asbestos carcinogenesis and mesothelioma (Carbone, Adusumilli et al. 2019).

In this chapter, we provide an overview of the current mechanisms underlying the development of mesothelioma, with a focus on the impact of carcinogenic mineral fibers on mesothelial cells, the related molecular responses, and how the environmental carcinogenic fibers can interact with human genes in regulating cancer predisposition, which is shown as the significance of gene-environment (G×E) interactions (Carbone, Arron et al. 2020).

5.2 ASBESTOS CARCINOGENESIS

Physicochemical characteristics of the fibers play a crucial role in determining their carcinogenic potential. Previous studies have shown that fiber dimensions, durability, and dose (referred to as the "three D's") and their physical properties are critical factors (Stanton, Laynard et al. 1977; Mossman 1990; Huang, Jaurand et al. 2011). Fiber dimensions are associated with durability and dose, affecting the bioavailability after inhalation. Longer and thinner fibers exhibit higher cytotoxicity and mutagenic potency. A meta-analysis has indicated that individuals exposed to fibers longer than 10 μm, or even 20μm, have a significantly increased risk of asbestos-related diseases (Barlow, Grespin et al. 2017). Macrophages struggle to efficiently engulf and clear larger and longer fibers, leading to repeated failed attempts of phagocytosis, referred to as "frustrated phagocytosis." This process triggers inflammatory cells surrounding the fibers to release reactive oxygen species (ROS) and reactive nitrogen species (RNS), which may exert mutagenic activity (Huang, Jaurand et al. 2011; Carbone, Ly et al. 2012). The World Health Organization (WHO) operationally distinguishes asbestos fibers into two groups, as short asbestos fibers (SAF) with a length <5 μm and long asbestos fibers (LAF) with a length >5 μm, diameter <3 μm, and length-diameter ratio >3, which are the focus of current regulatory rules (Boulanger, Andujar et al. 2014). Furthermore, variations in the biopersistence of fibers after exposure have an impact on tumorigenesis. For instance, serpentine chrysotile fibers, characterized by shorter biopersistence compared to amphiboles and erionite, exhibit a lower carcinogenic potential (Bernstein, Donaldson et al. 2008). However, prolonged exposure to chrysotile fibers leads to equivalent transformation of mesothelial cells (Qi, Okimoto et al. 2013). Conversely, palygorskite, a fibrous silicate mineral that is abundant in southern Nevada, lacks the ability to induce carcinogenesis in vivo due to reduced cytotoxicity and biopersistence in vitro. This diminished carcinogenic effect is attributed to its significantly reduced ability to induce inflammation compared to carcinogenic fibers (Larson, Powers et al. 2016).

5.3 CELL TRANSFORMATION IS ASSOCIATED WITH FIBER EXPOSURE

The mechanisms underlying asbestos-induced carcinogenesis have long been elusive, and the initial hypothesis of fiber-induced mechanical interference with cell division has been definitively dismissed (Carbone, Adusumilli et al. 2019). Some studies have suggested that the chemical structure of fibers, particularly the presence of iron as an impurity or component, may contribute to the carcinogenic process induced by asbestos and erionite (Croce, Allegrina et al. 2015). The deposition of asbestos fibers in tissues provides a surface where iron-rich macromolecular aggregates, known as asbestos bodies, facilitate the development of chronic inflammation (Nagai, Ishihara et al. 2011). Furthermore, asbestos-activated macrophages have been found to release ROS, which can indirectly cause DNA damage by forming 8-hydroxy-2'-deoxyguanosine (8-OHdG) adducts (Xu, Wu et al. 1999). Recent studies on iron-catalyzed ROS production suggest that a form of iron-dependent, non-apoptotic cell death called ferroptosis may be involved in asbestos-related carcinogenesis (Ramos-Nino, Blumen et al. 2008; Toyokuni 2019).

It has been proposed that asbestos carcinogenesis is associated with the accumulation of iron-induced by asbestos exposure, leading to ferroptosis-resistant mesothelial cells subjected to oxidative DNA damage and genomic alterations. The proposed mechanism involves ferroptosis-dependent extracellular vesicles, whose major components are ferritin heavy/light chains, transporting iron from ferroptotic macrophages to mesothelial cells, capable of internalizing these extracellular vesicles, particularly when in the S and G2/M mitotic phases, thereby contributing to asbestos-induced mesothelial carcinogenesis (Ito, Kato et al. 2021). Interestingly, the knockdown of poly(rC)-binding protein 2 (PCBP2), a cytosolic Fe(II) chaperone, led to decreased expression of transferrin receptor 1 (TfR1) and ferritin heavy chain (FTH), disrupting intracellular iron transport, and leading to inhibited mesothelial cell proliferation. This evidence suggested a possible role of PCBP2 in regulating ferroptosis resistance during mesothelial carcinogenesis (Yue, Luo et al. 2022). Furthermore, in a rat model with mutated BRCA1 (L63X/+), partially reproducing human mesothelioma characteristics, the intraperitoneal injection of chrysotile or crocidolite asbestos induced mesothelioma only in BRCA1 haploinsufficient, but not in wild type animals. The mutant rats exhibited dysregulation of iron metabolism, with increased catalytic iron levels, elevated Ki67-index, and resistance to ferroptosis as well (Luo, Akatsuka et al. 2023). An alternative hypothesis comes from the chemical analyses of ferruginous protein bodies extracted from lung tissues of Japanese patients that revealed anomalously high concentrations of radioactive radium, reaching millions of times higher concentrations than that of seawater. It has been proposed that continuous and prolonged internal exposure to hotspot ionizing radiation from radium and its daughter nuclides could cause DNA damage and cancer, including malignant mesothelioma (Nakamura, Makishima et al. 2009).

Additionally, it has been suggested that the hepatocyte growth factor (HGF) may play a role in asbestos-induced carcinogenesis by activating the PI3K/MEK5/Fra-1 axis (Broaddus, Yang et al. 1996; Ramos-Nino, Blumen et al. 2008). Also, downregulation of the insulin-like growth factor 1 (IGF1) prevented mesothelioma in a hamster model (Pass, Mew et al. 1996). The relevance of any of these mechanisms to asbestos-induced human mesothelioma remains to be demonstrated.

What is well established is that exposure to asbestos fibers causes death in human mesothelial cells, a cell type particularly susceptible to fiber cytotoxicity. Asbestos cytotoxicity was initially attributed to apoptosis (Broaddus, Yang et al. 1996). Subsequently, asbestos pathogenesis has been largely associated with TNF-α, a mediator of inflammation (Yang, Bocchetta et al. 2006) and with programmed necrosis (Yang, Rivera et al. 2010).

Exposure to asbestos drives mesothelial cells to release inflammatory cytokines, such as IL-1β IL-6, and IL-8 which play a role in mesothelial cell transformation (Rosenthal, Germolec et al. 1994; Chen, Gaudino et al. 2017). IL-6 is related to the JAK-STAT3 pathway, critical for inflammation-driven tumor growth. Within this inflammatory pathway, the pharmacological inhibition of the interaction between glycoprotein 130 (gp130) and the IL-6 receptor (IL6R), by using the gp130 inhibitor SC144, suppressed STAT3 downstream signaling in cells of the mesothelial lineage. In a mouse model of asbestos-induced cancer, SC144, along with the NSAID sulindac and the IL-1 receptor antagonist, anakinra, prolonged mice survival after asbestos exposure (Kadariya, Sementino et al. 2022).

Moreover, microRNAs (miRNAs), small RNA molecules regulating gene expression and recently linked to cancer have been investigated in relation to asbestos-induced carcinogenesis. An in vivo study investigated miRNAs and gene expression in lung tissues of mice exposed to asbestos administered intratracheally, by microarray analysis, real-time PCR, Western blotting, and immunohistochemistry (Hiraku, Watanabe et al. 2021). Fourteen miRNAs were significantly changed by asbestos exposure, including miR-21, known as highly oncogenic (Calin and Croce 2006), which was upregulated by both chrysotile and crocidolite. By RNA signature analysis, miR-21 was predicted to target and shown by Western blotting and immunohistochemistry to downregulate the tumor suppressor genes, Pdcd4 and Reck. These findings suggest that miR-21 upregulation could be an early response to asbestos exposure, that facilitates mesothelial transformation, via upregulation of oncogenes and downregulation of tumor suppressor genes (Hiraku, Watanabe et al. 2021).

5.4 HMGB1, CHRONIC INFLAMMATION, AND MESOTHELIOMA

Persistent inflammation plays a pivotal role in the development and progression of asbestos-induced pathogenesis and tumorigenesis (Yang, Bocchetta et al. 2006; Hillegass, Shukla et al. 2010; Yang, Rivera et al. 2010). The generation of a pro-inflammatory microenvironment at the fiber deposition sites, involving both human mesothelial cells (HM) and macrophages, combined with the enduring presence of numerous mineral fibers, provides certain HMs with the means to evade cell death and subsequently undergo oncogenic transformation (Carbone and Yang 2017). Investigations have unveiled that a significant proportion of HMs exposed to crocidolite asbestos (Yang, Rivera et al. 2010), chrysotile asbestos (Qi, Okimoto et al. 2013), and erionite fibers (Carbone, Baris et al. 2011) experience cell death through a variant of regulated necrosis termed programmed cell necrosis (Yang, Rivera et al. 2010). This form of necrosis is recognized by the passive release of high mobility group box 1 (HMGB1) from necrotic HMs at fiber deposition sites. HMGB1, a damage-associated molecular pattern (DAMP), fosters the attraction of macrophages which in turn release HMGB1 and several cytokines, thereby starting and perpetuating—because of the persistence of asbestos fibers in tissue—the chronic inflammatory process (Yang, Rivera et al. 2010; Kadariya, Menges et al. 2016). Because of the field effect of asbestos, multiple foci of chronic inflammation around asbestos deposits and related mesothelial hyperplasia may develop, accordingly, mesothelioma is often a polyclonal malignancy (Comertpay, Pastorino et al. 2014).

HMGB1 binds to several cell membrane receptors, including RAGE, priming macrophages for inflammasome activation, which occurs through the assembly of NLRP3 inflammasome via oligomerization of inactive NLRP3, apoptosis-associated speck-like protein (ASC), and procaspase-1. The NLRP3 inflammasome then triggers the release of IL-1β, IL-18, IL-1α, IL-8, and HMGB1, establishing an autocrine chronic inflammatory process (Thompson, Shukla et al. 2018). During this process, TNF-α is secreted, activating NF-κB and promoting the survival of HMs exposed to asbestos fibers. These surviving HMs may continue to proliferate and accumulate genetic mutations (Carbone and Yang 2017). Ranpirnase, a drug that downregulates NF-κB, has been tested in clinical trials and has had some beneficial effects in a small fraction of mesothelioma patients (Goparaju, Blasberg et al. 2011; Nasu, Carbone et al. 2011). The role of HMGB1 and related chronic inflammation in asbestos carcinogenesis is supported by findings that HMGB1 inhibitors or antagonists significantly inhibit asbestos-induced malignant transformation. Moreover, aspirin, which targets HMGB1 activities and inflammation, has both, a preventive effect on mesothelioma, and also an antitumor activity observed in mesothelioma xenograft models treated with aspirin (Yang, Pellegrini et al. 2015). Furthermore, both in vitro and in vivo studies have shown that ethyl pyruvate, an inhibitor of HMGB1 release and a suppressor of the expression of the RAGE receptor, inhibits the growth of mesothelioma cells, further supporting the key role of HMGB1 in mesothelioma pathogenesis (Pellegrini, Xue et al. 2017).

The increased expression and release of HMGB1 into the extracellular environment, as observed in mesothelioma cells compared to HM, along with the evidence demonstrating the growth-delaying effect of competitive HMGB1 inhibitors on mesothelioma xenografts, provide a mechanistic rationale for the anticancer potential of aspirin and some other anti-inflammatory drugs. While HMGB1 predominantly localizes to the nucleus in HMs and in other cell types, HMGB1 is observed in both the nucleus and cytosol in mesothelioma cells (Jube, Rivera et al. 2012). The cellular distribution of HMGB1 hinges on the equilibrium between histone acetyltransferase (HAT) and histone deacetylase (HDAC) activities, which modulate the acetylation status of HMGB1 (Bonaldi, Talamo et al. 2003); Evankovich, Cho et al. 2010). Additionally, poly(ADP-ribose) polymerase-1 (PARP-1) has a role in regulating this acetylation status (Yang, Li et al. 2014). In the context of mesothelioma, HMGB1 is actively released with hyper-acetylation into the extracellular milieu. There, it establishes an autocrine mechanism involving RAGE and TLR receptors, thereby stimulating proliferation, motility, and survival, ultimately contributing to the progression of mesothelioma (Jube, Rivera et al. 2012).

Moreover, we recently discovered that the translocation of HMGB1 from the nucleus to the cytoplasm upon asbestos exposure triggers autophagy, a pro-survival mechanism, fostering a greater proportion of HMs to survive asbestos-induced cell death. Silencing HMGB1 hindered autophagy and intensified asbestos-triggered HM cell death, thereby reducing asbestos-induced HM transformation. Both the cytoplasmic and the extracellular fractions of HMGB1 prompted autophagy through engagement with the RAGE receptor, the mTOR-ULK pathway and Beclin 1 phosphorylation, facilitating malignant transformation and malignant cell growth, while nuclear HMGB1 did not contribute to these processes. Notably, Inhibitors of autophagy, namely chloroquine and desmethylclomipramine, which is an antidepressant drug, amplified cell death and reduced the development of asbestos-driven foci (Xue, Patergnani et al. 2020) A diagram demonstrating some of the main mechanisms of asbestos carcinogenesis, especially the role of HMGB1 in mesothelioma development is presented in Figure 5.1.

To identify whether the main source of extracellular HMGB1 that drives asbestos carcinogenesis derives from mesothelial cells, from inflammatory cells, or both, we conducted a comprehensive study using two unique mouse models: the conditional mesothelial HMGB1-knockout ($Hmgb1^{\Delta pMeso}$) and the conditional myelomonocytic-lineage HMGB1-knockout ($Hmgb1^{\Delta Mylc}$). We demonstrated that HMGB1 was mainly released by mesothelial cells in the early stages of the inflammation resulting from asbestos exposure. This inflammatory process causes atypical mesothelial hyperplasia near asbestos deposits, and over the years, this process progresses into mesothelioma. The mesothelial HMGB1 knockout ($Hmgb1^{\Delta pMeso}$) exhibited significantly reduced inflammatory responses to asbestos, with low to undetectable levels of TNF-α nearby asbestos deposits. Additionally, in these mice, a higher proportion of M1-polarized macrophages compared to M2-macrophages was detected in the peritoneal lavage and the tissue microenvironment of areas with asbestos deposits. These $Hmgb1^{\Delta pMeso}$ mice, lacking HMGB1 production in mesothelial cells, showed a delayed and decreased incidence of mesothelioma and improved survival, which further validated the role of HMGB1 as an essential driver of asbestos-induced mesothelioma (Suarez, Novelli et al. 2023).

5.5 GENE × ENVIRONMENT INTERACTIONS

Asbestos fibers primarily induce necrotic cell death in HM, with additional contributions from other cell death mechanisms (Yang, Rivera et al. 2010; Affar and Carbone 2018). Carcinogenesis is often associated with somatic gene mutations that affect DNA repair mechanisms, leading to the accumulation of DNA damage and an increased fraction of cells with damaged DNA. When these cells acquire mechanisms of survival, such as those facilitated by the HMGB1 pathway in mesothelioma, cancer can develop. Inherited mutations in DNA repair and other genes may further enhance susceptibility to environmental carcinogens (Carbone, Amelio et al. 2018). To investigate gene-environment interactions, the current approach combines genetic and environmental studies (Carbone, Adusumilli et al. 2019).

Chromothripsis is a catastrophic and random event in which a single—or multiple—chromosome shatters and randomly reassembles, causing incorrect rearrangements or deletions of DNA sequences, and has been linked to increased mutational levels in cancer cell genomes. Chromothripsis may be facilitated by the accumulation of genetic damage associated with aging and/or by exposure to carcinogens. Chromothripsis causes significant genome alterations which may result in the activation of oncogenes and loss of tumor suppressor genes and may precipitate cancer development (Ly and Cleveland 2017). In 2016; Yoshikawa Y, et al., discovered chromothripsis in the majority of human mesotheliomas they studied. Specifically, Yoshikawa et al. discovered non-contiguous biallelic genome alterations in DNA from human mesothelioma biopsies, which could only be accounted for by the chromothripsis process (Yoshikawa, Emi et al. 2016). These findings were supported by several research teams that proposed that chromothripsis resulted in the formation of neo-antigens and that some of them could be targeted using immunotherapy (Yoshikawa, Emi et al. 2016; Mansfield, Peikert et al. 2019; Oey, Daniels et al. 2019).

Multiple tumor suppressors involved in DNA repair, cell cycle control and apoptosis can be found mutated in human mesothelioma. The most common somatic mutations in mesothelioma are biallelic inactivation of the *BAP1* gene, resulting in loss of nuclear staining by immunohistochemistry in over 60% of mesotheliomas (Nasu, Emi et al. 2015). Initially, NGS and Sanger sequencing were used to detect somatic *BAP1* mutations. These studies underestimated their true incidence to about 22% (Bott, Brevet et al. 2011; Testa, Cheung et al. 2011). In subsequent studies using an integrated approach that included MLPA, high-density CGH arrays, and immunohistochemistry, together with NGS and Sanger sequencing, 60% or more of BAP1 inactivation was discovered. The detection difference resulted from DNA deletions of about 300 to 3000 kb that could not be detected by Sanger and NGS, techniques developed to identify nucleotide-level mutations (i.e., point mutations). These deletions were detected by MLPA and high-density CGH-arrays, techniques that in turn missed the inactivating point mutations. Remarkably the most reliable methodology to detect *BAP1* mutations was immunohistochemistry as over 90% of *BAP1* inactivating mutations result from truncating mutations (Nasu, Emi et al. 2015). Since the nuclear localization signal is located at the carboxy-terminus of the BAP1 protein, almost all mutations result in the loss of nuclear BAP1 staining (Carbone, Harbour et al. 2020). Indeed, BAP1 immunostaining is nowadays used in all pathology laboratories to aid in the diagnosis of mesothelioma (Carbone, Shimizu et al. 2016; Carbone, Pass et al. 2022).

The second most common genetic alteration in mesothelioma is the homozygous deletion of the 9p21 locus, affecting the transcription of two tumor suppressors: p16INK4a and p14ARF. Loss of p16INK4a blocks cell division, while loss of p14ARF inhibits p53 ubiquitination, promoting apoptosis in $NF2^{+/-}$ knockout mice (Altomare, Vaslet et al. 2005). Deletion of the 9p21 region or *CDKN2A/p16INK4a* has been reported in up to 45% of primary pleural mesothelioma by whole-exome sequencing (Guo, Chmielecki et al. 2015). The consequent inactivation of the p16 gene has been associated with a poor clinical outcome (Singhi, Krasinskas et al. 2016). Transgenic mice with reduced p14ARF levels exhibit increased susceptibility to asbestos-induced carcinogenesis (Jongsma, van Montfort et al. 2008).

Alterations within the Hippo signaling pathway intermediates are notably prevalent in cases of mesothelioma. Neurofibromatosis type 2 (NF2)/Merlin, a regulatory element situated upstream in the Hippo pathway, is inactivated in up to 50% of malignant mesotheliomas (Lo Iacono, Monica et al. 2014; Guo, Chmielecki et al. 2015). However, 92% of the NF2-mutated mesothelioma biopsies studied by Lo Iacono et al., expressed NF2 by immunohistochemistry raising concerns about the possible biological significance of NF2 mutations (Carbone, Gaudino et al. 2015). On the other hand, heterozygous $NF2^{+/-}$ mice display heightened susceptibility to asbestos exposure and demonstrate expedited tumorigenesis when contrasted with their wild-type counterparts. The dysfunction of NF2 leads to the accumulation of Yes-Associated Protein (YAP) and WW domain-containing transcription regulator (WWTR1 or TAZ) within the nucleus as part of the Hippo pathway. Under inflammatory circumstances triggered by asbestos fibers, the assembly of the YAP/TAZ complex within the nucleus was further enhanced, bolstering the expression of multiple proto-oncogenes and fostering the survival of cancer cells (Altomare, Vaslet et al. 2005; Rehrauer, Wu et al. 2018; Sato and Sekido 2018). In mesothelioma cells, TAZ is more active than in mesothelial cells. Silencing TAZ in mesothelioma cells significantly inhibited cell growth, motility, and invasion that were induced in mesothelial cells transduced with active TAZ. Interleukin 1 (IL-1) signaling was necessary for TAZ-promoted proliferation and IL-1 inactivation, by knockdown or by an antagonist drug, reversed the tumor phenotype (Matsushita, Sato et al. 2019). Recently, it has been shown that NF2 is involved in the mechanosensory component of the Hippo pathway in mesothelial cells and that its loss leads to YAP/TAZ-driven anchorage-independent cell growth (Cunningham, Jia et al. 2023). Several other genes have also been implicated in mesothelioma progression (Ivanov, Miller et al. 2009).

5.6 THE ROLE OF THE *BAP1* GENE

Epidemiological studies have shown that up to 5–10% of individuals with heavy and prolonged asbestos exposure develop mesothelioma (Carbone, Adusumilli et al. 2019; Carbone, Yang et al. 2023). The study of mesothelioma epidemics in Cappadocia, Turkey, where villagers had high exposure to erionite fibers and an exceptionally high incidence of mesothelioma—~50% of the population in these villages developed and died of mesothelioma—revealed the transmission of mesothelioma susceptibility through Mendelian autosomal dominant inheritance. Further, studies on two unrelated US families with a similarly high incidence of mesothelioma and no occupational asbestos exposure identified frequent alterations on chromosome 3p21, leading to the discovery of germline BAP1 mutations associated with autosomal dominant transmission of mesothelioma and uveal melanoma (Roushdy-Hammady, Siegel et al. 2001; Carbone, Emri et al. 2007; Testa, Cheung et al. 2011; Wiesner, Obenauf et al. 2011) as well as MBAITs that were later identified as melanocytic BAP1 associated intradermal tumors, because of their histological and molecular characteristics setting them apart from other spitzoid nodules (Carbone, Ferris et al. 2012).

Animal studies using $Bap1^{+/-}$ heterozygous mice demonstrated that these animals developed mesothelioma with much higher incidence compared to wild-type Bap1 mice and that they developed mesothelioma even when they were exposed to much lower doses of asbestos fibers that normally do not induce mesothelioma in Bap1 wild-type mice (Napolitano, Pellegrini et al. 2016). This study clearly showed that the loss of BAP1 can increase the susceptibility to asbestos carcinogenesis.

Initially characterized as a nuclear protein with deubiquitylase activity, BAP1 plays a role in chromatin remodeling, DNA double-strand repair, and auto-deubiquitylation to promote its own nuclear localization. Recent studies have shown that BAP1 has dual activity in the nucleus and cytoplasm. BAP1 is part of multiprotein transcriptional regulators involved in metabolism, mitochondrial function, and cell proliferation, which contributes to tumor suppression. In the cytoplasm, BAP1 deubiquitylates and stabilizes the type 3 inositol-1,4,5-trisphosphate receptor (IP3R3), leading to the release of Ca^{2+} from the endoplasmic reticulum into the mitochondrial space, ultimately inducing apoptosis. Reduced BAP1 levels impair DNA repair and apoptotic response, selecting cells with oncogenic mutations and promoting tumorigenesis. Additionally, reduced cytoplasmic BAP1 levels induce the Warburg effect, a metabolic shift to aerobic glycolysis, which may accelerate tumorigenesis (Carbone, Yang et al. 2013; Ismail, Davidson et al. 2014; Lee, Lee et al. 2014; Yu, Pak et al. 2014; Bononi, Giorgi et al. 2017; Bononi, Yang et al. 2017).

Inherited *BAP1* mutations have been linked to an elevated susceptibility to several tumor types, including, in order of frequency, mesothelioma, uveal melanoma, cutaneous melanoma, renal cell carcinoma of the clear cell type, breast cancer, basal cell carcinoma, cholangiocarcinoma, a particular type of aggressive meningioma known as rhabdoid meningioma (Hu, Miettinen et al. 2022), and others (Carbone, Harbour et al. 2020). About 25% of carriers of BAP1 mutations develop multiple cancers which characteristically are much less aggressive than their sporadic counterparts (Carbone, Pass et al. 2022). A comprehensive global genomic investigation of germline *BAP1* mutations and the clinical manifestations of the BAP1 cancer syndrome has unveiled that core syndrome-associated tumors are prevalent within a substantial portion of the analyzed families (Carbone, Ferris et al. 2012; Njauw, Kim et al. 2012; Pena-Llopis, Vega-Rubin-de-Celis et al. 2012; Popova, Hebert et al. 2013) (Abdel-Rahman, Pilarski et al. 2011; Murali, Wilmott et al. 2013; Pilarski, Cebulla et al. 2014; Baumann, Buck et al. 2015; de la Fouchardiere, Cabaret et al. 2015; Wadt, Aoude et al. 2015; Rai, Pilarski et al. 2016; Shankar, Abedalthagafi et al. 2017; Kittaneh and Berkelhammer 2018; Panou, Gadiraju et al. 2018; Walpole, Pritchard et al. 2018) (Carbone, Flores et al. 2015).

5.7 HMGB1 AND BAP1 COOPERATE TOWARD TUMORIGENESIS

It was recently discovered that BAP1—the most frequently inactivated gene in mesothelioma—interacts with HMGB1, the protein that plays a critical role in mesothelioma induced by asbestos.

It was found that BAP1 forms a trimeric protein complex with HMGB1 and HDAC1. Proximity ligation assay (PLA) comparing primary fibroblasts from carriers of *BAP1*$^{+/-}$ with those from individuals with normal *BAP1* alleles revealed an interaction between BAP1 and HMGB1 within the cell nucleus. Coimmunoprecipitation, SPR, and computational modeling further validated the BAP1-HMGB1 interaction through specific BAP1 domain and demonstrated that BAP1 also plays a role in deubiquitylating and stabilizing HDAC1, which in turn regulates HMGB1 acetylation and cellular localization as well as its activity. Finally, it was found that BAP1 bound both HMGB1 and HDAC1 in a DNA-independent manner (Novelli, Bononi et al. 2021). Furthermore, *BAP1*$^{+/-}$ fibroblasts exhibited significantly increased extranuclear acetylated HMGB1 and decreased nuclear HMGB1 levels compared to fibroblasts with normal BAP1. Similar results were observed in THP-1 differentiated macrophages. Elevated levels of acetylated HMGB1 in cells with BAP1 mutations promoted malignant transformation and tumorigenesis. Reduced BAP1 levels enhanced asbestos-induced HM transformation in vitro, demonstrating a gene-environment interaction. Notably, BAP1 did not deubiquitylate HMGB1 and did not affect total HMGB1 protein, mRNA levels, or stability, while decreased nuclear activity of HDAC1 in *BAP1*$^{+/-}$ cells led to hyperacetylation and release of HMGB1.

In conclusion, BAP1 interacts with both HMGB1 and HDAC1 simultaneously, promoting the stable assembly of the trimeric complex. Reduced BAP1 levels due to germline mutations lead to elevated HDAC1 ubiquitylation and degradation, increasing acetylated HMGB1 release that promotes inflammation and mesothelial cell transformation (Novelli, Bononi et al. 2021).

This finding substantiates the mechanistic basis for the gene-environment (G×E) interaction involving BAP1 mutations, asbestos-induced chronic inflammation, and mesothelioma.

5.8 OTHER GENES PREDISPOSING TO ASBESTOS CARCINOGENESIS AND MESOTHELIOMA

Subsequent investigations have been carried out to analyze the genotypes of cancer patients, particularly those with a heightened susceptibility to familial inheritance, aiming to detect hereditary modifications in other genes that might play a role in mesothelioma and other cancers (Yoshikawa, Sato et al. 2015; Panou, Gadiraju et al. 2018; Pastorino, Yoshikawa et al. 2018).

We identified two families with a high occurrence of mesothelioma and whole-genome sequencing was performed on 10 mesothelioma patients from four Turkish families with multiple cases of the disease. In one family, both the mother and son had a rare genetic mutation of the Bloom syndrome gene (*BLM*) (c.569_570del;p.R191Kfs*4) with subsequent loss of the BLM protein in cancer cells, indicating inactivation of both alleles. Affected family members developed mesothelioma. Another family from the United States had a different rare *BLM* mutation (c.569_570del;p.R191Kfs*4). This mutation was found in a patient and two of her siblings. Both mutations were predicted to be pathogenic based on computational analysis (Bononi, Goto et al. 2020). Bloom syndrome is characterized by growth deficiency, sensitivity to sunlight, type 2 diabetes, and a significantly higher risk of various cancers. BLM functions as a RecQ helicase involved in DNA replication, double-strand break (DSB) DNA repair, and apoptosis triggered by the p53 pathway. Biallelic mutations in *BLM* cause an autosomal-recessive condition that increases susceptibility to tumors because DNA repair and apoptosis are impaired (Carbone, Arron et al. 2020).

Heterozygous BLM mutations in vitro caused genomic instability. Mesothelial cells from mice with one functional BLM allele accumulated more micronuclei when exposed to asbestos. In HM, BLM silencing and exposure to asbestos hindered H2A.X phosphorylation, a marker of DNA damage, leading to DNA DSBs, due to impaired repair mechanisms. Interestingly, in BLM-silenced macrophages, the release of TNF-α increased as well as in *Blm*$^{+/-}$ mice injected with asbestos, which also displayed a larger presence of M1 macrophages in the peritoneal cavity. In summary, evidence suggests that heterozygous BLM mutations increase the risk of mesothelioma, either due to asbestos exposure or potentially independently of it, as observed in patients (Bononi, Goto et al. 2020).

More recently, germline analysis of 264 patients with sporadic mesothelioma revealed the occurrence of eight different likely pathogenic variants of the BARD1 gene associated with mesothelioma. Decreased BARD1 levels or expression of mutated BARD1 in cells exposed to asbestos fibers enhance genomic instability and DNA damage, as well as protect cells against cell death. These results indicate that heterozygous BARD1 germline mutations may predispose individuals to mesothelioma and increase susceptibility to asbestos-induced carcinogenesis (Novelli, Yoshikawa et al. 2024).

Additional germline mutations with a high CADD score (>15) and therefore likely to be pathogenic, have been detected in patients with mesothelioma. These include pathogenic mutations of BRCA1, BRCA2, TP53, ATM, etc., which are well-known tumor suppressor genes that when mutated predispose to various cancer types, as well as many others whose clinical significance remains to be validated by functional analyses (Betti, Aspesi et al. 2016; Betti, Aspesi et al. 2018; Panou, Gadiraju et al. 2018; Pastorino, Yoshikawa et al. 2018; Hassan, Morrow et al. 2019; Panou and Roe 2020; Mitchell, Gilliam et al. 2023). At times multiple germline mutations are present in the same patient, raising the issue of G×G interactions in the pathogenesis of these mesothelioma. Moreover, as shown for carriers of pathogenic germline TP53 mutations, radiation, including therapeutic radiation and imaging-based radiation (i.e., CT scans), may increase the risk of developing cancer including mesothelioma, in carriers of pathogenic mutations of BAP1 and of other genes involved with DNA repair (G×E interaction). Also, infection with the SV40 virus together with asbestos exposure significantly increased asbestos carcinogenesis in a hamster model and in vitro malignant transformation of human mesothelial cells, evidence of co-carcinogenesis among a biological infectious agent and asbestos (Kroczynska, Cutrone et al. 2006; Qi, Carbone et al. 2011). The possible significance of these findings to the development of human mesothelioma has been hypothesized but remains to be demonstrated (Carbone, Rizzo et al. 2000; Carbone and Pass 2004; Carbone, Gazdar et al. 2020).

5.9 CONCLUSION

Mesothelioma originates from transformed mesothelial cells that form the membranes that cover the body cavities and is largely linked to asbestos exposure. The regulatory term "asbestos" covers six minerals, yet around 400 similar minerals exist, some may be even more carcinogenic, like erionite (Carbone, Baris et al. 2011; Baumann, Ambrosi et al. 2013). Several mechanisms have been proposed for asbestos-induced carcinogenesis, based on the chemical composition of the fibers. The content of iron in asbestos bodies may contribute to carcinogenesis by facilitating chronic inflammation (Nagai, Ishihara et al. 2011). Asbestos-activated macrophages release ROS, forming 8-OHdG adducts (Xu, Wu et al. 1999).

TNF-α mediates inflammation-related asbestos pathogenesis (Yang, Bocchetta et al. 2006) and leads to HM survival from programmed cell necrosis, which contribute to mesothelioma development (Yang, Rivera et al. 2010). Moreover, asbestos exposure induces IL-1β and IL-6 release, associated with murine mesothelial transformation. IL-6's JAK-STAT3 pathway supports inflammation-driven tumor growth. This hypothesis is supported by the observation that inhibition of IL-1 and IL6R pathways extends mouse survival after asbestos exposure (Kadariya, Sementino et al. 2022). Experiments using human cells are required to validate the clinical significance of the experiments in mice.

Chronic inflammation is a critical driver of asbestos pathogenesis and tumorigenesis. At fiber deposition sites, a pro-inflammatory microenvironment forms involving HMs and macrophages. The ensuing chronic inflammation, supported by the persistence of mineral fibers in tissue, occasionally allows some HMs to evade cell death and these damaged cells may undergo oncogenic transformation (Carbone and Yang 2017). Crocidolite-, chrysotile-, and erionite-exposed HMs undergo programmed cell necrosis, releasing high mobility group box 1 (HMGB1), a damage-associated molecular pattern (DAMP) that initiates the inflammatory response. This prompts macrophage attraction and perpetuation of chronic inflammation (Yang, Rivera et al. 2010; Kadariya, Menges et al. 2016). This process involves the formation of the NLRP3 inflammasome by bringing together inactive NLRP3, apoptosis-associated speck-like protein (ASC), and procaspase-1. As a result, the NLRP3 inflammasome prompts the secretion of IL-1β, IL-18, IL-1α, IL-8, and HMGB1, setting off a self-sustaining chronic inflammation process within the cell (Thompson, Shukla et al. 2018). In mesothelioma, HMGB1 is hyper-acetylated and therefore it is released from the nucleus into the cytoplasm where it induces autophagy (Xue, Patergnani et al. 2020) and extracellularly where HMGB1 activates the RAGE and TLR receptors, promoting cell proliferation, motility, and survival (Jube, Rivera et al. 2012).

Aspirin's anti-HMGB1 function and its preventive effect on mesothelioma and antitumor activity in xenograft models support the role of HMGB1-related inflammation in the pathogenesis of mesothelioma (Yang, Pellegrini et al. 2015). Ethyl pyruvate, inhibiting HMGB1 release and suppressing RAGE, also prevents the growth of mesothelioma (Pellegrini, Xue et al. 2017), findings based on experiments in primary human mesothelial cells and validated in mouse models. Mesothelial HMGB1 knockout mice further supported HMGB1's role in mesothelioma, because the KO mice displayed reduced inflammation and reduced TNFα levels, altered macrophage profiles, as well as delayed and reduced mesothelioma incidence and improved survival (Suarez, Novelli et al. 2023).

The development of mesothelioma may also involve intricate interplay between genetics and the environment (G×E interactions) because inherited DNA repair gene mutations can increase the susceptibility to environmental carcinogens, both asbestos and therapeutic radiation (Carbone, Adusumilli et al. 2019). Accordingly, carriers of germline BAP1 mutations should be screened preferentially with ultrasonography and MRI for early cancer detection rather than with CT scans because, similarly to carriers of germline TP53 mutations, they may be at higher risk of radiation-induced malignancies.

Accumulation of genetic damage may favor chromothripsis, which may either cause cell death—the most likely outcome—or occasionally generate a malignant cell clone. Non-contiguous biallelic genome alterations with a chromothripsis pattern have been detected in the majority of mesotheliomas, suggesting that chromothripsis may be a common mechanism that drives the development of mesothelioma. Studies are in progress to see whether it is possible to target therapeutically the neoantigens created by chromothripsis (Yoshikawa, Emi et al. 2016; Mansfield, Peikert et al. 2019).

Epidemiology clearly indicates that only a small proportion of individuals with prolonged asbestos exposure develop mesothelioma, indicating that inheritance of mesothelioma susceptibility exists (Roushdy-Hammady, Siegel et al. 2001). As a matter of fact, high mesothelioma incidence in two US families with no occupational asbestos exposure was demonstrated and these were causally linked to inherited germline *BAP1* mutations, transmitted in an autosomal dominant fashion because of haplotype insufficiency (Testa, Cheung et al. 2011). BAP1 is a multifunctional deubiquitylase active in the nucleus and the cytoplasm regulating transcription, metabolism, and DNA repair (Carbone, Yang et al. 2013). When BAP1 levels are reduced by germline truncating mutations, DNA repair (Ismail, Davidson et al. 2014; Yu, Pak et al. 2014) and Ca^{2+} release from mitochondria are impaired, which causes the suppression of apoptotic response and induction of tumorigenesis (Bononi, Giorgi et al. 2017). Decreased cytoplasmic BAP1 levels also induce the Warburg effect, enhancing aerobic glycolysis (Bononi, Yang et al. 2017).

Therefore, a strong body of evidence points at BAP1 and HMGB1 as key players in the process of mesothelial transformation and onset of mesothelioma upon asbestos exposure. Interestingly, BAP1 orchestrates the formation of a stable trimeric complex with HMGB1 and HDAC1, and mutations reducing BAP1 levels cause increased ubiquitylation and degradation of HDAC1, with the consequence of increased HMGB1 acetylation and release that in turn promotes asbestos-driven inflammation and transformation of mesothelial cells (Novelli, Bononi et al. 2021; Carbone, Minaai et al. 2023).

Hereditary alterations in other genes, possibly contributing to susceptibility for mesothelioma, were investigated by a genetic profiling study. Whole-genome sequencing conducted on patients from families with multiple cases of mesothelioma revealed other rare heterozygous pathogenic mutations that are linked to mesothelioma predisposition, such as the *BLM* gene (Bononi, Goto et al. 2020). With more ongoing continuous studies, there will be more genetic factors discovered later that may contribute to the risk of mesothelioma (Bononi, Goto et al. 2020).

In addition to BAP1, several tumor suppressor genes involved in DNA repair, cell cycle regulation, and apoptosis are commonly mutated in mesothelioma. The deletion of the 9p21 locus, affecting p16INK4a and p14ARF tumor suppressors, is a prevalent genetic alteration. Loss of p16INK4a halts cell division, while p14ARF loss hampers p53 ubiquitination, promoting apoptosis (Altomare, Menges et al. 2011). Mesotheliomas often lack p16INK4a, correlating with poorer clinical outcomes. Altered p14ARF levels in transgenic mice impact asbestos-induced carcinogenesis (Jongsma, van Montfort et al. 2008; Husain, Colby et al. 2018).

Neurofibromatosis type 2 (NF2)/Merlin, a regulator of Hippo pathway signaling is frequently altered in mesothelioma, often inactivated. Experiments in rodent cells revealed that NF2 dysfunction, as well as inflammatory conditions induced by asbestos, lead to the accumulation of yes-associated protein (YAP) and WW domain-containing transcription regulator (TAZ), promoting tumor cell survival (Altomare, Vaslet et al. 2005; Rehrauer, Wu et al. 2018; Sato and Sekido 2018). Moreover, NF2 has been linked to the mechanosensory aspect of the Hippo pathway in mesothelial cells, and its loss triggers YAP/TAZ-driven anchorage-independent cell growth (Cunningham, Jia et al. 2023). However, the persistent expression of NF2 detected by immunohistochemistry in 92% of NF2-mutated biopsies, raises concerns about the clinical significance of NF2 mutations in human mesothelioma (Lo Iacono, Monica et al. 2014). Functional studies in human mesothelioma are needed to address this issue.

In summary, most mesotheliomas have been caused by exposure to asbestos or less frequently to other carcinogenic mineral fibers. Asbestos and mineral fibers carcinogenesis has been strongly linked to the chronic inflammatory reaction that develops at sites of asbestos deposits and that is driven by HMGB1 released extracellularly. In addition to its extracellular activity, cytoplasmic HMGB1 activates autophagy, a survival mechanism that allows some mesothelial cells to survive asbestos exposure. These cells accumulate genetic damage that may ensue in chromothripsis and occasionally, especially when BAP1 and or CDKN2A are inactivated, in the emergence of a malignant clone. Germline mutations of BAP1 and less frequently of other tumor suppressor genes cause familial mesothelioma and when these individuals are exposed to asbestos or therapeutic radiation, mesothelioma may develop in the contest of G×E interaction.

Asbestos fibers cause mesothelial cells to undergo programmed cell necrosis, which leads to the release of HMGB1 to the extracellular space, where HMGB1 acts as a pro-inflammatory factor recruiting macrophages and other inflammatory cells. Macrophages with activated NLRP3 inflammasome secrete cytokines, such as TNF-α and IL-1β, thus propagating inflammation around asbestos deposits and activating NF-κB pathway that helps mesothelial cells survive. Moreover, asbestos induces HMGB1 cytoplasmic translocation that induces autophagy, which also increases the pool of proliferating mesothelial cells carrying genetic damages caused by asbestos, a process that over time may lead to malignant transformation and mesothelioma development.

REFERENCES

Abdel-Rahman, M. H., R. Pilarski, C. M. Cebulla, J. B. Massengill, B. N. Christopher, G. Boru, P. Hovland and F. H. Davidorf (2011). "Germline BAP1 mutation predisposes to uveal melanoma, lung adenocarcinoma, meningioma, and other cancers." *J Med Genet* 48(12): 856–859.

Affar, E. B. and M. Carbone (2018). "BAP1 regulates different mechanisms of cell death." *Cell Death Dis* 9(12): 1151.

Altomare, D. A., C. W. Menges, J. Xu, J. Pei, L. Zhang, A. Tadevosyan, E. Neumann-Domer, Z. Liu, M. Carbone, I. Chudoba, A. J. Klein-Szanto and J. R. Testa (2011). "Losses of both products of the Cdkn2a/

Arf locus contribute to asbestos-induced mesothelioma development and cooperate to accelerate tumorigenesis." *PLoS One* 6(4): e18828.

Altomare, D. A., C. A. Vaslet, K. L. Skele, A. De Rienzo, K. Devarajan, S. C. Jhanwar, A. I. McClatchey, A. B. Kane and J. R. Testa (2005). "A mouse model recapitulating molecular features of human mesothelioma." *Cancer Res* 65(18): 8090–8095.

Barlow, C. A., M. Grespin and E. A. Best (2017). "Asbestos fiber length and its relation to disease risk." *Inhal Toxicol* 29(12–14): 541–554.

Baumann, F., J. P. Ambrosi and M. Carbone (2013). "Asbestos is not just asbestos: An unrecognised health hazard." *Lancet Oncol* 14(7): 576–578.

Baumann, F., B. J. Buck, R. V. Metcalf, B. T. McLaurin, D. J. Merkler and M. Carbone (2015). "The presence of asbestos in the natural environment is likely related to mesothelioma in young individuals and women from Southern Nevada." *J Thorac Oncol* 10(5): 731–737.

Baumann, F. and M. Carbone (2016). "Environmental risk of mesothelioma in the United States: An emerging concern-epidemiological issues." *J Toxicol Environ Health B* 19(5–6): 231–249.

Bernstein, D. M., K. Donaldson, U. Decker, S. Gaering, P. Kunzendorf, J. Chevalier and S. E. Holm (2008). "A biopersistence study following exposure to chrysotile asbestos alone or in combination with fine particles." *Inhal Toxicol* 20(11): 1009–1028.

Betti, M., A. Aspesi, A. Biasi, E. Casalone, D. Ferrante, P. Ogliara, L. C. Gironi, R. Giorgione, P. Farinelli, F. Grosso, R. Libener, S. Rosato, D. Turchetti, A. Maffe, C. Casadio, V. Ascoli, C. Dianzani, E. Colombo, E. Piccolini, M. Pavesi, S. Miccoli, D. Mirabelli, C. Bracco, L. Righi, R. Boldorini, M. Papotti, G. Matullo, C. Magnani, B. Pasini and I. Dianzani (2016). "CDKN2A and BAP1 germline mutations predispose to melanoma and mesothelioma." *Cancer Lett* 378(2): 120–130.

Betti, M., A. Aspesi, D. Ferrante, M. Sculco, L. Righi, D. Mirabelli, F. Napoli, M. Rondon-Lagos, E. Casalone, F. Vignolo Lutati, P. Ogliara, P. Bironzo, C. L. Gironi, P. Savoia, A. Maffe, S. Ungari, F. Grosso, R. Libener, R. Boldorini, M. Valiante, B. Pasini, G. Matullo, G. Scagliotti, C. Magnani and I. Dianzani (2018). "Sensitivity to asbestos is increased in patients with mesothelioma and pathogenic germline variants in BAP1 or other DNA repair genes." *Genes Chromosomes Cancer* 57(11): 573–583.

Bonaldi, T., F. Talamo, P. Scaffidi, D. Ferrera, A. Porto, A. Bachi, A. Rubartelli, A. Agresti and M. E. Bianchi (2003). "Monocytic cells hyperacetylate chromatin protein HMGB1 to redirect it towards secretion." *EMBO J* 22(20): 5551–5560.

Bononi, A., C. Giorgi, S. Patergnani, D. Larson, K. Verbruggen, M. Tanji, L. Pellegrini, V. Signorato, F. Olivetto, S. Pastorino, M. Nasu, A. Napolitano, G. Gaudino, P. Morris, G. Sakamoto, L. K. Ferris, A. Danese, A. Raimondi, C. Tacchetti, S. Kuchay, H. I. Pass, E. B. Affar, H. Yang, P. Pinton and M. Carbone (2017). "BAP1 regulates IP3R3-mediated Ca(2+) flux to mitochondria suppressing cell transformation." *Nature* 546(7659): 549–553.

Bononi, A., K. Goto, G. Ak, Y. Yoshikawa, M. Emi, S. Pastorino, L. Carparelli, A. Ferro, M. Nasu, J. H. Kim, J. S. Suarez, R. Xu, M. Tanji, Y. Takinishi, M. Minaai, F. Novelli, I. Pagano, G. Gaudino, H. I. Pass, J. Groden, J. J. Grzymski, M. Metintas, M. Akarsu, B. Morrow, R. Hassan, H. Yang and M. Carbone (2020). "Heterozygous germline BLM mutations increase susceptibility to asbestos and mesothelioma." *Proc Natl Acad Sci U S A* 117(52): 33466–33473.

Bononi, A., H. Yang, C. Giorgi, S. Patergnani, L. Pellegrini, M. Su, G. Xie, V. Signorato, S. Pastorino, P. Morris, G. Sakamoto, S. Kuchay, G. Gaudino, H. I. Pass, A. Napolitano, P. Pinton, W. Jia and M. Carbone (2017). "Germline BAP1 mutations induce a Warburg effect." *Cell Death Differ* 24(10): 1694–1704.

Bott, M., M. Brevet, B. S. Taylor, S. Shimizu, T. Ito, L. Wang, J. Creaney, R. A. Lake, M. F. Zakowski, B. Reva, C. Sander, R. Delsite, S. Powell, Q. Zhou, R. Shen, A. Olshen, V. Rusch and M. Ladanyi (2011). "The nuclear deubiquitinase BAP1 is commonly inactivated by somatic mutations and 3p21.1 losses in malignant pleural mesothelioma." *Nat Genet* 43(7): 668–672.

Boulanger, G., P. Andujar, J. C. Pairon, M. A. Billon-Galland, C. Dion, P. Dumortier, P. Brochard, A. Sobaszek, P. Bartsch, C. Paris and M. C. Jaurand (2014). "Quantification of short and long asbestos fibers to assess asbestos exposure: A review of fiber size toxicity." *Environ Health* 13: 59-76.

Broaddus, V. C., L. Yang, L. M. Scavo, J. D. Ernst and A. M. Boylan (1996). "Asbestos induces apoptosis of human and rabbit pleural mesothelial cells via reactive oxygen species." *J Clin Invest* 98(9): 2050–2059.

Calin, G. A. and C. M. Croce (2006). "MicroRNA signatures in human cancers." *Nat Rev Cancer* 6(11): 857–866.

Carbone, M., P. S. Adusumilli, H. R. J. Alexander, P. Baas, F. Bardelli, A. Bononi, R. Bueno, E. Felley-Bosco, F. Galateau-Salle, D. Jablons, A. S. Mansfield, M. Minaai, M. de Perrot, P. Pesavento, V. Rusch, D. T. Severson, E. Taioli, A. Tsao, G. Woodard, H. Yang, M. G. Zauderer and H. I. Pass (2019). "Mesothelioma: Scientific clues for prevention, diagnosis, and therapy." *CA Cancer J Clin* 69(5): 402–429.

Carbone, M., I. Amelio, E. B. Affar, J. Brugarolas, L. A. Cannon-Albright, L. C. Cantley, W. K. Cavenee, Z. Chen, C. M. Croce, A. Andrea, D. Gandara, C. Giorgi, W. Jia, Q. Lan, T. W. Mak, J. L. Manley, K. Mikoshiba, J. N. Onuchic, H. I. Pass, P. Pinton, C. Prives, N. Rothman, S. M. Sebti, J. Turkson, X. Wu, H. Yang, H. Yu and G. Melino (2018). "Consensus report of the 8 and 9th Weinman Symposia on Gene x Environment Interaction in carcinogenesis: Novel opportunities for precision medicine." *Cell Death Differ* 25(11): 1885–1904.

Carbone, M., S. T. Arron, B. Beutler, A. Bononi, W. Cavenee, J. E. Cleaver, C. M. Croce, A. D'Andrea, W. D. Foulkes, G. Gaudino, J. L. Groden, E. P. Henske, I. D. Hickson, P. M. Hwang, R. D. Kolodner, T. W. Mak, D. Malkin, R. J. Monnat Jr., F. Novelli, H. I. Pass, J. H. Petrini, L. S. Schmidt and H. Yang (2020). "Tumour predisposition and cancer syndromes as models to study gene-environment interactions." *Nat Rev Cancer* 20(9): 533–549.

Carbone, M., Y. I. Baris, P. Bertino, B. Brass, S. Comertpay, A. U. Dogan, G. Gaudino, S. Jube, S. Kanodia, C. R. Partridge, H. I. Pass, Z. S. Rivera, I. Steele, M. Tuncer, S. Way, H. Yang and A. Miller (2011). "Erionite exposure in North Dakota and Turkish villages with mesothelioma." *Proc Natl Acad Sci U S A* 108(33): 13618–13623.

Carbone, M., S. Emri, A. U. Dogan, I. Steele, M. Tuncer, H. I. Pass and Y. I. Baris (2007). "A mesothelioma epidemic in Cappadocia: Scientific developments and unexpected social outcomes." *Nat Rev Cancer* 7(2): 147–154.

Carbone, M., L. K. Ferris, F. Baumann, A. Napolitano, C. A. Lum, E. G. Flores, G. Gaudino, A. Powers, P. Bryant-Greenwood, T. Krausz, E. Hyjek, R. Tate, J. Friedberg, T. Weigel, H. I. Pass and H. Yang (2012). "BAP1 cancer syndrome: Malignant mesothelioma, uveal and cutaneous melanoma, and MBAITs." *J Transl Med* 10: 179-185.

Carbone, M., E. G. Flores, M. Emi, T. A. Johnson, T. Tsunoda, D. Behner, H. Hoffman, M. Hesdorffer, M. Nasu, A. Napolitano, A. Powers, M. Minaai, F. Baumann, P. Bryant-Greenwood, O. Lauk, M. B. Kirschner, W. Weder, I. Opitz, H. I. Pass, G. Gaudino, S. Pastorino and H. Yang (2015). "Combined genetic and genealogic studies uncover a large BAP1 cancer syndrome kindred tracing back nine generations to a common ancestor from the 1700s." *PLoS Genet* 11(12): e1005633.

Carbone, M., G. Gaudino and H. Yang (2015). "Recent insights emerging from malignant mesothelioma genome sequencing." *J Thorac Oncol* 10(3): 409–411.

Carbone, M., A. Gazdar and J. S. Butel (2020). "SV40 and human mesothelioma." *Transl Lung Cancer Res* 9(Suppl 1): S47–S59.

Carbone, M., J. W. Harbour, J. Brugarolas, A. Bononi, I. Pagano, A. Dey, T. Krausz, H. I. Pass, H. Yang and G. Gaudino (2020). "Biological mechanisms and clinical significance of BAP1 mutations in human cancer." *Cancer Discov* 10(8): 1103–1120.

Carbone, M., B. H. Ly, R. F. Dodson, I. Pagano, P. T. Morris, U. A. Dogan, A. F. Gazdar, H. I. Pass and H. Yang (2012). "Malignant mesothelioma: Facts, myths, and hypotheses." *J Cell Physiol* 227(1): 44–58.

Carbone, M., M. Minaai, Y. Takinishi, I. Pagano and H. Yang (2023). "Preventive and therapeutic opportunities: Targeting BAP1 and/or HMGB1 pathways to diminish the burden of mesothelioma." *J Transl Med* 21(1): 749–757.

Carbone, M. and H. I. Pass (2004). "Multistep and multifactorial carcinogenesis: When does a contributing factor become a carcinogen?" *Semin Cancer Biol* 14(6): 399–405.

Carbone, M., H. I. Pass, G. Ak, H. R. Alexander Jr.,, P. Baas, F. Baumann, A. M. Blakely, R. Bueno, A. Bzura, G. Cardillo, J. E. Churpek, I. Dianzani, A. De Rienzo, M. Emi, S. Emri, E. Felley-Bosco, D. A. Fennell, R. M. Flores, F. Grosso, N. K. Hayward, M. Hesdorffer, C. D. Hoang, P. A. Johansson, H. L. Kindler, M. Kittaneh, T. Krausz, A. Mansfield, M. Metintas, M. Minaai, L. Mutti, M. Nielsen, K. O'Byrne, I. Opitz, S. Pastorino, F. Pentimalli, M. de Perrot, A. Pritchard, R. T. Ripley, B. Robinson, V. Rusch, E. Taioli, Y. Takinishi, M. Tanji, A. S. Tsao, A. M. Tuncer, S. Walpole, A. Wolf, H. Yang, Y. Yoshikawa, A. Zolondick, D. S. Schrump and R. Hassan (2022). "Medical and surgical care of patients with mesothelioma and their relatives carrying germline BAP1 mutations." *J Thorac Oncol.* 17(7): 873–889.

Carbone, M., P. Rizzo and H. Pass (2000). "Simian virus 40: The link with human malignant mesothelioma is well established." *Anticancer Res* 20(2A): 875–877.

Carbone, M., D. Shimizu, A. Napolitano, M. Tanji, H. I. Pass, H. Yang and S. Pastorino (2016). "Positive nuclear BAP1 immunostaining helps differentiate non-small cell lung carcinomas from malignant mesothelioma." *Oncotarget* 7(37): 59314–59321.

Carbone, M. and H. Yang (2017). "Mesothelioma: Recent highlights." *Ann Transl Med* 5(11): 238–244.

Carbone, M., H. Yang, H. I. Pass, T. Krausz, J. R. Testa and G. Gaudino (2013). "BAP1 and cancer." *Nat Rev Cancer* 13(3): 153–159.

Carbone, M., H. Yang, H. I. Pass and E. Taioli (2023). "Did the ban on asbestos reduce the incidence of mesothelioma?" *J Thorac Oncol* 18(6): 694–697.

Chen, Z., G. Gaudino, H. I. Pass, M. Carbone and H. Yang (2017). "Diagnostic and prognostic biomarkers for malignant mesothelioma: An update." *Transl Lung Cancer Res* 6(3): 259–269.

Comertpay, S., S. Pastorino, M. Tanji, R. Mezzapelle, O. Strianese, A. Napolitano, F. Baumann, T. Weigel, J. Friedberg, P. Sugarbaker, T. Krausz, E. Wang, A. Powers, G. Gaudino, S. Kanodia, H. I. Pass, B. L. Parsons, H. Yang and M. Carbone (2014). "Evaluation of clonal origin of malignant mesothelioma." *J Transl Med* 12: 301-309.

Croce, A., M. Allegrina, C. Rinaudo, G. Gaudino, H. Yang and M. Carbone (2015). "Numerous iron-rich particles lie on the surface of erionite fibers from Rome (Oregon, USA) and Karlik (Cappadocia, Turkey)." *Microsc Microanal* 21(5): 1341–1347.

Cunningham, R., S. Jia, K. Purohit, O. Salem, N. S. Hui, Y. Lin, N. O. Carragher and C. G. Hansen (2023). "YAP/TAZ activation predicts clinical outcomes in mesothelioma and is conserved in in vitro model of driver mutations." *Clin Transl Med* 13(2): e1190.

de la Fouchardiere, A., O. Cabaret, L. Savin, P. Combemale, H. Schvartz, C. Penet, V. Bonadona, N. Soufir and B. Bressac-de Paillerets (2015). "Germline BAP1 mutations predispose also to multiple basal cell carcinomas." *Clin Genet* 88(3): 273–277.

Evankovich, J., S. W. Cho, R. Zhang, J. Cardinal, R. Dhupar, L. Zhang, J. R. Klune, J. Zlotnicki, T. Billiar and A. Tsung (2010). "High mobility group box 1 release from hepatocytes during ischemia and reperfusion injury is mediated by decreased histone deacetylase activity." *J Biol Chem* 285(51): 39888–39897.

Goparaju, C. M., J. D. Blasberg, S. Volinia, J. Palatini, S. Ivanov, J. S. Donington, C. Croce, M. Carbone, H. Yang and H. I. Pass (2011). "Onconase mediated NFKbeta downregulation in malignant pleural mesothelioma." *Oncogene* 30(24): 2767–2777.

Guo, G., J. Chmielecki, C. Goparaju, A. Heguy, I. Dolgalev, M. Carbone, S. Seepo, M. Meyerson and H. I. Pass (2015). "Whole-exome sequencing reveals frequent genetic alterations in BAP1, NF2, CDKN2A, and CUL1 in malignant pleural mesothelioma." *Cancer Res* 75(2): 264–269.

Hassan, R., B. Morrow, A. Thomas, T. Walsh, M. K. Lee, S. Gulsuner, M. Gadiraju, V. Panou, S. Gao, I. Mian, J. Khan, M. Raffeld, S. Patel, L. Xi, J. S. Wei, M. Hesdorffer, J. Zhang, K. Calzone, A. Desai, E. Padiernos, C. Alewine, D. S. Schrump, S. M. Steinberg, H. L. Kindler, M. C. King and J. E. Churpek (2019). "Inherited predisposition to malignant mesothelioma and overall survival following platinum chemotherapy." *Proc Natl Acad Sci U S A* 116(18): 9008–9013.

Hillegass, J. M., A. Shukla, S. A. Lathrop, M. B. MacPherson, S. L. Beuschel, K. J. Butnor, J. R. Testa, H. I. Pass, M. Carbone, C. Steele and B. T. Mossman (2010). "Inflammation precedes the development of human malignant mesotheliomas in a SCID mouse xenograft model." *Ann N Y Acad Sci* 1203: 7–14.

Hiraku, Y., J. Watanabe, A. Kaneko, T. Ichinose and M. Murata (2021). "MicroRNA expression in lung tissues of asbestos-exposed mice: Upregulation of miR-21 and downregulation of tumor suppressor genes Pdcd4 and Reck." *J Occup Health* 63(1): e12282.

Hu, Z. I., M. Miettinen, M. Quezado, A. P. Lebensohn, K. Aldape, M. Agra, C. Wagner, Y. Mallory, R. Hassan and A. Ghafoor (2022). "Meningiomas in patients with malignant pleural mesothelioma harboring germline <em>BAP1</em> mutations." *J Thorac Oncol* 17(3): 461–466.

Huang, S. X., M. C. Jaurand, D. W. Kamp, J. Whysner and T. K. Hei (2011). "Role of mutagenicity in asbestos fiber-induced carcinogenicity and other diseases." *J Toxicol Environ Health B* 14(1–4): 179–245.

Husain, A. N., T. V. Colby, N. G. Ordonez, T. C. Allen, R. L. Attanoos, M. B. Beasley, K. J. Butnor, L. R. Chirieac, A. M. Churg, S. Dacic, F. Galateau-Salle, A. Gibbs, A. M. Gown, T. Krausz, L. A. Litzky, A. Marchevsky, A. G. Nicholson, V. L. Roggli, A. K. Sharma, W. D. Travis, A. E. Walts and M. R. Wick (2018). "Guidelines for pathologic diagnosis of malignant mesothelioma 2017 update of the consensus statement from the international mesothelioma interest group." *Arch Pathol Lab Med* 142(1): 89–108.

Ismail, I. H., R. Davidson, J. P. Gagne, Z. Z. Xu, G. G. Poirier and M. J. Hendzel (2014). "Germline mutations in BAP1 impair its function in DNA double-strand break repair." *Cancer Res* 74(16): 4282–4294.

Ito, F., K. Kato, I. Yanatori, T. Murohara and S. Toyokuni (2021). "Ferroptosis-dependent extracellular vesicles from macrophage contribute to asbestos-induced mesothelial carcinogenesis through loading ferritin." *Redox Biol* 47: 102174.

Ivanov, S. V., J. Miller, R. Lucito, C. Tang, A. V. Ivanova, J. Pei, M. Carbone, C. Cruz, A. Beck, C. Webb, D. Nonaka, J. R. Testa and H. I. Pass (2009). "Genomic events associated with progression of pleural malignant mesothelioma." *Int J Cancer* 124(3): 589–599.

Jongsma, J., E. van Montfort, M. Vooijs, J. Zevenhoven, P. Krimpenfort, M. van der Valk, M. van de Vijver and A. Berns (2008). "A conditional mouse model for malignant mesothelioma." *Cancer Cell* 13(3): 261–271.

Jube, S., Z. S. Rivera, M. E. Bianchi, A. Powers, E. Wang, I. Pagano, H. I. Pass, G. Gaudino, M. Carbone and H. Yang (2012). "Cancer cell secretion of the DAMP protein HMGB1 supports progression in malignant mesothelioma." *Cancer Res* 72(13): 3290–3301.

Kadariya, Y., C. W. Menges, J. Talarchek, K. Q. Cai, A. J. Klein-Szanto, R. A. Pietrofesa, M. Christofidou-Solomidou, M. Cheung, B. T. Mossman, A. Shukla and J. R. Testa (2016). "Inflammation-related IL-1beta/IL-1R signaling promotes the development of asbestos-induced malignant mesothelioma." *Cancer Prev Res (Phila)* 9(5): 406–414.

Kadariya, Y., E. Sementino, U. Shrestha, G. Gorman, J. M. White, E. A. Ross, M. L. Clapper, N. Neamati, M. S. Miller and J. R. Testa (2022). "Inflammation as a chemoprevention target in asbestos-induced malignant mesothelioma." *Carcinogenesis* 43(12): 1137–1148.

Kittaneh, M. and C. Berkelhammer (2018). "Detecting germline BAP1 mutations in patients with peritoneal mesothelioma: Benefits to patient and family members." *J Transl Med* 16(1): 194–200.

Kroczynska, B., R. Cutrone, M. Bocchetta, H. Yang, A. G. Elmishad, P. Vacek, M. Ramos-Nino, B. T. Mossman, H. I. Pass and M. Carbone (2006). "Crocidolite asbestos and SV40 are cocarcinogens in human mesothelial cells and in causing mesothelioma in hamsters." *Proc Natl Acad Sci U S A* 103(38): 14128–14133.

Larson, D., A. Powers, J. P. Ambrosi, M. Tanji, A. Napolitano, E. G. Flores, F. Baumann, L. Pellegrini, C. J. Jennings, B. J. Buck, B. T. McLaurin, D. Merkler, C. Robinson, P. Morris, M. Dogan, A. U. Dogan, H. I. Pass, S. Pastorino, M. Carbone and H. Yang (2016). "Investigating palygorskite's role in the development of mesothelioma in southern Nevada: Insights into fiber-induced carcinogenicity." *J Toxicol Environ Health B* 19(5–6): 213–230.

Lee, H. S., S. A. Lee, S. K. Hur, J. W. Seo and J. Kwon (2014). "Stabilization and targeting of INO80 to replication forks by BAP1 during normal DNA synthesis." *Nat Commun* 5: 5128.

Lo Iacono, M., V. Monica, L. Righi, F. Grosso, R. Libener, S. Vatrano, P. Bironzo, S. Novello, L. Musmeci, M. Volante, M. Papotti and G. V. Scagliotti (2014). "Targeted next-generation sequencing of cancer genes in advanced stage malignant pleural mesothelioma: A retrospective study." *J Thorac Oncol* 10(3): 492–499.

Luo, Y., S. Akatsuka, Y. Motooka, Y. Kong, H. Zheng, T. Mashimo, T. Imaoka and S. Toyokuni (2023). "BRCA1 haploinsufficiency impairs iron metabolism to promote chrysotile-induced mesothelioma via ferroptosis resistance." *Cancer Sci* 114(4): 1423–1436.

Ly, P. and D. W. Cleveland (2017). "Rebuilding chromosomes after catastrophe: Emerging mechanisms of Chromothripsis." *Trends Cell Biol* 27(12): 917–930.

Mansfield, A. S., T. Peikert, J. B. Smadbeck, J. B. M. Udell, E. Garcia-Rivera, L. Elsbernd, C. L. Erskine, V. P. Van Keulen, F. Kosari, S. J. Murphy, H. Ren, V. V. Serla, J. L. Schaefer Klein, G. Karagouga, F. R. Harris, C. Sosa, S. H. Johnson, W. Nevala, S. N. Markovic, A. O. Bungum, E. S. Edell, H. Dong, J. C. Cheville, M. C. Aubry, J. Jen and G. Vasmatzis (2019). "Neoantigenic potential of complex chromosomal rearrangements in mesothelioma." *J Thorac Oncol* 14(2): 276–287.

Matsushita, A., T. Sato, S. Mukai, T. Fujishita, E. Mishiro-Sato, M. Okuda, M. Aoki, Y. Hasegawa and Y. Sekido (2019). "TAZ activation by Hippo pathway dysregulation induces cytokine gene expression and promotes mesothelial cell transformation." *Oncogene* 38(11): 1966–1978.

Mitchell, O. D., K. Gilliam, D. Del Gaudio, K. E. McNeely, S. Smith, M. Acevedo, M. Gaduraju, R. Hodge, A. S. S. Ramsland, J. Segal, S. Das, F. Hathaway, D. S. Bryan, S. Tawde, S. Galasinski, P. Wang, M. Y. Tjota, A. N. Husain, S. G. Armato, J. Donington, M. K. Ferguson, K. Turaga, J. E. Churpek, H. L. Kindler and M. W. Drazer (2023). "Germline variants incidentally detected via tumor-only genomic profiling of patients with mesothelioma." *JAMA Netw Open* 6(8): e2327351.

Mossman, B. T. (1990). "In vitro studies on the biologic effects of fibers: Correlation with in vivo bioassays." *Environ Health Perspect* 88: 319–322.

Murali, R., J. S. Wilmott, V. Jakrot, H. A. Al-Ahmadie, T. Wiesner, S. W. McCarthy, J. F. Thompson and R. A. Scolyer (2013). "BAP1 expression in cutaneous melanoma: A pilot study." *Pathology* 45(6): 606–609.

Nagai, H., T. Ishihara, W. H. Lee, H. Ohara, Y. Okazaki, K. Okawa and S. Toyokuni (2011). "Asbestos surface provides a niche for oxidative modification." *Cancer Sci* 102(12): 2118–2125.

Nakamura, E., A. Makishima, K. Hagino and K. Okabe (2009). "Accumulation of radium in ferruginous protein bodies formed in lung tissue: Association of resulting radiation hotspots with malignant mesothelioma and other malignancies." *Proc Jpn Acad B* 85(7): 229–239.

Napolitano, A., L. Pellegrini, A. Dey, D. Larson, M. Tanji, E. G. Flores, B. Kendrick, D. Lapid, A. Powers, S. Kanodia, S. Pastorino, H. I. Pass, V. Dixit, H. Yang and M. Carbone (2016). "Minimal asbestos exposure in germline BAP1 heterozygous mice is associated with deregulated inflammatory response and increased risk of mesothelioma." *Oncogene* 35(15): 1996–2002.

Nasu, M., M. Carbone, G. Gaudino, B. H. Ly, P. Bertino, D. Shimizu, P. Morris, H. I. Pass and H. Yang (2011). "Ranpirnase interferes with NF-kappaB pathway and MMP9 activity, inhibiting malignant mesothelioma cell invasiveness and xenograft growth." *Genes Cancer* 2(5): 576–584.

Nasu, M., M. Emi, S. Pastorino, M. Tanji, A. Powers, H. Luk, F. Baumann, Y. A. Zhang, A. Gazdar, S. Kanodia, M. Tiirikainen, E. Flores, G. Gaudino, M. J. Becich, H. I. Pass, H. Yang and M. Carbone (2015). "High Incidence of Somatic BAP1 alterations in sporadic malignant mesothelioma." *J Thorac Oncol* 10(4): 565–576.

Njauw, C. N., I. Kim, A. Piris, M. Gabree, M. Taylor, A. M. Lane, M. M. DeAngelis, E. Gragoudas, L. M. Duncan and H. Tsao (2012). "Germline BAP1 inactivation is preferentially associated with metastatic ocular melanoma and cutaneous-ocular melanoma families." *PLoS One* 7(4): e35295.

Novelli, F., A. Bononi, Q. Wang, F. Bai, S. Patergnani, F. Kricek, E. Haglund, J. S. Suarez, M. Tanji, R. Xu, Y. Takanishi, M. Minaai, S. Pastorino, P. Morris, G. Sakamoto, H. I. Pass, H. Barbour, G. Gaudino, C. Giorgi, P. Pinton, J. N. Onuchic, H. Yang and M. Carbone (2021). "BAP1 forms a trimer with HMGB1 and HDAC1 that modulates gene × environment interaction with asbestos." *Proc Natl Acad Sci U S A* 118(48): e2111946118.

Novelli, F., Y. Yoshikawa, V.A.M. Vitto, L. Modesti, M. Minaai, M. Emi, S. Pastorino, J-H. Kim, F. Kricek, J. Onuchic, A. Bononi, J.S. Suarez, M. Tanji, C. Favaron, A. Zolondick, R. Xu, Y. Takanishi, Z. Wang, G. Sakamoto, G. Gaudino, J. Grzymski, F Grosso, H.I. Pass, R Hassan, D. Schrump, M-C. King, C Giorgi, P. Pinton, H Yang, and M. Carbone (2024). "Germline BARD1 mutations variants predispose to mesothelioma by affecting DNA repair and Calcium metabolism. predisposing to malignant mesothelioma."*Proc Natl Acad Sci* in press.

Oey, H., M. Daniels, V. Relan, T. M. Chee, M. R. Davidson, I. A. Yang, J. J. Ellis, K. M. Fong, L. Krause and R. V. Bowman (2019). "Whole-genome sequencing of human malignant mesothelioma tumours and cell lines." *Carcinogenesis* 40(6): 724–734.

Panou, V., M. Gadiraju, A. Wolin, C. M. Weipert, E. Skarda, A. N. Husain, J. D. Patel, B. Rose, S. R. Zhang, M. Weatherly, V. Nelakuditi, A. Knight Johnson, M. Helgeson, D. Fischer, A. Desai, N. Sulai, L. Ritterhouse, O. D. Roe, K. K. Turaga, D. Huo, J. Segal, S. Kadri, Z. Li, H. L. Kindler and J. E. Churpek (2018). "Frequency of germline mutations in cancer susceptibility genes in malignant mesothelioma." *J Clin Oncol* 36(28): 2863–2871.

Panou, V. and O. D. Roe (2020). "Inherited genetic mutations and polymorphisms in malignant mesothelioma: A comprehensive review." *Int J Mol Sci* 21(12). 4327–4343.

Pass, H. I., D. J. Mew, M. Carbone, W. A. Matthews, J. S. Donington, R. Baserga, C. L. Walker, M. Resnicoff and S. M. Steinberg (1996). "Inhibition of hamster mesothelioma tumorigenesis by an antisense expression plasmid to the insulin-like growth factor-1 receptor." *Cancer Res* 56(17): 4044–4048.

Pastorino, S., Y. Yoshikawa, H. I. Pass, M. Emi, M. Nasu, I. Pagano, Y. Takinishi, R. Yamamoto, M. Minaai, T. Hashimoto-Tamaoki, M. Ohmuraya, K. Goto, C. Goparaju, K. Y. Sarin, M. Tanji, A. Bononi, A. Napolitano, G. Gaudino, M. Hesdorffer, H. Yang and M. Carbone (2018). "A subset of mesotheliomas with improved survival occurring in carriers of BAP1 and other germline mutations." *J Clin Oncol* 36(35): 3485–3494.

Pellegrini, L., J. Xue, D. Larson, S. Pastorino, S. Jube, K. H. Forest, Z. S. Saad-Jube, A. Napolitano, I. Pagano, V. S. Negi, M. E. Bianchi, P. Morris, H. I. Pass, G. Gaudino, M. Carbone and H. Yang (2017). "HMGB1 targeting by ethyl pyruvate suppresses malignant phenotype of human mesothelioma." *Oncotarget* 8(14): 22649–22661.

Pena-Llopis, S., S. Vega-Rubin-de-Celis, A. Liao, N. Leng, A. Pavia-Jimenez, S. Wang, T. Yamasaki, L. Zhrebker, S. Sivanand, P. Spence, L. Kinch, T. Hambuch, S. Jain, Y. Lotan, V. Margulis, A. I. Sagalowsky, P. B. Summerour, W. Kabbani, S. W. Wong, N. Grishin, M. Laurent, X. J. Xie, C. D. Haudenschild, M. T. Ross, D. R. Bentley, P. Kapur and J. Brugarolas (2012). "BAP1 loss defines a new class of renal cell carcinoma." *Nat Genet* 44(7): 751–759.

Pilarski, R., C. M. Cebulla, J. B. Massengill, K. Rai, T. Rich, L. Strong, B. McGillivray, M. J. Asrat, F. H. Davidorf and M. H. Abdel-Rahman (2014). "Expanding the clinical phenotype of hereditary BAP1 cancer predisposition syndrome, reporting three new cases." *Genes Chromosomes Cancer* 53(2): 177–182.

Popova, T., L. Hebert, V. Jacquemin, S. Gad, V. Caux-Moncoutier, C. Dubois-d'Enghien, B. Richaudeau, X. Renaudin, J. Sellers, A. Nicolas, X. Sastre-Garau, L. Desjardins, G. Gyapay, V. Raynal, O. M. Sinilnikova, N. Andrieu, E. Manie, A. de Pauw, P. Gesta, V. Bonadona, C. M. Maugard, C. Penet, M. F. Avril, E. Barillot, O. Cabaret, O. Delattre, S. Richard, O. Caron, M. Benfodda, H. H. Hu, N. Soufir, B. Bressac-de Paillerets, D. Stoppa-Lyonnet and M. H. Stern (2013). "Germline BAP1 mutations predispose to renal cell carcinomas." *Am J Hum Genet* 92(6): 974–980.

Qi, F., M. Carbone, H. Yang and G. Gaudino (2011). "Simian virus 40 transformation, malignant mesothelioma and brain tumors." *Expert Rev Respir Med* 5(5): 683–697.

Qi, F., G. Okimoto, S. Jube, A. Napolitano, H. I. Pass, R. Laczko, R. M. Demay, G. Khan, M. Tiirikainen, C. Rinaudo, A. Croce, H. Yang, G. Gaudino and M. Carbone (2013). "Continuous exposure to chrysotile asbestos can cause transformation of human mesothelial cells via HMGB1 and TNF-alpha signaling." *Am J Pathol* 183(5): 1654–1666.

Rai, K., R. Pilarski, C. M. Cebulla and M. H. Abdel-Rahman (2016). "Comprehensive review of BAP1 tumor predisposition syndrome with report of two new cases." *Clin Genet* 89(3): 285–294.

Ramos-Nino, M. E., S. R. Blumen, T. Sabo-Attwood, H. Pass, M. Carbone, J. R. Testa, D. A. Altomare and B. T. Mossman (2008). "HGF mediates cell proliferation of human mesothelioma cells through a PI3K/MEK5/Fra-1 pathway." *Am J Respir Cell Mol Biol* 38(2): 209–217.

Rehrauer, H., L. Wu, W. Blum, L. Pecze, T. Henzi, V. Serre-Beinier, C. Aquino, B. Vrugt, M. de Perrot, B. Schwaller and E. Felley-Bosco (2018). "How asbestos drives the tissue towards tumors: YAP activation, macrophage and mesothelial precursor recruitment, RNA editing, and somatic mutations." *Oncogene* 37(20): 2645–2659.

Rosenthal, G. J., D. R. Germolec, M. E. Blazka, E. Corsini, P. Simeonova, P. Pollock, L. Y. Kong, J. Kwon and M. I. Luster (1994). "Asbestos stimulates IL-8 production from human lung epithelial cells." *J Immunol* 153(7): 3237–3244.

Roushdy-Hammady, I., J. Siegel, S. Emri, J. R. Testa and M. Carbone (2001). "Genetic-susceptibility factor and malignant mesothelioma in the Cappadocian region of Turkey." *Lancet* 357(9254): 444–445.

Sato, T. and Y. Sekido (2018). "NF2/merlin inactivation and potential therapeutic targets in mesothelioma." *Int J Mol Sci* 19(4): 988–1005.

Shankar, G. M., M. Abedalthagafi, R. A. Vaubel, P. H. Merrill, N. Nayyar, C. M. Gill, R. Brewster, W. L. Bi, P. K. Agarwalla, A. R. Thorner, D. A. Reardon, O. Al-Mefty, P. Y. Wen, B. M. Alexander, P. van Hummelen, T. T. Batchelor, K. L. Ligon, A. H. Ligon, M. Meyerson, I. F. Dunn, R. Beroukhim, D. N. Louis, A. Perry, S. L. Carter, C. Giannini, W. T. Curry Jr., D. P. Cahill, F. G. Barker 2nd, P. K. Brastianos and S. Santagata (2017). "Germline and somatic BAP1 mutations in high-grade rhabdoid meningiomas." *Neuro Oncol* 19(4): 535–545.

Singhi, A. D., A. M. Krasinskas, H. A. Choudry, D. L. Bartlett, J. F. Pingpank, H. J. Zeh, A. Luvison, K. Fuhrer, N. Bahary, R. R. Seethala and S. Dacic (2016). "The prognostic significance of BAP1, NF2, and CDKN2A in malignant peritoneal mesothelioma." *Mod Pathol* 29(1): 14–24.

Stanton, M. F., M. Laynard, A. Tegeris, E. Miller, M. May and E. Kent (1977). "Carcinogenicity of fibrous glass: Pleural response in the rat in relation to fiber dimension." *J Natl Cancer Inst* 58(3): 587–603.

Suarez, J. S., F. Novelli, K. Goto, M. Ehara, M. Steele, J.-H. Kim, A. A. Zolondick, J. Xue, R. Xu, M. Saito, S. Pastorino, M. Minaai, Y. Takanishi, M. Emi, I. Pagano, A. Wakeham, T. Berger, H. I. Pass, G. Gaudino, T. W. Mak, M. Carbone and H. Yang (2023). "HMGB1 released by mesothelial cells drives the development of asbestos-induced mesothelioma " *Proc Natl Acad Sci U S A* 120(39): e2307999120.

Testa, J. R., M. Cheung, J. Pei, J. E. Below, Y. Tan, E. Sementino, N. J. Cox, A. U. Dogan, H. I. Pass, S. Trusa, M. Hesdorffer, M. Nasu, A. Powers, Z. Rivera, S. Comertpay, M. Tanji, G. Gaudino, H. Yang and M. Carbone (2011). "Germline BAP1 mutations predispose to malignant mesothelioma." *Nat Genet* 43(10): 1022–1025.

Thompson, J. K., A. Shukla, A. L. Leggett, P. B. Munson, J. M. Miller, M. B. MacPherson, S. L. Beuschel, H. I. Pass and A. Shukla (2018). "Extracellular signal regulated kinase 5 and inflammasome in progression of mesothelioma." *Oncotarget* 9(1): 293–305.

Toyokuni, S. (2019). "Iron addiction with ferroptosis-resistance in asbestos-induced mesothelial carcinogenesis: Toward the era of mesothelioma prevention." *Free Radic Biol Med* 133: 206–215.

Wadt, K. A., L. G. Aoude, P. Johansson, A. Solinas, A. Pritchard, O. Crainic, M. T. Andersen, J. F. Kiilgaard, S. Heegaard, L. Sunde, B. Federspiel, J. Madore, J. F. Thompson, S. W. McCarthy, A. Goodwin, H. Tsao, G. Jonsson, K. Busam, R. Gupta, J. M. Trent, A. M. Gerdes, K. M. Brown, R. A. Scolyer and N. K. Hayward (2015). "A recurrent germline BAP1 mutation and extension of the BAP1 tumor predisposition spectrum to include basal cell carcinoma." *Clin Genet* 88(3): 267–272.

Walpole, S., A. L. Pritchard, C. M. Cebulla, R. Pilarski, M. Stautberg, F. H. Davidorf, A. de la Fouchardiere, O. Cabaret, L. Golmard, D. Stoppa-Lyonnet, E. Garfield, C. N. Njauw, M. Cheung, J. A. Turunen, P. Repo, R. S. Jarvinen, R. van Doorn, M. J. Jager, G. P. M. Luyten, M. Marinkovic, C. Chau, M. Potrony, V. Hoiom, H. Helgadottir, L. Pastorino, W. Bruno, V. Andreotti, B. Dalmasso, G. Ciccarese, P. Queirolo, L. Mastracci, K. Wadt, J. F. Kiilgaard, M. R. Speicher, N. van Poppelen, E. Kilic, R. T. Al-Jamal, I. Dianzani, M. Betti, C. Bergmann, S. Santagata, S. Dahiya, S. Taibjee, J. Burke, N. Poplawski, S. J.

O'Shea, J. Newton-Bishop, J. Adlard, D. J. Adams, A. M. Lane, I. Kim, S. Klebe, H. Racher, J. W. Harbour, M. L. Nickerson, R. Murali, J. M. Palmer, M. Howlie, J. Symmons, H. Hamilton, S. Warrier, W. Glasson, P. Johansson, C. D. Robles-Espinoza, R. Ossio, A. de Klein, S. Puig, P. Ghiorzo, M. Nielsen, T. T. Kivela, H. Tsao, J. R. Testa, P. Gerami, M. H. Stern, B. B. Paillerets, M. H. Abdel-Rahman and N. K. Hayward (2018). "Comprehensive study of the clinical phenotype of germline BAP1 variant-carrying families worldwide." *J Natl Cancer Inst*110(12): 1328–1341.

Wiesner, T., A. C. Obenauf, R. Murali, I. Fried, K. G. Griewank, P. Ulz, C. Windpassinger, W. Wackernagel, S. Loy, I. Wolf, A. Viale, A. E. Lash, M. Pirun, N. D. Socci, A. Rutten, G. Palmedo, D. Abramson, K. Offit, A. Ott, J. C. Becker, L. Cerroni, H. Kutzner, B. C. Bastian and M. R. Speicher (2011). "Germline mutations in BAP1 predispose to melanocytic tumors." *Nat Genet* 43(10): 1018–1021.

Xu, A., L. J. Wu, R. M. Santella and T. K. Hei (1999). "Role of oxyradicals in mutagenicity and DNA damage induced by crocidolite asbestos in mammalian cells." *Cancer Res* 59(23): 5922–5926.

Xue, J., S. Patergnani, C. Giorgi, J. Suarez, K. Goto, A. Bononi, M. Tanji, F. Novelli, S. Pastorino, R. Xu, N. Caroccia, A. U. Dogan, H. I. Pass, M. Tognon, P. Pinton, G. Gaudino, T. W. Mak, M. Carbone and H. Yang (2020). "Asbestos induces mesothelial cell transformation via HMGB1-driven autophagy." *Proc Natl Acad Sci U S A* 117(41): 25543–25552.

Yang, H., M. Bocchetta, B. Kroczynska, A. G. Elmishad, Y. Chen, Z. Liu, C. Bubici, B. T. Mossman, H. I. Pass, J. R. Testa, G. Franzoso and M. Carbone (2006). "TNF-alpha inhibits asbestos-induced cytotoxicity via a NF-kappaB-dependent pathway, a possible mechanism for asbestos-induced oncogenesis." *Proc Natl Acad Sci U S A* 103(27): 10397–10402.

Yang, H., L. Pellegrini, A. Napolitano, C. Giorgi, S. Jube, A. Preti, C. J. Jennings, F. De Marchis, E. G. Flores, D. Larson, I. Pagano, M. Tanji, A. Powers, S. Kanodia, G. Gaudino, S. Pastorino, H. I. Pass, P. Pinton, M. E. Bianchi and M. Carbone (2015). "Aspirin delays mesothelioma growth by inhibiting HMGB1-mediated tumor progression." *Cell Death Dis* 6(6): e1786.

Yang, H., Z. Rivera, S. Jube, M. Nasu, P. Bertino, C. Goparaju, G. Franzoso, M. T. Lotze, T. Krausz, H. I. Pass, M. E. Bianchi and M. Carbone (2010). "Programmed necrosis induced by asbestos in human mesothelial cells causes high-mobility group box 1 protein release and resultant inflammation." *Proc Natl Acad Sci U S A* 107(28): 12611–12616.

Yang, Z., L. Li, L. Chen, W. Yuan, L. Dong, Y. Zhang, H. Wu and C. Wang (2014). "PARP-1 mediates LPS-induced HMGB1 release by macrophages through regulation of HMGB1 acetylation." *J Immunol* 193(12): 6114–6123.

Yoshikawa, Y., M. Emi, T. Hashimoto-Tamaoki, M. Ohmuraya, A. Sato, T. Tsujimura, S. Hasegawa, T. Nakano, M. Nasu, S. Pastorino, A. Szymiczek, A. Bononi, M. Tanji, I. Pagano, G. Gaudino, A. Napolitano, C. Goparaju, H. I. Pass, H. Yang and M. Carbone (2016). "High-density array-CGH with targeted NGS unmask multiple noncontiguous minute deletions on chromosome 3p21 in mesothelioma." *Proc Natl Acad Sci U S A* 113(47): 13432–13437.

Yoshikawa, Y., A. Sato, T. Tsujimura, T. Otsuki, K. Fukuoka, S. Hasegawa, T. Nakano and T. Hashimoto-Tamaoki (2015). "Biallelic germline and somatic mutations in malignant mesothelioma: Multiple mutations in transcription regulators including mSWI/SNF genes." *Int J Cancer* 136(3): 560–571.

Yu, H., H. Pak, I. Hammond-Martel, M. Ghram, A. Rodrigue, S. Daou, H. Barbour, L. Corbeil, J. Hebert, E. Drobetsky, J. Y. Masson, J. M. Di Noia and B. el Affar (2014). "Tumor suppressor and deubiquitinase BAP1 promotes DNA double-strand break repair." *Proc Natl Acad Sci U S A* 111(1): 285–290.

Yue, L., Y. Luo, L. Jiang, Y. Sekido and S. Toyokuni (2022). "PCBP2 knockdown promotes ferroptosis in malignant mesothelioma." *Pathol Int* 72(4): 242–251.

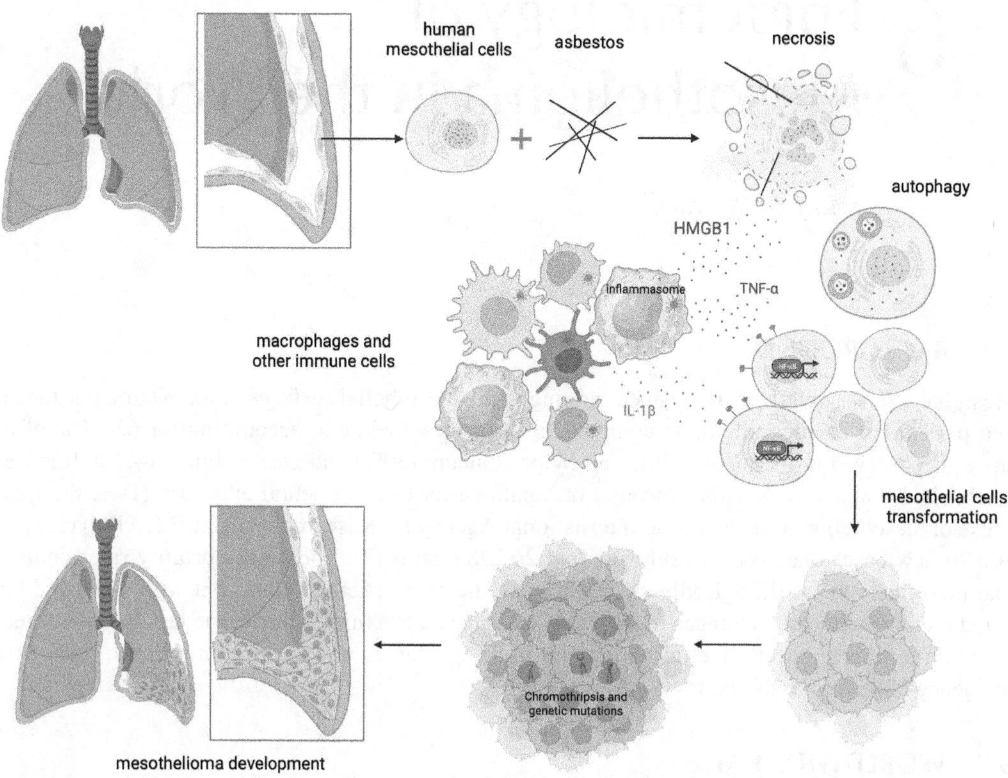

FIGURE 5.1 Diagram showing the mechanisms of asbestos carcinogenesis and the role of HMGB1 in mesothelioma development. Figure was created with BioRender.com.

6 Epidemiology of Mesothelioma in the World

Emanuela Taioli

6.1 BACKGROUND

Mesothelioma is a relatively rare cancer arising in the mesothelial surfaces of the pleura, peritoneal, and pericardial cavities; the most common form of mesothelioma, accounting for 65–70% of all cases, is observed in the pleura, followed by peritoneum (30%) and pericardium (1–2%). It is well established that asbestos, either through occupational or environmental exposure (1), is the main cause of mesothelioma. In 2020, the International Agency for Research on Cancer (IARC) reported 30,870 new cases diagnosed worldwide, and 26,278 deaths (2). The high mortality rates confirm that mesothelioma is still a deadly cancer, despite the many attempts to treat it with novel and targeted therapies. Because changes in mortality rates have been minimal over the last 50 years, much attention has been placed on eliminating and limiting sources of exposure, in order to reduce the incidence of the disease.

6.2 WORLDWIDE RATES

GLOBOCAN, an online database providing global cancer statistics and estimates of incidence and mortality in 185 countries for 36 types of cancer, regularly publishes mesothelioma rates from registries around the world. The most recent publications include incidence rates in 2020 (Figure 6.1), and show that new cases are mostly concentrated in Europe, Australia, New Zealand, and Southern Africa. Another observation from the GLOBOCAN statistics is that incidence and mortality go hand in hand all over the world, confirming the deadly nature of this cancer in both developed and developing countries. In fact, the ratio of incidence to mortality rates is close to 1 in most of the geographic areas. Survival rates for mesothelioma are low, with an estimated median survival of 9–12 months.

6.3 SEX DIFFERENCES

When incidence rates are analyzed according to sex, it appears that the ratio of males to females is in favor of males globally; this is partly explained by the fact that males are historically holding jobs associated with asbestos exposure, such as shipyard workers or pipefitters. The male-to-female ratio varies greatly across the globe, and while in most geographic areas it is a 3:5 ratio in favor of males, there are notable exceptions in Central/Eastern Europe, Northern Africa and Melanesia where the ratio is close to 1 (Figure 6.2). Reasons for this variation could be an incomplete system of data collection on mesothelioma cases, an imprecise pathological diagnosis, and the substantial presence of environmental exposure to asbestos and asbestos-like fibers in the general population (1), along with exposure in family members of occupationally exposed workers. It is also possible that biological and genetic factors (3) differ with sex across geographic areas, and this reflects on the observed incidence rates.

Despite the uncertainties described above around a correct mesothelioma diagnosis and a complete evaluation of asbestos exposure from both conventional and less conventional sources (4), one

DOI: 10.1201/9781003431909-6

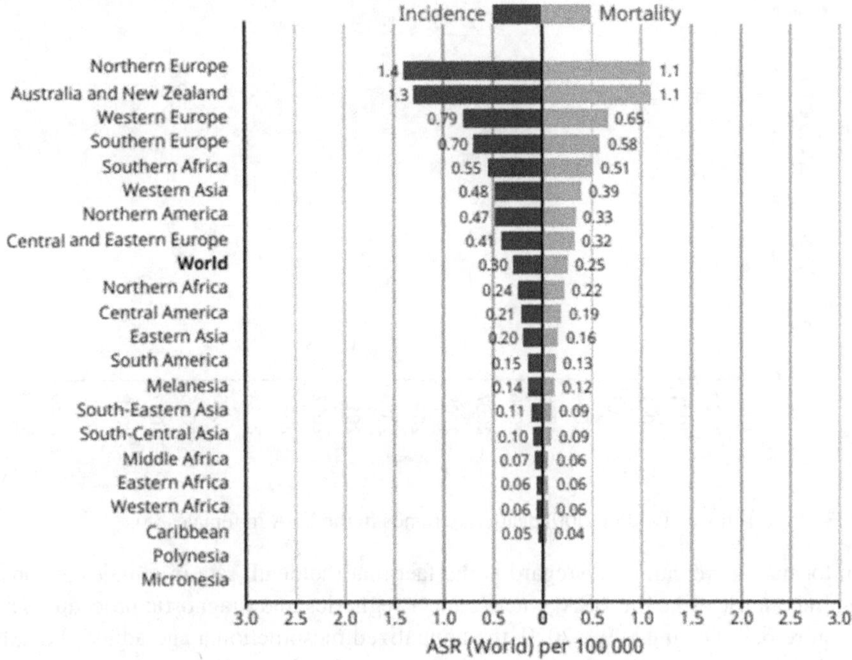

FIGURE 6.1 Age-standardized (world) incidence and mortality rates, GLOBOCAN 2020 (2).

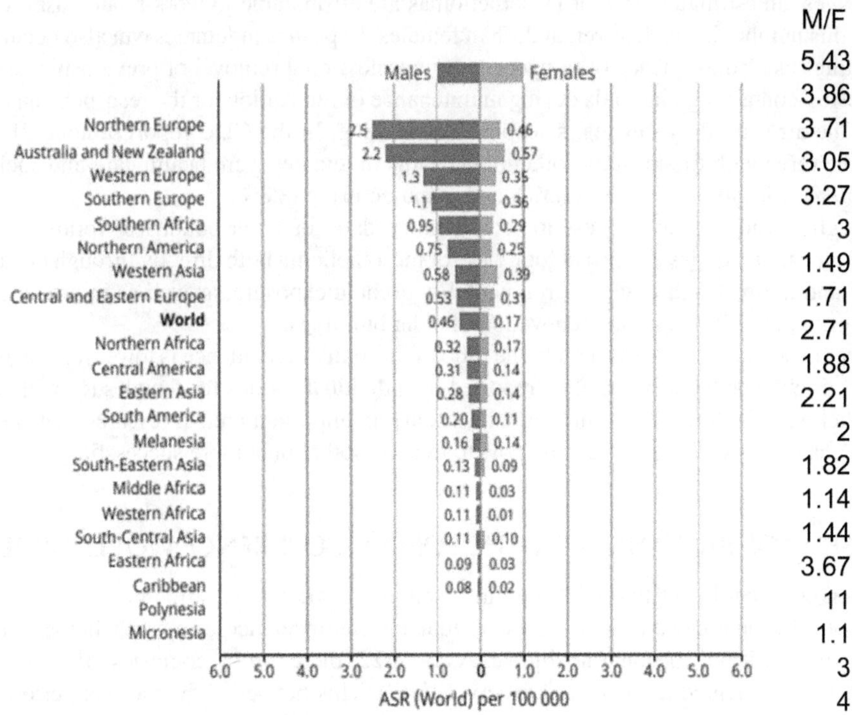

FIGURE 6.2 Age-standardized (world) incidence rates by sex, GLOBOCAN 2020 (2).

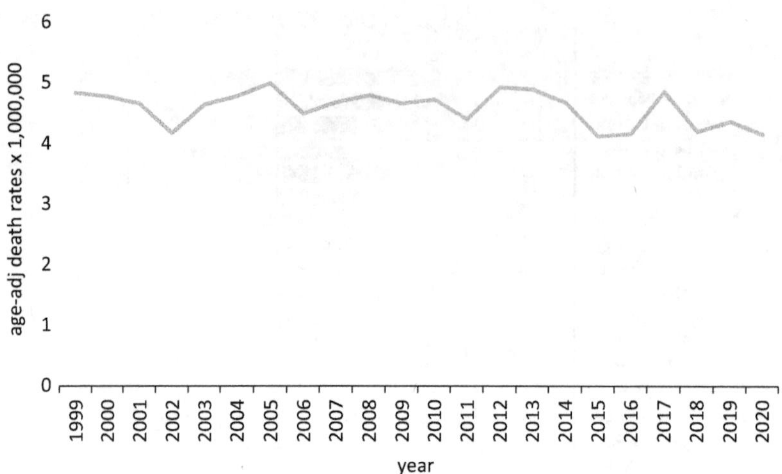

FIGURE 6.3 Age-adjusted (×1,000,000) death rate trends in the USA in females (5).

piece of information we cannot disregard is the fact that the death rate in females is constant and plateauing in countries like the USA, where cancer registries and diagnostic procedures are pretty reliable (Figure 6.3). During 1999–2020, the annualized mesothelioma age-adjusted death rate by state exceeded 6.0 per 1 million females in seven states: Louisiana, Maine, Minnesota, Montana, Oregon, Washington, and Wisconsin (5). The persistent occurrence of new cases in females clearly reflects exposure to sources of asbestos that are difficult to pinpoint, and suggest that studies should focus on this vulnerable section of the population.

The most recent Centers for Disease Control and Prevention (CDC) report (5) indicates that among males, an estimated 85% of mesotheliomas are attributable to work-related asbestos exposure, but this number is much lower, at 23% in females. Exposure in females can also occur in other work settings as a consequence of tampering or unprofessional removal of previously installed friable asbestos-containing materials during maintenance or renovation, or the resuspension of settled fibers in the air caused by dusting, sweeping, or cleaning. In the CDC report, among 21 industry groups, the three with the most mesothelioma deaths in females were health care and social assistance (15.7%), education services (11.3%), and manufacturing (8.8%).

Although we do not have access to such detailed data for other countries worldwide, we can safely assume that females are still at high risk for mesothelioma both directly through occupational exposure and indirectly through environmental/household exposure, as well as improper handling of asbestos material in repair and renovation of older buildings.

Another observation is that generally the ratio of mortality to incidence is lower for females globally, reflecting the better survival often reported by individual studies for females (6) with all forms of mesothelioma. Differences in survival with sex are an important area of research that needs to be expanded, as it may give novel clues on how to treat mesothelioma more successfully.

6.4 ASBESTOS BAN AND MESOTHELIOMA OCCURRENCE WORLDWIDE

It has been common belief that with the introduction of asbestos bans, the production and use of asbestos will become close to zero, and consequently the incidence of mesothelioma will gradually decline until it will become negligible. As of 2022, there are 69 countries all over the world which have implemented a complete asbestos ban (7). This happened over a long period of time, with the first bans occurring in the early 1980s (Norway), and the latest as recent as 2018 (Canada). However, even in those countries with complete ban, exemptions for minor uses are permitted in some of them. Although the USA banned some forms of asbestos in 1973, and attempted to ban most asbestos-containing products in 1989 through the Toxic Substances Control Act, the ban was overturned in 1991 (8).

Despite the common knowledge that asbestos causes mesothelioma, and the legislative attempts to control its production and use, as of today, it is very difficult to estimate how much asbestos is produced and used worldwide. In previous work, we have reported that the apparent consumption (kg/year) of asbestos in the USA and Europe has declined from 1980 to 2007, the same period when the bans were introduced in various countries (6).

However, according to the U.S. Geological Survey Mineral Commodity Summaries (January 2022), the estimated worldwide consumption of asbestos fiber only decreased from approximately 2 million tons in 2010 to roughly 1.2 million tons per year in the past several years. Asbestos-cement products, such as corrugated roofing tiles, pipes, and wall panels, are expected to continue to be the leading global market for asbestos.

The worldwide production of asbestos remains high according to the same agency (U.S. Geological Survey, Mineral Commodity Summaries, January 2023) at 1.3 Million tons in 2022. Major mine producers are (in order) Brazil, China, Kazakhstan, Russia, and Zimbabwe (9).

The continued mining, export, and use of large quantities of asbestos around the world make it unlikely that mesothelioma will decrease or disappear in the near future. As an example, data from the U.S. Census Bureau (2018) indicate that the U.S. imports for internal use several manufactured products containing asbestos (10) (Table 6.1). This isolated statistic seems to indicate that several products containing asbestos regularly enter the USA, despite the internal limitations imposed on extraction, production, and use. As the COVID-19 pandemic taught us, in a global market it is hard to trace and identify the manufacturer origin for every product, and it is even harder to impose blocks on asbestos-contaminated products.

A study conducted on global data (12) shows that mesothelioma rates in those countries that introduced a complete ban keep climbing for years after the ban, and seem to reach a flat line after 20 or more years after the ban (Figure 6.4).

TABLE 6.1
Asbestos-containing products imported into the USA.

Category	Quantity (Metric Tons)	US Custom Value	Major Sources
Asbestos-cement products	48	$97,800	China
Crocidolite products (except footwear)	52	26,400	China, Italy*
Clothing (except footwear)	1	42,800	Germany,* Spain*
Paper, millboard, and felt	NA	25,200	India, Germany,* France*
Compressed asbestos fiber joint	NA	38,500	China, India
Yarn and thread	51	410,000	Mexico
Cords and string	(10)	2500	Japan*
Products for use in civil aircraft	NA	9090	China, Israel,* Canada
Gaskets, packing, and seals	8	310,000	Japan,[8] Guatemala, Taiwan, Germany*
Building materials	NA	248,000	Canada
Asbestos articles not specified	NA	340,000	China
Brake linings and pads, civil aircraft	NA	370,000	Japan*
Brake linings and pads, other	NA	2,990,000	China
Friction materials, civil aircraft	NA	12,400	France*
Other friction materials	NA	6,450,000	Japan*
	160	11,400,000	

*Countries with asbestos ban; material may have been trans-shipped (11).

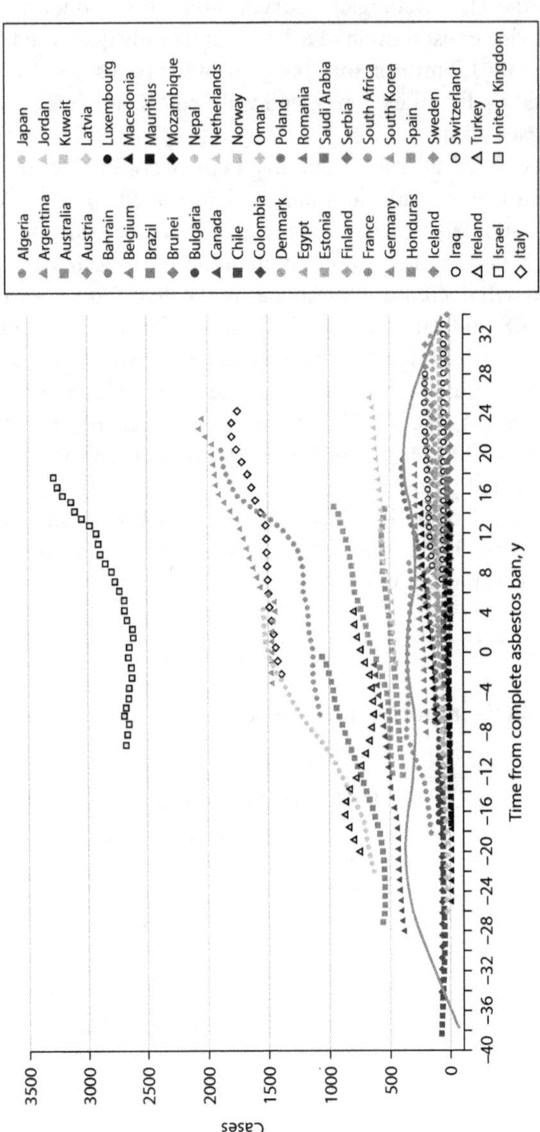

FIGURE 6.4 Mesothelioma trends in 47 countries with complete asbestos ban.

The same study found a temporal increase in mesothelioma cases in females and in those aged >70 years. The statistics suggest that an asbestos ban alone cannot contain mesothelioma rates in the immediate future, given the long latency of mesothelioma occurrence, and the ubiquitous presence of asbestos in our surroundings from before the ban.

6.5 GLOBAL TRENDS

A recent study (13) reported global mesothelioma trends based on national cancer registries, and calculated annual percentage change from 1990 to 2019 according to several variables. The study suggests a global annual decrease of –0.36% in mesothelioma incidence, mostly attributable to decrease in females rather than in males (–1.02 versus –0.15%). According to the same publication, the decrease is present across geographic areas, with some exceptions: High income in Asia-Pacific areas, Western Europe, Southern and Central Latin America, Central Europe, South Asia, and Oceania, where the rates instead increased over time.

One consideration when interpreting these worldwide trends is the importance of latency, and the role that latency plays in calculating any expected future mesothelioma rates. It has been reported (14) that latency between exposure and mesothelioma occurrence is around 34 years, and that latency is shorter for those who worked in production of asbestos-containing items or in asbestos factories. In addition, the same publication suggested that age at initial exposure was negatively correlated with the latency period. These results highlight the fact that different types of exposure to asbestos, occurring at different times during the life course could be one further contributing factor to the heterogeneity in mesothelioma occurrence and trends that we observe around the world, as well as in age at disease occurrence.

A global study (15) suggests an almost linear relationship between country-specific asbestos consumption and mesothelioma mortality. An additional relevant information from this study is that there is inconsistency/lack of data on mesothelioma mortality in those countries where asbestos use is the greatest. This result underlines, once more, the need for appropriate epidemiologic surveillance systems in order to estimate correctly the health effects of asbestos exposure globally (16). We have summarized the status of cancer registries worldwide, and noticed that five countries have a mesothelioma-specific registry: Italy, France, the UK, Australia, and South Korea, all created in response to the emerging needs of occupationally exposed cases and workers compensation. The registries have limited information on treatment, quality of life, and other patient-centered outcomes such as symptoms and pain management. We concluded that to thoroughly collect exposure data, "real-time" enrollment is preferable; to maximize the capture of mesothelioma cases, optimal coverage, and a simplified consent process are needed (16).

6.6 TEMPORAL TRENDS

A recently published paper (14) has addressed some of the challenges described in this chapter by reporting the number of mesothelioma cases recorded by each country in the world according to the commonly accepted 2019–2020 World Bank "National Income Categories." The authors show that roughly half of all countries reported mesothelioma deaths to the WHO, and of these, more than half were in the high-income category, more than a third in the upper middle income, and only one-tenth could be defined as lower middle-income countries. About two thirds of high-income (68%) and upper middle income (65%) countries reported mesothelioma deaths, whereas the majority (86%) of low middle income countries did not. The gradient in the reporting status of mesothelioma by national income likely reflects the gradient in the level of medical resources; for example, the pathological confirmation of a mesothelioma diagnosis requires the proper use of a panel of immunohistochemical markers, and this option is often unavailable in resource-poor countries.

Another relevant phenomenon is that the global volume of asbestos consumption peaked in 1980, declined rapidly between 1980 and 1995, remained stable until around 2012, and thereafter declined further. The rapid decline around 1980–1995 may be attributed to changes first in high-income countries, where most of the bans were introduced, and subsequently in upper-middle income countries. In contrast, low middle-income countries have increased their volume and share in recent years. Since the last decade, almost no consumption has been recorded by high-income countries, while the global asbestos consumption is now shared almost solely by upper and lower middle-income countries. We can reasonably expect that the burden of new cases and deaths will almost completely move to low-income countries soon.

Three countries with known high asbestos use are likely to impact the global future mesothelioma burden, due to their large populations: China, Russia, and India. China used 207,000 metric tons of asbestos per year, Russia 840,000 metric tons per year during 1970–1980, the most relevant period that could account for the recent mesothelioma rates; however, epidemiologic data on mesothelioma incidence and death are non-existent in these countries.

In summary, currently the global mesothelioma burden is mostly shouldered by high-income countries. Based on recorded historical, recent, and current use of asbestos, however, mesothelioma burdens will likely become an important problem in upper and lower middle-income countries, where health-care resources and novel diagnostics are scarce, asbestos production and use is not regulated, and incidence and death records are not available , therefore cannot be monitored.

6.7 UNCERTAINTY IN MESOTHELIOMA STATISTICS AND EXPOSURE ASSESSMENT

We have listed in Table 6.2 some of the factors that can contribute to making the overall picture about mesothelioma incidence and mortality more precise and reliable, and could help predict with some confidence future trends worldwide. One important piece is an accurate assessment and measurement of exposure. This information will help predict where and who will likely experience some health consequences associated with asbestos and asbestos-like fibers. Another element is the appropriateness of a mesothelioma diagnosis. Novel immunohistochemical markers are crucial for pathologists in order to more reliably distinguish mesothelioma from other malignancies (17). For example, recently it was discovered that lack of BAP1 nuclear staining combined with FISH analyses for biallelic loss of CDKN2A allow to distinguish mesothelioma from benign reactive mesothelial proliferations. Because these immunohistochemical techniques are not readily available worldwide, when cases are reviewed by an expert team of pathologists, many of the diagnoses are incorrect and need to be reclassified. This happened in France in 2018, when 14% of 5258 mesotheliomas diagnosed made in recent years were changed to benign lesions, primary pleural or lung sarcomas invading the pleura, metastases from various carcinomas, or direct pleural invasion by lung cancer (17). The rate of errors is much higher in developing countries, where it can approach 50% due to lack of trained pathologists, of standardized methods for staining and lack of

TABLE 6.2
Factors Involved in a Correct Definition of Asbestos-Mesothelioma Association

Variable	Determinants	Contributing Factors
Incidence	Exposure	Length of exposure, time of first exposure, protective equipment, other asbestos like exposures, environmental exposures
	Diagnosis	Country average income, SDI, quality of pathology, presence cancer of registry
Mortality	Incidence	
	Health-care quality	Country average income, SDI, registry
	Access to novel therapy/clinical trials	

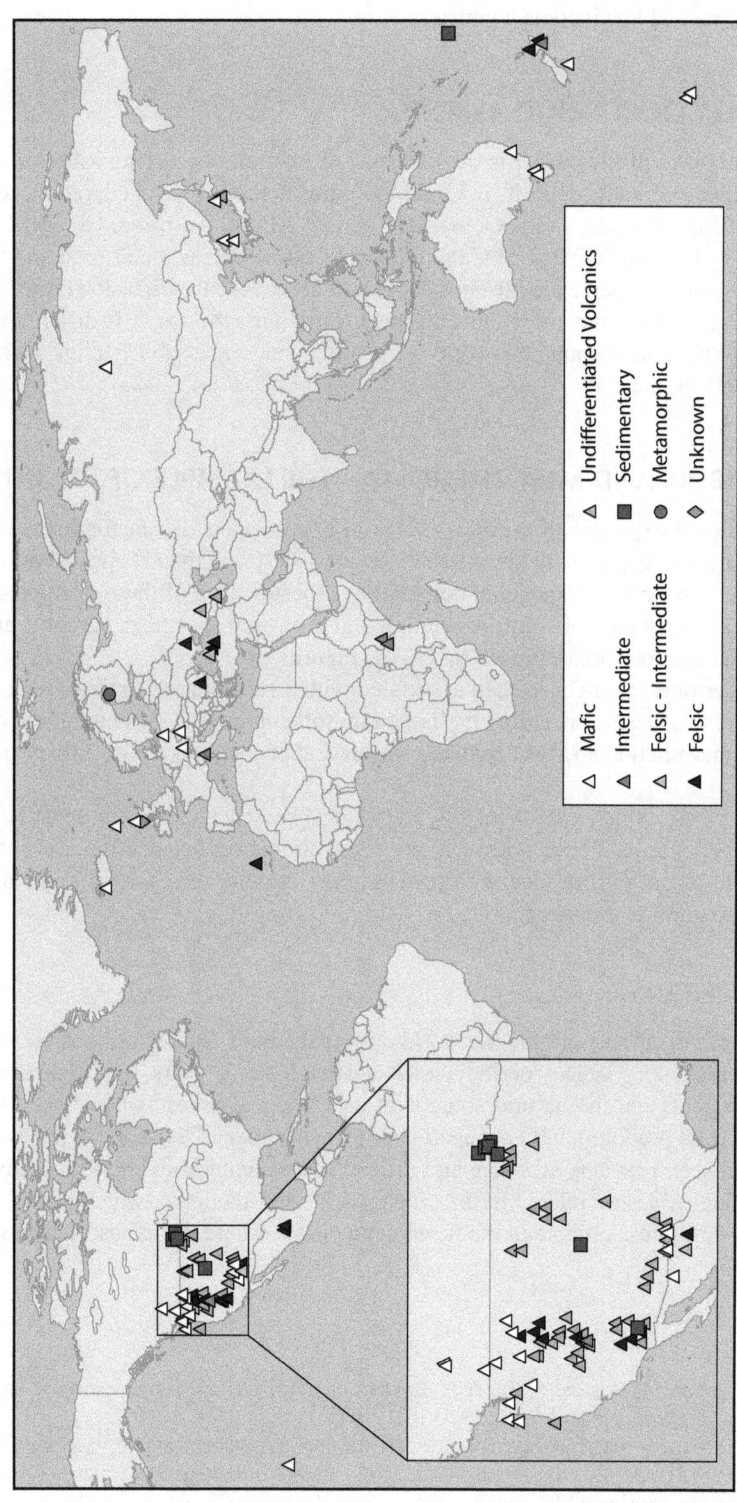

FIGURE 6.5 Erionite presence in the world.

availability of testing for novel markers (18). Therefore, disparities in access to proper diagnostic tools, together with poor measurement of exposure, may widen the gap in mesothelioma burden between high income and low income countries.

6.8 NATURALLY OCCURRING ASBESTOS

Another important piece of the puzzle is the presence of naturally occurring asbestos in the environment, for example chrysotile deposits in Ural Mountains in the Russian Federation, Appalachian Mountains in the USA, Canada, India, China, Italy, South Africa, Australia, Greece, Cyprus, and other countries (19). Human activity, rain, and other processes such as major road and bridge constructions may move and disperse the asbestos deposits and provoke the diffusion of inhalable fibers in the environment. Because the soil is not routinely tested for asbestos, it is difficult to map this natural presence of the fibers around the world, and consequently to establish a link with new cases of malignant mesothelioma.

6.9 OTHER FIBERS AND MESOTHELIOMA—THE EXAMPLE OF ERIONITE

Although occupational exposure to asbestos is a well-documented risk factor for mesothelioma, there are other sources of exposure to fibers that resemble asbestos in their shape and properties, and therefore may have the same carcinogenic potential as asbestos. One of these examples is erionite (20), a naturally occurring fiber of volcanic origin found in several specific geographic areas worldwide, and classified as group 1 carcinogen by IARC (Figure 6.5)

When inhaled, erionite fibers have been associated with effects similar to those seen as a consequence of exposure to asbestos, including malignant mesothelioma (21). Erionite fibers were linked to the malignant mesothelioma (MM) epidemic in the Cappadocia region of Turkey in the 1970s (22).

These geographic areas that are plagued by the natural presence of erionite must be monitored closely for mesothelioma incidence rates, age at mesothelioma occurrence in cases, and possible familial clusters in those with residence in proximity of erionite deposits, in order to intervene immediately where sentinel events occur.

6.10 CONCLUSION

Mesothelioma is still occurring around the world despite the bans and restrictions on asbestos use. Reasons for this are the long latency period, which can reach 40–50 years, the persistence of asbestos in the environment, and the natural sources of asbestos and asbestos-like fibers. Changes in type of exposure, from predominantly occupational to environmental, have made the assessment of the association between previous exposure and disease more complex and hard to establish. There are also methodological issues related to the diagnosis of mesothelioma, which make statistics on incidence and mortality less reliable in the developing world, where the exposure is more likely to still occur.

REFERENCES

1. Liu B, van Gerwen M, Bonassi S, Taioli E. Epidemiology of environmental exposure and malignant mesothelioma. *J. Thorac. Oncol.* 2017; 12(7):1031–1045
2. https://gco.iarc.fr/today/data/factsheets/cancers/18-Mesothelioma-fact-sheet.pdf (accessed 5/4/2023)
3. Carbone M, Pass HI, Ak G, et al. Medical and surgical care of patients with mesothelioma and their relatives carrying germline BAP1 mutations. *J. Thorac. Oncol.* 2022; 17(7):873–889
4. Carbone M, Yang H, Pass HI, Taioli E. Did the ban on asbestos reduce the incidence of mesothelioma? *J. Thorac. Oncol.* 2023; 18(6):694–697

5. Mazurek JM, Blackley DJ, Weissman DN. Malignant mesothelioma mortality in women — United States, 1999–2020. *MMWR* 71(19), 19
6. Alpert N, van Gerwen M, Taioli E. Epidemiology of mesothelioma in the 21st century in Europe and the United States, 40 years after restricted/banned asbestos use. *Transl. Lung Cancer Res.* 2020; 9(Suppl 1):S28–S38
7. http://www.ibasecretariat.org/alpha_ban_list.php (accessed 5/4/2023)
8. https://www.epa.gov/asbestos/epa-actions-protect-public-exposure-asbestos (accessed 5/4/2023)
9. https://pubs.usgs.gov/periodicals/mcs2023/mcs2023-asbestos.pdf (accessed 5/4/2023)
10. https://www.usgs.gov/centers/national-minerals-information-center/asbestos-statistics-and-information (accessed 5/4/2023)
11. https://d9-wret.s3.us-west-2.amazonaws.com/assets/ palladium/production/atoms/files/myb1-2018-asbes.pdf (accessed 5/4/2023)
12. Zhai Z, Ruan J, Zheng Y, Xiang D, Li N, Hu J, Shen J, Deng Y, Yao J, Zhao P, Wang S, Yang S, Zhou L, Wu Y, Xu P, Lyu L, Lyu J, Bergan R, Chen T, Dai Z. Assessment of global trends in the diagnosis of mesothelioma from 1990 to 2017. *JAMA Netw. Open* 2021; 4(8):e2120360
13. Han Y, Zhang T, Chen H, Yang X. Global magnitude and temporal trend of mesothelioma burden along with the contribution of occupational asbestos exposure in 204 countries and territories from 1990 to 2019: Results from the Global Burden of Disease Study 2019. *Crit. Rev. Oncol. Hematol.* 2022; 179:103821
14. Chimed-Ochir O, Arachi D, Driscoll T, Lin RT, Takala J, Takahashi K. Burden of mesothelioma deaths by national income category: Current status and future implications. *Int. J. Environ. Res. Public Health* 2020; 17(18):6900
15. Gariazzo C, Gasparrini A, Marinaccio A. Asbestos consumption and malignant mesothelioma mortality trends in the major user countries. *Ann. Glob. Health* 2023; 89(1):1–11
16. van Gerwen M, Alpert N, Flores R, Taioli E. An overview of existing mesothelioma registries worldwide, and the need for a US Registry. *Am. J. Ind. Med.* 2020; 63(2):115–120
17. Carbone M, Adusumilli PS, Alexander HR Jr., et al. Mesothelioma: Scientific clues for prevention, diagnosis, and therapy. *CA Cancer J. Clin.* 2019; 69(5):402–429
18. Guo Z, Carbone M, Zhang X, et al. Improving the accuracy of mesothelioma diagnosis in China. *J. Thorac. Oncol.* 2017; 12(4):714–723
19. Ricchiuti C, Bloise A, Punturo R. Occurrence of asbestos in soils: State of the art. *Episodes* 2020; 43(3):881–891
20. Patel JP, Brook MS, Kah M, Hamilton A. Global geological occurrence and character of the carcinogenic zeolite mineral, erionite: A review. *Front. Chem.* 2022; 10:1066565
21. Beaucham C, King B, Feldmann K, Harper M, Dozier A. Assessing occupational erionite and respirable crystalline silica exposure among outdoor workers in Wyoming, South Dakota, and Montana. *J. Occup. Environ. Hyg.* 2018; 15(6):455–465
22. Bariş YI, Artvinli M, Sahin AA. Environmental mesothelioma in Turkey. *Ann. N. Y. Acad. Sci.* 1979; 330:423–432

7 Environmental Exposure to Asbestos and Cancer

Francine Baumann

7.1 WHAT IS "ASBESTOS"?

"Asbestos" is a commercial and legal name given to fibrous minerals that were used by industry, and that caused mesothelioma and other cancers. Asbestos has been known for its fire-resistant qualities and its woven ability for over 5000 years, and from the 1880s has been used in a wide range of products (Alleman & Mossman, 1997) including insulation, fireproofing, brake linings, and paving materials. Numerous occupational studies have shown that inhalation of asbestos can cause malignant mesothelioma (MM), asbestosis, and lung cancers, resulting in the implementation of regulations that limit its use.

In fact, approximately 400 minerals can occur naturally in a fibrous habit, but most are very rare. Only six of these have been used commercially or have been associated with other commercially used minerals; these six have been referred to as "asbestos." Diseases related to asbestos have been studied in numerous papers that analyzed cohorts of workers exposed to these fibers. The potential for asbestos fibers to cause cancer is related to fiber shape (Case et al., 2011), usually defined as elongated mineral particles (EMPs) with length ≥5 μm, an aspect ratio (length to width) of 3:1 or greater, and parallel sides. In the USA, asbestos was first regulated by OSHA in 1971. Since 1977, all asbestos fibers have been declared carcinogenic by the International Agency for Research on Cancer (IARC, 1977). However, the statutory definition of asbestos designates as "asbestos" only the six fibrous minerals that are largely present in the industry: five amphiboles (tremolite, actinolite, crocidolite, anthophyllite, amosite) and the serpentine chrysotile.

Asbestos minerals have been extensively exploited commercially throughout the world, causing mesothelioma and lung cancer epidemic, especially in occupationally exposed workers. They have been progressively regulated and eventually banned in the western world in the 1980s and 1990s (Carbone et al., 2016). However, asbestos is still mined in Russia, China, Kazakhstan, Brazil, and Zimbabwe. It is massively used in India and other developing countries (Franck & Joshi, 2014).

7.1.1 Various Definitions of "Asbestos"

In 1971, the National Academy of Sciences defined "asbestos" as "a generic term for a number of hydrated silicates that, when crushed or processed, separate into flexible fibers made up of fibrils. Although there are many asbestos minerals, only six are of commercial importance" (Committee on Biologic Effects of Atmospheric Pollutants, 1971). Thus, this definition encompasses all asbestiform minerals, including the non-commercial fibrous minerals.

From a public health and media's perception, the generic term "asbestos" refers to a group of fibrous minerals associated with asbestosis, MM and other cancers. In fact "asbestos" has multiple definitions based on context (Skinner et al., 1988): the commercial definition is based on its industrial properties; mineralogical and geological definitions distinguish "asbestos" from other particles according to their shape, chemical composition and their physical properties; regulatory definitions identify minerals to be regulated for the protection of workers; and analytical definitions describe the rules that must be followed in order to characterize and count mineral fibers (Glenn et al., 2008).

DOI: 10.1201/9781003431909-7

Geologic and commercial definitions of "asbestos" involve the six natural fibrous minerals that are mined for their extraordinary fire-resistant properties, high tensile strength, low heat conductivity and their resistance to chemicals. Chrysotile represents 95% of all asbestos industrial production (OECD, 1984), while crocidolite (a mineral variety of riebeckite) and amosite account for the remaining 5% (Gibbs, 1990). Other three amphiboles anthophyllite, actinolite and tremolite have been used in very small quantities but are regulated because they often contaminate other industrially used minerals (Gunter et al., 2007). This definition based on commercial use is totally inconsistent since it does not consider the obvious toxicity of other fibrous minerals (Egilman et al., 2019).

Chemically speaking, "asbestos" are hydrated silicates with mainly magnesium, iron, calcium and sodium, and other minor elements (<~2%) (Wachowski & Domka, 2000), which would include many minerals that may not occur with a fibrous habit, e.g. some minerals from the mica group or the pyroxene group. This definition does not distinguish commercial asbestos from other fibrous minerals or even non-fibrous minerals. In addition, some minerals may occur in different habits (Middendorf et al., 2007) including for example, flattened prismatic, acicular (needle-shape), elongated or fibrous, all common habits for tremolite. Several groups of silicate minerals may show a fibrous habit, including serpentine, amphibole, zeolite, or clay (Skinner et al., 1988). The term "asbestos" has been used widely to indicate fibers that possess similar properties of tensile strength, flexibility, and durability, as commercial asbestos, regardless of whether they belong to the six "asbestos" types. Adding to the confusion, some minerals are designated under multiple nomenclatures. For example, amosite is a commercial term for either the asbestos form of cummingtonite or the fibrous variety grunerite. Lastly, the mineralogical nomenclature has been re-evaluated over time: for example, amphibole nomenclature has been revised three times since 1978 (Case et al., 2011), leading to a change in status of certain fibers from regulated to non-regulated (Meeker et al., 2003).

The Center for Disease Control and Prevention (CDC) website defined "asbestos" as a group of minerals having long, thin and separable fibers, which can be inhaled and can cause cancer and other lung disease. The World Health Organization (WHO) expanded the definition of "asbestos" to include all fibers that possess the physical and chemical properties of commercial asbestos (2000). However, regulatory health agencies recognize only the six commercial varieties of asbestos, as does the U.S. Department of the Interior, the American Council on Science and Health (Kava, 2007) and its French equivalent the Haute Autorité de Santé (2009). This limited regulation leads the general population as well as most physicians and scientists to believe that only the six mineral fibers that are called "asbestos" are hazardous, and that the ~390 remaining are not (Baumann et al., 2013).

7.1.2 Mineral Fibers or Cleavage Fragments?

Commonly, "fiber" refers to a thin elongated particle, having a high length/diameter (aspect) ratio. Non-mineralogists use the term "mineral fiber" to designate elongated mineral particles that may be asbestiform, acicular, or cleavage fragments (NIOSH, 2011). Mineralogists define the term "mineral fiber" as the smallest elongated crystalline unit that can be separated from a bundle or appears to have grown individually, and that exhibits an organic fiber appearance and by extension a long thin thread or threadlike solid with distinctive elongated shape (Millette & Bandli, 2005). In 1958, the Association for Research on Cancer (ARC) set the limit of aspect ratio of fibers to 3:1; some authors have recommended increasing this ratio to 10:1 (NIOSH, 1989) or even 20:1 (Lee, 2008). Only particles longer than or equal to 5 μm fall under the analytical definition of a fiber (Strohmeier et al., 2010) because shorter fibers are not visible by standard optical microscope, and because experiments in rats suggested that longer fibers were more carcinogenic (Dunnigan, 1984). On the other hand, several studies showed that short fibers are also involved in the induction of MM (Carbone et al., 2011; Godleski, 2004).

Asbestos naturally exists as bundles of thin and long fibrils running parallel to the main axis, which can be easily separated from one another and split at the ends (Figure 7.1). When the length is extremely long compared to the width, the crystal is called "asbestiform," otherwise the general term "acicular" may be used (Virta, 2001; Ross et al., 2008).

Cleavage refers to breakage of a mineral (Veblen & Wylie, 1993). Asbestiform crystals are produced by fibers growing along their main crystallographic axis leading to a fibrous or needle-like structure, while cleavage fragments are produced by breakage of crystals in directions that are related to crystal structure along cleavage planes (Aust et al., 2011). When a mineral possesses two coaxial cleavage planes, fragments are acicular; when it has only one cleavage plane, fragments are planar. The strength and flexibility of cleavage fragments depend on the crystal they originate from. Cleavage fragments are considered asbestiform when they possess a small diameter, a high aspect ratio, a high tensile strength, and when they are flexible (NRC, 1984).

There is no consensus about the harmful potential of cleavage fragments. Some reports have suggested that cleavage fragments are less hazardous than asbestos fibers because of their large diameter and short length (Ilgren, 2004). In the USA, the Occupational Safety and Health Administration (OSHA) and the Mine Safety and Health Administration (MSHA) have distinguished between fibers and cleavage fragments coming from the same minerals since 1992. However, the NIOSH recommended including the acicular analogs of asbestos minerals in the definition of asbestos (2011), and the EPA does not distinguish between fibers and cleavage fragments having the same chemical composition, the same shape, and the same size (Van Orden et al., 2008). All mineral particles having a high aspect ratio and dimensions making them breathable should be considered potentially hazardous.

7.1.3 The Geological Sources of Asbestos

Asbestos minerals are present in many geological formations throughout the world, but few deposits are commercially exploitable (Nicholson & Pundsack, 1973). Asbestos-bearing rock is most associated with either ultramafic rocks such as peridotite, pyroxenite, dunite, serpentinite or metamorphic rocks including amphibolite, marble, calc-silicate, quartzite, and schists (Schreier, 1989). Soils resulting from the weathering of these rocks may contain asbestos.

Asbestos present in rocks is not hazardous unless crushing or weathering release fibers. Macroscopic fibers disintegrate into micro fibrils (diameter <0.3 μm) that are released into the environment. These fibrils form a stable suspension in the air, which may spread out over considerable distances from the source of emission, due to their aerodynamic properties. The rate and direction of fiber dispersion depend upon atmospheric conditions, such as nebulosity, rainfall, strength and direction of wind, and temperature. Airborne fibers are very resistant; atmosphere cleanup only occurs with the intervention of precipitation (Wachowski & Domka, 2000). Airborne asbestos may become a public health problem as populations are exposed to airborne mineral fibers because of natural erosion or human activities producing dust, such as mines, quarries, roads, and outside activities (Carbone et al., 2016).

7.2 ASBESTOS AND CANCER

7.2.1 Asbestos-Related Diseases

Experimental and epidemiological studies showed that inhalation of asbestos fibers may cause asbestosis, pleural fibrosis, lung and laryngeal cancers, pleural and peritoneal mesothelioma, possibly other cancers (Franck & Joshi, 2014), and non-neoplastic pleural pathologies (pleural plaques, pleural effusion, diffuse pleural thickening, and rounded atelectasis). All forms of asbestos are proven carcinogens, and there is no safe level of exposure (Franck & Joshi, 2014).

Because MM is only due to the inhalation of mineral fibers, this cancer is a marker of exposure to asbestos or asbestos-like fibers. Asbestos may cause a higher number of lung cancers than of MMs (McCormack et al., 2012). For example, linear relations between asbestos exposure indexes (based on dust concentration multiplied by exposure duration) and lung cancers and asbestosis have been demonstrated in occupational studies (McDonald et al., 1980). But the confounding factor of smoking makes it difficult to estimate the risk of lung and other cancers attributable to asbestos (WHO, 2000).

The relationship between asbestos exposure and disease is particularly difficult to study because of the several decades' latency between initial asbestos exposure and disease. Moreover, the precise assessment of the overall exposure of a given individual to different types of fibers is very difficult. In addition, environmental exposure is generally involuntary and unknown.

7.2.2 Mechanisms of Toxicity of Asbestos Fibers

Mineral fibers present in the air are inhaled and trapped in the lungs where, using lymphatic vessels, they may reach the pleura (Mutti et al., 2018). It has been suggested that penetration of fibers into the lung is possible only if the fiber diameter is below 1 μm (Wylie et al., 1993). These fibers may also reach the abdominal lymph nodes, mesentery, and omentum, where they can cause peritoneal mesothelioma (Carbone et al., 2012a). More rarely, asbestos also caused mesothelioma of the pericardium and mesothelioma of the tunica vaginalis testis (Dodson et al., 2001).

Because asbestos is also associated with cancers of the digestive tract, it has been suggested that asbestos fibers present in water might be digested and, likewise inhaled fibers in the lung, deposited in stomach or colorectum and cause cancer (Di Ciaula, 2017). To reduce the risk of human contamination, U.S. Environmental Protection Agency (U.S. EPA) defined a maximum contaminant level of asbestos in drinking water of 7.10^6 f/L (U.S. EPA, 2004).

Once trapped in the body, mineral fibers cause inflammation, which can lead to cancer (Yang et al., 2022). This mechanism mobilizes mesothelial cells and macrophages, which gather around fiber deposits. These cells produce different molecules, including high mobility group box 1 (HMGB1) and other cytokines, reactive oxygen species, and growth factors responsible for inflammation, DNA damage and abnormal cell growth, leading to fibrosis and/or carcinogenesis (Carbone et al., 2016).

Respirable fibers (diameter <3 μm) may persist for decades in the lung (Kuempel et al., 2006). Clearance mechanisms depend on length, diameter, and chemical composition of the fibers. Although asbestos carcinogenesis appears to increase with fiber length, a precise threshold cannot be established for the minimum fiber length associated with cancer risk. Short fibers (<5 μm) constitute most fibers in the lung (Aust et al., 2011), but there is controversy on their role in producing disease because they are cleared more easily (Mossman et al., 2011). Yet a review of animal models concluded that fibers of all lengths induce pathological responses (Dodson et al., 2003).

In conclusion, the main factors that influence asbestos fibers toxicity are fiber dose, dimensions, and biopersistence (Lippmann, 1990; Hillerdal, 2003).

7.2.3 Cancers Due To Asbestos Exposure

Numerous studies of asbestos-exposed workers demonstrated the link between exposure to asbestos and cancer. Because exposure is generally via the air, inhalation of asbestos fibers increases the risk of lung cancer. The risk of lung cancer after exposure to asbestos is at least twice the risk of MM. Lung cancer develops several decades after first exposure to asbestos. When the person exposed to asbestos is also a smoker, these two factors have a synergetic (more than additive) effect on the risk of developing lung cancer (Klebe et al., 2019).

Mesothelioma is a very rare cancer of the pleura, and even rarer cancer of the peritoneum, the pericarditis or the tunica vaginalis of the testis. Because exposure to asbestiform mineral fibers is the only known causing factor of MM, it is considered a marker of exposure to these fibers.

Exposure to asbestos has also been linked to cancers of the larynx and pharynx, of ovaries, of the stomach, colon, and rectum. For these three last cases, a way of exposure could be by swallowing asbestos fibers.

Recently, some studies have also found higher rates of breast cancer among women previously exposed to asbestos fibers. It is possible that inflammation caused by asbestos participates in the development of breast cancer (Danforth, 2021).

7.3 NON-REGULATED FIBROUS MINERALS MAY ALSO CAUSE CANCER

The risk posed by mineral fibers from the natural environment has long been hidden by the occupational exposure to asbestos. Actually, several groups of silicate minerals may show a fibrous habit, including serpentines, amphiboles, zeolites, and some clay minerals (Skinner et al., 1988). Approximately 400 minerals can occur naturally in a fibrous habit (Table 7.1), but only five amphiboles (tremolite, actinolite, crocidolite, anthophyllite, and amosite) and the serpentine chrysotile have been used by the industry and are regulated under the term "asbestos" (Baumann et al., 2013).

Some studies showed that MM and asbestos-related diseases are also caused by non-regulated fibers (Below et al., 2011). The carcinogenicity of "asbestos" minerals has been largely demonstrated in occupational and experimental studies and is linked to their fibrous shape. Thus, unregulated mineral fibers that share similar properties to regulated asbestos fibers may cause similar hazards, and specifically MM (Baumann et al., 2013). However, the restricted definition of "asbestos" can lead people to believe that only the six regulated minerals can cause MM and other asbestos-related diseases (Baumann et al., 2013).

In addition to the regulated asbestos minerals, non-regulated amphiboles may also crystallize in asbestiform habit and are suspected to present the same risks as commercial asbestos (Lee et al., 2008). Many non-regulated fibrous minerals are potentially as dangerous as asbestos because of their similar physical and chemical properties; epidemiological studies and *in vivo* experiments have demonstrated their toxicity (Wachowski & Domka, 2000).

The term *naturally occurring asbestos* (NOA) has been created to describe potentially hazardous asbestos-like fibrous minerals that are present in rocks and soils, may or may not fit the regulatory or industrial definitions of asbestos, and may become airborne mineral fibers after being released in the air by erosion or human activity (Harper, 2008).

The rising awareness about the risk due to NOA environmental exposure motivated investigations and research on non-regulated mineral fibers (Bailey & Kalika, 2020). In Italy, a field survey found the presence of several asbestiform minerals, such as asbestiform antigorite, asbestiform diopside, asbestiform carlosturanite, asbestiform forsterite, asbestiform sepiolite, asbestiform balangeroite, asbestiform talc, asbestiform erionite, asbestiform offretite, and asbestiform fluoro-edenite (Belluso et al., 2020).

Following epidemiological and geological studies that found a probable source of environmental MM in desertic rocks in Southern Nevada, USA, experiments were carried out to study the toxicity of fibrous palygorskite (Larson et al., 2016). Similarly, fibrous glaucophane was found to be common in California, USA, raising concerns about its potential toxicity (Di Giuseppe et al., 2019). Nanoparticles with high aspect ratio are also suspected to cause mesothelioma (Andujar et al., 2016)

The increased risk of disease has been described in individuals exposed to NOA minerals in Turkey (erionite), Italy (fluoro-edenite), and the United States (winchite/richterite). In New Caledonia, an increased incidence of mesothelioma was correlated with the natural occurrence of fibrous antigorite in outcrops, roadways, and soils (Baumann & Ambrosi, 2015).

7.3.1 Winchite and Richterite Amphiboles Caused MM in the USA

Asbestiform varieties of winchite and richterite minerals contaminated the vermiculite mined from Libby, Montana (USA) (Sullivan, 2007). Winchite and richterite minerals may produce plentiful thin fibers when subjected to abrasion or crushing (Meeker et al., 2003). They were originally identified as tremolite-actinolite; later, electron microscopy with X-ray analysis revealed the amphibole composition of winchite and richterite (Bandli & Gunter, 2006). These amphiboles were associated with MM, lung cancer and asbestosis among the inhabitants of Libby and the mining and milling workers of vermiculite (Sullivan, 2007; McDonald et al., 1986; Amandus & Wheeler, 1987; Peipins et al., 2003; Miller et al., 2018). *In vitro* tests have demonstrated the toxic and mutagenic effect of richterite (Collan et al., 1986). Vermiculite contaminated with these minerals was used in construction, agricultural, industrial and many consumer products in the USA and other countries (Sullivan, 2007), exposing millions of people to these carcinogenic fibers.

7.3.2 Erionite Is Highly Carcinogenic and Is Present in U.S. Soils

Erionite refers to naturally occurring fibrous minerals that belong to the zeolite group. Electron microscopy analyses of erionite samples revealed a microstructure of bundles of fibers that were less than 1 μm in diameter (Dogan, 2003; Dogan et al., 2008) (Figure 7.1b).

In three villages of Cappadocia, Turkey, houses were built from volcanic stones containing erionite and roads were paved with erionite-containing gravel (Baris et al., 1978; Artvinli & Baris, 1979). Inhabitants were exposed to high concentrations of erionite fibers, causing a MM epidemic (Baris et al., 1978; Carbone et al., 2007, 2011). A prospective study from 1979 through 2003 in those Turkish villages with high levels of erionite exposure revealed that 44.5% of all deaths were due to MM (Baris & Grandjean, 2006). The follow-up of a Turkish emigrant cohort from one of these villages showed that 78% of deaths were due to MM (Boman et al., 1982; Metintas et al., 1999).

The extremely carcinogenic properties of erionite have been demonstrated in numerous *in vivo* and *in vitro* experiments (Maltoni et al., 1982; Johnson et al., 1984; Fraire et al., 1997; Carbone et al., 2012b). In particular, the risk of MM in rats is higher in erionite-treated groups compared to "asbestos" fiber-treated groups (Carthew et al., 1992; Wagner et al., 1985). Erionite fibers accumulate iron on the surface (Eborn & Aust, 1995; Fach et al., 2002) and are genotoxic (Poole et al., 1983; Okayazu et al., 1999). Erionite induces macrophages and polymorphonuclear lymphocytes to generate mutagenic reactive oxygen metabolites (Urano et al., 1991), and transforms human mesothelial cells *in vitro* (Bertino et al., 2007). The strong correlation that has been demonstrated between exposure to erionite fibers and the development of MM led WHO to classify erionite as a group 1 carcinogen (IARC, 1987).

Deposits of fibrous erionite are present in volcanic tuffs of the western USA (Forsman, 1986). In North Dakota, erionite-contaminated gravel has been used during the past three decades to pave hundreds of miles of roads, parking lots, and playgrounds. The levels of erionite exposure inside cars and school buses transiting on these roads are comparable to those detected in some of the MM villages in Turkey (Carbone et al., 2011). A U.S. EPA study showed asbestos-like radiographic pleural changes among workers employed in road maintenance or gravel pits in Dunn County (Ryan et al., 2011). MM cases caused by erionite have recently been reported in the USA (Kliment et al., 2009). In Southern Nevada, USA, amphiboles and erionite deposits cover large desert areas and off-road activities may release those carcinogenic fibers into the air, exposing the local population (Baumann et al., 2015). Erionite deposits are found in many parts of the western U.S. (Van Gosen et al., 2013).

7.3.3 Fibrous Antigorite Induces Cancer and Asbestosis

Antigorite appears as a lamellar greenish mineral. It belongs to the serpentine group, which includes chrysotile and lizardite. Chrysotile, lizardite, and antigorite have the same generic chemical formulae but different crystallographic structure and Mg/Fe ratio (Dodony et al., 2002). Like amphiboles, antigorite may have massive, acicular, fibrous or asbestiform habits according to its geological formation condition. When asbestiform, antigorite aggregates consist of bundles of fibers that split into very thin needles (Fitz Gerald et al., 2010) (Figure 7.1c).

Serpentinites (rocks made of serpentine minerals) are very common in mafic and ultramafic massifs and their soils throughout the world. The unsuspected presence of fibrous antigorite may constitute a hazard where populations are exposed to airborne fibers by human activities producing dust from these soils. For example, in Montgomery County, Maryland, serpentinite used to pave roads was found to contain fibrous antigorite; air analyses highlighted a high concentration of mineral fibers in areas close to unsealed roads (Rohl et al., 1977).

In Poland, fibrous antigorite in lateritic nickel ores was identified as the likely cause of 25 cases of asbestosis among the workers in a nickel metallurgic plant (Wozniak et al., 1988). The level of environmental exposure to breathable antigorite fibers among a population living near a serpentinite mine and a processing mill was estimated to be well above the established thresholds for regulated asbestos (Wozniak et al., 1993, 1994). Experiments in rats demonstrated that antigorite induces MM; the carcinogenic and mutagenic effects of fibrous antigorite were shown to be comparable to the effects of crocidolite (Wozniak, 1999).

In Australia, antigorite was mined from the late 1940s to 1978 in the Rowland Flat quarry, north of Adelaide (Fitz Gerald et al., 2010). A mixture of talc and antigorite was extracted and milled for use as fibrous mineral filler. This "asbestos" was first described as an amphibole, and then as a chrysotile. It was correctly identified as antigorite decades later during a study for the rehabilitation of abandoned mining sites (Keeling et al., 2010).

In the Piemonte Alps, Italy, serpentinites present a carcinogenic risk (Harf et al., 1993), because of the abundance of fibrous antigorite (Bandli & Gunter, 2001). Asbestiform antigorite was also described in Elba (Viti & Mellini, 1996), and in serpentinite veins of the ultramafic massif of Lanzo, Italy, manifested as bundles of rigid and brittle fibers with a length of 14–20 μm and a diameter of 0.08–0.4 μm (Groppo & Compagnoni, 2007). *In vitro* studies showed that the toxicity and cellular response to fibrous antigorite were comparable with those of regulated asbestos. Antigorite fibers induced chronic inflammation, increased immune cell activity and stimulated the formation of new blood vessels, leading to the malignant transformation of lung cells (Pugnaloni et al., 2008). Toxicity tests showed that mesothelial cells exposed to antigorite fibers released ROS and RNS, which contribute to MM pathogenesis (Cardile et al., 2007).

In New Caledonia, exceptional MM incidences were highlighted in tribal areas (Baumann et al., 2011; Baumann, 2011). These MM cases were first thought to be due to the former white-washing of dwellings using tremolite-containing whitewash (Luce et al., 2000). This first study included only 15 MM cases; information on the whitewashing was reported by the patients only, and no verification of the whitewash composition was done (Luce et al., 2000). In a study including all 109 MM cases recorded at the Cancer registry of New Caledonia from 1984 to 2008, the MM clusters did not correlate with the tremolite-whitewashing locations but were instead significantly linked with the geographical distribution of serpentinite occurrences (Baumann et al., 2007, 2011; Baumann, 2011). Serpentinite outcrops were sampled and analyzed; they contained antigorite fibers. Previous air samples from these areas did not show any fibers because the laboratories did not check for any fibers other than the six regulated "asbestos." The authors then checked for the possible presence of additional types of mineral fibers in air samples; antigorite was identified (Baumann et al., 2011; Baumann, 2011). It was discovered that antigorite-containing serpentinite was mined from multiple quarries and used to cover the roads in some tribal areas (Baumann et al., 2011; Baumann, 2011) (Figure 7.2). An ecological analysis showed that these serpentinite-paved roads were the main source of environmental exposure to mineral fibers and fibrous antigorite was significantly related to the distribution of MM in New Caledonia (Baumann et al., 2011). These results led local authorities to regulate the use of antigorite, similarly to asbestos. New experiments showed that the alteration of fibro-lamellar antigorite causes the emission of asbestos-like fibers in the air. A recent study demonstrated the toxic potential of antigorite from New Caledonia (Petriglieri et al., 2020).

7.3.4 There Are Numerous Examples of Carcinogenic Non-regulated Mineral Fibers

Among other non-regulated natural fibers that have been associated with MM are: arfvedsonite mined in the Ural Mountains, Russia; balangeroite and carlosturanite in Piemont, Italy (Groppo et al., 2005); and the amphibole fluoro-edenite, which is extracted from a volcanic material of Etna in Biancavilla, Italy, and used in building construction (Paoletti et al., 2000; Comba et al., 2003; Bruni et al., 2006). *In vitro* and *in vivo* experiments have confirmed the potential of fluoro-edenite to cause MM (Cardile et al., 2004; Soffritti et al., 2004). Fluoro-edenite fibers are acicular and are very similar to the particles of tremolite, winchite and richterite (Gianfagna et al., 2003). Additional mineral fibers suspected to be hazardous in the USA include fibrous and asbestiform grunerite, a widespread mineral that is present for example in some taconite ores mined in Minnesota (Nelson, 2009); phyllosilicates sepiolite and palygorskite that are found in the dust from southern Nevada (Soukup et al., 2011); fibrous varieties of the hornblende minerals series; serpentine antigorite; and zeolites mordenite and erionite (Table 7.1) (NIOSH, 2011). In addition, man-made fibers, including manufactured nanoparticles that are thin enough to be breathable, also raise some health concerns because of their biopersistence (Bernstein, 2007).

7.4 WHAT IS ENVIRONMENTAL EXPOSURE?

Public health problems caused by exposure to asbestiform fibers from the natural environment have been studied only within the last two decades. In fact, no known exposure to asbestos is found in about 20% of all MM cases, and in over 80% of cases in women (Spirtas et al., 1994; Lacourt et al., 2014; Linton et al., 2012; Rake et al., 2009). These non-occupational cases were likely exposed to carcinogenic fibers dispersed from the environment, either from indoor asbestos, from industrial sources of asbestos, or from natural sources (outcrops, soils, deposits) that were disturbed by weathering or human activities (Baumann et al., 2015). Similarly, former asbestos mines, plants and shipyards may also be a source of environmental exposure (Hansen et al., 1993; Magnani et al., 2001; Reid et al., 2007; Tarres et al., 2013). These exposures are predicted to account for an increasing proportion of asbestos-related diseases (Robinson et al., 2005).

Environment is a generic term that may include indoor and outdoor environments, as well as occupational and non-occupational environments. After a brief description of the different types of exposure to asbestos and asbestos-like fibers, we will develop more specifically the particularities of non-occupational exposure to fibers from the natural environment.

7.4.1 Occupational Exposure

Occupational exposure to asbestos affects mostly workers in construction (particularly insulators), manufactories (brakes, asbestos-textile, fiber cement pipes, …), mining and quarrying, and electricity, gas, steam and air conditioning supply. Between 1940 and 1980, about 27,500,000 workers have been potentially exposed to asbestos (Nicholson et al., 1982). Numerous occupational studies demonstrated the causal links between asbestos exposure and cancer and other respiratory diseases, mostly in men. Because of regulation and eventually ban of asbestos, this exposure decreased since the 1970s in the Western countries, resulting in the decrease of MM in men after the year 2000. However, asbestos is still used in Russia, China, India and other developing countries.

7.4.2 Para-occupational or Familial Exposure

There is an increased risk of MM among family members of individuals occupationally exposed to asbestos (Miller, 2005). Workers may bring asbestos in their hair and work clothes, and thus secondary expose their family members to hazardous fibers (D'Agostin et al., 2018). Ferrante et al. (2016) showed that having a family member occupationally exposed to asbestos doubled the risk of MM.

7.4.3 Indoor or Domestic Exposure

Domestic exposure occurs when people have asbestos-containing materials installed at home, such as insulation, paints, some cements, and jointing compounds, or when people handle those materials during home repairs. Once asbestos fibers are released at home, they may spread in all rooms, and it is impossible to remove them even with a vacuum cleaner. The risk associated with domestic exposure due to the use of asbestos-containing tools or the presence of asbestos-containing materials at home was estimated to increase the MM risk by a factor of about three (Ferrante et al., 2016).

7.4.4 Urban Exposure

In cities the air may contain asbestos fibers released from buildings, in particular during demolition work, or from brake pads of cars and trucks, or from the industry.

7.4.5 Exposure from the Natural Environment

Fibrous minerals are present in many geological formations that are widespread throughout the world (Nicholson & Pundsack, 1973; Schreier, 1989). Mineral fibers present in rocks are not hazardous unless crushing or weathering releases them. Soils resulting from the eroding of these rocks may also contain mineral fibers (Baumann & Ambrosi, 2015). Macroscopic fibers disintegrate into micro fibrils that are released into the environment and may travel for kilometers (Baumann et al., 2015). Thus, humans are exposed to these fibers when natural events or human activities such as mining, quarrying, roadwork, and outside recreational activities produce dust (Baumann et al., 2015).

For example, in California, USA, Pan et al. (2005) showed that the risk of MM decreased by 6% for every addition of 10 km distance from a natural asbestos source.

In New Caledonia, the presence of antigorite fibers in serpentinite rocks used to pave roads had a spatial association with MM incidence (Baumann et al., 2011), leading the local authorities to add antigorite to the list of regulated asbestos.

In Turkey, exposure to erionite fibers present in rocks used to construct some villages has been related to exceptionally high MM rates in the general population (Carbone et al., 2007). In the USA, a concern arose because roads were constructed in North Dakota with crushed stone containing erionite, exposing construction workers and the local population to these carcinogenic fibers (Carbone et al., 2011).

7.4.6 Exposure from Environment Contaminated by Past Use of Asbestos And Asbestiform Minerals

Past asbestos use may also become a source of environmental exposure. Former quarries and factories may be contaminated by fibers for decades and cause MM and other cancers (Ripabelli et al., 2018). Shipyards were also an important source of contamination in the UK (McElvenny et al., 2005), Italy (Fazzo et al., 2012) and the USA (Case et al., 2011). For example, the state of Louisiana, USA, presents significantly high MM rates because of asbestos and vermiculite that was used in both shipyards and former plants (Case et al., 2011). In these facilities, soils have been contaminated for years, causing the exposure of the neighborhood to carcinogenic mineral fibers. Similarly, in Casale Monferrato, Italy, MM risk was associated with decreasing distance to a large asbestos-cement factory (Magnani et al., 2001; Maule et al., 2007). In Biancavilla, Sicily, an environmental exposure to fluoro-edenite fibers present in stones used to build houses caused a local epidemic of MM (Paoletti et al., 2000; Comba et al., 2003; Bruni et al., 2006). In the UK, Howel et al. (1999) found a strong association of MM with residential proximity to an asbestos exposure source.

In addition, mineral fibers coming from mines, quarries, roads, factories, asbestos-contaminated waste, …, may pollute water in rivers and lakes, then migrate airborne after water vaporization (Avataneo et al., 2022), creating a new risk for humans and the environment. Waterborne fibers may also be generated by natural processes when surface and deep waters flow into rock formations containing fibrous minerals, and by weathering of these rocks (Avataneo et al., 2022). For example, presence of airborne asbestos fibers was noticed during agricultural activities in the surrounding of a former asbestos mine in Italy. Asbestos fibers were detected in samples of the stream water draining the former mine, and this water was used to irrigate the field (Turci et al., 2016). Transport of fibers by water may result in airborne diffusion of this pollutant far from the source of contamination.

Thus, asbestos removal and remediation of all contaminated sites are necessary, in addition to clear information, in order to prevent environmental exposure and disease.

7.5 ANALYTICAL METHODS USED TO ASSESS ENVIRONMENTAL EXPOSURE TO MINERAL FIBERS

The presence of mineral fibers in rocks and soils may be assessed by conducting an analysis of samples of these rocks and soils. Similarly, the presence of fibers in the air is assessed by analyzing air samples.

Analytical methods used to analyze samples were devised to regulate occupational exposure to asbestos. Because asbestos toxicity is related to the length and diameter of fibers, analytical methods must be able to determine the size, concentration, and type of mineral fibers. Phase-contrast microscopy (PCM) has been used for more than 50 years to check for the presence of asbestos fibers in the work environment (Edwards & Lynch, 1968); all observed fibers were counted (Walton, 1982). PCM presents several advantages: it allows for the exclusion of non-fibrous particles, it provides an estimate of risk, it is cost-effective, analysis is quick and can be conducted on site, and this "old" technique enables direct comparisons between current and past data. The main disadvantages of PCM are that it is not possible to distinguish between regulated asbestos and other mineral fibers, and that PCM cannot be used to observe fibers shorter than 5 μm. This threshold in detection may introduce significant bias to exposure analysis.

For these reasons, in 2000 the WHO stated that electron microscopy was the most reliable technique for the detection and identification of asbestos fibers (WHO, 2000). Electron microscopy is sometimes used in combination with X-ray diffraction analysis (Van Orden et al., 2008). These methods are expensive and require technically qualified staff. Transmission electron microscopy (TEM) can be used to identify asbestos fibers collected from air samples and for lung content analyses. This method allows for the identification of very small fibers (Walton, 1982), but fibers longer than 10 μm are sometimes overlooked, and cleavage fragments may be mistaken for asbestiform amphiboles (Lee et al., 2008). Scanning electron microscopy (SEM) allows for the examination of surface details and particle morphology (Figure 7.1) and may be coupled with different spectrometers to obtain semi-quantitative chemistry of individual particles (Middleton, 1982). There are very few standards for SEM asbestos analysis and there may be differences in sample preparation methods (Frasca et al., 2000).

Aside from TEM, the most common method for fiber analysis is polarized light microscopy (PLM) (Santee & Lott, 2003; Gunter, 2004). Spindle stage-assisted PLM method allows for a better description of particle morphology (Bandli & Gunter, 2001; Millette & Bandli, 2005).

Raman microspectroscopy may also be used to distinguish between the regulated amphibole and serpentine minerals (Rinaudo et al., 2003, 2004). The accuracy of this method to discriminate fibrous and non-fibrous forms has been investigated (Bard et al., 1997; Petry et al., 2006); its use is currently limited to the analysis of fiber bundles (Stromeier et al., 2010). Progress in this area of spectroscopy is moving rapidly and the reliability of this technique is improving.

In summary, the methods used for the identification of mineral fibers vary. Sampling and analytical methods need to be well defined and standardized in order to reduce inter-operator and inter-laboratory variability. Moreover, most of the laboratories that analyze air samples for fiber diagnosis only look for the six regulated asbestos. Yet there is evidence that short fibers (<5 μm long), thin fibers (<0.2 μm wide), some asbestos-like fibers, and asbestiform cleavage fragments affect human health (Egilman, 2019). Assessing exposure to NOA requires testing for all potentially harmful fibrous minerals, not just those subject to national/local regulation (Carbone et al., 2016). In order to be able to assess for exposure to mineral fibers from the natural environment, new procedures are urgently needed, including the use of detailed geological models that allow for the identification of potential presence of fibrous minerals, and analytical methods that allow identification of any kind of mineral fiber (Turci et al., 2020).

7.6 EPIDEMIOLOGICAL CHARACTERISTICS OF ENVIRONMENTAL MESOTHELIOMA

MM is generally diagnosed 30–60 years after exposure to mineral fibers. For this reason, assessing the source and level of exposure is very difficult. Adding to the difficulties, in the case of an environmental source of fibers, people are not aware of the exposure. Consequently, ecological studies are more fitted to analyze the relationship between environmental exposure and disease (Baumann et al., 2011), rather than case-control studies.

In the past century, MM was largely caused by occupational exposure to asbestos. Thus, considering the long latency of this cancer, the mean age at death for MM was about 70 years with a male to female ratio of about 4:1 (Delgermaa et al., 2011; Binazzi et al., 2022; Mazurez et al., 2017). For instance, in the USA, the mean age was 72.8 years, and the male-to-female ratio was 4.2:1 for the 1994–2008 period (Delgermaa et al., 2011) and 4:1 for the 1999–2015 period (Mazurez et al., 2017). In Italy, between 1993 and 2018, about 70% of MM cases were occupationally exposed. Mean age at diagnosis was 70 years (Binazzi et al., 2022). Because of the decreased use of asbestos, MM incidence rate decreased in males older than 45 years between 2003 and 2008, but it remained stable in women (Weill et al., 2004; Moolgavkar et al., 2009; Henley et al., 2013).

When the source of exposure to mineral fibers is not occupational, both genders and all age groups are exposed (D'Agostin et al., 2018). In this case, MM distribution by gender and age shows a pattern that is different from occupational MM: the M:F sex ratio is ~1:1 and the mean age at diagnosis is of ~60 years (Baris et al., 1978; Metintas et al., 2002; Metintas et al., 2008; Bruno et al., 2014). For example, in New Caledonia we showed that outside the main city, Nouméa, MM was diagnosed from the age of 35 years, and was as frequent in women as in men, indicating a probable environmental source of exposure (Baumann et al., 2007). Mesothelioma deaths occurring in individuals less than 55 years old suggest that they are non-occupationally exposed to asbestiform fibers (Mazurek et al., 2017).

7.6.1 A Higher Proportion of Female and Young MM Cases May Be Used as Indicators of Environmental Exposure to Carcinogenic Fibers

The geographic distribution of total MM mortality reflects both occupational and environmental exposures. Because an environmental source of fibers may expose both genders from a very young age, while occupational exposure concerns mostly men over 18 years old, it is possible to differentiate areas having environmental sources of exposure from areas with occupational exposure only, by studying the spatial distribution of the proportion of female and young MM cases (Baumann et al., 2015a, 2015b; Baumann, 2016; Baumann & Carbone, 2016).

For example, in New Caledonia, in areas where there was no occupational exposure to asbestos, we found significant MM spatial clusters grouping some Melanesian tribes. The sex ratio close to 1 and the high percentage of young cases in those tribal areas were consistent with environmental exposure (Baumann et al., 2011). Our ecological analysis identified the serpentinite present on roads as the main source of environmental exposure, and antigorite as a "new" carcinogenic fiber. This study demonstrated that cluster analysis and ecological studies at a small geographic scale are useful tools to identify areas with environmental exposure.

Similarly, an ecological study integrating individual data about asbestos exposure in Italy found that the percentage of female cases among MM clusters was explained by type and sources of exposure (Corfiati et al., 2015). Another recent study in Sicily showed that the MM risk ratio was the most sensitive in females and in young age groups exposed to an environmental source of fibers (Bruno et al., 2014).

7.6.2 Spatial Disparities Due To Environmental Exposure May Be Identified Only at Small Geographic Scale

As explained above, in countries where asbestos has been used, most MM cases are caused by occupational exposure. These occupational cases hide MM cases that are due to a source of environmental exposure, which is limited to a specific area, and which intensity is generally lower than the intensity of occupational exposure. For example, in Nevada, USA, the analysis of MM at the scale of the state did not allow to identify any risk of environmental exposure (Baumann et al., 2015b). Just the opposite, an analysis at a smaller geographic scale than the whole state allowed to identify a pattern of MM that suggested an environmental exposure in Southern Nevada (Baumann et al., 2015a). Compared to the rest of the USA, a significantly lower M:F sex ratio was found in Clark and Nye counties, where geological investigations discovered deposits of different types of fibrous minerals (Baumann et al., 2015a).

Indeed, in places where occupational exposure was important, cases due to an environmental source of exposure may be diluted among occupational cases. They become impossible to distinguish in a large area such as the entire state. In fact, an environmental source of exposure to mineral fibers, such as a quarry, a road, a mine, or a factory, causes a MM risk spatially limited to a small area, which can be identified only by studying small areas.

Studying MM mortality rates in females only, even at a small geographic scale, would not help identifying places with environmental exposure. Indeed, counties with high MM mortality in women may include both places associated with past asbestos industry (and high MM rates in males), and places with no asbestos use (thus low MM rates in males) but an environmental source of exposure. On the contrary, a higher proportion of females among MM cases suggests an exposure that is not limited to males, thus a probable non-occupational source of exposure. Similarly, a higher proportion of young cases indicates exposure at a very young age, thus, again, a non-occupational source of exposure.

7.7 CONCLUSION

"Asbestos" is an imprecise and confusing term that includes only some of the carcinogenic mineral fibers. Epidemiological and experimental data show that the risk of mineral fiber-related diseases is largely dependent on the physical characteristics of the fibers. The regulations implemented to limit or ban the use of commercial asbestos in most industrialized countries have resulted in great benefit to human health and are expected to prevent thousands of workers from developing MM and other asbestos-associated malignancies. On the other hand, MM incidence has not decreased in women, and some MMs—the so-called non-asbestos related MMs—may be caused by increasing environmental exposure to non-commercial mineral fibers.

Like the tragic story of the vermiculite mined in Libby, Montana, both examples of erionite and antigorite illustrate the problem of underestimating the risk of mineral fiber carcinogenesis, due to the restrictive regulatory definition of "asbestos" that is limited to only six of the almost 400 mineral fibers that may be present in nature. Because people are not aware of being exposed in the natural environment, cancer due to this type of exposure is very difficult to prevent. To the best of our knowledge there is no natural occurring mineral fiber that has been shown not to be carcinogenic in animal and tissue culture experiments. Even if some of these fibrous minerals are rare, the use/disturbance of all proven carcinogenic mineral fibers should be regulated in the same way as "asbestos," and the use of other mineral fibers should be dependent on proving that they do not cause disease and cancer, as for any other suspected carcinogen (Carbone et al., 2004). Undoubtedly, the categorization of more minerals as regulated would have an economic impact (Harper, 2008); nevertheless, the exclusion of hazardous fibers may result in underestimation of the risk for non-informed exposed cohorts.

Because of the long latency and the involuntary nature of environmental exposures, accurate reconstruction of personal exposure is impossible. Therefore, classical epidemiology methods, such as case-control studies, cannot be used. Environmental spatial epidemiology, which analyzes geographical units rather than individuals, is more appropriate to study environmental disease. In countries where a past occupational exposure to asbestos exists, classical epidemiologic rates such as MM incidence or standard mortality ratio do not allow to detect a possible environmental exposure to carcinogenic mineral fibers. Environmental risk of MM can be studied only at a small geographic scale. Increased proportions of MM in women and in young individuals are good indicators of environmental exposure to carcinogenic mineral fibers.

Finally, to protect the general population, it is important that the assessment of exposure to any NOA may be carried out using a proper methodology and analytical technologies that are able to detect all types of mineral fibers.

REFERENCES

Alleman JE, Mossman BT. 1997. Asbestos revisited. *Sci Am* 277(1):70–75.

Amandus HE, Wheeler R. 1987. Morbidity and mortality of vermiculite miners and millers exposed to tremolite-actinolite. *Am J Ind Med* 11(1):15–26.

Andujar P, Lacourt A, Brochard P, Pairon JC, Jaurand MC, Jean D. 2016. Five years update on relationships between malignant pleural mesothelioma and exposure to asbestos and other elongated mineral particles. J Toxicol Environ Health B Crit Rev 19(5):151–172.

Artvinli M, Baris YI. 1979. Malignant mesothelioma in a small village in the Anatolian region of Turkey: An epidemiologic study. *J Nat Cancer Inst* 63:17–23.

Aust A, Cook P, Dodson R. 2011. Morphological and chemical mechanisms of elongated mineral particle toxicities. *J Toxicol Environ Health B* 14(1–4):40–75.

Avataneo C, Petriglieri JR, Capella S, Tomatis M, Luiso M, Marangoni G, Lazzari E, Tinazzi S, Lasagna M, De Luca DA, Bergamini M, Belluso E, Turci F. 2022. Chrysotile asbestos migration in air from contaminated water: An experimental simulation. *J Hazard Mater* 424(C):127528.

Bailey RM, Kalika S. 2020. Foreword to the environmental & engineering geoscience special edition on naturally occurring asbestos. *Environ Eng Geosci* 26(1):1–2. https://doi.org/10.2113/EEG-26-01-07

Bandli BR, Gunter ME. 2001. Identification and characterization of mineral and asbestos particles using the spindle stage and the scanning electron microscope: The Libby, Montana, USA amphibole-asbestos an example. *Microscope* 49:191–199.

Bandli BR, Gunter ME. 2006. A review of scientific literature examining the mining history, geology, mineralogy, and amphibole asbestos health effects of the rainy creek igneous complex, Libby, Montana, USA. *Inhal Toxicol* 18(12):1–14.

Bard D, Yarwood J, Tylee B. 1997. Asbestos fiber identification by Raman microspectroscopy. *J Raman Spectrosc* 28(10):803–809.

Baris YL, Sahin AA, Orezmi M, Kerse I, Ozen E, Kolacan B, Altinörs M, Göktepeli A. 1978. An outbreak of pleural mesothelioma and chronic fibrosing pleurisy in the village of Karain/Urgüp in Anatolia. *Thorax* 33(2):181–192.

Baris YL, Grandjean P. 2006. Prospective study of mesothelioma mortality in Turkish villages with exposure to fibrous zeolite. *J Natl Cancer Inst* 98(6):414–417.

Baumann F, Rougier Y, Ambrosi JP, Robineau B. 2007. Pleural mesothelioma in New Caledonia: An acute environmental concern. *Cancer Detect Prev* 31(1):70–76.

Baumann F, Maurizot P, Mangeas M, Ambrosi JP, Douwes J, Robineau B. 2011. Pleural mesothelioma in New Caledonia: Associations with environmental risk factors. *Environ Health Perspect* 119(5):695–700.

Baumann F. 2011. *Facteurs de Risque d'Exposition à l'Amiante Naturel: Analyse Spatiale et Déterminants Environnementaux du Mésothéliome Malin Pleural en Nouvelle-Calédonie* [in French]. Saarbrucken, Germany: Edition Universitaires Europeennes.

Baumann F, Ambrosi JP, Carbone M. 2013. Asbestos is not just asbestos: An unrecognized health hazard. *Lancet Oncol* 14(7):576–578. PMID: 23725699.

Baumann F, Ambrosi JP. 2015. Environmental non-asbestos related causes of malignant pleural mesothelioma. In *Book: Malignant Pleural Mesothelioma: Present Status and Future Directions*, 129–147. https://doi.org/102174/9781681081946116010014.

Baumann F, Buck B, Metcalf R, McLaurin BT, Merkler D, Carbone M. 2015a. The presence of asbestos in the natural environment is likely related to mesothelioma in young individuals and women in Southern Nevada. *J Thorac Oncol* 10(5):731–737.

Baumann F, Buck B, Metcalf R, McLaurin BT, Merkler D, Carbone M. 2015b. Answer to the Letter to the Editor: No increased risk for mesothelioma in relation to natural-occurring asbestos in Southern Nevada. *J Thorac Oncol* 10(7):e64 (*Invited*).

Baumann F. 2016. Epidemiological patterns of environmental asbestos-related disease. Book chapter. In *Asbestos: Risk Assessment, Health Implications and Impacts on the Environment.* Nova Science Publishers. ISBN 13: 9781634853712.

Baumann F, Carbone M. 2016. Environmental risk of mesothelioma in the U.S.: An emerging concern - Epidemiological issues. *J Toxicol Environ Health A Curr Issues* 19(5–6):231–249.

Below J, Cox N, Fukagawa N, Hirvonen A, Testa J. 2011. Factors that impact susceptibility to fiber-induced health effects. *J Toxicol Environ Health B Crit Rev* 14(1–4):246–266.

Belluso E, Baronnet A, Capella S. 2020. Naturally occurring asbestiform minerals in Italian Western Alps and in other Italian sites. *Environ Eng Geosci* 26(1):39–46. https://doi.org/10.2113/EEG-2276.

Bernstein DM. 2007. Synthetic vitreous fibers: A review toxicology, epidemiology and regulations. *Crit Rev Toxicol* 37(10):839–886.

Bertino P, Marconi A, Palumbo L, Bruni BM, Barbone D, Dogan AU, Tassi GF, Porta C, Mutti L, Gaugino G. 2007. Erionite and asbestos differently cause transformation of human cells. *Int J Cancer* 121:12–20.

Binazzi A, Di Marzio D, Verardo M, Migliore E, Benfatto L, Malacarne D, Mensi C, Consonni D, Eccher S, Mazzoleni G, et al. 2022. Asbestos exposure and malignant mesothelioma in construction workers—Epidemiological remarks by the Italian national mesothelioma registry (ReNaM). *Int J Environ Res Public Health* 19(1):235. https://doi.org/10.3390/ijerph19010235.

Boman G, Schubert V, Svane B, Westerholm P, Bolinder E, Rohl AN, Fischbein A. 1982. Malignant mesothelioma in Turkish immigrants residing in Sweden. *Scand J Work Environ Health* 8(2):108–112.

Bruni BM, Pacella A, Mazziotti Tagliani S, Gianfagna A, Paoletti L. 2006. Nature and extent of the exposure to fibrous amphiboles in Biancavilla. *Sci Total Environ* 370(1):9–16.

Bruno C, Tumino R, Fazzo L, Cascone G, Cernigliaro A, De Santis M, Giurdanella MC, Nicita C, Rollo PC, Scondotto S, Spata E, Zona A, Comba P. 2014. Incidence of pleural mesothelioma in a community exposed to fibres with fluoro-edenitic composition in Biancavilla (Sicily, Italy). *Ann Ist Super Sanita Ist Super Sanità* 50(2):111–118.

Carbone M, Klein G, Gruber J, Wong M. 2004. Modern Criteria to establish Human Cancer Etiology. *Cancer Res* 64(15):5518–5524.

Carbone M, Emri S, Dogan AU, Steele I, Tuncer M, Pass HI, Baris YI. 2007. A mesothelioma epidemic in Cappadocia: Scientific developments and unexpected social outcomes. *Nat Rev Cancer* 7(2):147–154.

Carbone M, Baris YI, Bertino P, Brass B, Comertpay S, Dogan AU, Gaudino G, Jube S, Kanodia S, Partridge CR, Pass HI, Rivera ZS, Steele I, Tuncer M, Way S, Yang H, Miller A. 2011. Erionite exposure in North Dakota and Turkish villages with mesothelioma. *Proc Natl Acad Sci U S A* 108(33):13618–13623.

Carbone M, Ly B, Dodson R, Pagano I, Morris P, Dogan U, Gazdar A, Pass H, Yang H. 2012a. Malignant mesothelioma: Facts, myths and hypotheses. *J Cell Physiol* 227(1):44–58.

Carbone M, Yang H. 2012b. Molecular pathways : Targeting mechanisms of asbestos and erionite carcinogenesis in mesothelioma. *Clin Cancer Res* 18(3):598–604.

Carbone M, Chao A, Kanodia S, Miller A, Wali A, Weissman D, Adjei A, Baumann F et al. 2016. Consensus report of the 2015 Weinman international conference on mesothelioma. *J Thorac Oncol* 11(8):1246–1262.

Cardile V, Renis M, Scifo C, Lombardo L, Gulino R, Mancari B, Panico A. 2004. Behaviour of new asbestos amphibole fluoro-edenite in different lung cell systems. *Int J Biochem Cell Biol* 36(5):849–860.

Cardile V, Lombardo L, Belluso E, Panico A, Capella S, Balazy M. 2007. Toxicity and carcinogenicity mechanisms of fibrous antigorite. *Int J Environ Res Public Health* 4(1):1–9.

Carthew P, Hill RJ, Edwards RE, Lee PN. 1992. Intrapleural administration of fibers induces mesothelioma in rats in the same relative order of hazard as occurs in man after exposure. *Hum Exp Toxicl* 11(6):530–534.

Case BW, Abraham JL, Meeker G, Pooley FD, Pinkerton KE. 2011. Applying definitions of "asbestos" to environmental and "low-dose" exposure levels and health effects, particularly malignant mesothelioma. *J Toxicol Environ Health B* 14(1–4):3–39.

Collan Y, Kosma VM, Anttonen H, Kulju T. 1986. Toxicity of richterite in hemolysis tests and macrophage cultures. *Arch Toxicol Suppl* 9:292–295.

Comba P, Gianfagna A, Paoletti L. 2003. Pleural mesothelioma cases in Biancavilla are related to a new fluoro-edenite fibrous amphibole. *Arch Environ Health* 58(4):229–232.

Committee on Biologic Effects of Atmospheric Pollutants. 1971. *Asbestos: The Need for and Feasibility of Air Pollution Controls.* Washington, DC: National Academy of Sciences.

Corfiati M, Scarselli A, Binazzi A, Di Marzio D,Verardo M, Mirabelli D, Gennaro V, Mensi C, Schallemberg G, Merler E, Negro C, Romanelli A, Chellini E, Silvestri S, Cocchioni M, Pascucci C, Stracci F, Romeo E, Trafficante L, Angelillo I, Menegozzo S, Musti M, Cavone D, Cauzillo G, Tallarigo F, Tumino R, Melis M, Iavicoli S, Marinaccio A. 2015. Epidemiological patterns of asbestos exposure and spatial clusters of incident cases of malignant mesothelioma from the Italian national registry. *BMC Cancer* 15:1–14.

D'Agostin F, De Michieli P, Negro C. 2018. *J Lung Health Dis* 1(1):27–30.

Danforth DN. 2021. The role of chronic inflammation in the development of breast cancer. *Cancers* 3(15):3918. https://doi.org/10.3390/cancers13153918.

Delgermaa V, Takahashi K, Park EK, Vinh Le G, Haraa T, Sorahan T. 2011. Global mesothelioma deaths reported to the World Health Organization between 1994 and 2008. *Bull World Health Organ* 89(10):716–724C.

Di Ciaula A. 2017. Asbestos ingestion and gastrointestinal cancer: A possible underestimated hazard. *Expert Rev Gastroenterol Hepatol* 11(5):419–425.

Di Giuseppe D, Harper M, Bailey M, Erskine B, Della Ventura G, Ardit M, Pasquali L, Tomaino G, Ray R, Mason H, Dyar MD, Hanuskova M, Giacobbe C, Zoboli A, Gualtieri AF. 2019. Characterization and assessment of the potential toxicity/pathogenicity of fibrous glaucophane. Environ Res 178(2):108723.

Dodony I, Posfai M, Buseck PR. 2002. Revised structure models for antigorite: An HRTEM Study. *Am Mineral* 87(10):1443–1457.

Dodson RF, O'Sullivan MF, Brooks DR, Bruce JR. 2001. Asbestos content of omentum and mesentery in nonoccupationally exposed individuals. *Toxicol Ind Health* 17(4):138–143.

Dodson RF, Atkinson MA, Levin JL. 2003. Asbestos fiber length as related to potential pathogenicity: A critical review. *Am* J Int Med 44(3):291–297.

Dogan AU. 2003. Zeolite mineralogy and Cappadocian erionite. *Indoor Built Environ* 12(5):337–342.

Dogan AU, Dogan M, Hoskins JA. 2008. Erionite series minerals: Mineralogical and carcinogenic properties. *Environ Geochem Health* 30(4):367–381.

Dunnigan J. 1984. Biological effects of fibers: Stanton's hypothesis revisited. *Environ Health Perspect* 57:333–337.

Eborn SK, Aust AE. 1995. Effects of iron acquisition on induction of DNA single-strand breaks by erionite, a carcinogenic mineral fiber. *Arch Biochem Biophys* 316(1):507–514.

Edwards GH, Lynch JR. 1968. The method used by the US Public Health Service for enumeration of asbestos dust on membrane filters. *Ann Occup Hyg* 11(1):1–6.

Egilman D. 2019. Response to Paustenbach. *Am J Ind Med* 62(7):627–630.

Egilman D, Steffen JE, Triet TH, Longo W et al. 2019. Health effects of censored elongated mineral particles: A critical review. In *Book: Detection Limits in Air Quality and Environmental Measurements.* https://doi.org/10.1520/STP161820180080.

Fach E, Waldman WJ, Williams M, Long J, Meister RK, Dutta PK. 2002. Analysis of the biological and chemical reactivity of zeolite-based aluminosilicate fibers and particulates. *Environ Health Perspect* 110(11):1087–1096.

Fazzo L, De Santis M, Minelli G, Bruno C, Zona A, Marinaccio A, Conti S, Pirastu R, Comba P. 2012. Pleural mesothelioma mortality and asbestos exposure mapping in Italy. *Am J Ind Med* 55(1):11–24.

Ferrante D, Mirabelli D, Tunesi S, *et al.* 2016. Pleural mesothelioma and occupational and non-occupational asbestos exposure: A case-control study with quantitative risk assessment. *Occup Environ Med* 73(3):147–153.

Fitz Gerald JD, Eggleton RA, Keeling JL. 2010. Antigorite from Rowland Flat, South Australia: Asbestiform character. *Eurn J Mineral* 22(4):525–533.

Forsman NF. 1986. *Documentation and Diagnosis of Tuffs in the Kildeer Mountains, Dunn County, North Dakota.* Report of Investigation No. 87. North Dakota Geological Survey.

Fraire AE, Greenberg SD, Spjut HJ, Dodson RF, Williams G, Lach-Pasko E, Roggli VL. 1997. Effect of erionite on the Pleural mesothelium of the Fisher 344 Rat. *Chest* 111(5):1375–1380.

Franck AL, Joshi TK. 2014. The global spread of asbestos. *Ann Glob Health* 80(4):257–262.

Frasca P, De Malo R, Newton J, Goldale M. 2000. *Asbestos Analysis of Soil by Scanning Electron Microscopy and Energy Dispersive X-ray Spectroscopy*, Standard Operating Procedure: Report no. EPA-Libby-01. Washington, DC: US Environmental Protection Agency.

Gianfagna A, Ballirano P, Bellatreccia F, Bruni B, Paoletti L, Oberti R. 2003. Characterisation of amphibole fibers linked to mesothelioma in the area of Biancavilla, eastern Sicily, Italy. *Mineral Mag* 67(6):1221–1229.

Gibbs AR. 1990. Role of asbestos and other fibers in the development of diffuse malignant mesothelioma. *Thorax* 45(9):649–654.

Glenn RE, Lee RJ, Jastrem LM, Bunker KL, Van Orden DR, Strohmeier BR. 2008. Asbestos: By any other name, is it still? *Chem Regul Report* 32(21):22–33.

Godleski J. 2004. Role of asbestos in etiology of malignant pleural mesothelioma. *Thorac Surg Clins* 14(4):479–487.

Groppo C, Tomatis M, Turci F, Gazzano E, Ghigo D, Compagnoni R, Fubini R. 2005. Potential toxicity of nonregulated asbestiform minerals: Balangeroite from the western Alps. Part 1: Identification and characterization. *J Toxicol Environ Health A* 68(1):1–19.

Groppo R, Compagnoni R. 2007. Ubiquitous fibrous antigorite veins from the Lanzo ultramafic Massif, Internal Western Alps (Italy): Characterization and genetic conditions. *Period Mineral* 76:169–181.

Gunter ME. 2004. The polarized light microscope: Should we teach the use of a 19th century instrument in the 21st century? *J Geol Educ* 52(1):34–44.

Gunter ME, Belluso E, Mottana A. 2007. Amphiboles: Environmental and health concerns. *Rev Mineral Geochem* 67(1):453–516.

Hansen J, de Klerk NH, Eccles JL, Musk AW, Hobbs MST. 1993. Malignant mesothelioma after environmental exposure to blue asbestos. *Int J Cancer* 54(4):578–581.

Harf R, Laval I, Davezies P, Prost G. 1993. Unrecognized occupational risk of pleural mesothelioma. The example of the Rhone-Alps region. *Rev Mal Respir* 10(5):453–458.

Harper M. 2008. 10th Anniversary Critical Review: Naturally occurring asbestos. *J Environ Monit* 10(12):1394–1408.

Haute Autorité de Santé. 2009. *Synthèse Exposition Environnementale à l'Amiante : État des Données et Conduite à Tenir.* [in French]. Available at: http://www.has-sante.fr [Accessed 2 August 2012].

Henley SJ, Larson TC, Wu M, Antao VCS, Lewis M, Pinheiro GA, Eheman C. 2013. Mesothelioma incidence in 50 states and the District of Columbia, United States, 2003–2008. *Int J Occup Environ Health* 19(1):1–10.

Hillerdal G. 2003. Health problems related to environmental fibrous minerals. In Skinner HCW and Berger AR (Eds.), *Geology and Health: Closing the Gap*. New York: Oxford University Press, 113–118.

Howel D, Gibbs A, Arblaster L, *et al.* 1999. Mineral fibre analysis and routes of exposure to asbestos in the development of mesothelioma in an English region. *Occup Environ Med* 56(1):51–58. https://doi.org/10.1136/oem.56.1.51.

IARC. 1977. Asbestos. *IARC Monogr Eval Carcinog Risk Hum* 14:1–106.

IARC. 1987. Overall evaluations of the carcinogenicity: An updating of IARC Monographs volume 1 to 42. *IARC Monogr Eval Carcinog Risks Hum Suppl* 7:1–440.

Ilgren E. 2004. The biology of cleavage fragments: A brief synthesis and analysis of current knowledge. *Indoor Built Environ* 13(5):343–356.

Johnson NF, Edwards RE, Munday DE, Rowe N, Wagner JC. 1984. Pluripotential nature of mesothelioma induced by inhalation of erionite in rats. *Br J Exp Pathol* 65(3):377–388.

Kava R. 2007. Asbestos exposure: How risky is it? ACSH. Available at: http://www.acsh.org/docLib/20071015_Asbestos.pdf. [Accessed 21 April 2012].

Keeling JL, Raven MD, Self PG. 2010. Asbestiform antigorite – Implications for the risk assessment of fibrous silicates. Extended Abstracts, 21st Australian Clay Minerals Conference, Brisbane, Australia.

Klebe S, Leigh J, Henderson DW, Nurminen M. 2019. Asbestos, smoking, and lung cancer: An update. *Int J Environ Res Public Health* 17(1):258. https://doi.org/10.3390/ijerph17010258.

Kliment CR, Clemens K, Oury TD. 2009. North American erionite-associated mesothelioma with pleural plaques and pulmonary fibrosis: A case report. *Int J Clin Exp Pathol* 2(4):407–410.

Kuempel ED, Stayner LT, Dement JD, Gilbert SJ, Hein MJ. 2006. Fiber size-specific exposure estimates and updated mortality analysis of chrysotile asbestos textile workers. *Toxicologist* 90(1):71.

Lacourt A, Gramond C, Rolland P, Ducamp S, Audignon S, Astoul P, Chamming's S, Glig Soit Ilg S, Rinaldo M, Raherison C, Gallateau-Salle F, Imbernon E, Pairon JC, Goldberg M, Brochard P. 2014. Occupational and non-occupational attributable risk of asbestos exposure for malignant pleural mesothelioma. *Thorax* 69(6):532–539.

Larson D, Powers A, Ambrosi JP, Tanji M, Napolitano A, Flores EG, Baumann F, et al. 2016. Investigating palygorskite's role in the development of mesothelioma in southern Nevada: Insights into fiber-induced carcinogenicity. *J Toxicol Environ Health B Crit Rev* 19(5–6):213–230.

Lee R, Strohmeier BR, Bunker KL, Van Orden DR. 2008. Naturally occurring asbestos—A recurring public policy challenge. *J Hazard M* 153:1–21.

Linton A, Vardy J, Clarke S, Van Zandwijk N. 2012. The ticking time-bomb of asbestos: Its insidious role in the development of malignant mesothelioma. *Crit Rev Oncol Hematol* 84(2):200–212.

Lippmann M. 1990. Effects of fiber characteristics on lung deposition, retention, and disease. *Environ Health Perspect* 88:311–317.

Luce D, Bugel I, Goldberg P, Goldberg M, Salomon C, Billon-Galland MA, Nicolau J, Quenel P, Fevotte J, Brochard P. 2000. Environmental exposure to tremolite and respiratory cancer in New Caledonia: A case-control study. *Am J Epidemiol* 151(3):259–265.

Magnani C, Dalmasso P, Biggeri A, Ivaldi C, Mirabelli D, Terracini B. 2001. Increased risk of malignant mesothelioma of the pleura after residential or domestic exposure to asbestos: A case-control study in Casale Monferrato, Italy. *Environ Health Perspect* 109(9):915–919.

Maltoni C, Minardi F, Morisi L. 1982. Pleural mesothelioma in Sprague-Dawley rats by erionite: First experimental evidence. *Environ Res* 28(1):238–244.

Maule MM, Magnani C, Dalmasso P, Mirabelli D, Merletti F, Biggeri A. 2007. Modeling mesothelioma risk associated with environmental asbestos exposure. *Environ Health Perspect* 115(7):1066–1071.

Mazurek JM, Syamlal G, Wood JM, Hendricks SA, Weston A. 2017. Malignant mesothelioma mortality – United States, 1999–2015. *MMWR* 66(8):214–218.

McCormack V, Peto J, Byrmes G, Stralf K, Boffetta P. 2012. Estimating the asbestos-related lung cancer burden from mesothelioma mortality. *Br J Cancer* 106(3):575–584.

McDonald JC, Liddell FDK, Gibbes GW, Eyssen GE, McDonald AD. 1980. Dust exposure and mortality in chrysotile mining, 1910–1975. *Brit J Ind Med* 37:11–24.

McDonald JC, McDonald AD, Armstrong B, Sébastei P. 1986. Cohort study of mortality of vermiculite miners exposed to tremolite. *Br J Ind Med* 43(7):436–444.

McElvenny DM, Darnton AJ, Price MJ, Hodgson JT. 2005. Mesothelioma mortality in Great Britain from 1968 to 2001. *Occup Med (Lond)* 55(2):79–87.

Meeker GP, Bern AM, Brownfield IK, Lowers HA, Sutley SJ, Hoepen TM, Vance JS. 2003. The composition and morphology of amphibole from the Rainy Creek Complex, near Libby, Montana. *Am Mineral* 88(11–12):1955–1969.

Metintas M, Hillerdal G, Metintas S. 1999. Malignant mesothelioma due to environmental exposure to erionite: Follow-up of a Turkish emigrant cohort. *Eur Respir J* 13(3):523–526.

Metintas S, Metintas M, Ucgun I, Oner U. 2002. Malignant mesothelioma due to environmental exposure to asbestos: Follow-up of a Turkish cohort living in a rural area. *Chest* 122(6):2224–2229.

Metintas M, Metintas SG, Erginel S, Alatas F, Kurt E, Ucgun I, Yildirim H. 2008. Epidemiology of pleural mesothelioma in a population with non-occupational asbestos exposure. *Respirology* 13(1):117–121.

Middendorf P, Zumwalde R, Castellan R. 2007. *Asbestos and Other Mineral Fibers: A Roadmap for Scientific Research.* Washington, DC: National Institute for Occupational Safety and Health, NIOSH Mineral Fibers Working Group.

Middleton AP. 1982. Visibility of fine fibers of asbestos during routine electron microscopical analysis. *Annals of Occupational Hygiene* 25(1):53–62.

Miller A. 2005. Mesothelioma in household members of asbestos-exposed workers: 32 United States cases since 1990. *Am j Ind Med* 47(5):458–462. https://doi.org/10.1002/ajim.20167.

Millette JR, Bandli BR. 2005. Asbestos identification using available standard methods. *Microscope* 53:179–185.

Miller A, Szeinuk J, Noonan CW, Henschke CI, Pfau J, Black B, Yankelevitz DF, Liang M, Liu Y, Yip R, McNew T, Linker L, Flores R. 2018, February. Libby amphibole disease. Pulmonary function and CT abnormalities in vermiculite miners. *J Occup Environ Med* 60(2):167–173. https://doi.org/10.1097/JOM.0000000000001178.

Moolgavkar SH, Meza R, Turim J. 2009. Pleural and peritoneal mesotheliomas in SEER: Age effects and temporal trends, 1973–2005. *Cancer Causes Control* 20(6):935–944.

Mossman BT, Lippmann M, Hesterberg TW, Kelsey KT, Barchowsky A, Bonner JC. 2011. Pulmonary endpoints (lung carcinomas and asbestosis) following inhalation exposure to asbestos. *J Toxicol Environ Health B* 14(1–4):76–121.

Mutti L, Peikert T, Robinson BWS, et al. 2018. Scientific advances and new frontiers in mesothelioma therapeutics. *J Thorac Oncol* 13(9):1269–1283.

Nelson AR. 2009. *A Review of the NIOSH Roadmap for Research on Asbestos Fibers and Other Elongate Mineral Particles. Institute of Medicine and NRC.* National Academic Press.

Nicholson WJ, Pundsack FL. 1973. Asbestos in the environment. In Bogovski P, Gilson J, Timbrell V, Wagner JC (Eds.), IARC Scientific Publications 8, 126–131.

Nicholson WJ, Perkel G, Selikoff IJ. 1982. Occupational exposure to asbestos: Population at risk and projected mortality-1980–2030. *Am J Ind Med* 3(3):259–311. https://doi.org/10.1002/ajim.4700030305.

NIOSH. 1989. *Manual of Analytical Methods.* Asbestos TEM Method 7402.

NIOSH. 2011. Current intelligence Bulletin 62: Asbestos fibers and other elongate mineral particles: State of the science and roadmap for research. Version 4. http://www.cdc.gov/niosh/docket/archive/docket099C.html [Accessed 15 December 2011].

NRC. 1984. *Asbestiform Fibers: Non Occupational Health Risks.* Washington, DC: National Academy Press.

OECD. 1984. *Control of Toxic Substances in the Atmosphere: Asbestos. Environment Committee: Air Management.* Policy Group ENV/AIR/81.18, 2nd Revision. Paris: Organization for Economic Cooperation and Development.

Okayazu R, Wu L, Hei TK. 1999. Biological effects of naturally occurring and man-made fibres: In vivo cytotoxicity and mutagenesis in mammalian cells. *Br J Cancer* 79(9–10):1319–1324.

Pan X, Day H, Wang W, Beckett L, Schenker M. 2005. Residential proximity to naturally occurring asbestos and mesothelioma risk in California. *Am J Respir Crit Care Med* 172(8):1019–1025.

Paoletti L, Batisti D, Bruno C, Di Paola M, Gianfagna A, Mastrantonio M, Nesti M, Comba P. 2000. Unusually high incidence of malignant pleural mesothelioma in a town of eastern Sicily: An epidemiological and environmental study. *Arch Environ Health* 55(6):392–398.

Paoletti L, Batisti D, Bruno C, Di Paola M, Gianfagna A, Mastrantonio M, Nesti N, Comba P. 2000. Unusually high incidence of malignant pleural mesothelioma in a town of eastern Sicily: An epidemiological and environmental study. *Arch Environ Health* 55(6):392–398.

Peipins LA, Lewin M, Campolucci S, Lybarge JA, Miller A, Middleton D, Weiss C, Spence M, Black B, Kapi V. 2003. Radiographic abnormalities and exposure to asbestos-contaminated vermiculite in the community of Libby, Montana, USA. *Environ Health Perspect* 111(14):1753–1759.

Petriglieri JR, Laporte-Magoni C, Salvioli-Mariani E, Tomatis M, Gazzano E, Turci F, Cavallo A, Fubini B. 2020. Identification and preliminary toxicological assessment of a non-regulated mineral fiber: Fibrous antigorite from New Caledonia. *Environ Eng Geosci* 26(1):89–97. https://doi.org/10.2113/EEG-2274.

Petry R, Mastalerz R, Zah S, Mayerhöfer TG, Völksch G, Viereck-Götte L, Kreher- Hartmann B, Holz L, Lankers M, Popp J. 2006. Asbestos mineral analysis by UV Raman and Energy-dispersive X-ray spectroscopy. *Chem Phys Chem* 7(2):414–420.

Poole A, Brown RC, Turver CJ, Skidmore JW, Griffiths DM. 1983. In vitro genotoxic activities of fibrous erionite. *Br J Cancer* 47(5):697–705.

Pugnaloni A, Giantomassi F, Lucarini G, Capella S, Mattioli Belmonte M, Orciani M, Belluso E. 2008. Effects of asbestiform antigorite on human alveolar epithelial A549 cells: A morphological and immunohistochemical study. *Acta Histochem* 112(2):133–146.

Rake C, Gilham C, Hatch J, Darnton A, Hodgson J, Peto J. 2009. Occupational, domestic and environmental mesothelioma risks in the British population: A case–control study. *Br J Cancer* 100(7):1175–1183.

Reid A, Berry G, de Klerk N, Hansen J, Heyworth J, Ambrosini G, Fritschi L, Olsen N, Merler E, Musk AW. 2007. Age and sex differences in malignant mesothelioma after residential exposure to blue asbestos (crocidolite). *Chest* 131(2):376–382.

Rinaudo C, Gastaldi D, Belluso E. 2003. Characterization of chrysotile, antigorite and lizardite by FT Raman spectroscopy. *Can Mineral* 41(4):883–890.

Rinaudo C, Belluso E, Gastaldi D. 2004. Assessment of the use of Raman spectroscopy for the determination of amphibole asbestos. *Mineral Mag* 68(3):455–465.

Ripabelli G, Tamburro M, Di Tella D, Carrozza F, Sammarco ML. 2018. Asbestos exposures, mesothelioma incidence and mortality, and awareness by general practitioners in the Molise region, central Italy. *J Occup Environ Med* 60(2):e90–e97. https://doi.org/10.1097/JOM.0000000000001211.

Robinson BW, Lake RA. 2005. Advances in malignant mesothelioma. *N Engl J Med* 353:159 –603.

Rohl AN, Langer AM, Selikoff IJ. 1977. Environmental asbestos pollution related to use of quarried serpentine rock. *Science* 196(4296):1319–1322.

Ross M, Langer AM, Nord GL, Nolan RP, Lee RJ, Van Orden D, Addison J. 2008. The mineral nature of asbestos. *Regul Toxicol Pharmacol* 52(1):S26–S30.

Ryan PH, Dihle M, Griffin S, Partridge C, Hilbert TJ, Taylor R, Adjei S, Lockey JE. 2011. Erionite in road gravel associated with intersticial and pleural changes - An occupational hazard in western United States. *J Occup Environ Med* 53(8):892–898.

Santee K, Lott PF. 2003. Asbestos analysis: A review. *Appl Spectrosc Rev* 38(3):355–394.

Schreier H. 1989. *Asbestos in the Natural Environment.* Amsterdam, NY: Elsevier.

Skinner HCW, Ross M, Frondel C. 1988. *Asbestos and Other Fibrous Materials: Mineralogy, Crystal Chemistry and Health Effects.* New York, NY: Oxford University Press.

Soffritti M, Minardi F, Bua L, Degli Esposti D, Belpoggi F. 2004. First experimental evidence of peritoneal and pleural mesotheliomas induced by fluoro-edenite fibers present in Etnean volcanic material from Biancavilla (Sicily, Italy). *Eur J Oncol* 9(3):169–175.

Soukup D, Buck BJ, Goossens D, Teng Y, Baron D. 2011. Mineralogical composition of soil samples in the Nellis Dunes recreation area. In Goossens D, Buck BJ (Eds.), *Assessment of Dust Emissions, Chemistry, and Mineralogy for Management of Natural and Disturbed Surfaces at Nellis Dunes Recreation Area, Nevada*, Final Report to Bureau of Land Management for Task Agreement; Number FAA010017:171-187.

Spirtas R, Heineman EF, Bernstein L, Beebe GW, Keehn RJ, Stark A, Harlow BL, Benichou J. 1994. Malignant mesothelioma: Attributable risk of asbestos exposure. *Occup Environ Med* 51(12):804–811.

Strohmeier BR, Huntington JC, Bunker KL, Sanchez MS, Lee RJ. 2010. What is asbestos and why is it important? - The challenges of defining and characterizing asbestos. Int Geol Rev 7–8(52):801–872.

Sullivan P. 2007. Vermiculite, respiratory disease and asbestos exposure in Libby, Montana: Update of a cohort mortality study. *Environ Health Perspect* 115(4):579–585.

Tarres J, Alberti C, Martinez-Artes X, Rosell-Murphy M, García-Allas I, Krier I, Cantarell G, Gallego M, Canela-Soler J, Orriols R. 2013. Pleural mesothelioma in relation to meteorological conditions and residential distance from an industrial source of asbestos. *Occup Environ Med* 70(8):588–590.

Turci F, Favero-Longo SE, Gazzano C, Tomatis M, Gentile-Garofalo L, Bergamini M. 2016. Assessment of asbestos exposure during a simulate agricultural activity in the proximity of the former asbestos mine of Balangero, Italy. *J Hazard Mater* 308:321–327. https://doi.org/10.1016/j.jhazmat.2016.01.056.

Turci F, Avataneo C, Botta S, Marcelli I, Barale L, Tomatis M, Cossio R, Tallone S, Piana F, Compagnoni R. 2020. New tools for the evaluation of asbestos-related risk during excavation in an NOA-rich geological setting. *Environ Eng Geosci* 26(1):113–120. https://doi.org/10.2113/EEG-2272.

Urano N, Yano E, Evans PH. 1991. Reactive oxygen metabolites produced by carcinogenic fibrous mineral erionite. *Environ Res* 54(1):74–81.

U.S. EPA-Environmental Protection Agency. 2004. Safe drinking water act. EPA 816-F04-030. https://www.epa.gov/ground-water-and-drinking-water/national-primary-drinking-water-regulations#Inorganic [Accessed 10 September 2023].

Van Gosen BS, Blitz TA, Plumlee GS, Meeker GP, Pierson MP. 2013. Geologic occurrences of erionite in the United States: An emerging national public health concern for respiratory disease. *Environ Geochem Health* 35(4):419–430. https://doi.org/10.1007/s10653-012-9504-9.

Van Orden DR, Allison KA, Lee RJ. 2008. Differentiating amphibole asbestos in a complex mineral environment. *Indoor Built Environ* 17(1):58–68.

Veblen DR, Wylie AG. 1993. Mineralogy of amphiboles and 1:1 layer silicates. In Guthrie Jr GD, Mossman BT (Eds.), *Health Effects of Mineral Dusts: Reviews in Mineralogy*, 28, 61–137.

Virta RL. 2001. Some facts about asbestos. US Geological Survey. Fact Sheet FS-012-01.

Viti C, Mellini M. 1996. Vein antigorites from Elba Island, Italy. *Eur J Mineral* 8(2):423–434.

Wachowski L, Domka L. 2000. Sources and effects of asbestos and other mineral fibers present in ambient air. *Pol J Environ Stud* 9(6):443–454.

Wagner JC, Skidmore JW, Hill RJ, Griffiths DM. 1985. Erionite exposure and mesothelioma in rats. *Br J Cancer* 51(5):727–730.

Walton WH. 1982. The nature, hazards, and assessment of occupation exposure to airborne asbestos dust: A review. *Ann Occup Hyg* 25:115–247.

Weill H, Hughes JM, Churg AM. 2004. Changing trends in US mesothelioma incidence. *Occup Environ Med* 61(5):438–441.

WHO. Chapter 6.2 Asbestos. 2000. In *Air Quality Guidelines.* 2nd edition. Copenhagen and Denmark: WHO Regional Office for Europe.

Wozniak H. 1994. Respirable mineral fibers in atmospheric air of Wrocław. *Med Pr* 45(3):239 –47.

Wozniak H, Wiecek E, Stetkiewicz J. 1988. Fibrogenic and carcinogenic effects of antigorite. *Pol J Occup Med Environ Health* 1(3):192–202.

Wozniak H, Wiecek E, Stetkiewicz J. 1993. Experimental carcinogenicity and mutagenicity of non-asbestos natural fibers (Preliminary report). *Pol J Occup Med Environ Health* 6(1):55–60.

Wozniak H, Wiecek E, Pelc W, Dobrucka D, Król M, Opalska B. 1994. Respirable mineral fibers in atmospheric air of Wrocław. *Med Pr* 45(3):239–247.

Wozniak H. 1999. Dolomite: Occurrence, occupational exposure, biological effect, and maximum admissible concentrations. *Med Pr* 50(5):443–452.

Wylie AG, Bailey KF, Kelse JW, Lee RJ. 1993. The importance of width in asbestos fiber carcinogenicity and its implications for public policy. *Am Ind Hyg Assoc J* 54(5):239–252.

Yang H, Gaudino G, Bardelli F, Carbone M. 2022. Does the amount of asbestos exposure influence prognosis? *J Thorac Oncol* 17(8):949–952.

TABLE 7.1
Main Silicates with Possible Fibers, Fibrous or Asbestiform Habits, Geological Setting and Main Countries of Occurrence Based on Mineral Classification

Subclass GROUP, *subgroup* Mineral species	Chemical Formulae	Habits	Geological Setting *Past Name, Common Language*	Known Countries of Occurrence
Inosilicates subclass Carlosturite	$(MgFe^{2+}TiMn)_{21}(SiAl)_{12}O_{28}(OH)_{34}$	Fiber, fibrous, asbestiform	Veins in antigorite serpentinite, in an ophiolite	Italy, Sweden
GAGEITE GROUP Balangeroite	$(MgFe^{3+}Fe^{2+}Mn^{2+})_{42}Si_{16}O_{54}(OH)_{40}$	Fiber, fibrous, asbestiform	In schistose serpentinite, near ultramafic massif, asbestos mine	Italy
WOLLASTONITE GROUP Wollastonite	$CaSiO_3$	Massive, lamellar, fibrous, asbestiform	Common in skarns and contact metamorphic rocks, associated with tremolite	Worldwide according to geological context
AMPHIBOLE GROUP *Cummingtonite subgroup* Cummingtonite	$(MgFe^{2+})_7Si_8O_{22}(OH)_2$	Lamellar, columnar, fiber, fibrous	Common in contact and regional metamorphic rocks	Worldwide according to geological context
Grunerite *(Amosite)*	$(Fe^{2+}Mg)_7Si_8O_{22}(OH)$	Massive, columnar, fibers, fibrous, asbestiform	Second in asbestos production *amosite*, *cummingtonite asbestos*	Australia, Austria, Bolivia, Brazil, Cameroon, Canada, China, Czech Republic, Finland, France, Hungary, India, Japan, Madagascar, Mauritania, Norway, Portugal, Romania, Russia, Slovakia, South Africa, Spain, Swede, UK, Ukraine, USA
Anthophyllite subgroup Anthophyllite	$Mg_7Si_8O_{22}(OH)_2$	Massive, lamellar, fiber, fibrous, asbestiform	Metamorphic rocks, used as asbestos	Argentina, Australia, Austria, Bolivia, Brazil, Bulgaria, Burkina Faso, Canada, China, Colombia, Czech Republic, Egypt, Ethiopia, Finland, France, Germany, Greenland, Hungary, India, Indonesia, Italy, Japan, New Zealand, Norway, Poland, Russia, Slovakia, South Africa, Spain, Sweden, Switzerland, Taiwan, Tajikistan, UK, Ukraine, USA, Zambia, Zimbabwe

(*Continued*)

TABLE 7.1 (CONTINUED)
Main Silicates with Possible Fibers, Fibrous or Asbestiform Habits, Geological Setting and Main Countries of Occurrence Based on Mineral Classification

Subclass GROUP, *subgroup* Mineral species	Chemical Formulae	Habits	Geological Setting *Past Name, Common Language*	Known Countries of Occurrence
Tremolite subgroup Actinolite	$Ca_2(MgFe^{2+})_5Si_8O_{22}(OH)_2$	Prismatic, bladed, fiber, fibrous, asbestiform	Common in some metamorphic rocks *byssolite, nephrite jade, mountain leather*	Worldwide according to geological context
Fluoro-edenite	$NaCa_2Mg_5(Si_7Al)O_{22}(F,OH)_2$	Prismatic, acicular, fiber, fibrous	In altered hydrothermal lavas contaminate raw mineral materials	Austria, Burma, Finland, France, Italy, Japan, New Zealand, Romania, Russia, USA
Magnesio-hornblende	$Ca_2Mg_4(Al,Fe^{3+}](Si_7Al)O_{22}(OH)_2$	Massive, granular prismatic, acicular, fiber, fibrous	Igneous and metamorphic rocks *Actinolitic hornblende, tremolitic hornblende*	Australia, Austria, Brazil, Bulgaria, Canada, China, Cuba, Czech Republic, Egypt, Ethiopia, France, Germany, Greece, Greenland, Hungary, India, Italy, Japan, New Zealand, Norway, Pakistan, Poland, Portugal, Russia, Slovakia, Slovenia, South Africa, Spain, Sweden, Switzerland, Tanzania, UK, USA
Tremolite	$Ca_2Mg_5Si_8O_{22}(OH)_2$	Flattened prismatic, fibrous, asbestiform	Common in contact metamorphic Ca rocks *Mountain leather, mountain cork*	Worldwide according to geological context
Richterite subgroup Richterite	$(Na_2Ca)(Mg_3Fe^{2+}{}_2)Si_8O_{22}(OH)_2$	Massive, prismatic, thin tabular, asbestiform	Not common, as small constituent in contact metamorphosed limestones, ultramafic igneous extrusives, metasomatic deposits and alkaline rocks, contaminate raw mineral materials *Soda tremolite*	Afghanistan, Australia, Austria, Brazil, Bulgaria, Burma, Canada, China, Finland, France, Germany, Greenland, India, Italy, Japan, Kenya, Madagascar Namibia, New Zealand, Poland, Russia, Slovakia, South Africa, Spain, Sweden, Switzerland, Uganda, USA
Winchite	$(CaNa)Mg_4(Al,Fe^{3+})Si_8O_{22}(OH)_2$	Prismatic, asbestiform	Metamorphosed Mn deposits, contaminated raw mineral material	Afghanistan, Algeria, Australia, Canada, China, Czech Republic, Greece, India, Italy, Japan, Namibia, Oman, Poland, Romania, Russia, Slovakia, South Korea, Spain, Switzerland, UK, USA, Venezuela, Zimbabwe

(Continued)

TABLE 7.1 (CONTINUED)
Main Silicates with Possible Fibers, Fibrous or Asbestiform Habits, Geological Setting and Main Countries of Occurrence Based on Mineral Classification

Subclass GROUP, *subgroup* Mineral species	Chemical Formulae	Habits	Geological Setting *Past Name, Common Language*	Known Countries of Occurrence
Glaucophane subgroup Arfvedsonite	$Na_3(Fe^{2+}Mg)_4Fe^{3+}Si_8O_{22}(OH)_2$	Prismatic, acicular, lamellar, fibrous	Limited occurrence in peculiar igneous intrusion, mined in Russia *Soda hornblende*	Algeria, Argentina, Armenia, Australia, Brazil, Cameroon, Canada, Chile, China, Czech Republic, France, Germany, Greece, Greenland, Guinea, Guyana, Hungary, India, Italy, Japan, Kazakhstan, Kenya, Libya, Madagascar, Malawi, Mongolia, Morocco, Namibia, New Zealand, Niger, Nigeria, North Korea, Norway, Portugal, Romania, Russia, South Africa, Spain, Sweden, USA
Riebeckite *(Crocidolite)*	$Na_2(Fe^{2+}Mg)_3Fe^{3+}{}_2Si_8O_{22}(OH)_2$	Massive, striated fiber, fibrous, asbestiform	Third in asbestos production *Crocidolite, blue asbestos, riebeckite asbestos, tiger's eye, hawk's eye, falcon's eye*	Worldwide according to geological context
Phyllosilicates subclass SERPENTINE GROUP Antigorite	$(MgFe^{2+})_3Si_2O_5(OH)_4$	Massive, platy, fibrous, asbestiform	Common in metamorphosed serpentinite, asbestos mine *Baltimorite, bastard asbestos, bowensite, jenkensite, williamsite Andes jade, picrolite*	Worldwide according to geological context
Chrysotile	$Mg_3Si_2O_5(OH)_4$	Acicular, fibrous, asbestiform	95% of asbestos production *Asbestos, Canadian asbestos, white asbestos, bostonite, deweylite, mountain leather, serpentine*	Afghanistan, Argentina, Australia, Austria, Bolivia, Brazil, Canada, China, Cuba, Czech Republic, Egypt, Ethiopia, Finland, France, Germany, Greenland, Hungary, India, Indonesia, Italy, Jamaica, Japan, Madagascar, Mexico, Morocco, Namibia, New Caledonia, New Zealand, Norway, Oman, Pakistan, Poland, Romania, Russia, Slovakia, South Africa, Spain, Swaziland, Sweden, Switzerland, Turkey, UK, USA, Zimbabwe

(Continued)

TABLE 7.1 (CONTINUED)
Main Silicates with Possible Fibers, Fibrous or Asbestiform Habits, Geological Setting and Main Countries of Occurrence Based on Mineral Classification

Subclass GROUP, *subgroup* Mineral species	Chemical Formulae	Habits	Geological Setting *Past Name, Common Language*	Known Countries of Occurrence
Lizardite	$Mg_3Si_2O_5(OH)_4$	Massive, lamellar, bladed	low temperature serpentinization alteration of Mg silicates *Maufite, orthoantigorite, scyelite*	Argentina, Australia, Austria, Brazil, Canada, China, Cuba, Egypt, Ethiopia, Finland, France, Germany, Greece, Hungary, Indonesia, Israel, Italy, Jamaica, Japan, Morocco, New Zealand, Norway, Oman, Poland, Romania, Russia, Slovakia, South Africa, Spain, Sweden, Switzerland, UK, USA
PALYGORSKITE-SEPIOLITE GROUP *Palygorskite subgroup* Palygorskite (*Attapulgite*)	$(MgAl)_2Si_4O_{10}(OH){\bullet}4(H_2O)$	Massive, earthy, fibrous, fibrous, fine-grained forms	Hydrothermal deposit, fault lines, and soils overlaying occurrence *Attapulgite, mountain leather*	Australia, Austria, Bulgaria, Canada, Chile, China, Czech Republic, Ecuador, France, Germany, Iran, Iraq, Greenland, Hungary, Italy, Japan, Madagascar, Mexico, Morocco, Namibia, Norway, Peru, Poland, Russia, Senegal, Slovakia, Slovenia, Spain Sweden, Switzerland, Turkey, UK, Ukraine, USA, Uzbekistan
Yofortierite	$(MnMg)_5Si_8O_{20}(OH)_2{\bullet}8\text{-}9(H_2O)$	Acicular, fibrous	Relatively rare low stage hydrothermal mineral *Mn-sepiolite, Mn-palygorskite*	Canada, Greenland, Namibia, Russia, USA
Kalifersite	$(KNa)_5Fe^{3+}{}_7Si_{20}O_{50}(OH)_6{\bullet}12(H_2O)$	Fiber, fibrous, asbestiform	In hydrothermal altered pegmatite	Russia
Sepiolite subgroup Sepiolite	$Mg_4Si_6O_{15}(OH)_2{\bullet}6(H_2O)$	Massive, earthy, fiber, fibrous	Secondary minerals associated with serpentine. Can precipitate from alkaline water in arid environments *Sea foam, Meerschaum*	Australia, Austria, Brazil, Canada, China, Colombia, Czech Republic, Dominican Republic, France, Germany, Greece, Greenland, Hungary, Israel, Italy, Japan, Kenya, Madagascar, Malaysia, Mexico, Morocco, Norway, Poland, Romania, Russia, Slovakia, South Korea, Spain, Sweden, Switzerland, Turkey, UK, USA, Venezuela

(*Continued*)

TABLE 7.1 (CONTINUED)
Main Silicates with Possible Fibers, Fibrous or Asbestiform Habits, Geological Setting and Main Countries of Occurrence Based on Mineral Classification

Subclass GROUP, *subgroup* Mineral species	Chemical Formulae	Habits	Geological Setting *Past Name, Common Language*	Known Countries of Occurrence
Falcondoite	$(NiMg)_4Si_6O_{15}(OH)_2•6(H_2O)$	Earthy, microscopic crystals, fiber, fibrous	Laterite deposit, rare Ni analogue of sepiolite *Garnierite, genthite*	Australia, Dominican Republic
Loughlinite	$Na_2Mg_3Si_6O_{16}•8(H_2O)$	Massive, fibrous, fibrous fine-grained forms	In dolomitic oil-shale	Turkey, USA
Tectosilicates subclass ZEOLITE GROUP *Chabazite subgroup* *Erionite serie* Erionite -Na-Ca-K varieties	$Ca_3K_2Na_2[A_{110}Si_{26}O_{72}].30H_2O$	Fibrous, wool-like, asbestiform	Tuffs, basalts and other volcanic or sedimentary rocks	Antarctica, Australia, Austria, Bulgaria, Canada, Czech Republic, Denmark, France, Germany, Greece, Iceland, Italy, Japan, Kenya, New Zealand, Poland, Romania, Russia, Spain, Tanzania, Turkey, UK, Ukraine, USA
Mordenite subgroup Mordenite	$CaNa_2K_2[Al_2Si_{10}O_{24}]•7(H_2O)$	Acicular, fibrous asbestiform	Cavities in andesitic rocks, veins in igneous rocks *Arduinite, ashtonite, ptilolite, pseudonatrolite*	Antarctica, Argentina, Australia, Austria, Brazil, Bulgaria, Canada, China, Costa Rica, Cyprus, Czech Republic, Denmark, Ecuador, France, Germany, Greece, Greenland, Hungary, Iceland, India, Italy, Japan, Mexico, New Zealand, Nicaragua, Portugal Romania, Russia, Slovakia, South Africa, Spain, Turkey, UK, Ukraine, USA

Internet sources: ima.mineralogy.org; rruff.info/ima/; webmineral.com; mindat.com; mineralienatlas.de.

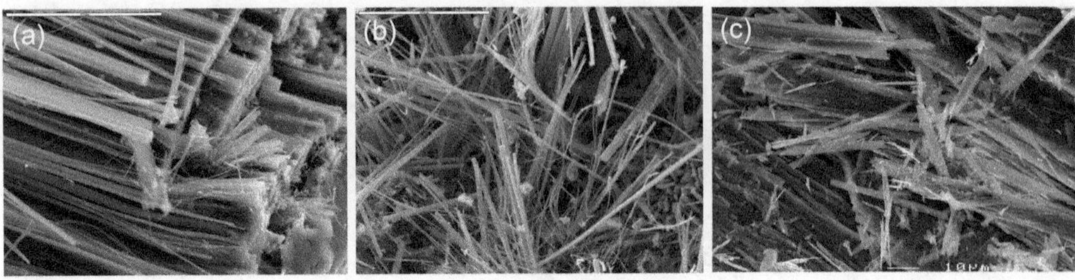

FIGURE 7.1 SEM imagery of a) crocidolite (amphibole group), South Africa; b) erionite (zeolite group), Turkey; and c) antigorite (serpentine group), New Caledonia.

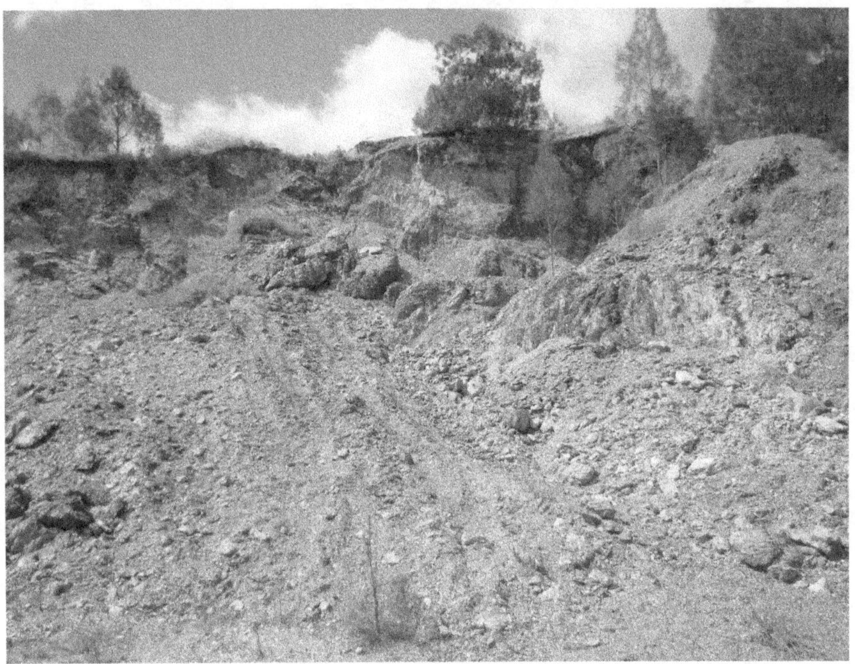

FIGURE 7.2 Photography of a serpentinite quarry in New Caledonia.

8 Asbestos and Immunity

Yasumitsu Nishimura

8.1 IMMUNE FUNCTIONS AND ASBESTOS-RELATED DISEASES

Inhalation exposure to asbestos causes various kinds of related diseases including asbestosis and malignant tumors, with mesothelioma being a characteristic example. Asbestosis is a type of pneumoconiosis caused by exposure to asbestos, where fibrosis of the lung progresses chronically following asbestos-induced inflammation, which is a representative relationship between asbestos exposure and immune functions. Alveolar macrophages, a population of phagocytes in the broncho-alveolar space, assist in the removal of various substances derived from the external environment, and can be induced to produce several cytokines including tumor necrosis factor alpha (TNF-α), interleukin 1 beta (IL-1β) and IL-6 (1, 2), as well as reactive oxygen species (ROS) and nitrogen species (RNS) (3). Additionally, crocidolite, with higher amounts of iron compared with chrysotile, can participate in Fenton-like reactions, which involve the iron-catalyzed oxidation of organic substrates to generate hydroxyl radicals (4, 5). Additionally, inhalation exposure to asbestos induces apoptosis of mesothelial cells as well as pulmonary cells (6–9). The aforementioned responses involving inflammatory cytokine production, ROS/RNS and free radical generation, and apoptotic cells contribute to triggering fibrogenic responses by surrounding fibroblasts, thereby leading to asbestosis (10), where it is generally known that alveolar macrophages play a significant role in inflammation. However, less information was known about the functional alterations in alveolar macrophages following the inflammatory response with asbestos exposure. Therefore, we focused on the role of alveolar macrophages in the fibrogenic response, and sought to determine whether transforming growth factor beta (TGF-β), a representative cytokine that induces the generation of the extracellular matrix comprising collagen and fibronectin, would be produced by alveolar macrophages without help from other cells. As alveolar macrophages can migrate to various areas, their functional alteration can broadly affect lung tissue. Additionally, since TGF-β is an immune-suppressive cytokine, aggressive production by alveolar macrophages would also contribute to a suppressed immune status, and is related with the development of malignant tumors following exposure to asbestos. Moreover, our interest turned to lymphocytes subjected to asbestos exposure. Inhaled asbestos fibers exit the broncho-alveolar space into the pleural cavity. It is known that asbestos fibers accumulate in the lungs and draining lymph nodes. In fact, a previous study reported that shipyard workers occupationally exposed to asbestos showed high amounts of asbestos in their lymph nodes as well as lung tissues and pleural plaques (PPs) (11), and that individuals previously defined as nonoccupationally exposed to asbestos showed asbestos in the nodes, which was heavier per gram compared with in the lungs (12). These findings indicate that lymphocytes may be exposed to accumulated asbestos in the draining lymph nodes, even if they are not attracted to the lungs by inflammatory responses caused by inhaled asbestos. This indicates that asbestos exposure has the potential to cause functional alterations in lymphocytes. This potential relationship between asbestos and lymphocytes is consistent with the accumulated knowledge pertaining to mesothelioma. Asbestosis is caused by high-dose exposure to asbestos, which usually occurs in occupational settings, whereas malignant mesothelioma is caused by relatively low- or middle-dose exposure to asbestos in occupational as well as environmental settings, and takes a very long period of over 40 years to develop following asbestos exposure (13). This indicates that mesothelioma could not be explained only by marked inflammation and mutagenic events resulting from exposure to asbestos,

DOI: 10.1201/9781003431909-8

but rather other events might contribute to the development of mesothelioma over a long period of time. Therefore, we hypothesized that immune-suppressive events might result from asbestos exposure and examined various kinds of lymphocyte functions associated with anti-tumor immunity, where natural killer cells, in addition to $CD4^+$ T helper and $CD8^+$ cytotoxic T lymphocytes, play a role in innate and acquired immunity. respectively. In our series of studies, we examined the effects of asbestos exposure using *in vitro* experiments with a human cell line or peripheral blood mononuclear cells (PBMCs) followed by analysis for immunological characteristics of peripheral blood obtained from patients with malignant mesothelioma and individuals positive for PPs (14). These studies revealed that exposure to asbestos caused functional alterations in those lymphocytes related to dysfunction of anti-tumor immunity, and that several characteristics of the altered functions were actually observed in peripheral blood specimens from mesothelioma patients and/or plaque-positive individuals. In the following paragraphs, our findings to date are introduced for each area investigated. These findings describe characteristics of cellular functional decline, in addition to referring to molecular mechanisms of the relationship between asbestos and lymphocytes. Moreover, recent investigative efforts regarding the potential restoration of asbestos-induced impairment in immune functions will also be discussed. Finally, we summarize our conclusions and discuss the relationship between the immunological effects of asbestos exposure and asbestos-related diseases.

8.2 FUNCTIONAL ALTERATION OF ALVEOLAR MACROPHAGES UPON EXPOSURE TO ASBESTOS

As mentioned above, alveolar macrophages produce inflammatory cytokines and ROS/RNS, in addition to undergoing apoptosis following exposure to asbestos. It is generally known that those inflammatory events result in a fibrogenic response, where fibroblasts or epithelial cells produce TGF-β which leads to the generation and accumulation of the extracellular matrix (ECM). Therefore, the pro-fibrogenic function of alveolar macrophages to produce TGF-β following asbestos exposure was examined by *in vivo* and *in vitro* experiments with rats (15). It was confirmed that intratracheal instillation with chrysotile asbestos resulted in increased levels of granulocytes and inflammatory cytokines such as TNF-α, IL-1β and IL-6 in broncho-alveolar lavage (BAL) analyses following one day of the instillation, while *in vitro* production of TNF-α in alveolar macrophages obtained by BAL from control rats treated with saline was also confirmed in the cell culture with chrysotile for one day. In contrast, BAL samples obtained from rats after 5 days of instillation with chrysotile showed high concentrations of TGF-β as well as increased levels of apoptotic cells testing positive for annexin V and low in DNA content. Additionally, alveolar macrophages obtained by BAL of rats after instillation with chrysotile showed higher amounts of TGF-β in the culture in the absence of chrysotile for 5 days compared with those from control rats. These findings indicate that alveolar macrophages generated high levels of TGF-β following production of inflammatory cytokines and apoptosis caused by exposure to asbestos. However, it was surprising that alveolar macrophages prepared from BAL of control rats also showed increased production of TGF-β in the culture upon exposure to chrysotile for 5 days, and that the increased concentration did not differ from the level shown by alveolar macrophages prepared from BAL of rats intratracheally instilled with chrysotile. Additionally, when apoptosis of alveolar macrophages in the culture with chrysotile was examined, and it was found that high doses ($\geq$12.5 μg/cm^2) of chrysotile caused clear apoptosis while low doses ($\leq$5 μg/cm^2) did not. Furthermore, alveolar macrophages derived from control rats showed a peak of TGF-β production in the culture with 2.5 μg/cm^2 of chrysotile, a dose which did not induce apoptosis as mentioned above. These findings indicate that alveolar macrophages acquire the ability to produce high levels of TGF-β without any other types of cells or apoptotic cells following exposure to asbestos. Moreover, these alveolar macrophages showed continuously high levels of TGF-β in fresh media for the secondary 3 days (day 5 to 8), and with much higher levels for the tertiary 3 days (day 8 to 10). Consistent with long-term survival, the alveolar macrophages cultured with chrysotile showed increased expression of Bcl-x_L, a representative anti-apoptotic gene. Taken together, these findings confirmed that alveolar macrophages autonomously acquire the ability to generate long-lasting high levels of TGF-β with prolonged survival. This suggests that this type of functional alteration in alveolar macrophages might contribute to lung fibrosis, separate from their role in inflammation, following exposure to asbestos. Additionally, TGF-β plays a role in immune suppression (16) in addition to its crucial role in inducing regulatory T cells (17). Therefore, these alveolar macrophages might also contribute to the development of tumor diseases following exposure to asbestos.

8.3 IMPAIRED CYTOTOXICITY OF NATURAL KILLER CELLS WITH ALTERED EXPRESSION OF ACTIVATING RECEPTORS FOLLOWING ASBESTOS EXPOSURE

Natural killer (NK) cells are able to respond quickly to the presence of abnormal cells following mutagenic stimuli because they do not require clonal selection or clonal proliferation, which differs from T lymphocytes. T cells recognize target cells with T cell receptor (TCR), whereas NK cells utilize various kinds of activating receptors which display no diversity unlike TCR (18, 19). When the activating receptors on the cell surface of NK cells ligate each ligand on the target cells, they transduce activating signals inside the cells, followed by ERK and JNK pathways, resulting in degranulation of cytotoxic granules including perforin and granzyme, which execute apoptosis of target cells. Thus, expression levels of activating receptors influence the target recognition and function of NK cells. Therefore, investigations were performed to determine whether exposure to asbestos affects target-lytic activity (cytotoxicity) of NK cells as well as cell surface expression of activating receptors. Cells of the human NK cell line YT-A1 were cultured with chrysotile asbestos at a concentration of 5 μg/mL for a prolonged period, and assayed periodically for cytotoxicity and expression of cell surface receptors. The asbestos-exposed subline (YT-CB5) showed a marked decline in cytotoxicity against K562 cells, representative targets recognized by human NK cells, after over four months (20). Furthermore, YT-CB5 showed decreased expression of NKG2D and 2B4 activating receptors. NKG2D is a member of the NKG2 family, which is a well-known group of NK cell receptors and characterized by a lectin-like domain. 2B4 is a receptor of the signaling lymphocytic activation molecule (SLAM) family. The NKG2 family includes members with activating and inhibitory functions such as NKG2D and NKG2A, respectively (18, 19). In contrast to NKG2D, YT-CB5 showed only a negligible change in expression levels of NKG2A and CD94, which consist of heterodimers that function as inhibitory receptors. Additionally, YT-CB5 showed decreased degranulation following stimulation with antibodies to NKG2D or 2B4. Consistent with these results, phosphorylation of ERK was low in YT-CB5 after incubation with K562 cells or stimulation with antibodies for NKG2D (21). These findings indicate that exposure to asbestos causes impaired cytotoxicity of NK cells with altered expression of activating receptors. It was then determined whether peripheral blood NK cells in patients with malignant mesothelioma showed altered expression of activating receptors as well as cytotoxicity. It was found that the NK cells showed decreased cytotoxicity as well as characteristic alterations in cell surface expression of receptors, where NKp46 levels were markedly lower compared with NK cells of healthy individuals, although expression levels of NKG2D and 2B4 were normal (20). NKp46 is a member of the natural cytotoxicity receptor (NCR) family, which plays a major role in the NK-mediated killing of most tumor cell lines (22, 23). Therefore, human PBMCs were cultured and then exposed to chrysotile asbestos in the media supplemented with IL-2, a cytokine that activates NK cells, for one week and assayed for cell surface expression of NKG2D, 2B4 and NKp46. It is interesting that NK cells in culture with asbestos showed a marked decrease in expression of NKp46, but not in NKG2D or 2B4, which is consistent with the results obtained from peripheral blood NK cells in mesothelioma patients (20). Additionally, exposure to glass wool, an asbestos substitute comprising man-made mineral fibers, did not cause such a decrease in NKp46 expression. Taken together, it was confirmed that exposure to asbestos causes functional failure in cytotoxicity and expression of activating receptors in NK cells, and in particular that low expression of NKp46 is a notable feature shared between the effects of asbestos exposure and patients with malignant mesothelioma.

8.4 CLARIFICATION OF DECREASE IN T HELPER 1 CELL FUNCTION CAUSED BY ASBESTOS EXPOSURE ON THE BASIS OF GENE EXPRESSION ANALYSIS

It is known that $CD4^+$ T helper cells play a pivotal role in guiding or regulating acquired immunity. T helper 1 (Th1) type effector cells were differentiated from naïve Th cell function in anti-tumor immunity (24). Th1 cells show stronger production of interferon gamma (IFN-γ) compared with Th2 cells, which support differentiation of effector cytotoxic T lymphocytes (CTL) from naïve $CD8^+$ T cells. The effect of long-term asbestos exposure on the function of Th cells was examined using the human T cell line MT-2, with a focus on Th1 function. *In vitro* exposure to chrysotile caused apoptosis of MT-2 cells in a dose-dependent manner, as confirmed by the TUNEL method. However, MT-2 subline cells continuously cultured with chrysotile (MT-2Rst) acquired resistance against asbestos-induced apoptosis after more than 8 months of culture. Interestingly, MT-2Rst showed low production of IFN-γ as well as high production of IL-10 with increased expression of the bcl-2 anti-apoptotic gene (25). These findings indicate that chronic exposure to asbestos caused decreased Th1 function with potency of long survival upon exposure to asbestos. Based on these results, the effects of chronic asbestos exposure on gene expression in Th cells were comprehensively examined. Six sublines of MT-2Rst (three exposed to chrysotile A and three exposed to chrysotile B) were prepared by continuous culture with these asbestos types, and analyzed for gene expression by DNA microarray analysis. Clustering analysis showed altered expression of 139 genes caused by long-term exposure to asbestos, and the profile was almost similar among the six sublines when compared with the original MT-2 cells (26). Additionally, pathway and network analysis showed suppression of the IFN-γ signaling pathway, where expression of IFN regulatory factor 9 (IRF9) and IFN-stimulated gene factor 3 (ISGF3) was significantly reduced in all six sublines. Moreover, network analysis identified decreased expression of CXCR3 in these sublines, which was regulated by IRF9. CXCR3 is a representative chemokine receptor that is expressed on Th1 cells and functions in the migration of effector cells to the periphery (27). Moreover, in an effort to confirm the impairment of Th1 function with asbestos exposure, peripheral blood $CD4^+$ T cells isolated from PBMCs of healthy volunteers and expanded upon stimulation with anti-CD3 and CD28 antibodies were cultured with chrysotile asbestos in the media supplemented with IL-2. Consistent with the results of MT-2Rsts, $CD4^+$ T cells exposed to asbestos showed decreased cell surface expression of CXCR3 and decreased intracellular expression and mRNA levels of IFN-γ (28). Furthermore, peripheral blood $CD4^+$ T cells in patients with malignant mesothelioma (MM) showed a lower percentage of $CXCR3^+$ cells and lower mRNA levels of IFN-γ compared with healthy volunteers (HV), while $CD4^+$ T cells in PP-positive individuals showed intermediate values of %$CXCR3^+$ cells, with HV>PP>MM (28). These results indicate that chronic exposure to asbestos altered gene expression in Th cells, where Th1 function was clearly suppressed with low production of IFN-γ and low expression of CXCR3. Interestingly, peripheral blood $CD4^+$ Th cells in patients with malignant mesothelioma also showed similar characteristics of impaired Th1 function as observed in cells chronically exposed to asbestos.

8.5 ENHANCED REGULATORY T CELL FUNCTION RESULTED FROM EXPOSURE TO ASBESTOS

As described in the above paragraph, MT-2 cells continuously cultured upon exposure to chrysotile asbestos showed decreased production of IFN-γ and increased production of IL-10 with high expression of the bcl-2 anti-apoptotic gene (25). It is known that the MT-2 cell line can be immortalized by human T-lymphotropic virus 1 (HTLV-1) with Treg-like features (29). Therefore, MT-2 cells exposed to asbestos were examined for Treg function. Treg cells control stimulation-induced immune responses by suppressing cell proliferation of responder T lymphocytes. MT-2Org, the original subline of MT-2 maintained without any exposure, suppressed cell proliferation of $CD4^+$ $CD25^-$ conventional T helper cells following stimulation with anti-CD3 antibody and induced dendritic cells in a dose-dependent manner. However, it was found that the sublines generated by continuous exposure to chrysotile asbestos showed enhancement in Treg function to suppress cell proliferation of conventional Th cells (30). Treg cells exert suppressive functionality by using cell surface molecules such as CTLA-4 as well as secreted cytokines such as IL-10 and TGF-β. It is known that adequate proliferation of T cells requires a signal via cell surface CD28 following ligation with CD80 and CD86 on antigen-presenting cells in addition to TCR signaling, which is inhibited by CTLA-4 with high affinity against those ligands in an antagonistic manner (31, 32). Both TGF-β and IL-10 are representative cytokines that function in immune suppression (33–35). The asbestos-exposed subline showed increases in cell surface expression of CTLA-4 and secreted production of IL-10 and TGF-β. Additionally, it was confirmed that gene knockdown of IL-10 or TGF-β resulted in a partial decrease in suppressive function of the asbestos-exposed subline, which indicates that the enhanced Treg function observed in the subline exposed to asbestos is due to secreted IL-10 and TGF-β as well as cell-cell contact via surface molecules such as CTLA-4. Moreover, the effect of asbestos exposure on cell cycle progression of Treg cells was examined by experiments with MT-2 cells. The results obtained from the experiments showed that cyclin D1 expression was markedly enhanced in all the asbestos-exposed sublines by 20- to 60-fold compared with MT-2Org, although cyclin A and B showed decreased expression in the sublines by a factor of 0.2- to 0.5-fold. Additionally, levels of cyclin-dependent inhibitors of p21 Cip1, p57 Kip2, p18 Ink4c and p16 Ink4d were reduced in sublines exposed to asbestos in the culture (36). Consistent with these results, when the cell cycle was examined by flow cytometry with BrdU incorporation and 7AAD staining to distinguish G1, S and G2/M phases, the sublines examined showed clear increases in the number of cells at the S phase. These findings indicate that continuous asbestos exposure caused enhancement of Treg function, mediated by cytokines and cell-cell contact, with accelerated cell cycle progression. Such enhanced Treg cell levels and functionality may contribute to reduced anti-tumor immunity in individuals exposed to asbestos.

8.6 UNCONTROLLED T HELPER 17 CELL FUNCTION IN ASBESTOS-EXPOSED TH CELLS

As described above, our studies have clarified the effects of asbestos exposure on Th cell functions. Exposure of cells to asbestos in the cultures resulted in decreased Th1 functionality of the MT-2 cell line or isolated peripheral blood $CD4^+$ T cells, together with decreased production of IFN-γ and low expression CXCR3, which are also observed in peripheral blood $CD4^+$ T cells of patients with malignant mesothelioma as well as individuals positive for PPs. Additionally, asbestos exposure augmented cell line Treg function to suppress cell proliferation of stimulated T cells with high production of TGF-β and IL-10 and high expression of cell surface CTLA-4. These findings indicate that asbestos exposure induces dominance of effector $CD4^+$ T cells with decreased Th1 and increased Treg functionality, which contribute to suppression of anti-tumor immunity. Next, our study focused on another population of effector Th cells induced following antigenic stimulation. Th17 cells represent a characteristic population of Th cells with high production of IL-17, which functions in inflammation and autoimmunity (37). Although the role of Th17 in the development of tumor diseases has been extensively examined (38–41), a consensus has yet to be reached regarding the question of whether Th17 cells are beneficial in anti-tumor immunity. In contrast, it is known that Th17 cells play a crucial role in the pathogenesis of autoimmune diseases (42). Therefore, an investigation was performed to determine whether exposure to chrysotile asbestos would influence Th17 functionality by culture experiments with isolated peripheral blood $CD4^+$ Th cells obtained from healthy volunteers. Freshly isolated $CD4^+$ Th cells were pre-cultured upon stimulation with anti-CD3 and CD28 antibodies and IL-2 prior to culture with asbestos. After 4 weeks of culture with asbestos, $CD4^+$ Th cells were harvested and assayed for IFN-γ and IL-17 mRNA levels, as well as T-bet and RORγT transcription factors, which control the development of Th1 and Th17, respectively. Cells exposed to asbestos showed decreased IFN-γ mRNA levels, which is consistent with the results found in our previous studies, whereas these cells showed increased IL-17 mRNA levels in a dose-dependent manner. However, T-bet and RORγT mRNA levels were unexpectedly not altered in the asbestos-exposed cells. These findings indicate that exposure to asbestos caused a decrease in Th1 function as well as increase in Th17 function. The observed augmented Th17 function upon exposure to asbestos may be related to the production of autoantibodies and the development of autoimmune disease occasionally caused by exposure to asbestos (43–45).

8.7 DECREASED INDUCTION AND PERFORMANCE OF EFFECTOR CYTOTOXIC T LYMPHOCYTES CAUSED BY ASBESTOS EXPOSURE

$CD8^+$ cytotoxic T lymphocytes (CTLs) play a key role in the elimination of tumor cells in acquired immunity (46). Naïve $CD8^+$ T cells differentiate into effector cells which have lytic activity against target cells following antigenic stimulation. The mixed lymphocyte reaction (MLR) of PBMCs with irradiated allogenic PBMCs is a convenient method to induce effector CTLs with lytic activity. Thus, investigations were performed to determine whether exposure to chrysotile asbestos in the culture of the MLR would interfere with the induction of effector CTLs. $CD8^+$ T cells isolated from the culture of the MLR upon exposure to asbestos clearly showed decreased cytotoxicity against allogenic targets (47). The cytotoxicity of CTLs is executed by degranulation of cytotoxic granules, whereby released granzymes and perforin cause apoptosis of target cells. The $CD8^+$ T cells isolated from the asbestos-exposed culture of the MLR showed decrease percentages of intracellular granzyme B as well as IFN-γ. TNF-α and IFN-γ are representative cytokines produced by effector CTLs (48). Additionally, cell proliferation of $CD8^+$ T cells induced by stimulation with allogenic PBMC was reduced upon exposure to chrysotile asbestos. These $CD8^+$ T cells also showed decreased cell surface expression of CD45RO and CD25, effector/memory and activation markers, respectively. Moreover, analyses of the production of cytokines in culture supernatants showed decreased secreted levels of IFN-γ as well as TNF-α in the culture of the MLR upon exposure to asbestos. These findings indicate that exposure to asbestos suppressed differentiation of naïve $CD8^+$ T cells into effector CTLs with decreased cell proliferation and production of cytokines. Then, the properties of peripheral blood $CD8^+$ T cells were examined and compared between patients with malignant mesothelioma (MM) and individuals positive for pleural plaques (PL). There was no difference in the percentage of $CD3^+$ $CD8^+$ cells in PBMCs among healthy volunteers (HV), PL and MM, although the total number of PBMCs in the PL and MM groups was lower compared with HV. Interestingly, $CD8^+$ T cells of MM patients showed reduced intracellular perforin levels after stimulation with PMA/ionomycin compared with PP-positive individuals (49). Although the reduction in perforin levels reflects suppressed cytotoxicity, the results obtained from the experiments with the MLR with exposure to asbestos did not show a reduction in perforin levels. Furthermore, the effect of long-term asbestos exposure on the function of effector CTLs remained to be determined. Hence, investigations were performed in an effort to determine whether chronic exposure to asbestos would result in functional impairment of the human cell line EBT-8 with characteristics of effector CTLs. EBT-8 cells were continuously cultured in media supplemented with IL-2 and exposed to chrysotile asbestos for more than 1 month, and assayed for intracellular granzyme B and perforin levels in addition to examining the production of IFN-γ. Exposure to chrysotile at 5 or 30 μg/mL did not result in a decrease in intracellular granzyme B levels. In contrast, the percentage of intracellular perforin-positive cells decreased in the cell line continuously exposed to chrysotile (50), similar to peripheral blood $CD8^+$ T cells in patients with mesothelioma. The subline continuously exposed to asbestos also showed decreased levels of secreted IFN-γ following stimulation with anti-CD3 antibodies. Taken together, the results obtained from the culture experiments with PBMCs and the cell line and analyses for $CD8^+$ cells in MM patients indicate that exposure to asbestos suppresses stimulation following induction of effector CTLs and maintenance of their functions, and that certain characteristics of $CD8^+$ T cells in patients with mesothelioma resemble that of cells chronically exposed to asbestos.

8.8 AUGMENTED MIGRATORY ACTIVITY WITH HIGH EXPRESSION OF MATRIX METALLOPROTEINASE 7 IN T CELL LINE CONTINUOUSLY EXPOSED TO ASBESTOS

As already mentioned, MT-2 sublines continuously exposed to chrysotile asbestos showed augmented Treg function as well as suppressed Thl function. Our studies also revealed several other facts of asbestos-induced functional alterations related to those characteristics. Augmented expression of matrix metalloproteinase 7 (MMP-7) in MT-2 sublines continuously exposed to chrysotile or crocidolite asbestos was an important feature to note, which was identified by cDNA microarray analysis. It is known that Treg cells migrate to tumor microenvironments and act as a shield against tumor-attacking T cells (51, 52). Fibronectin is a component of extracellular matrix (ECM), upregulation of which is associated with pro-tumoral reprogramming of the stroma (53), and MMP-7 can cleave ECM and basement membrane proteins such as fibronectin (54). Therefore, investigations were performed in an effort to determine whether MT-2 sublines exposed to asbestos would show alterations in migratory activity in the culture environment with fibronectin. Although the sublines showed no alterations in Treg function, their passage through a fibronectin-coated filter was greater compared with cells of the original MT-2 cell line (55). It is known that Treg cells exert an immune-suppressive role on the basis of the following three considerations; (1) cell-cell contact, (2) production of soluble factors such as IL-10 and TGF-β, and (3) the tumor microenvironment (56, 57). Findings pertaining to MMP-7 and migratory activity indicate augmentation of Treg function related to the third consideration above, which suggests that asbestos-exposed Treg cells function to provide protection from tumor-attacking immune cells. Taken together, a series of our studies demonstrated that exposure to asbestos caused augmentation of Treg functions with respect to all three considerations above, which may contribute to suppression of anti-tumor immunity in individuals exposed to asbestos.

8.9 PRODUCTION OF REACTIVE OXYGEN SPECIES AND FUNCTION OF ANTI-OXIDATIVE STRESS IN T CELL LINE CONTINUOUSLY EXPOSED TO ASBESTOS

Experiments using the MT-2 T cell line revealed various features in cells continuously exposed to asbestos as described above. It is known that generation of ROS and RNS are key events in carcinogenesis following exposure to asbestos (58, 59). Thus, investigations were performed to determine whether the expression of genes and molecules related to anti-oxidative stress would be altered in asbestos-exposed MT-2 sublines, and complexes related to oxidative phosphorylation were also examined with regard to the production of ROS. Sublines continuously exposed to chrysotile or crocidolite showed decreased expression of thioredoxin. It is interesting that nicotinamide nucleotide transhydrogenase (NNT) expression was markedly enhanced in those sublines, while production of ROS observed in the MT-2 original subline was suppressed in an asbestos dose-dependent manner (60). Although knockdown of NNT did not interfere with proliferation or apoptosis of the asbestos-exposed sublines, it resulted in recovery of ROS production in those sublines. Additionally, the production of ROS in the sublines continuously exposed to chrysotile or crocidolite increased following treatment with the NNT-inhibitor palmitoyl CoA-K. These findings indicate that continuous exposure to asbestos caused alterations in anti-oxidative stress functionality with increased expression of NNT, which might be related to functional alterations in asbestos-exposed MT-2 subline cells.

8.10 ALTERATION OF CYTOSKELETAL MOLECULES IN THE T CELL LINE CONTINUOUSLY EXPOSED TO ASBESTOS

Our studies revealed many aspects of the immunological effects of asbestos exposure on lymphocytes, and showed that the lymphocytes adhered onto asbestos without being subjected to phagocytosis as is the case with macrophages. Thus, investigations were performed in an effort to identify any alterations in protein expression among the six sublines of the MT-2 T cell line continuously exposed to chrysotile asbestos using ProteinChip and two-dimensional fluorescence difference gel electrophoresis (2D-DIGE) assays. The results indicated that there were characteristic differences in 2D-DIGE images between the asbestos-exposed subline and original MT-2 cells, and subsequent analysis by peptide sequencing using liquid chromatography electrospray ionization tandem mass spectrometry (LC-ESI-MS/MS) revealed that one spot in the gel images was identified as β-actin, which indicated that changes in these cells includes post-translational modification of β-actin in the chrysotile-exposed subline (61). The results obtained from immunoprecipitation by anti-β-actin antibody and immunoblotting using anti-phospho-β-actin antibody showed phosphorylation of β-actin in the subline exposed to chrysotile asbestos, unlike the case with the original MT-2 cell line. These findings indicate that asbestos caused alterations in the control of cytoskeleton, and raised the possibility that asbestos may bind directly to cytoskeletal molecules on the cell surface related to upregulation and phosphorylation of β-actin. Thus, direct binding between chrysotile fibers and original MT-2 cells or a subline continuously exposed to chrysotile was examined. Four chrysotile-bound proteins, myosin-9, vimentin, tubulin-β2 and β-actin, were identified by ESI-MS analysis. Taken together, these results indicate that the cell surface cytoskeleton may play an important role in inducing the cellular changes caused by asbestos in immune cells, as asbestos fibers are not incorporated into the lymphocytes.

8.11 POTENTIAL RESTORATION OF ASBESTOS-INDUCED ALTERATIONS IN IMMUNE FUNCTIONS BY SUPPLEMENTATION WITH CYTOKINES AND NATURAL COMPOUNDS

Our studies also examined the possibility of restoring immune functions adversely affected by asbestos exposure. As described above, exposure to asbestos suppressed the stimulation-induced differentiation of naïve $CD8^+$ T cells into effector CTLs with decreases in cell proliferation and production of IFN-γ and TNF-α. Decreased cell proliferation suggested insufficient production of IL-2, a representative regulator of T lymphocyte proliferation and activation, which may have contributed to suppressed differentiation of effector CTLs following stimulation. Although the assay for secreted IL-2 in the culture of the MLR showed no difference between control cells and those exposed to asbestos, the concentration of IL-2 was very low (less than 10 pg/mL), and may support the notion of insufficient production of IL-2 as being pivotal following exposure of cells to asbestos. Thus, the effect of exogenously added IL-2 into the culture following exposure to chrysotile asbestos was examined. The addition of IL-2 on the second day of the MLR did not restore asbestos-induced decreases in cell proliferation or percentage of $CD25^+$ and $CD45RO^+$ cells in $CD8^+$ T cells, but did partially recover the decrease in percentage of granzyme B^+ cells. Additionally, $CD8^+$ T cells isolated from the culture with asbestos showed the same degree of cytotoxicity against target cells as those in cultures without asbestos (62). These findings demonstrated that insufficient production of IL-2 was not the primary cause for the observed suppression of effector CTL induction upon exposure to asbestos. However, the results also indicated the potential recovery of asbestos-induced suppression of effector CTL induction. Then, the effect of supplementation with IL-15 into the culture with asbestos was examined since IL-15 has a similar function to IL-2 but with greater effectiveness on the functional acquisition of effector CTLs (63, 64). The amount of IL-15 determined in the cultures of the MLR was negligible, even under conditions without asbestos (65). However, since IL-15 binds to IL-15Rα on one cell and stimulates another cell via IL-2Rβ-γc in the manner of a membrane-bound ligand (66), it could not be discounted that the asbestos-induced decrease in effector CTL function may be due to insufficient levels of IL-15. The addition of IL-15 partially reversed the decrease in the number of $CD3^+$ $CD8^+$ cells and completely restored the percentage decrease of granzyme B+ cells, although the percentage decreases of $CD25^+$ and $CD45RO^+$ cells were not restored by IL-15 addition (65). These results indicate that supplementation with IL-15 is more effective in the recovery of asbestos-induced suppression of effector CTL induction compared with IL-2. Taken together, these findings regarding supplementation with IL-2 or IL-15 demonstrated the possible recovery of asbestos-induced suppression in anti-tumor immunity.

In another study, the potential of natural compounds to restore asbestos-induced alterations in the function of $CD4^+$ T cells with decreased Th1 function and increased Treg function was examined, where trehalose (Treh) and hesperidin (Hesp) were selected as potential candidate compounds for investigation. Treh is a compound present in some bacteria, fungi, plants and invertebrate animals that can act as a source of energy in these organisms to facilitate survival under freezing and water shortage conditions (67, 68). The compound is now used as an ingredient in the food, cosmetics and pharmaceutical industries following mass production of Treh by Hayashibara Co. Ltd.. In the medical field, Treh has been reported to display neuroprotective activity in the treatment of Parkinson's disease (69) as well as to improve glucose tolerance (70). Hesp is a flavanone glycoside found in citrus fruit (71, 72) and has been reported to play a role in protecting plants from external toxins, and also displays antioxidant properties (73). Pharmacological effects have also been investigated in terms of inflammation, hypertension, dyslipidemia, allergy, anxiety and cancer prevention (74, 75). Hayashibara Co. Ltd. has also succeeded in producing glycosyl hesperidin (gHesp) with increased water solubility (76, 77). Thus, investigations were performed to determine whether Treh and gHesp could restore asbestos-induced functional alterations in $CD4^+$ T cells. Isolated $CD4^+$ T cells from PBMCs were cultured with IL-2 and anti-CD3 and -CD28 antibodies for a week, and then cultured with IL-2 upon exposure to chrysotile asbestos for 4 weeks in the presence of Treh or gHesp. After harvesting, cells were stored for 6 hours in the absence or presence of medium containing PMA/ionomycin and then assayed for mRNA levels of several genes by RT-qPCR. It was found that addition of Treh or gHesp blocked asbestos-induced alterations in expression of MMP-7, NNT and IL-17A (78). These results suggest that the supplements or foods examined might contribute to the attenuation of asbestos-induced reduction in anti-tumor immunity.

8.12 CONCLUSION

As described above, our studies clarified several findings pertaining to the effects of asbestos exposure on immune function in innate immunity as well as in acquired immunity, where various characteristics related to functional alterations were observed in alveolar macrophages, NK, $CD4^+$ T and $CD8^+$ T lymphocytes (Figure 8.1). Observations included high production of TGF-β by alveolar macrophages and increased expression of anti-apoptotic gene functions such as profibrogenic as well as tumor-promoting processes related to pneumoconiosis and malignant diseases. Impaired cytotoxicity of NK and $CD8^+$ CTLs together with decreased Th1 function and increased Treg function results in reduction of anti-tumor immunity, which allows for immune escape of asbestos-induced abnormal cells, leading to development of malignant diseases. Augmentation of Th17 function may contribute to occasional onset of autoimmune disease caused by asbestos exposure. Taken together, these findings showed that several common characteristics were observed in cell cultures exposed to asbestos as well as in peripheral blood specimens of patients with malignant mesothelioma. These findings include decreased levels of NKp46 in NK cells, decreased levels of IFN-γ and CXCR3 in $CD4^+$ T cells and decreased levels of perforin in $CD8^+$ T cells under stimulation. These data suggest a correlation between the immune-suppressive effects of asbestos and malignant mesothelioma since accumulated asbestos in regional lymph nodes might gradually cause this type of suppressed immune function in local areas. Our study also identified a possible machinery involving the binding of asbestos to cell surface cytoskeleton that may trigger functional alterations in lymphocytes. Furthermore, it was also demonstrated that asbestos-induced functional alterations may be reversed, which might form the basis of future strategies involving the prevention and treatment of malignant mesothelioma in individuals exposed to asbestos. To date, the discovery of immune checkpoint inhibitors such as nivolumab and ipilimumab is drastically affecting therapeutic strategies pertaining to mesothelioma. Further immunological studies concerning the effects of asbestos exposure and malignant mesothelioma should yield greater benefits for individuals suffering from asbestos-related diseases.

REFERENCES

1. Li XY, Lamb D, Donaldson K. The production of TNF-alpha and IL-1-like activity by bronchoalveolar leucocytes after intratracheal instillation of crocidolite asbestos. *Int J Exp Pathol* 1993;74(4):403–10.
2. Lemaire I, Ouellet S. Distinctive profile of alveolar macrophage-derived cytokine release induced by fibrogenic and nonfibrogenic mineral dusts. *J Toxicol Environ Health* 1996;47(5):465–78.
3. Kamp DW, Graceffa P, Pryor WA, Weitzman SA. The role of free radicals in asbestos-induced diseases. *Free Radic Biol Med* 1992;12(4):293–315.
4. Jackson JH. Potential molecular mechanisms of oxidant-induced carcinogenesis. *Environ Health Perspect* 1994;102(Suppl 10):155–7.
5. Rihn B, Coulais C, Kauffer E, Bottin MC, Martin P, Yvon F, et al. Inhaled crocidolite mutagenicity in lung DNA. *Environ Health Perspect* 2000;108(4):341–6.
6. Broaddus VC, Yang L, Scavo LM, Ernst JD, Boylan AM. Asbestos induces apoptosis of human and rabbit pleural mesothelial cells via reactive oxygen species. *J Clin Invest* 1996;98(9):2050–9.
7. Panduri V, Weitzman SA, Chandel NS, Kamp DW. Mitochondrial-derived free radicals mediate asbestos-induced alveolar epithelial cell apoptosis. *Am J Physiol Lung Cell Mol Physiol* 2004;286(6):L1220–7.
8. Hamilton RF, Iyer LL, Holian A. Asbestos induces apoptosis in human alveolar macrophages. *Am J Physiol* 1996;271(5 Pt 1):L813–9.
9. Aljandali A, Pollack H, Yeldandi A, Li Y, Weitzman SA, Kamp DW. Asbestos causes apoptosis in alveolar epithelial cells: Role of iron-induced free radicals. *J Lab Clin Med* 2001;137(5):330–9.
10. Mossman BT, Churg A. Mechanisms in the pathogenesis of asbestosis and silicosis. *Am J Respir Crit Care Med* 1998;157(5 Pt 1):1666–80.
11. Dodson RF, Williams MG Jr., Corn CJ, Brollo A, Bianchi C. A comparison of asbestos burden in lung parenchyma, lymph nodes, and plaques. *Ann N Y Acad Sci* 1991;643:53–60.
12. Dodson RF, Huang J, Bruce JR. Asbestos content in the lymph nodes of nonoccupationally exposed individuals. *Am J Ind Med* 2000;37(2):169–74.
13. Bohlig H, Otto H. *Asbest unt Mesotheliom: Fakten, Fragen, Umweltprobleme*. Stuttgart: G. Thieme, 1975.
14. Nishimura Y, Kumagai-Takei N, Lee S, Yoshitome K, Ito T, Otsuki T. Asbestos fiber and immunological effects: Do immunological effects play any role in asbestos-related diseases? In Kijima T, Nakano T, eds. *Malignant Pleural Mesothelioma; Advances in Pathogenesis, Diagnosis, and Treatments. Respiratory Disease Series: Diagnostic Tools and Disease Managements*. 1st ed. Berlin: Springer, 2021, pp. 33–41.
15. Nishimura Y, Nishiike-Wada T, Wada Y, Miura Y, Otsuki T, Iguchi H. Long-lasting production of TGF-beta1 by alveolar macrophages exposed to low doses of asbestos without apoptosis. *Int J Immunopathol Pharmacol* 2007;20(4):661–71.
16. Shull MM, Ormsby I, Kier AB, Pawlowski S, Diebold RJ, Yin M, et al. Targeted disruption of the mouse transforming growth factor-beta 1 gene results in multifocal inflammatory disease. *Nature* 1992;359(6397):693–9.
17. Chen ZM, O'Shaughnessy MJ, Gramaglia I, Panoskaltsis-Mortari A, Murphy WJ, Narula S, et al. IL-10 and TGF-beta induce alloreactive CD4+CD25- T cells to acquire regulatory cell function. *Blood* 2003;101(12):5076–83.

18. Moretta L, Moretta A. Unravelling natural killer cell function: Triggering and inhibitory human NK receptors. *EMBO J* 2004;23(2):255–9.
19. Yokoyama WM, Plougastel BF. Immune functions encoded by the natural killer gene complex. *Nat Rev Immunol* 2003;3(4):304–16.
20. Nishimura Y, Miura Y, Maeda M, Kumagai N, Murakami S, Hayashi H, et al. Impairment in cytotoxicity and expression of NK cell- activating receptors on human NK cells following exposure to asbestos fibers. *Int J Immunopathol Pharmacol* 2009;22(3):579–90.
21. Nishimura Y, Maeda M, Kumagai N, Hayashi H, Miura Y, Otsuki T. Decrease in phosphorylation of ERK following decreased expression of NK cell-activating receptors in human NK cell line exposed to asbestos. *Int J Immunopathol Pharmacol* 2009;22(4):879–88.
22. Moretta A, Bottino C, Vitale M, Pende D, Cantoni C, Mingari MC, et al. Activating receptors and coreceptors involved in human natural killer cell-mediated cytolysis. *Annu Rev Immunol* 2001;19:197–223.
23. Sivori S, Pende D, Bottino C, Marcenaro E, Pessino A, Biassoni R, et al. NKp46 is the major triggering receptor involved in the natural cytotoxicity of fresh or cultured human NK cells. Correlation between surface density of NKp46 and natural cytotoxicity against autologous, allogeneic or xenogeneic target cells. *Eur J Immunol* 1999;29(5):1656–66.
24. Li T, Wu B, Yang T, Zhang L, Jin K. The outstanding antitumor capacity of CD4(+) T helper lymphocytes. *Biochim Biophys Acta Rev Cancer* 2020;1874(2):188439.
25. Miura Y, Nishimura Y, Katsuyama H, Maeda M, Hayashi H, Dong M, et al. Involvement of IL-10 and Bcl-2 in resistance against an asbestos-induced apoptosis of T cells. *Apoptosis* 2006;11(10):1825–35.
26. Maeda M, Nishimura Y, Hayashi H, Kumagai N, Chen Y, Murakami S, et al. Reduction of CXC chemokine receptor 3 in an in vitro model of continuous exposure to asbestos in a human T-cell line, MT-2. *Am J Respir Cell Mol Biol* 2011;45(3):470–9.
27. Nagarsheth N, Wicha MS, Zou W. Chemokines in the cancer microenvironment and their relevance in cancer immunotherapy. *Nat Rev Immunol* 2017;17(9):559–72.
28. Maeda M, Nishimura Y, Hayashi H, Kumagai N, Chen Y, Murakami S, et al. Decreased CXCR3 expression in CD4+ T cells exposed to asbestos or derived from asbestos-exposed patients. *Am J Respir Cell Mol Biol* 2011;45(4):795–803.
29. Chen S, Ishii N, Ine S, Ikeda S, Fujimura T, Ndhlovu LC, et al. Regulatory T cell-like activity of Foxp3+ adult T cell leukemia cells. *Int Immunol* 2006;18(2):269–77.
30. Ying C, Maeda M, Nishimura Y, Kumagai-Takei N, Hayashi H, Matsuzaki H, et al. Enhancement of regulatory T cell-like suppressive function in MT-2 by long-term and low-dose exposure to asbestos. *Toxicology* 2015;338:86–94.
31. Bron PA, van Baarlen P, Kleerebezem M. Emerging molecular insights into the interaction between probiotics and the host intestinal mucosa. *Nat Rev Microbiol* 2012;10(1):66–U90.
32. McGuirk P, Mills KHG. Pathogen-specific regulatory T cells provoke a shift in the Thl/Th2 paradigm in immunity to infectious diseases. *Trends Immunol* 2002;23(9):450–5.
33. Yoshimura A, Muto G. TGF-beta function in immune suppression. *Curr Top Microbiol Immunol* 2011;350:127–47.
34. Rubtsov YP, Rudensky AY. TGFbeta signalling in control of T-cell-mediated self-reactivity. *Nat Rev Immunol* 2007;7(6):443–53.
35. Alhakeem SS, McKenna MK, Oben KZ, Noothi SK, Rivas JR, Hildebrandt GC, et al. Chronic lymphocytic leukemia–derived IL-10 suppresses antitumor immunity. *J Immunol* 2018;200(12):4180–9.
36. Lee S, Matsuzaki H, Maeda M, Yamamoto S, Kumagai-Takei N, Hatayama T, et al. Accelerated cell cycle progression of human regulatory T cell-like cell line caused by continuous exposure to asbestos fibers. *Int J Oncol* 2017;50(1):66–74.
37. Singh RP, Hasan S, Sharma S, Nagra S, Yamaguchi DT, Wong DTW, et al. Th17 cells in inflammation and autoimmunity. *Autoimmun Rev* 2014;13(12):1174–81.
38. Bailey SR, Nelson MH, Himes RA, Li Z, Mehrotra S, Paulos CM. Th17 cells in cancer: The ultimate identity crisis. *Front Immunol* 2014;5:276.
39. Lakshmi Narendra B, Eshvendar Reddy K, Shantikumar S, Ramakrishna S. Immune system: A double-edged sword in cancer. *Inflamm Res* 2013;62(9):823–34.
40. Alizadeh D, Katsanis E, Larmonier N. The multifaceted role of Th17 lymphocytes and their associated cytokines in cancer. *Clin Dev Immunol* 2013;2013:957878.
41. Zou W, Restifo NP. T(H)17 cells in tumour immunity and immunotherapy. *Nat Rev Immunol* 2010;10(4):248–56.
42. Yang J, Sundrud MS, Skepner J, Yamagata T. Targeting Th17 cells in autoimmune diseases. *Trends Pharmacol Sci* 2014;35(10):493–500.

43. Zebedeo CN, Davis C, Pena C, Ng KW, Pfau JC. Erionite induces production of autoantibodies and IL-17 in C57BL/6 mice. *Toxicol Appl Pharmacol* 2014;275(3):257–64.
44. Pfau JC, Serve KM, Noonan CW. Autoimmunity and asbestos exposure. *Autoimmune Dis* 2014;2014:782045.
45. Serve KM, Black B, Szeinuk J, Pfau JC. Asbestos-associated mesothelial cell autoantibodies promote collagen deposition in vitro. *Inhal Toxicol* 2013;25(14):774–84.
46. Raskov H, Orhan A, Christensen JP, Gögenur I. Cytotoxic CD8+ T cells in cancer and cancer immunotherapy. *Br J Cancer* 2021;124(2):359–67.
47. Kumagai-Takei N, Nishimura Y, Maeda M, Hayashi H, Matsuzaki H, Lee S, et al. Effect of asbestos exposure on differentiation of cytotoxic T lymphocytes in mixed lymphocyte reaction of human peripheral blood mononuclear cells. *Am J Respir Cell Mol Biol* 2013;49(1):28–36.
48. Harty JT, Tvinnereim AR, White DW. CD8+ T cell effector mechanisms in resistance to infection. *Annu Rev Immunol* 2000;18:275–308.
49. Kumagai-Takei N, Nishimura Y, Maeda M, Hayashi H, Matsuzaki H, Lee S, et al. Functional properties of CD8(+) lymphocytes in patients with pleural plaque and malignant mesothelioma. *J Immunol Res* 2014;2014:10–20.
50. Kumagai-Takei N, Nishimura Y, Matsuzaki H, Lee S, Yoshitome K, Otsuki T. Decrease in intracellular perforin Levels and IFN-γ Production in Human CD8+ T cell Line following Long-Term Exposure to asbestos Fibers. *J Immunol Res* 2018;2018:1–10.
51. Wang Y, Ma Y, Fang Y, Wu S, Liu L, Fu D, Shen X. Regulatory T cell: A protection for tumour cells. *J Cell Mol Med* 2012;16(3):425–36.
52. Gajewski TF, Meng Y, Blank C, Brown I, Kacha A, Kline J, Harlin H. Immune resistance orchestrated by the tumor microenvironment. *Immunol Rev* 2006;213:131–45.
53. Efthymiou G, Saint A, Ruff M, Rekad Z, Ciais D, Van Obberghen-Schilling E. Shaping up the tumor microenvironment with cellular fibronectin. *Front Oncol* 2020;10:641.
54. Wilson CL, Matrisian LM. Matrilysin: An epithelial matrix metalloproteinase with potentially novel functions. *Int J Biochem Cell Biol* 1996;28(2):123–36.
55. Lee S, Yamamoto S, Srinivas B, Shimizu Y, Sada N, Yoshitome K, et al. Increased production of matrix metalloproteinase-7 (MMP-7) by asbestos exposure enhances tissue migration of human regulatory T-like cells. *Toxicology* 2021:152717.
56. Harjunpaa H, Llort Asens M, Guenther C, Fagerholm SC. Cell adhesion molecules and their roles and regulation in the immune and tumor microenvironment. *Front Immunol* 2019;10:1078.
57. Tanaka A, Sakaguchi S. Regulatory T cells in cancer immunotherapy. *Cell Res* 2017;27(1):109–18.
58. Toyokuni S. Iron addiction with ferroptosis-resistance in asbestos-induced mesothelial carcinogenesis: Toward the era of mesothelioma prevention. *Free Radic Biol Med* 2019;133:206–15.
59. Kamp DW. Asbestos-induced lung diseases: An update. *Transl Res* 2009;153(4):143–52.
60. Yamamoto S, Lee S, Matsuzaki H, Kumagai-Takei N, Yoshitome K, Sada N, et al. Enhanced expression of nicotinamide nucleotide transhydrogenase (NNT) and its role in a human T cell line continuously exposed to asbestos. *Environ Int* 2020;138:105654.
61. Maeda M, Chen Y, Kumagai-Takei N, Hayashi H, Matsuzaki H, Lee S, et al. Alteration of cytoskeletal molecules in a human T cell line caused by continuous exposure to chrysotile asbestos. *Immunobiology* 2013;218(9):1184–91.
62. Kumagai-Takei N, Nishimura Y, Matsuzaki H, Lee S, Yoshitome K, Hayashi H, et al. The suppressed induction of human mature cytotoxic T lymphocytes caused by asbestos is not due to interleukin-2 insufficiency. *J Immunol Res* 2016;2016:10.
63. Weng NP, Liu K, Catalfamo M, Li YU, Henkart PA. IL-15 is a growth factor and an activator of CD8 memory T cells. *Ann N Y Acad Sci* 2006;975(1):46–56.
64. Schluns KS, Williams K, Ma A, Zheng XX, Lefrançois L. Cutting edge: Requirement for IL-15 in the generation of primary and memory antigen-specific CD8 T cells. *J Immunol* 2002;168(10):4827–31.
65. Kumagai-Takei N, Nishimura Y, Matsuzaki H, Lee S, Yoshitome K, Ito T, et al. Effect of IL-15 addition on asbestos-induced suppression of human cytotoxic T lymphocyte induction. *Environ Health Prev Med* 2021;26(1):50.
66. Leonard WJ, Lin J-X, O'Shea JJ. The γc family of cytokines: Basic biology to therapeutic ramifications. *Immunity* 2019;50(4):832–50.
67. Higashiyama T. Novel functions and applications of trehalose. *Pure Appl Chem* 2002;74(7):1263–9.
68. Richards AB, Krakowka S, Dexter LB, Schmid H, Wolterbeek AP, Waalkens-Berendsen DH, et al. Trehalose: A review of properties, history of use and human tolerance, and results of multiple safety studies. *Food Chem Toxicol* 2002;40(7):871–98.

69. Khalifeh M, Barreto GE, Sahebkar A. Trehalose as a promising therapeutic candidate for the treatment of Parkinson's disease. *Br J Pharmacol* 2019;176(9):1173–89.
70. Zhang Y, DeBosch BJ. Using trehalose to prevent and treat metabolic function: Effectiveness and mechanisms. *Curr Opin Clin Nutr Metab Care* 2019;22(4):303–10.
71. Roohbakhsh A, Parhiz H, Soltani F, Rezaee R, Iranshahi M. Neuropharmacological properties and pharmacokinetics of the citrus flavonoids hesperidin and hesperetin--A mini-review. *Life Sci* 2014;113(1–2):1–6.
72. Parhiz H, Roohbakhsh A, Soltani F, Rezaee R, Iranshahi M. Antioxidant and anti-inflammatory properties of the citrus flavonoids hesperidin and hesperetin: An updated review of their molecular mechanisms and experimental models. *Phytother Res* 2015;29(3):323–31.
73. Iranshahi M, Rezaee R, Parhiz H, Roohbakhsh A, Soltani F. Protective effects of flavonoids against microbes and toxins: The cases of hesperidin and hesperetin. *Life Sci* 2015;137:125–32.
74. Chikara S, Nagaprashantha LD, Singhal J, Horne D, Awasthi S, Singhal SS. Oxidative stress and dietary phytochemicals: Role in cancer chemoprevention and treatment. *Cancer Lett* 2018;413:122–34.
75. Tejada S, Pinya S, Martorell M, Capo X, Tur JA, Pons A, et al. Potential anti-inflammatory effects of hesperidin from the genus citrus. *Curr Med Chem* 2018;25(37):4929–45.
76. Miwa Y, Yamada M, Sunayama T, Mitsuzumi H, Tsuzaki Y, Chaen H, et al. Effects of glucosyl hesperidin on serum lipids in hyperlipidemic subjects: Preferential reduction in elevated serum triglyceride level. *J Nutr Sci Vitaminol (Tokyo)* 2004;50(3):211–8.
77. Yamada M, Tanabe F, Arai N, Mitsuzumi H, Miwa Y, Kubota M, et al. Bioavailability of glucosyl hesperidin in rats. *Biosci Biotechnol Biochem* 2006;70(6):1386–94.
78. Yamamoto S, Lee S, Ariyasu T, Endo S, Miyata S, Yasuda A, et al. Ingredients such as trehalose and hesperidin taken as supplements or foods reverse alterations in human T cells, reducing asbestos exposure-induced antitumor immunity. *Int J Oncol* 2021;58(4):1.

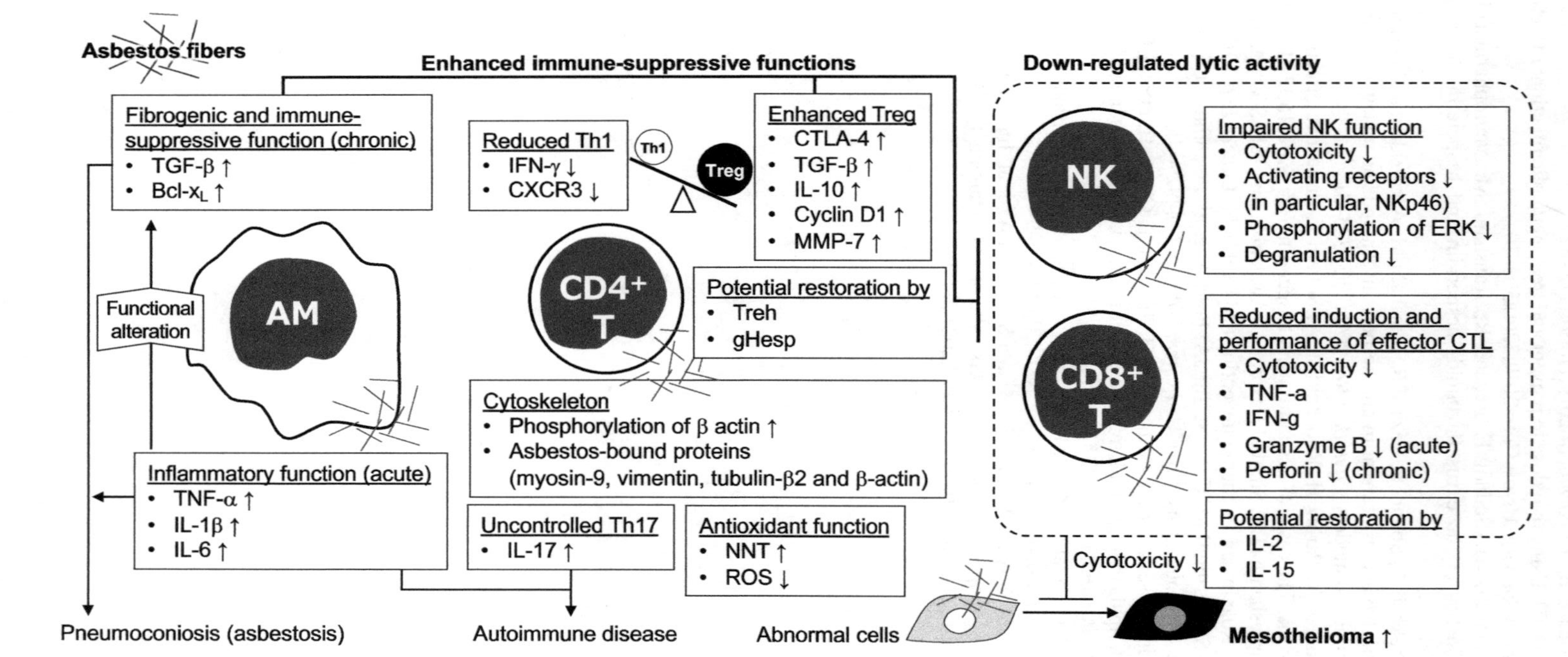

FIGURE 8.1 Summarized illustration of asbestos-caused functional alterations in immune cells related with malignant mesothelioma, as well as asbestosis and autoimmune disease, clarified by our studies.

9 Medical Findings Related to Asbestos Exposure

Yosuke Miyamoto and Nobukazu Fujimoto

9.1 INTRODUCTION

Asbestos exposure is associated with several benign lung or pleural diseases, including asbestos pleurisy, diffuse pleural thickening, and asbestosis. Exposure to asbestos can also cause a spectrum of malignant diseases [1–3]. The major thoracic malignancies associated with asbestos are lung cancer and malignant pleural mesothelioma. In a previous cross-sectional study of 2132 subjects with past asbestos exposure, a pathological diagnosis of lung cancer was confirmed in 45 cases (2.1%), and malignant pleural mesothelioma in 7 cases (0.3%) [4].

There is a close correlation between asbestos-related benign diseases and malignancy, likely because similar exposure levels are required to produce benign disease or malignant conditions. Evidence of asbestos exposure can be revealed by a subject's occupational or environmental history, the demonstration of asbestos fibers or bodies in lung tissue sections, or the presence of pleural plaques [3].

In this chapter, we present an overview of the association between asbestos-related medical imaging results and the risk of lung cancer or malignant pleural mesothelioma, focusing on imaging findings, such as asbestosis and pleural plaques.

9.2 ASBESTOSIS

Asbestosis is the interstitial pneumonitis and fibrosis caused by inhalation of asbestos fibers. The diagnosis of asbestosis should be based on an accurate exposure history that defines the duration, intensity, time of onset, and setting of exposure. The initial radiographic presentation of asbestosis is small, primarily irregular, parenchymal opacities in the bilateral lower lobes of the lungs (Figure 9.1). Over time, the distribution and density of opacities may spread throughout the middle and upper lung zones. In cases of mild or early asbestosis, a plain chest X-ray is limited in terms of sensitivity and specificity. One study showed that among individuals with asbestosis confirmed by histopathologic findings, 15–20% had no radiographic evidence of parenchymal fibrosis [5]. Compared to chest films, conventional computed tomography (CT) is superior for identifying parenchymal lesions [6], and high-resolution CT (HRCT) is much more sensitive for detecting asbestosis [6, 7]. Among asbestos-exposed individuals with unremarkable chest X-ray findings (International Labour Organization profusion score of 0/0 or 0/1), HRCT revealed that 34% had findings suggestive of asbestosis [8]. The HRCT findings in asbestosis are typically bilateral, and include evidence of fibrosis—such as intralobular interstitial thickening and interlobular septal thickening, subpleural dot-like opacities, subpleural lines (Figure 9.2), and parenchymal bands, sometimes ground-glass opacity, and honeycombing in advanced disease [9, 10]. It is often difficult to distinguish between asbestosis and other pulmonary fibrosis, but subpleural dot-like opacities and subpleural lines are considered more specific to asbestosis than to other types of pulmonary fibrosis [11, 12].

DOI: 10.1201/9781003431909-9

9.3 ASBESTOSIS AND ASSOCIATED RISKS OF LUNG CANCER AND MESOTHELIOMA

Multiple studies have demonstrated a clear association between asbestosis and increased risk of malignancy [13, 14]. One recent study assessed the association between asbestosis and the risk of lung cancer, and found that lung cancer mortality was increased by asbestos exposure alone among non-smokers (rate ratio = 3.6; 95% confidence interval (CI), 1.7–7.6), by asbestosis among non-smokers (rate ratio = 7.40; 95% CI: 4.0–13.7), and by smoking without asbestos exposure (rate ratio = 10.3; 95% CI: 8.8–12.2). The joint effect of smoking and asbestos alone was additive (rate ratio = 14.4; 95% CI: 10.7–19.4) and with asbestosis was supra-additive (rate ratio = 36.8; 95% CI: 30.1–45.0) [14]. In another study, former workers and residents of Wittenoom, Australia, with known asbestos exposure were monitored with chest X-ray and provided smoking information in a cancer prevention program. The results showed that smoking status was the strongest predictor of lung cancer, with the greatest risk among current smokers (odds ratio (OR) = 26.5; 95% CI: 3.5–198). Increased risk of lung cancer was also significantly associated with radiographic asbestosis (OR = 1.94; 95% CI: 1.09–3.46) and asbestos exposure (OR = 1.21 per fiber/mL-year; 95% CI: 1.02–1.42). This study concluded that asbestosis is not a mandatory precursor for asbestos-related lung cancer, and these findings support the hypothesis that the presence of asbestos fiber can lead to lung cancer development, with or without the presence of asbestosis [15].

Overall, the available evidence indicates that asbestos exposure alone increases lung cancer mortality among non-smokers, and adds to smoking-associated lung cancer risk. Asbestosis further increases the lung cancer risk, and has a supra-additive effect when considered jointly with smoking.

Few reports have focused on the association between asbestosis and risk of malignant pleural mesothelioma. One study demonstrated that up to 15% of patients with asbestosis developed malignant mesothelioma [16].

9.4 PLEURAL PLAQUES

Pleural plaques are circumscribed and discrete areas of hyaline or calcified fibrosis, which are localized on the parietal pleura of the lateral chest wall, the diaphragm, or the mediastinum [17]. The most common sites are the dorsolateral chest wall at the level of the 7–10th ribs, the anterolateral 6–9th ribs, the diaphragmatic dome, and the paravertebral regions—but not usually at the apex of the lung or diaphragmatic angle of the ribs [18]. Typical pleural plaques can be easily identified on plain chest X-ray based on sharp often-foliate borders, and a raised straight surface with clear cut-off edges when viewed face on, and irregular margins when viewed in profile on the chest wall or diaphragm (Figure 9.3). Pleural plaques are frequently documented on plain chest X-ray, but CT is more sensitive for their detection (Figure 9.4). In particular, non-calcified pleural plaques are difficult to identify on chest X-ray, with a detection rate of only about 14–54% [19, 20]. CT is a more accurate method of detecting circumscribed plaques [21–23]. Less-typical plaques on the diaphragm may be difficult to detect, and should be distinguished from atelectatic streaks, visceral folds, or diaphragmatic straightening caused by bullae [3]. Pleural plaques consistent with asbestos exposure appear in the chest films of 2.3% of U.S. males, and this percentage has been remarkably stable both within the general population in the early 1970s, and among veterans in the 1990s [24, 25]. The prevalence of pleural plaques is directly related to the duration since the first asbestos exposure. The extent of plaque formation is not correlated with cumulative asbestos exposure, and thus cannot be used to estimate the degree of exposure [26].

9.5 PLEURAL PLAQUES AND ASSOCIATED RISKS OF LUNG CANCER AND MESOTHELIOMA

Pleural plaques are indicators of exposure to asbestos, and are the most common manifestation of the inhalation, retention, and biologic effects of asbestos. Asbestos exposure is dose-dependently associated with risk of lung cancer. Among persons with comparable histories of asbestos exposure, the presence of plaques is reportedly associated with greater risks of mesothelioma and lung cancer compared to in subjects without plaques [27, 28]. However, these associations have mainly been established by a small number of studies based on chest X-ray, with limited numbers of subjects. There is no known biological activity or mechanism through which pleural plaques could promote carcinogenesis.

Pairon et al. reported a 6-year follow-up study of lung cancer mortality in an asbestos-related disease screening program in France. They found that lung cancer mortality was significantly associated with pleural plaques, in terms of both the unadjusted hazard ratio of 2.91 (95% CI: 1.49–5.70) and the adjusted hazard ratio of 2.41 (95% CI: 1.21–4.85). Based on these results, they concluded that pleural plaques may be an independent risk factor for lung cancer-related death among asbestos-exposed workers [29]. In a recent analysis of follow-up data from that study cohort, lung cancer incidence was significantly associated with pleural plaques, only among non-smokers after adjustment [30].

In another recent report, the presence of pleural plaques on radiologic imaging did not confer any additional increase of the lung cancer risk [31]. In that study, subjects from two cohorts underwent an annual examination by chest X-ray or low-dose CT scan, and outcome linkage was performed using national cancer and mortality registry data. The risk of lung cancer increased with cumulative exposure to cigarettes, asbestos, and presence of asbestosis, while the presence of pleural plaques did not confer any additional lung cancer risk. They concluded that asbestos exposure itself conferred a risk of lung cancer, not the presence of pleural plaques. According to these findings, smoking, and the history of occupational asbestos exposure itself appear to be major risk factors for developing lung cancer, and pleural plaques might be an additional risk factor among non-smokers.

An association between pleural plaques and pleural mesothelioma has been reported in some consensus statements [3, 32]. Two Swedish studies among asbestos-exposed shipyard or construction workers reported associations between pleural plaques and malignant pleural mesothelioma [33, 34]. Other authors have also reported an excess of mesothelioma linked to the observation of pleural plaques [28, 35, 36]. However, in two of these studies, subjects with pleural plaques were compared to the general population without asbestos exposure. Moreover, radiological assessments in these studies were performed using chest X-ray, which has poor sensitivity and specificity for the detection of pleural plaques [37].

In four regions of France, a large-scale screening program for asbestos-related diseases was initiated for workers previously exposed to asbestos [38]. Retired or unemployed workers who had previous occupational exposure to asbestos were invited to participate in the program to be screened for asbestos-related diseases, including by CT scan. A 7-year follow-up study was conducted among the 5287 male subjects for whom chest CT scans were available. The results showed a significant association between mesothelioma and pleural plaques [unadjusted hazard ratio (HR) = 8.9; 95% CI: 3.0–26.5; adjusted HR = 6.8; 95% CI: 2.2–21.4], after adjustment for time since first exposure and cumulative exposure index to asbestos [39].

9.6 CONCLUSION

Despite stringent regulation of asbestos use, asbestos-related disease is still a primary concern in the developed world. People face the risk of asbestos exposure in the workforce—for example, when removing insulation and other asbestos-containing products, or during the renovation and demolition of structures containing asbestos in developed countries. Persons identified as having a significant asbestos exposure history should be informed of the risk of progression of asbestos-related diseases, including the risk of malignancy, and especially the interaction between smoking and asbestos exposure in enhancing the risk of lung cancer.

Pleural plaques are very frequently observed in asbestos-exposed subjects. We have described several recent studies that have indicated associations between pleural plaques and risks of lung cancer and pleural mesothelioma. However, most subjects with pleural plaques or asbestosis do not develop cancer, and the risk of cancer is also relevant in persons exposed to asbestos without obvious signs of nonmalignant asbestos-related disease. At this time, it is considered reasonable and proper to monitor subjects with past asbestos exposure by regular medical check-ups, using chest X-ray and CT imaging, regardless of the presence or absence of imaging findings, such as pleural plaques or asbestosis.

REFERENCES

1. Becklake MR, Bagatin E, Neder JA. Asbestos-related diseases of the lungs and pleura: Uses, trends and management over the last century. *Int J Tuberc Lung Dis* 2007;11(4):356–69.
2. Jamrozik E, de Klerk N, Musk AW. Asbestos-related disease. *Intern Med J* 2011;41(5):372–80.
3. American Thoracic Society. Diagnosis and initial management of nonmalignant diseases related to asbestos. *Am J Respir Crit Care Med* 2004;170(6):691–715.
4. Kato K, Gemba K, Ashizawa K, Arakawa H, Honda S, Noguchi N, Honda S, Fujimoto N, Kishimoto T. Low-dose chest computed tomography screening of subjects exposed to asbestos. *Eur J Radiol* 2018;101:124–8.
5. Kipen HM, Lilis R, Suzuki Y, Valciukas JA, Selikoff IJ. Pulmonary fibrosis in asbestos insulation workers with lung cancer: A radiological and histopathological evaluation. *Br J Ind Med* 1987;44(2):96–100.
6. Gevenois PA, De Vuyst P, Dedeire S, Cosaert J, Vande Weyer R, Struyven J. Conventional and high-resolution CT in asymptomatic asbestos-exposed workers. *Acta Radiol* 1994;35(3):226–9.
7. Neri S, Boraschi P, Antonelli A, Falaschi F, Baschieri L. Pulmonary function, smoking habits, and high resolution computed tomography (HRCT) early abnormalities of lung and pleural fibrosis in shipyard workers exposed to asbestos. *Am J Ind Med* 1996;30(5):588–95.
8. Staples CA, Gamsu G, Ray CS, Webb WR. High resolution computed tomography and lung function in asbestos-exposed workers with normal chest radiographs. *Am Rev Respir Dis* 1989;139(6):1502–8.
9. Gevenois PA, de Maertelaer V, Madani A, Winant C, Sergent G, De Vuyst P. Asbestosis, pleural plaques and diffuse pleural thickening: Three distinct benign responses to asbestos exposure. *Eur Respir J* 1998;11(5):1021–7.
10. Staples CA. Computed tomography in the evaluation of benign asbestos-related disorders. *Radiol Clin North Am* 1992;30(6):1191–207.
11. Akira M, Morinaga K. The comparison of high-resolution computed tomography findings in asbestosis and idiopathic pulmonary fibrosis. *Am J Ind Med* 2016;59(4):301–6.
12. Arakawa H, Kishimoto T, Ashizawa K, Kato K, Okamoto K, Honma K, Hayashi S, Akira M. Asbestosis and other pulmonary fibrosis in asbestos-exposed workers: High-resolution CT features with pathological correlations. *Eur Radiol* 2016;26(5):1485–92.
13. Warnock ML, Isenberg W. Asbestos burden and the pathology of lung cancer. *Chest* 1986;89(1):20–6.
14. Markowitz SB, Levin SM, Miller A, Morabia A. Asbestos, asbestosis, smoking, and lung cancer. New findings from the North American insulator cohort. *Am J Respir Crit Care Med* 2013;188(1):90–6.
15. Reid A, de Klerk N, Ambrosini GL, Olsen N, Pang SC, Berry G, Musk AW. The effect of asbestosis on lung cancer risk beyond the dose related effect of asbestos alone. *Occup Environ Med* 2005;62(12):885–9.
16. Selikoff IJ, Lilis R, Nicholson WJ. Asbestos disease in United States shipyards. *Ann N Y Acad Sci* 1979;330:295–311.
17. American Thoracic Society. Medical section of the American lung association: The diagnosis of nonmalignant diseases related to asbestos. *Am Rev Respir Dis* 1986;134(2):363–8.
18. Peacock C, Copley SJ, Hansell DM. Asbestos-related benign pleural disease. *Clin Radiol* 2000;55(6):422–32.
19. Hourihane DO, Lessof L, Richardson PC. Hyaline and calcified pleural plaques as an index of exposure to asbestos. *Br Med J* 1966;1(5495):1069–74.
20. al Jarad N, Poulakis N, Pearson MC, Rubens MB, Rudd RM. Assessment of asbestos-induced pleural disease by computed tomography--Correlation with chest radiograph and lung function. *Respir Med* 1991;85(3):203–8.
21. Aberle DR, Gamsu G, Ray CS, Feuerstein IM. Asbestos-related pleural and parenchymal fibrosis: Detection with high-resolution CT. *Radiology* 1988;166(3):729–34.
22. Begin R, Boctor M, Bergeron D, Cantin A, Berthiaume Y, Peloquin S, Bisson G, Lamoureux G. Radiographic assessment of pleuropulmonary disease in asbestos workers: Posteroanterior, four view films, and computed tomograms of the thorax. *Br J Ind Med* 1984;41(3):373–83.

23. Katz D, Kreel L. Computed tomography in pulmonary asbestosis. *Clin Radiol* 1979;30(2):207–13.
24. Rogan WJ, Gladen BC, Ragan NB, Anderson HA. US prevalence of occupational pleural thickening. A look at chest X-rays from the first National Health and Nutrition Examination Survey. *Am J Epidemiol* 1987;126(5):893–900.
25. Miller JA, Zurlo JV. Asbestos plaques in a typical Veteran's hospital population. *Am J Ind Med* 1996;30(6):726–9.
26. Van Cleemput J, De Raeve H, Verschakelen JA, Rombouts J, Lacquet LM, Nemery B. Surface of localized pleural plaques quantitated by computed tomography scanning: No relation with cumulative asbestos exposure and no effect on lung function. *Am J Respir Crit Care Med* 2001;163(3 Pt 1):705–10.
27. Hillerdal G, Henderson DW. Asbestos, asbestosis, pleural plaques and lung cancer. *Scand J Work Environ Health* 1997;23(2):93–103.
28. Hillerdal G. Pleural plaques and risk for bronchial carcinoma and mesothelioma. A prospective study. *Chest* 1994;105(1):144–50.
29. Pairon JC, Andujar P, Rinaldo M, Ameille J, Brochard P, Chamming's S, Clin B, Ferretti G, Gislard A, Laurent F, Luc A, Wild P, Paris C. Asbestos exposure, pleural plaques, and the risk of death from lung cancer. *Am J Respir Crit Care Med* 2014;190(12):1413–20.
30. Gallet J, Laurent F, Paris C, Clin B, Gislard A, Thaon I, Chammings S, Gramond C, Ogier G, Ferretti G, Andujar P, Brochard P, Delva F, Pairon JC, Lacourt A *et al.* Pleural plaques and risk of lung cancer in workers formerly occupationally exposed to asbestos: Extension of follow-up. *Occup Environ Med* 2022 Aug 3;oemed-2022-108337.
31. Brims FJH, Kong K, Harris EJA, Sodhi-Berry N, Reid A, Murray CP, et al. Pleural plaques and the risk of lung cancer in asbestos-exposed subjects. *Am J Respir Crit Care Med* 2020;201(1):57–62.
32. Banks DE, Shi R, McLarty J, Cowl CT, Smith D, Tarlo SM, Franklin PJ, Musk AB, de Klerk NH. American College of Chest Physicians consensus statement on the respiratory health effects of asbestos. Results of a Delphi study. *Chest* 2009;135(6):1619–27.
33. Sanden A, Jarvholm B. A study of possible predictors of mesothelioma in shipyard workers exposed to asbestos. *J Occup Med* 1991;33(7):770–3.
34. Koskinen K, Pukkala E, Martikainen R, Reijula K, Karjalainen A. Different measures of asbestos exposure in estimating risk of lung cancer and mesothelioma among construction workers. *J Occup Environ Med* 2002;44(12):1190–6.
35. Karjalainen A, Pukkala E, Kauppinen T, Partanen T. Incidence of cancer among Finnish patients with asbestos-related pulmonary or pleural fibrosis. *Cancer Causes Control* 1999;10(1):51–7.
36. Reid A, de Klerk N, Ambrosini G, Olsen N, Pang SC, Musk AW. The additional risk of malignant mesothelioma in former workers and residents of Wittenoom with benign pleural disease or asbestosis. *Occup Environ Med* 2005;62(10):665–9.
37. Aberle DR, Balmes JR. Computed tomography of asbestos-related pulmonary parenchymal and pleural diseases. *Clin Chest Med* 1991;12(1):115–31.
38. Paris C, Thierry S, Brochard P, Letourneux M, Schorle E, Stoufflet A, et al. Pleural plaques and asbestosis: Dose- and time-response relationships based on HRCT data. *Eur Respir J* 2009;34(1):72–9.
39. Pairon JC, Laurent F, Rinaldo M, Clin B, Andujar P, Ameille J, Conso F, Pairon JC. Pleural plaques and the risk of pleural mesothelioma. *J Natl Cancer Inst* 2013;105(4):293–301.

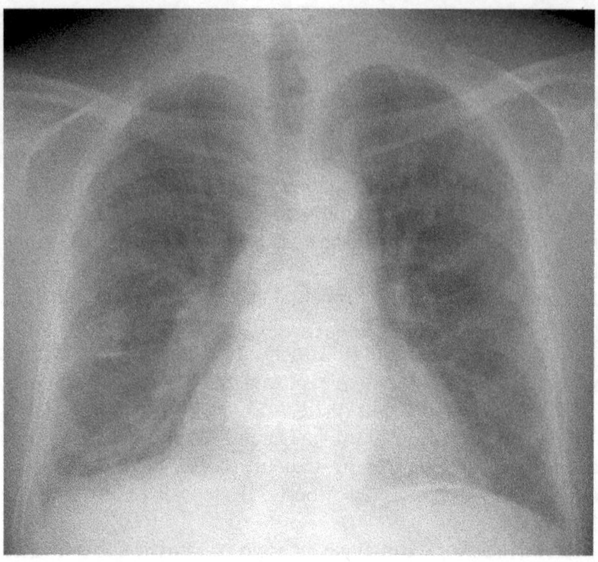

FIGURE 9.1 Radiographic image of asbestosis, presenting bilateral small irregular parenchymal opacities in the bilateral lower lobes of the lungs.

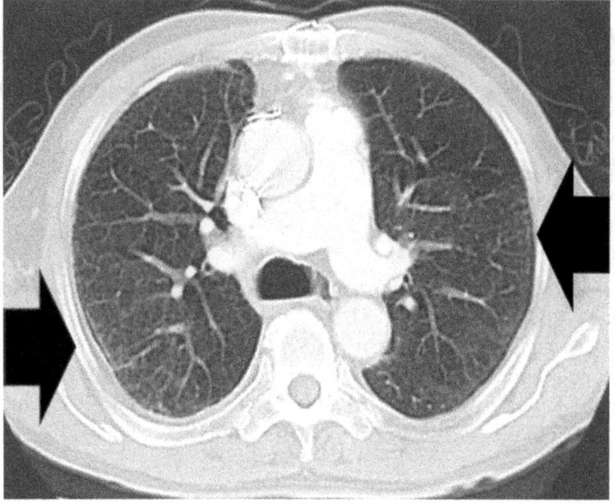

FIGURE 9.2 Computed tomography (CT) findings in asbestosis, presenting subpleural dot-like opacities and subpleural lines.

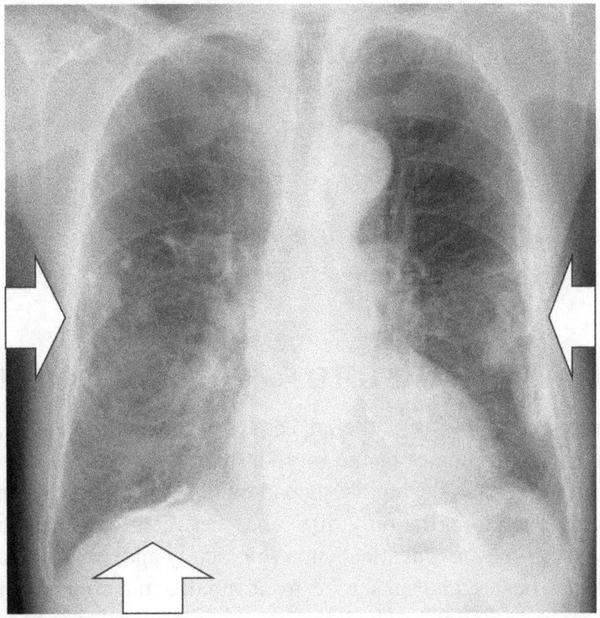

FIGURE 9.3 Typical pleural plaques on plain chest X-ray, presenting on the chest wall and diaphragm.

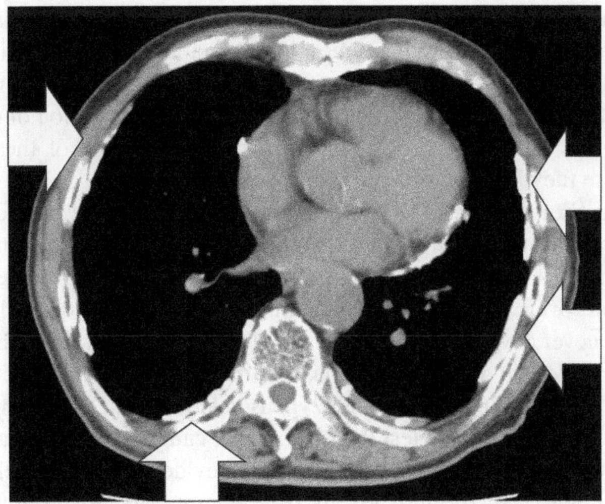

FIGURE 9.4 Typical pleural plaques on chest computed tomography (CT).

10 Mesothelioma in 2024
What's New?

Lydia Giannakou, Haining Yang, and Michele Carbone

10.1 MESOTHELIOMA: A NAME USED FOR THREE VERY DIFFERENT DISEASES

Mesothelioma originates from the mesothelial cells that form the pleura and the peritoneum. Mesothelial cells are the last remnant of the mesoderm that covers the celomic cavity, which is divided by the septum transversum during the second month of gestation to form the future thoracic and abdominal cavities. Therefore, the only difference between the pleura and the peritoneum is what they are exposed to, as they are identical embryologically and histologically. Since most mesotheliomas are caused by asbestos, and since asbestos is inhaled, pleural mesothelioma is much more frequent than peritoneal mesothelioma. The latter can however develop in heavily exposed asbestos workers as in these individuals asbestos may reach the peritoneal cavities in sufficient amounts to cause inflammation and mesothelioma.

Based on the "2021 WHO Classification of Tumors of the Pleura" [1], mesothelioma can be divided into three major types: mesothelioma in situ, localized mesothelioma, and diffuse mesothelioma (formerly called diffuse malignant mesothelioma). Moreover, there are three major histotypes used to characterize diffuse mesothelioma: epithelioid, sarcomatoid, and biphasic. Accurate diagnosis by adequate sampling from multiple areas, correct identification of cellular morphology, and immunohistochemical staining are important for the distinction of these different types of mesothelioma because they have very different prognoses.

Mesothelioma In Situ (MIS): MIS has been recently recognized as a distinct entity and is regarded as a precursor to invasive mesothelioma. A median time of 60 months for progression to invasive mesothelioma has been reported, but the significance of this example to the rest of mesotheliomas remains unproven. In other words, how many people are there who have in situ mesotheliomas and who will never develop mesotheliomas? The definition of MIS is that it is a noninvasive layer of mesothelial cells with a cuboidal shape, and inconspicuous nucleoli, that are negative for nuclear BAP1 or MTAP staining or show homozygous deletion of CDKN2A by Fluorescent In Situ Sybridization (FISH) (a more reliable test than MTAP). It can be present in patients with recurrent pleural effusions, without thoracoscopic, or radiographic evidence of mesothelioma. The diagnosis requires multiple samples (100–200 mm^2) from different areas to rule out invasion, in addition to clinical and radiologic information. The diagnosis of mesothelioma in situ is not reliable in carriers of germline BAP1 mutations, because in these patients the MIS lesions are always present, and are multiple, yet they rarely progress to invasive mesothelioma (Carbone et al., unpublished observations).

Localized Mesothelioma: This is an unusual form of mesothelioma that can be surgically resected and is associated with a better prognosis because when the tumor is entirely removed these patients are cured. It presents as a solitary, localized mass in imaging, and as a tumor with well-circumscribed borders in surgical specimens. Histologically, it has the same features as diffuse mesothelioma, but for the fact that it is contained in a defined region, without further spread [2]. This form of mesothelioma is often misdiagnosed, because histologically it is identical to diffuse mesothelioma, and therefore it is diagnosed as "mesothelioma". Unless the surgeon underscores the fact that the lesion is localized and the rest of the pleura or peritoneum is free of tumor, it will be

 DOI: 10.1201/9781003431909-10

assumed that mesothelioma means diffuse malignant mesothelioma, rather than the rare (although due to misdiagnosis is probably less rare than we think) localized form of mesothelioma. This is very unfortunate because these patients can be cured by surgical resection if the tumor is removed before it invades nearby tissues.

Diffuse Pleural Mesothelioma: Diffuse pleural mesothelioma presents as a pleural thickening or unequivocal tumor nodules visible on imaging that characteristically invade nearby tissues and organs. It has a diffuse pattern i.e. the disease is diffuse all over the right or left pleura or the peritoneum. According to data from the Surveillance, Epidemiology, and End Results (SEER) database and the National Cancer Database, the most common histologic type is epithelioid mesothelioma, which affects 68–69% of patients and is associated with a median survival of 9–14 months. Biphasic mesothelioma affects 12–13% of patients, with a median overall survival of about 10 months, and sarcomatoid mesothelioma, with a frequency of 18–19% of mesothelioma patients, is associated with a dismal median survival of 4–6 months [3, 4].

Epithelioid mesothelioma is composed of round, epithelioid cells with uniform architecture. Cellular characteristics that are associated with favorable prognosis are low nuclear grade, tubulopapillary, trabecular, or adenomatoid architectural patterns, and the presence of myxoid stroma. On the contrary, micropapillary or solid architecture, rhabdoid or pleomorphic cytologic features, and the presence of necrosis are associated with a worse prognosis. However, the differences in prognosis within the epithelioid group based on architectural patterns are measured in weeks to a few months, do not influence therapy, and the reliability at the single-patient level is minimal.

It has been proposed that the nuclear grade may be a predictor of prognosis, independent of age, procedural type, growth pattern, necrosis, and atypical mitosis [5]. Combining nuclear grade and the presence of necrosis, epithelioid mesothelioma is distinguished into four different groups with different prognoses, nuclear grade I tumors without necrosis (29 months median survival), nuclear grade I tumors with necrosis and grade II tumors without necrosis (16 months), nuclear grade II tumors with necrosis (10 months), and nuclear grade III tumors (8 months) [6]. In the latest update in 2020, the European Reference Network for Rare Solid Adult Cancers (EURACAN) and the International Association for the Study of Lung Cancer (IASLC) introduced a grading system for epithelioid diffuse pleural mesothelioma [7]. This system assigned tumors to low or high grade, taking into account nuclear features, mitotic rate, and necrosis. The value of this information is debatable, as the reliability at the single-patient level is minimal: whether a patient has a nuclear grade I, II, or III will not influence therapy.

On the other hand, it is important to identify sarcomatoid mesotheliomas, as these patients do not benefit from surgery or chemotherapy but may instead benefit from immunotherapy [8, 9]. Sarcomatoid mesothelioma is composed of elongated/spindle cells (length/width >2) arranged in solid sheets within a fibrous stroma. The so-called transitional architecture, comprising of cells that appear to be transitioning from epithelioid to spindle form and can be visualized well with a reticulin stain, is now included with the sarcomatoid mesotheliomas as it shares a similar poor prognosis [10]. Similarly, rhabdoid and pleomorphic features identify mesotheliomas that should be classified as sarcomatoid mesotheliomas as they share the same dismal prognosis.

Biphasic mesothelioma is composed of both epithelioid and sarcomatoid components. A minimum of 10% of either epithelioid or sarcomatoid component is usually considered the diagnostic criterion for biphasic mesothelioma in definitive surgical specimens. In the past it was 5%, showing how these criteria have a wide margin of error and depend on the rules we define. Practically speaking these mesotheliomas do almost as bad as sarcomatoid mesotheliomas, and a rule of thumb is that the more abundant the spindle component is, the worse the prognosis.

As a final comment, in recent years pathologists have managed to complicate an already complicated diagnosis adding architectural and nuclear requirements to the pathology report that do not influence therapy and that are unreliable as prognosticators at an individual level.

10.2 MESOTHELIOMA PATHOGENESIS

The factors that contribute to mesothelioma development have been extensively studied through the years. Until the end of the past century, mesothelioma was considered to be linked almost exclusively to asbestos exposure. Asbestos is the name used to identify 6 among over 400 mineral fibers present in nature, that were used for commercial purposes. Because these fibers were used commercially, millions of individuals worldwide were exposed. For regulatory purposes they were all named "asbestos" and their use was banned or strictly regulated in the Western world [11]. However, the remaining 390+ fibers present in nature can be carcinogenic to a greater or sometimes lesser extent than commercial asbestos [12]. Asbestos is a human carcinogen and the mechanisms through which asbestos and other fibers, such as erionite [13, 14], cause mesothelioma have been identified and are discussed in detail in a separate chapter in this book. Briefly, asbestos carcinogenesis has been linked to its deposition in the pleura and peritoneum where asbestos causes the release of HMGB1, a DAMP that kickstarts a chronic inflammatory process driven by HMGB1 that induces NFkB activation and TNF-alpha secretion. This process over time may promote the growth of mesothelioma [15–21]. NFkB was identified as a potential molecular target for mesothelioma therapy in 2011. Ranpirnase, with the commercial name Onconase, was the first cytotoxic ribonuclease ever discovered and developed for chemotherapy purposes. It targeted NFkB and showed some promising effects in a fraction of mesothelioma patients [22, 23]. However, a proposed target RNA therapy was still ahead of its time, and it took years until similar therapies were adopted.

As of 2019, 67 countries worldwide have implemented a complete ban on asbestos to eliminate occupational exposure that can cause mesothelioma [24]. Despite these measures, asbestos is still responsible for a high percentage of mesothelioma cases often among former asbestos workers. In addition, in many resource-limited countries, the asbestos ban has not been applied yet or the compliance rates are not satisfactory, leading to persistent exposure [25–28]. Even with a complete ban on occupational exposure to commercial asbestos, environmental exposure to asbestos and asbestos-like fibers is difficult to control and is often under-reported. Patients may be exposed in areas with naturally occurring fibers, in residential areas with proximity to industrial sources of asbestos, or in their household, if family members are occupationally exposed [27–29]. It would be helpful to standardize the reporting methods of asbestos exposure, so that reliable exposure information can be collected, and reliable conclusions on the true incidence of asbestos-related mesothelioma can be drawn [27, 28].

The appearance of clustered mesothelioma cases within the same families led to the discovery of germline mutations in BAP1 and later of other tumor suppressor genes that when mutated may cause the development of mesotheliomas, which characteristically are less aggressive than asbestos-induced mesothelioma (see below). Further research on the genetic background of tumors and their microenvironment revealed important genomic alterations and interactions that play an important role in the biological behavior of these tumors [27]. Studies have also revealed the causative effect of radiation and chronic inflammation on mesothelioma growth, while some cases have also been attributed to "spontaneous" tumor development [30, 31].

10.2.1 RADIATION

Radiation therapy for solid tumors and lymphomas has been associated with the development of mesothelioma. Exposure to both lower doses of radiation for a prolonged period or higher doses for a shorter period has been linked with a significantly increased risk for mesothelioma development. An analysis of SEER data on mesothelioma patients that had received external beam radiation for previous malignancies failed to reveal a dose–response relationship between exposure and mesothelioma development [32]. This may be attributed to the variability of dose distribution from different sources of exposure that may not allow for a precise calculation. The different energy deposition at the cell level can affect genetic damage and carcinogenesis [33]. The observed effect can also be explained by the limitations of the SEER database, which only provided follow-up data for 20 years. This does not allow for the assessment of relative risk in longer latency periods that could reveal a linear relationship between exposure and mesothelioma development, following the same trend with asbestos exposure. Furthermore, it appears likely that individuals carrying germline mutations of DNA repair genes – ATM, BAP1, BLM, BRCA1/2, TP53, etc. – are more susceptible than others to the carcinogenic effects of radiation. Radiation-induced mesothelioma presents in younger patients compared to asbestos-induced mesothelioma, in equal ratios between male and female patients, and a recorded latency period varying from about 5–50 years. It has a significantly better prognosis than asbestos-induced mesothelioma (median survival 32.5 versus 12.7 months). It often presents with unusual histologic types (pleomorphic, myxoid, clear cell, or signet ring cell) in up to 32% of these patients [34, 35]. In a Dutch study of patients who were treated for Hodgkin's lymphoma, mesothelioma risk was further increased in patients who had received both chemotherapy and radiotherapy [36]. Occupational radiation exposure was also linked to mesothelioma in patients working at atomic energy facilities, and radiation technologists [35]. However, studies on occupational radiation and asbestos exposure found that asbestos could be a confounding factor, responsible for some of these cases [35, 37].

10.2.2 The Role of Genetic and BAP1 Mutations in Mesothelioma Causation

The role of genetics was discovered at the beginning of this century by Carbone and collaborators as they studied families in Cappadocia, Turkey, in which 50% of all deaths were caused by mesothelioma. These rates were significantly higher than what was observed in heavily exposed asbestos workers which at most had an incidence of 5–8%. In these families, mesotheliomas appeared at a younger age and presented a 1:1 male-to-female ratio, and susceptibility to mesothelioma was transmitted in a Mendelian fashion [38]. This led to the hypothesis of the existence of a predisposing inherited mutation [38]. This hypothesis was later proved by the same team of researchers who identified inactivating truncating BAP1 germline mutations in all affected family members in two US families with a very high incidence of mesothelioma and no history of occupational exposure to asbestos [39]. Subsequent studies revealed that all carriers of heterozygous germline BAP1 mutations have developed some type of cancer, mesothelioma developing in 30% of mutation carriers [40–42]. In addition to mesothelioma, the most frequent malignancies in carriers of germline BAP1 mutations are uveal and cutaneous melanoma, while clear cell renal cell carcinoma bladder and breast carcinomas are also frequent. This novel medical condition has been named the "BAP1 cancer syndrome", to distinguish it from tumor predisposition syndromes in which only a fraction of affected individuals develop cancer [43]. These patients characteristically have much improved survival compared to sporadic mesothelioma [41, 43, 44].

BAP1 is a deubiquitylase, that is localized in the nucleus and the cytoplasm [40, 45].

BAP1 modulates the activities of multiple proteins and thus BAP1 simultaneously regulates cell proliferation, differentiation and cell death, and has an important role in metabolic processes. In the nucleus, BAP1 modulates gene expression, DNA replication, and DNA repair processes [46]. In the cytoplasm, BAP1 modulates Ca^{2+} signaling in the Endoplasmic Reticulum (ER), where it binds to and deubiquitilates type 3 inositol 1,4,5-trisphosphate receptor (IP3R3), regulating Ca^{2+} release into the cytosol and mitochondria, promoting apoptosis. The importance of this interaction is evident in cells with BAP1 mutations. These cells, upon exposure to asbestos, radiation, and other carcinogens, or during cell division, accumulate DNA damage due to loss of BAP1 DNA repair function and, at the same time, cannot undergo apoptosis, due to reduced BAP1 cytoplasmic function. As a result, these cells keep accumulating genetic damage and are prone to subsequent malignant transformation [47]. Heterozygous BAP1 mutations induce a Warburg effect, in other words, these cells switch their metabolism from Oxidative Phosphorylation (OXPHOS) to glycolysis, to sustain their growth [48]. This is unusual as a Warburg effect is characteristic of tumor cells that switch their metabolism to survive in hypoxia. Instead, normal cells from individuals carrying germline BAP1 mutations derive a large part of their energy through aerobic glycolysis even in the presence of oxygen. Specifically, cells with reduced or absent BAP1 levels show reduced mitochondrial OXPHOS and increased aerobic glycolysis and lactate production. The increased levels of secreted lactate create a cancer-growth-promoting environment, while this property of mutant cells can favor their survival during metabolic stress [48]. Recent work demonstrated that BAP1 binds and stabilizes the hypoxia-induced factors (HIF1-alpha) thus modulating cellular responses to hypoxia. Cells with reduced BAP1 levels exhibited significantly reduced activity of HIFs, a finding that may be linked to the reduced aggressiveness and the improved prognosis of mesotheliomas in patients with BAP1 mutations [49].

Moreover, BAP1 modulates the secretion of HMGB1 in the extracellular space. HMGB1 has been identified as an important regulator for mesothelioma development that can serve as a biomarker and a potential therapeutic target [50]. BAP1 forms a trimer with the Histone Deacetylase 1 (HDAC1) and HMGB1, regulating the stability of the complex and retaining HMGB1 in the nucleus [51]. In cells with reduced BAP1 levels, HDAC1 is degraded and HMGB1 becomes acetylated and released in the extracellular space, promoting inflammation that favors mesothelioma growth. Increased secretion of HMGB1 from BAP1 mutant cells induced malignant transformation of cells exposed to asbestos, in the presence of TNFα. Accordingly, patients carrying BAP1 mutations showed increased levels of circulating HMGB1 and these levels further increased when patients developed mesothelioma [44, 51].

10.2.3 Additional Factors Linked to Mesothelioma

The SV40 DNA tumor virus is a potent carcinogen that causes malignant transformation of human mesothelial cells and mesothelioma when injected into hamsters [52, 53]. In tissue culture, SV40 is much more potent than asbestos in inducing human mesothelial cell transformation, being capable of immortalizing these cells, which grow into cell lines that cause cancer when injected into nude mice [54–56]. Moreover, SV40 and asbestos synergized in causing malignant transformation of human mesothelial cells in tissue culture [57]. Since infectious SV40 contaminated human polio vaccines until 1963 in the USA and until the late 1970s in the countries that formed the former Soviet Union, there was reason for concern [58–61]. However epidemiological studies were inconclusive, because it was not possible to establish who had received and who had not received contaminated polio vaccines and therefore a panel of the Institute of Medicine (IOM), now renamed the US National Academy of Medicine concluded that it was not possible to definitively decide if SV40-infected polio vaccines had contributed to mesothelioma and the development of other cancers in humans [62].

10.2.4 Genomic Alterations in Mesothelioma

Studies on two Italian cohorts with a total of 89 mesothelioma patients, revealed that these patients carried germline mutations in BAP1, CDKN2A, and also in several DNA repair genes. The authors proposed that these mutations contributed to the development of mesothelioma upon low asbestos exposure, supporting the hypothesis of gene–environment interaction in mesothelioma [63, 64], originally proposed by studies in mice [65]. In patients carrying mutations in these genes, cells can accumulate more DNA damage after shorter exposure to lower asbestos concentration leading to mesothelioma development. For example, it was proved that mutations in Brca1 in rats caused impaired iron metabolism and ferroptosis resistance, and facilitated the development of mesothelioma after asbestos exposure. Brca1 mutant animals also had a higher rate of chromosomal deletions in CDKN2a/2b [66]. Studies in animals have helped elucidate the role of genetics and the interplay with asbestos exposure in mesothelioma carcinogenesis. A recently reported case of mesothelioma clustering in the same bovine herd, in senile animals without asbestos exposure, raised suspicion for familial germline genetic alterations in animals that lead to increased incidence of this rare cancer [67].

As for somatic genetic damage (acquired DNA damage after birth, most prominent in cancer cells), Guo et al. reported frequent genetic alterations in BAP1, CDKN2A, and NF2. Remarkably they reported a very low number of mutations, comparable to pediatric tumors, and somewhat unexpected in a malignancy associated with exposure to a human carcinogen [68]. Similar results were reported by Lo Iacono et al., who identified genetic variations in p53/DNA repair and phosphatidylinositol 3-kinase pathways, using a targeted NGS panel [69, 70] Subsequently, a comprehensive mesothelioma genomic analysis by Bueno et al., reported the inactivation of tumor suppressor genes with distinct expression patterns between mesothelioma sub-types and showed that combination of methods for detection of genomic alterations increases the mutation discovery rate and provides accurate results [71]. This study characterized copy number alterations, gene fusions, and splicing alterations as mechanisms leading to inactivation of tumor suppressor genes. A study confirming these results showed that mesothelioma had a very low somatic mutation burden, with a rate of <2 non-synonymous mutations per megabase. The copy number variations comprised mostly of deletions rather than amplifications, showing that mesothelioma development is driven largely by loss of function in tumor suppressor genes [72].

Using targeted NGS in a Japanese cohort of mesothelioma patients, Yoshikawa et al., found frequent somatic mutations in genes involved in DNA repair and chromatin-remodeling. The most commonly mutated genes were BAP1, CDKN2A, PBRM1, CHEK2, PALB2, SMARCC1, BRCA2, MLH1, POT1, MRE11A, NF2, TP53, LATS2, SETD2, and SETDB1 [73, 74]. Yoshikawa et al., found that the mechanisms responsible for the inactivation of NF2, BAP1, and SETD2 were gene fusions and splice alterations. In a separate study, gene fusions between the DNA repair and cellular aging gene EWSR1 and ATF-1 were detected in a subset of younger mesothelioma patients without asbestos exposure and with retained BAP1. These fusions were correlated with distinct phenotypes and epithelioid morphology fields[75]. In a cohort of 79 mesothelioma patients, Sanger sequencing and targeted NGS revealed mutations in genes implicated in tumor suppression, chromatin regulation, homologous recombination, transcriptional regulation, and RNA processing [74, 76]. A cohort of 88 mesothelioma patients that were tested with NGS revealed similar results, with the discovery of mutations in genes implicated in DNA repair during oxidative stress (RECQL4), mismatch repair (MSH3), and double-strand break repair (BARD1) [77]. Heterozygous BLM gene mutations, that cause the Bloom syndrome when biallelic, have also been linked to increased susceptibility to mesothelioma [78].

In 2016, Yoshikawa et al., discovered that mesotheliomas contained a high number of genetic rearrangements caused by chromothripsis. Specifically, the authors reported a high rate of deletions in chromosome 3p21, where the BAP1 locus is located, using comparative high-density genomic hybridization arrays (aCGH) and targeted NGS on mesothelioma biopsies. They found that the somatic alterations detected were produced by chromothripsis [79]. Subsequent studies proposed that chromothripsis in mesothelioma resulted in the creation of neo-antigens that enhanced the clonal expansion of tumor-infiltrating T cells, contributing to higher tumor immunogenicity [80–82].

The Hippo pathway has been investigated in various studies and alterations of this pathway have been linked to mesothelioma. Key regulators of the Hippo pathway are LATS1/2 kinases that phosphorylate downstream effector yes-associated protein (YAP) and TAZ and control cell growth, mobility, and invasion. Moreover, BAP1 regulates the Hippo pathway in the development of pancreatic adenocarcinoma [83]. Inactivation of the pathway leads to the accumulation of YAP in the nucleus and the upregulation of oncogenes. Amplification of YAP locus 11q22 has been observed in mesothelioma biopsies, and expression of constitutively active YAP in mesothelial cell lines was linked with augmented in vitro growth and tumor formation after cell injection in mice [84]. In a study using WES and RNA sequencing, a chromosomal translocation leading to a novel fusion of LATS1 and PSEN1 genes was identified, and the fusion could no longer phosphorylate YAP and suppress mesothelioma cell growth. Through pathway-targeted NGS, somatic mutations in the Hippo pathway genes (NF2, LATS2, RASSF1, and SAV1) were identified [85]. NF2 is an important component of the Hippo pathway, and it regulates the activity of LATS1/2. NF2 loss through mutations in the 22q12 coding region post-translational modifications is found in a high percentage of mesothelioma tumors [86]. NF2 also activates mTORC1 signaling, and staining of human mesothelioma samples revealed hyperactivation of mTORC1 [86, 87]. However, 90% of mesothelioma with NF2 genetic mutations express normal NF2 levels by immunohistochemistry: this raises concerns about the biological and clinical significance of these mutations [69, 70].

10.2.5 Germline Genetic Testing

Mesothelioma patients benefit from genetic testing because the detection of pathogenic mutations will influence their management and surveillance strategy. Carriers of germline mutations in BAP1 have significantly better prognosis than patients who develop sporadic mesothelioma, with recent studies showing a median 5–7 years overall survival, significantly higher than the control mesothelioma population [76, 88]. Physicians should be aware of the characteristics that create a high suspicion for inheritance of mesothelioma predisposing mutations. Members of families with BAP1 associated cancers clustering, patients with multiple malignancies or family history of mesothelioma, or patients who develop mesothelioma at a younger age, women with peritoneal mesothelioma – a type of mesothelioma presently rarely associated with asbestos exposure – should be referred for genetic testing [27, 41]. The testing panel should cover BAP1 as well as other DNA repair and tumor suppressor genes known to cause other cancer or tumor predisposition syndromes. All first-degree relatives of patients carrying germline BAP1 mutations or mutations of other tumor predisposing genes should be tested, and included in early detection screening programs. To identify the patients carrying BAP1 germline mutations, a family history of MM, BAP1-associated cancers, multiple malignancies, or age younger than 50 years are useful clues that can guide physicians to the correct diagnosis. In a cohort of 79 patients with mesothelioma that met these criteria, only 28% reported asbestos exposure, while half of them had germline BAP1 mutations, and their median age at diagnosis and median survival was 54 years and 5–7 years, respectively [76, 89]. In a recent preliminary study, researchers applied selection criteria to identify mesothelioma patients carrying BAP1 germline mutations. These criteria were based on age at diagnosis, presence of BAP1 syndrome-related cancers in patients or their family members, and clinical prognostic factors and they were able to correctly identify all patients in the cohort carrying BAP1 mutations [89]. Surveillance programs have been proven to be both accurate and cost-effective, leading to early diagnosis and improved survival of cancer patients, and to lower overall healthcare costs [90]. Early detection of cancer is not only linked to significantly improved overall survival but it can also make the patients and their affected relatives eligible for more effective therapeutic options or for enrollment in clinical trials. About 8% of carriers of germline BAP1 mutations develop meningiomas, often rhabdoid meningiomas which are a rare form of aggressive meningiomas that require therapy because they may cause the patient's demise [91].

10.2.6 In Vitro Studies

BAP1 loss has been associated with resistance to gemcitabine, but variable sensitivity to platinum chemotherapy and BAP1 status may also predict the sensitivity to PARP inhibitors [92, 93]. In vitro studies on mesothelioma cells with BAP1 mutation or BAP1 siRNA treatment revealed decreased sensitivity to gemcitabine. Further analysis revealed that gemcitabine-induced apoptosis was much faster in the wild-type cells and that DNA double-strand breaks were significantly decreased in mutant and silenced cells [94]. Recent studies identified RRM1 and RRM2, both parts of the ribonucleotide reductase complex as possible gene targets to increase lethality in BAP1-proficient cells. This work also showed that loss of BAP1 catalytic activity in mesothelioma cells induces chemoresistance to gemcitabine and hydroxyurea, both selective inhibitors of RRM1 and RRM2 [92, 93]. A retrospective cohort that performed genomic analysis on samples collected from patients with resectable mesothelioma who received chemotherapy revealed that BAP1 status is a potential biomarker for chemotherapy resistance. The predictive ability was also confirmed in in vitro studies of mesothelioma cells silenced for BAP1 that displayed increased cisplatin chemoresistance [95].

10.2.7 Genomic Testing of Mesotheloma DNA

The identification of specific mutations in the mesothelioma DNA can help physicians choose the right therapy for each patient. In a retrospective cohort from Denmark that was independently validated in a cohort from Australia, researchers proved the beneficial effect of BAP1 loss on the survival of patients treated with standard chemotherapy. The Denmark cohort revealed a survival benefit of 20.1 months in patients with somatic BAP1 loss in tumors versus 7.3 months in patients that retained BAP1 in tumors, after treatment with cisplatin-pemetrexed. The respective comparison in the Australian cohort resulted in 19.6 versus 11.1 in the two groups. In a combined cohort of mesothelioma patients from the Thoracic Medical Oncology Clinic of the National Cancer Institute (NCI) and from the University of Chicago, germline mutations of BAP1, CHEK2, PALB2, BRCA2, MLH1, POT1, TP53, and MRE11A were linked to increased sensitivity to platinum chemotherapy. Median survival was longer in patients carrying germline mutations in the identified genes and remained significant when adjusting for gender and age at diagnosis [96–98]. The effect of mutations in DNA repair genes on drug sensitivity was further investigated in a study where NGS analysis with a targeted panel of 107 cancer-predisposing genes was conducted in mesothelioma patients. The analysis revealed pathogenic variants in genes involved in DNA repair (BRCA1, BRIP1, CHEK2, SLX4, FLCN, and BAP1). To reveal the significance of these mutations, a 3D mesothelioma cell model with defective ATM expression was created to test synthetic lethality after treatment with tazemetostat, a selective inhibitor of EZH2. EZH2 is part of the polycomb repressive complex 2, is overexpressed in mesothelioma, and is important in cancer development, progression, and metastasis [99]. Targeting EZH2 in a context of defective DNA repair, created through ATM loss, led to increased DNA damage, and significantly reduced size and viability of the 3D cell spheroids [74].

The map of genes affecting mesothelioma patient's survival was further expanded with a study that identified a genomic signature of 48 genes, predictive of response to therapy and survival outcomes. In this study, genomic sequencing was performed on patients' blood and tumor tissues and transcriptomic analysis was conducted on the tumor immune microenvironment samples. The increased expression of 48 genes was associated with poorer survival, and the results were validated through two independent cohorts. Enrichment analysis of these genes revealed their implication in cell cycle processes, DNA repair, chromosome organization, telomere organization, and proliferation. On this dataset, researchers applied the SELECT approach, a valuable tool that uses transcriptomic data to predict the drug response of a given cancer, and effectively predicted the response to PD-1 inhibition [100, 101].

10.3 INCIDENCE TRENDS IN THE LAST DECADE

In 2020, the latest year for which incidence data are available, in the United States, 2,681 new cases of mesothelioma were reported, of which 1,900 were men, and 781 were women. In the same year, 2,376 people died of mesothelioma [102]. Based on data retrieved from the National Cancer Database, from 2004 to 2020, the absolute number of diagnoses is increasing, but the incidence rate presents a decreasing trend.

The mean age at diagnosis of mesothelioma in the last decade was 60–70 years, and the majority of patients were male, white, with no other reported comorbidities. A total of 78.5% had epithelioid malignancies and most cases were diagnosed at Stage III (62.3%), or Stage IV (37.7%), although in the last decade there was an increase in patients diagnosed at Stage I, from 13.5% to 15.6%. A large percentage of samples did not report the histologic subtype, however, this percentage is significantly improved compared to the last decade. The percentage of patients who were offered some type of treatment was 73.9%, a significant increase compared to previous cohorts: most of them (50.5%)

received chemotherapy, 27.6% had surgery, and 8.6% of them received additional radiation. In 5.4% of them, immunotherapy was also included in the therapeutic strategy. It is noted that more patients in the last decade were referred to palliative care programs (8.8% in 2004, and 13.4% in 2020). The median overall survival was 10.3 months and it notably increased to 12.1 months in the last three years of the cohort compared to data from the previous decade, where median survival was 8.97 months. A total of 38.7% of the cases had reported asbestos exposure prior to diagnosis [103, 104]. A study published in 2023, using data from the Global Cancer Observatory, Cancer Incidence in Five Continents Plus, and Global Burden of Disease calculated the epidemiological trends for mesothelioma. Globally, there were 30,870 cases reported, with a significant geographic disparity, and an overall decreasing trend in incidence, especially in the population group of 15–49 years. In accordance with these numbers, a study based on 47 registries in the US, covering almost 97% of the population, reported an overall decreased incidence, with variations between age groups. Higher rates were observed in patients over 85 years old, whereas incidence was decreased in younger patients. Pleural mesothelioma was reported in 84.9% of cases, and peritoneal mesothelioma in 7.2% of them [105]. It is important to note however, that this number may be an underestimation of the true disease incidence, due to the inaccuracy of the available diagnostic measures, the misclassification of cases, and the under-reporting in some developing countries, due to low coverage and analytical capacities of registries [106]. In general, diagnoses of mesothelioma from developing countries, especially countries in which immunohistochemistry is not used routinely, are unreliable [27]. Rates of misdiagnosis of about 50% from some countries have been reported; therefore, outside of the so-called "Western World" it is not possible to accurately estimate the incidence of mesothelioma [107, 108].

Based on the reported data, male patients were more frequently affected, however, an increase in the overall trend in female patients was observed. In the US, an increase in the annual number of deaths in female patients was reported in 2020, compared to 1999 [109]. Female patients were younger, with mostly epithelioid histology and better overall survival. The percentage of female patients who received cancer-directed surgery or chemotherapy was lower than male patients [110, 111]. Based on these retrospective data, overall, older age, male gender, histological grade, histotype, advanced stage at diagnosis, treatment at non-academic facilities relative to academic facilities, Medicaid insurance relative to commercial insurance, and greater comorbidities were, as expected, correlated with worse outcomes. Higher income, receipt of cancer-directed surgery, and receipt of chemotherapy were associated with better survival outcomes. It is worth noting however that surgical treatment is an approach with a debatable beneficial effect, that historically has been proved to be useful for only selected patients [104, 112, 113].

Higher incidence was observed in more developed regions and the areas with the highest age-standardized rate were Australia and New Zealand, Northern, Western and Southern Europe, and Southern Africa [103]. On the contrary, Caribbean, Eastern, Central, and Western Africa and South-Central Asia had lower incidence rates. Mesothelioma incidence was positively correlated with male sex and asbestos exposure, and countries with high human development index and higher gross domestic product per capita had higher incidence rates [114, 115].

The high incidence rates in developed regions may be linked to previous asbestos use during the industrialization of these countries and to more accurate diagnosis. Differences in incidence also reflect different access to healthcare across regions, and different diagnostic accuracy between healthcare centers. The definitive histological diagnosis of mesothelioma requires a complex panel of immunohistochemical markers that may not be available in medical centers of low-income countries.

The increased knowledge of the carcinogenic effect of asbestos led to improved regulations on asbestos use in the last decades, however, despite asbestos being characterized as a group 1 carcinogen by WHO, not all forms of asbestos are regulated. Indeed, in developing countries asbestos is still being produced. Moreover, the actual effect of asbestos regulation will be more evident in the future decades, due to the known latency between asbestos exposure and mesothelioma development. According to a projection based on data from the Global Burden of Disease Database, the age-standardized incidence and mortality rates are predicted to decrease over the next two decades [106, 114, 115].

Regarding the difference in incidence between the two sexes, it was shown that the male population was mostly part of the industrial mining, shipbuilding, and construction settings, and was affected by occupational asbestos exposure in the past century. A decreasing trend in males reflects the decrease of asbestos usage in these settings and, on the other hand, the increase in female patients affected can be attributed primarily to genetics, and in some cases also to non-occupational, environmental exposure, and or genetics, as well as to prior radiation therapy for gynecological malignancies. Patients may be exposed to an asbestos-containing environment, or have second-hand exposure from their familial and domestic environment. For this reason, it is useful to include the work history of a partner or household member who has lived with the mesothelioma patient in the work history questionnaire that tries to identify exposure to asbestos [116].

It is also important to take into account the overall aging of the population and the shift of population age pyramids in modern industrialized countries. Life expectancy is rising in most countries, mostly due to the overall improved quality of life and public health services. Due to the accumulation of genetic damage with older age, the cancer rates, mesothelioma included, inevitably increase [117, 118].

10.4 CLINICAL PRESENTATION AND DIAGNOSTIC WORKUP

The most common clinical symptoms of mesothelioma patients are cough, shortness of breath, fatigue, and weight loss. Chest discomfort may present due to the development of pleural effusions, disease progression, and encasement of the pleural cavity by the tumor. Approximately 70% of patients in an early stage will present with dyspnea due to pleural effusions. Unresolved pleural effusions, especially hemorrhagic effusions, are a warning sign of malignancy, and a patient with pleural effusions and a history of asbestos exposure should be closely monitored, because early diagnosis of the disease is linked with improved prognosis. Invasion of the chest wall in advanced stages may cause secondary bone pain or neuropathic pain, and difficulty breathing from damage to the intercostal nerves. Cough and hemoptysis may also present in bronchial involvement, and further progression may lead to superior vena cava compression. Bloating and abdominal discomfort may present in patients who develop ascites due to secondary dissemination of pleural mesothelioma or from primary peritoneal mesothelioma. Many patients may be asymptomatic and the diagnosis of the disease may occur as an incidental finding during imaging studies for another condition.

10.4.1 Imaging Modalities

The first diagnostic step in a patient with suspected pleural effusion is investigation with a chest X-ray and a computed tomography (CT) scan. After thoracentesis and drainage of the pleural effusion, cytologic analysis is performed on the collected fluid. However, for a definitive diagnosis of pleural mesothelioma a histologic sample is most often needed [27, 103, 118].

Chest X-Ray (CXR) has a limited role in the workup of mesothelioma diagnosis and is mostly used to exclude other diagnoses. The appearance of unilateral pleural effusion with ipsilateral lung volume loss and pleural thickening is characteristic of a malignancy, but is an indication of advanced disease. Useful findings of CXR in early stages that raise the suspicion for mesothelioma can be a drug-resistant unilateral pleural effusion, unilateral lobulated pleural thickening, or multiple peripherally distributed intrathoracic masses. The British Thoracic Society, suggests that a physician should keep a high level of suspicion in patients with clinical symptoms and a history of asbestos exposure, even in the absence of X-ray findings, and should refer the patients for further investigation [119].

The most important imaging tool for the diagnosis, staging, and follow-up of mesothelioma patients is computed tomography (CT). Characteristic findings in the CT are unilateral pleural effusion, circumferential pleural thickening, mediastinal pleura thickening, interlobular septal thickening, or mediastinal/pericardial/chest wall infiltration, lymphadenopathy and benign calcified or non-calcified plaques, indicating asbestosis. A circumferential or nodular pleural thickening, a large parietal thickening, and the involvement of the mediastinal pleura are findings that lead the physician to suspect a malignant cause rather than a benign one. Sometimes, the distinction of the malignant tumor from the surrounding normal structures may be challenging, as the tumor has similar attenuation with the surrounding tissue [120]. To avoid inaccuracies in pre-operative staging, an intravenous contrast agent is administered. The typical delay time between contrast administration and image acquisition is 40–60s, however, a recent imaging clinical trial revealed an optimal delay interval of 230–300s for CT image capture. This change in time interval reveals the importance of timing for the limitation of inaccurate staging estimation [121].

Magnetic Resonance Imaging (MRI), especially with contrast-enhanced T1 sequences with fat suppression, is superior to CT in identifying infiltration of the chest wall, mediastinal space and nerve structures, and involvement of bones, muscles, cardiac tissues, or endothoracic fascia. The administration of IV contrast is preferred, with studies reporting an ideal interval from administration to image acquisition of 150–300s[121]. MRI, together with 18-Fluorodeoxyglucose positron-emission tomography CT (FDG PET/CT) are especially useful in the pre-operative evaluation of surgical candidates, to better define anatomic planes and characterize cellularity, vascularity, and metabolic activity of the tumor [120, 122].

Volumetric analysis, is an important evaluation, since data has shown that overall survival is negatively correlated with tumor volumes. Tumor volume can be assessed by CT, PET/CT, or MRI, however, Diffusion Weighted Imaging (DWI) through MRI is the preferred modality to estimate tumor volume and is used to identify short- or long-term overall survivors [120]. MRI volumetric analysis models have been proven to be quicker and more reproducible than CT models, and they have correctly predicted overall patient survival based on tumor volumes, in pilot studies. The predictive strength of the models was further increased when patients with metastatic disease were excluded [123, 124]. Volumetric analysis can also be used for therapeutic planning and monitoring disease progression.

Positron-emission tomography (PET) with 18F-FDG offers higher sensitivity and lower intra-observer variability for staging, however it underestimates staging, and it needs careful standardization in order for it to be reliable and reproducible, especially in the clinical trial setting [120]. The same imaging protocol should be applied to all patients, with the same camera and the same reconstruction algorithms. In that way, the researchers can ensure the high quality and comparability of the collected data. Moreover, the exact dose of the FDG that is administered should be calculated based on body weight or body surface area, and both dose and timing of administration should be recorded. Strict recording and regulation of pre-imaging glucose blood levels should be applied to all patients. The suggested timing of imaging after FDG administration is 60 minutes. A non-enhanced CT scan should be acquired first, from head to proximal thighs, and the PET scan should follow immediately, with the patient remaining in the same position throughout the whole procedure. Timing and image capture intervals should be specified and remain constant, so that the total acquisition times will not vary between patients [122].

PET scan has proved to be a valuable prognostic tool, with higher uptake being correlated with overall worse survival. Using PET scan, volumetric parameters like Metabolic Tumor Volume showed better performance in predicting survival than the typically used Standardized Uptake Volume, the most common measure of tumor activity in clinical practice. FDG uptake has also been associated with higher expression of GLUT-1 transporters that reflect increased glucose metabolism, and upregulation of angiogenesis, proliferation, cell cycle regulation, and hypoxia-related factors. In order to establish a reliable predictive protocol, a stricter standardization process needs to be applied, for the definition of the uptake cut-off values and the limitation of heterogeneity of results [125].

PET scan images can be subjected to radiomics, a recently established mathematics analysis of tumor characteristics such as shape, intensity, and texture. The analysis normalizes the heterogenic biologic characteristics of the tumors, and offers more information on the biologic behavior of the tumors. Recently tested radiomics prognostic models have shown good discriminative power in predicting patient overall survival and characterizing the levels of tumor control [125, 126].

Another important application of PET scan is in the setting of preclinical research. This field is particularly important for the understanding of tumor biology, growth patterns, and interaction with the tumor microenvironment. It can also be used in the development of new therapeutic agents. More specifically, the distribution, metabolism, and therapeutic effect of new agents can be tested in vivo. Animal models can be also used for the creation of xenograft tumors, through cell implantation and the study of tumor development. 18-FDG PET using a small animal PET camera is the most ideal tool for monitoring tumor growth and response to therapy in preclinical studies. 18-F-fluoromisonidazole (FMISO) PET scan can be also used in the preclinical setting for monitoring hypoxia in tumors, and changes in intra-tumor drug efficacy through hypoxia modulation [121].

The latest advance in imaging modalities is the use of Convolutional Neural Networks (CNN) for the automatic segmentation of tumors based on annotated CT scan images. The purpose of these deep-learning models is to create a high-resolution assembly of the tumor structure, predicting the missing pixels using mirroring of the input images. A newly tested CNN model showed significant overlap with previous segmentation methods, using a smaller number of images for training and providing very accurate segmentations [127].

10.4.2 Staging

Attention should be given to the recent changes in the tumor staging system based on imaging findings. In the eighth edition of mesothelioma TNM staging [128], there were significant modifications in the distinctions of tumor and lymph node staging, based on the analysis of survival data from the IASLC database. Since there were no differences in survival of patients with tumors restricted in the parietal pleura or tumors invading the visceral pleura as well, the distinction between these two types was abolished, with T1a and T1b merging into the T1 category. When it comes to lymph node involvement, previously categorized N3 lymph nodes are now considered N2, and N1–N2 categories were combined into one. Important results of the lymph node status analysis revealed that survival was more affected by the number of involved nodes rather than the exact location of them. When it comes to distant metastases, based on the last staging system, only M1 is now considered Stage IV disease. The presence of pleural thickening and average tumor thickness were correlated with poor survival outcomes and are considered for evaluation in the next edition of staging criteria [121, 129].

10.4.3 Cytology Diagnosis

Most of the time, pleural fluid is the first available specimen for the physician to examine. Cytologic examination of the pleural fluid is a method with high intra-observer variability, with recent studies reporting that sensitivity is dependent on the primary malignancy that causes the effusion [130]. In our experience, the accuracy of cytological diagnosis of mesothelioma is high when performed by a very experienced cytopathologist and quite unreliable otherwise. The highest sensitivity was reported for adenocarcinomas and breast cancer, and the lowest sensitivity was seen in patients with mesothelioma [130]. Specific factors related to higher chances of false negative cytopathology results were pleural thickening on CT, asbestos exposure, and small effusion volumes. Lower odds of false negative results were correlated with cloudy or yellow-appearing pleural fluid, whereas fluid biochemical characteristics did not influence the performance of the diagnostic method. The mesothelioma histotype can influence results, as the sarcomatoid type rarely sheds cells in the fluid and therefore it is difficult to diagnose with cytology, resulting in false negative results [27]. The pathologist should be aware of the patients' clinical history and the atypical cytological presentations of mesothelioma, and confirm with the right histological markers in order to correctly identify the disease and differentiate from metastatic extrapleural disease or inflammatory reaction.

The differential diagnosis with a metastatic carcinoma is relatively simple using immunohistochemistry that will reveal the presence of cells that stain positive for epithelial markers, evidence for a metastatic carcinoma. More difficult is to distinguish cytologically malignant versus benign reactive mesothelial cells. The most reliable cytological evidence of mesothelioma is the presence of three-dimensional cell structures, the so-called "cannon-balls": when they are found in larger numbers and bigger size, they suggest the diagnosis of malignancy. The cytological diagnosis of mesothelioma should be validated by correlating the results with imaging and should be confirmed histologically [27]. Recent advances in Immunohistochemistry (IHC) have rendered the differential diagnosis among benign and malignant mesothelial proliferation more reliable, as over 90% of mesotheliomas will show loss of BAP1 by IHC, or of CDKN2A tested directly by FISH analyses or indirectly by testing by IHC the nearby MTAP gene. In a study published in 2022, IHC staining of cytology samples with a combination of BAP1 and MTAP offered a diagnosis of malignancy with 100% concordance with the IHC results of the respective histopathologic samples. The combination of the two markers performed with high sensitivity in differentiating all three histologic mesothelioma types from benign proliferations [131].

10.4.4 Histopathology Diagnosis

Histological evaluation of adequate samples retrieved through thoracoscopy gives the final diagnosis of mesothelioma. Video-Assisted Thoracoscopy (VATS) or CT/US-guided thoracoscopy should be used. In cases of circumferential thickening that doesn't allow thoracoscopy to be performed, ultrasound has been successfully used as a tool to guide extrapleural biopsies. Recent studies highlighted the importance of ultrasound as a faster and cheaper tool than CT that can accurately assess the exact location, nature, and extent of the tumor with high sensitivity rates and strong positive and negative predictive value. The procedures guided by the US were correlated with less adverse effects, like pneumothorax, hemorrhage, infection, and hemoptysis [132]. Recent guidelines recommend against thoracentesis for diagnostic purposes, as this method presents a higher risk of permeation metastasis. At least three sites should be sampled to ensure an accurate diagnosis and grading [133].

The immunohistochemical staining panel should include Cam5.2 (pankeratin), calretinin, WT1, and several markers, targeted for differential diagnosis from suspected malignancies based on the patient's background, clinical presentation, and medical history. BAP1 immunostaining helps to distinguish benign chronic pleuritis (positive nuclear stain) from mesothelioma (usually negative nuclear stain) and from metastatic lung cancer to the pleura (positive BAP1 nuclear staining) [107, 134]. Mesothelioma should present positive staining for Cam5.2 and for both mesothelial markers WT1 and calretinin, and negative staining for Claudin 4, a pan-carcinoma marker, and specific carcinoma markers depending on the differential [135]. To separate mesothelioma from benign mesothelial proliferations, BAP1 IHC and detection of CDKN2A homozygous deletion by FISH, offer excellent specificity [136]. According to the latest National Comprehensive Cancer Network (NCCN) guidelines on pathologic diagnosis of mesothelioma, only BAP1, MTAP IHC, and CDKN2A (p16) FISH have sufficient reproducibility of results to be considered established markers [9]. If CDKN2a deletion cannot be assessed by FISH analyses, cytoplasmic loss of MTAP expression is a reliable alternative due to the proximity of the two genes. A recent study proposed that a panel consisting of BAP1, MTAP, and Merlin offered high sensitivity and specificity in identifying mesothelioma [137].

The panel of markers should be adjusted based on the suspected malignancy. The markers most commonly used for differential diagnosis are presented in Table 10.1. TTF1 and p40 negativity help rule out adenocarcinoma and squamous cell carcinoma of the lung metastasizing to the pleura. More recently Claudin 4 membranous and cytoplasmic staining has shown high sensitivity (77–100%) and specificity (99–100%) for distinction from lung adenocarcinoma [138, 139]. ER and PAX8 negativity helps distinguish mesothelioma from gynecological malignancy and PAX8 from renal cell carcinomas [140].

Sarcomatoid mesothelioma identification is more challenging and different markers should be used. Loss of BAP1 is less common and these tumors stain reliably only with pancytokeratin, for this reason we prefer to use CAM5.2. GATA3 has been suggested as a marker for sarcomatoid mesothelioma, as it offers high sensitivity [141, 142]. However, its specificity is low, and various sarcomas also stain positive for GATA3. To differentiate between sarcomatoid mesothelioma and other spindle cell tumors, a wide panel of markers should be used, and a definitive reliable diagnosis may not always be possible [119, 135, 138, 143–145].

10.5 EMERGING BIOMARKERS

An accurate and timely mesothelioma diagnosis plays an important role in determining the survival outcomes of mesothelioma patients [146]. Correct identification of mesothelioma sub-types, and characterization of distinct molecular signatures can contribute to the stratification of patients to the correct therapeutic plans and can help predict patient prognosis. At the molecular levels, differentially expressed genes, cell surface proteins, and microenvironment proteins have shown a prognostic value and have been used as biomarkers to improve the accuracy of diagnostic tools. The levels of circulating proteins are also being evaluated as diagnostic biomarkers, in an attempt to create less-invasive and more accurate diagnostic techniques that will be able to detect mesothelioma tumors in early stages where the correct intervention may be life-saving. The advances in the field of biomarker research are further explained in the chapter "Biomarkers of Asbestos Exposure and Mesothelioma".

10.6 ADVANCES IN THERAPEUTIC MANAGEMENT

10.6.1 The Role of Surgery

Up to date, there is no class I evidence that supports surgical therapy as the treatment of choice for mesothelioma. On the contrary, the results of the most recent randomized MARS 2 clinical trial, which was reported in September of 2023 at the IASLC meeting in Singapore, are not in favor of the use of surgery, even though surgical interventions have been historically used in a multimodal setting.

The goal of surgical therapy is macroscopic complete resection of the tumor, defined as leaving no visible or palpable tumor residues [147, 148]. The surgical techniques that are mainly used are extrapleural pneumonectomy (EPP) and lung-sparing procedures such as partial pleurectomy, pleurectomy-decortication (P/D), and extended pleurectomy-decortication ((e)P/D). EPP has been linked with higher complication rates and perioperative mortality, making P/D the most widely used technique, although most of the studies comparing the two approaches are characterized by significant heterogeneity of results [148]. Significant advantages of PD are its better post-operative outcomes and its applicability to patients with worse performance status. There are however important limitations of PD, as there is a greater variability in the qualitative assessment of the "complete" resection and the procedure may leave behind a higher burden of microscopic disease. There is no standardization of the technique between medical practitioners. It takes longer to perform, and it is frequently linked to post-operative air-leaks [149].

Although the inclusion of P/D combined with chemotherapy is mentioned in the latest National Comprehensive Cancer Network guidelines, it may only be beneficial for selected patients with early-stage disease, retained in the pleural cavity without N2 lymph node involvement, with epithelioid histology. In patients with progressed disease, however, surgical intervention should only be considered in the setting of clinical trials [9]. The American Society of Clinical Oncology and the European Society of Medical Oncology recommended only using EPP in carefully selected patients, in expertise medical centers, and suggested the use of lung-sparing procedures when possible, combined with chemotherapy pre- or post-operatively [133, 150]. Factors related to poorer overall survival and higher rates of perioperative mortality are male sex, higher age at diagnosis, advanced stage, lymph node involvement, and non-epithelioid histology, while the inclusion of chemotherapy and immunotherapy in the therapeutic plan was related to improved outcomes [104, 151]. At the same time, in an effort to standardize surgical techniques, a universal reporting system that provides details on the procedure and patients' characteristics was recommended [149].

The addition of intraoperative therapies has been tested in an attempt to improve surgical outcomes. The intracavity administration of chemotherapeutic agents with hyperthermia has offered enhanced cytoreduction, allowing for lung-preserving therapies, good tolerability, and rapid post-operative recovery in selected patients, and lower systemic toxicity compared to traditional chemotherapy [152]. Indeed, in a recent retrospective cohort, hyperthermic intrathoracic chemotherapy (HITHOC) with cisplatin improved survival, especially in patients with later disease stage [153]. A newly tested protocol of lung-preserving surgery, HITHOC, and adjuvant chemotherapy, applied from 2005 to 2014, also showed promising results. In patients with epithelioid, biphasic, or sarcomatoid mesothelioma, 5-year survival of 79.6%, 45.7%, and 9.9% for each type was observed, without post-operative complications [154]. A retrospective analysis comparing patients with localized epithelioid mesothelioma who received three different therapeutic plans, namely chemotherapy alone, EPP and adjuvant chemotherapy, and EPD with HITHOC followed by chemotherapy, proved that EPD/HITHOC group had a significantly longer overall survival of 38 months, with lower perioperative morbidity [151]. However, this method requires a more complex and long surgical and anesthesiological procedure with high morbidity rates and it can be accompanied by serious adverse effects. Recent studies are testing the combination of cisplatin with other chemotherapeutic agents, or with vehicles that can enhance the therapeutic effect and the tissue distribution, while limiting the toxicities. A single-institution phase I clinical trial testing the addition of gemcitabine in HITHOC with cisplatin established a maximum tolerated dose of gemcitabine and assessed the adverse-effect profile of the combination of the two agents. A small advantage of overall survival in the group that received the drug combination was observed, however there were still high recurrence rates and serious adverse effects [155]. Combination of cisplatin with fibrin gel carrier in patients who underwent induction chemotherapy and (e)P/D showed 0% 30- and 90-day mortality rate and no dose-limiting toxicities, with only 1/3 of the patients developing major adverse effects. In this study, cisplatin-fibrin was applied on the surgical surfaces and lung tissue, and the drug levels remained constant locally, even on the highest doses. Preliminary survival data of this cohort also showed significant survival benefits of the patients who received this regimen [156].

However, by comparing patients in different treatment plans, many studies presented a bias in patient selection, as it was evident in the results showing significantly improved survival in patients with good performance status, favorable histology, and the physical reserve to be able to undergo the trimodality treatments. Most of the studies were retrospective, and there is a lack of randomized trials that can eliminate confounding factors and offer reliable conclusions. The latest randomized trials comparing the surgical interventions failed to reveal a beneficial effect of surgery in mesothelioma treatment. MARS 1 feasibility study revealed that EPP not only did not offer a survival benefit, but it harmed patients. The results of the multicenter, randomized MARS 2 study revealed 28% reduced survival and a much higher rate of complications in the surgical group, supporting the results of the MARS 1 trial. MesoVATS trial showed that partial pneumonectomy could not improve patients' survival either, and only offered a limited improvement in the quality of life [113, 157, 158]. These studies support the argument against the use of surgery in the mesothelioma therapeutic plan, as a method that conveys a significant risk for mortality and adverse effects, and should only be used in a palliative setting [113]. In summary, the future of surgery to treat patients affected by mesothelioma is presently dubious. We anticipate that the role of surgery will be reduced in the coming years and will target specific subsets of patients for which a benefit is possible.

10.6.2 Radiotherapy

In the treatment plan of mesothelioma patients, radiotherapy is used in an adjuvant, neo-adjuvant, or palliative setting. Analysis of SEER data and the National Cancer Database revealed that the addition of radiotherapy in the trimodality therapy led to significantly improved survival outcomes, especially in the earlier stage patients [159, 160]. However, radiotherapy is usually accompanied by high rates of serious and life-threatening adverse effects and there have been controversial results regarding its safety and effectiveness.

According to the most recent NCCN guidelines, adjuvant radiotherapy can be recommended to selected patients with resectable tumors for local disease control, with the minimum radiation dose used, when possible. After EPP, adjuvant radiotherapy should be considered only in patients with good performance status, preserved kidney function, and absence of disseminated disease. The use of Intensity-Modulated Radiotherapy (IMRT) after lung-sparing procedures, showed better survival results and was linked with fewer adverse effects and can be performed in specific settings, in expertise centers [9, 161]. American Society of Clinical Oncology (ASCO) also suggests the use of 3D or IMRT for local disease, in the adjuvant or neoadjuvant setting [150]. There are studies that tried to compare 3D-conformal radiotherapy with IMRT techniques, with IMRT showing relatively better local control, however no survival advantages have been found, and the serious adverse-effect rates remain high for both methods [162, 163]. In the case of macroscopically visible residual tumors, higher doses could be administered, with consideration of the maximum dosage that the surrounding tissues can tolerate. In the palliative setting, guidelines suggest the use of IMRT, 2D, or 3D radiotherapy, to better control the administered dosage and provide adequate symptom control, however the optimal dosage has not been clearly determined yet.

The need to limit the serious adverse effects of radiotherapy led to the study of more techniques that showed promising results. Photodynamic Therapy (PDT) is a nonionizing radiation therapeutic technique that uses a laser beam to target a photosensitized drug and produce free oxygen radicals and reactive oxygen species that cause tumor cell death. PDT can be used with EPP or P/D, when a macroscopically complete resection has been achieved [164]. In a cohort from 2005 to 2010 where patients received radical pleurectomy and PDT, a median survival of 31.7 months was achieved. Patients with epithelial tumors had a median survival of 41.2 months [165]. Current technological advances offer the option to better control the light delivery to the thoracic cavity. A navigation system that was recently developed provides real-time guidance through 3D scanners that capture the pleural surface topography. This way, the target surface can be identified and the light distribution can be limited to the desired area [166]. PDT has also been combined with proton therapy, in another attempt to improve local control and safety of radiation treatment. Proton therapy has been proven to be superior to IMRT in reducing radiation delivery to local tissues and limiting toxicities. In a study conducted from 2011 to 2015, where patients with epithelioid mesothelioma received PT after (e)P/D and PDT, the median survival was 19.5 months. The 1-year and 2-year survival was 58% and 29%, respectively, and no patient developed serious or life-threatening adverse effects [167]. The encouraging results of proton therapy led to the suggestion of this intervention in the latest ASCO guidelines, if it can be performed in selected centers of expertise, especially in clinical trials that can help identify the best approach in the field of radiation therapy [150].

10.6.3 Chemotherapy-Immunotherapy

The current recommended first-line regimen for mesothelioma treatment is systemic cisplatin-pemetrexed in 4–6 cycles, with the concurrent administration of folic acid and vitamin B12 [9, 133, 150]. Systemic therapy alone is recommended only for patients with advanced stages and inoperable tumors, or for patients with biphasic and sarcomatoid histology, due to the inefficiency of surgical approach in these patients [168]. The identification of molecular pathways responsible for mesothelioma pathogenesis, and the characterization of the tumor microenvironment components, initiated the search for the right targeted therapeutic compounds. In the past decade, a wide number of studies have tested immunotherapy agents, anti-angiogenic regimens, and molecular targeted therapies. However, only a few agents proved to be safe although minimally effective in increasing the survival rates of patients with mesothelioma [169].

In an attempt to target the rapid mitotic activity of the tumors, the recently published phase II STELLAR trial tested the therapeutic effects of Tumor Treating Fields (TTF) when combined with platinum-based chemotherapy. The regimen used, NovoTTF-100L, is an anti-cancer agent that uses specifically tuned electric fields to disrupt tumor cell division. Patients with unresectable mesothelioma received TTF through a portable medical device and specific dermal transducers placed near the tumors and experienced a median overall survival of 18.2 months [170].

The hypothesis that mesothelioma is an immunogenic disease led researchers to assess the efficacy of immune checkpoint inhibitors on the tumors. The Japanese MERIT phase II trial tested the safety and efficacy of nivolumab, an immune checkpoint inhibitor targeting PD-1. In this study, patients with unresectable, advanced, or metastatic chemoresistant mesothelioma received nivolumab 240 mg intravenously every 2 weeks, with the purpose of assessing the response rate and the adverse effects. Patients with epithelioid, biphasic, and sarcomatoid tumors had 26%, 25%, and 67% response rates, respectively, with 11.1 months median duration of response and 17.3 months overall survival. A 68% disease control rate was observed, and the objective response rate was dependent on the PD-L1 expression of the tumors. Nivolumab also showed a manageable adverse-effect profile, meeting the primary endpoints for its use as a second- or third-line treatment [171].

The phase III CheckMate 743 trial, tested the combination of nivolumab plus ipilimumab as a first-line regimen in treatment naïve unresectable mesotheliomas, versus standard chemotherapy. The study showed a significantly improved median survival of 18.1 months, versus 14.1 months in the chemotherapy group [8]. In the 3-year follow-up, there was an overall survival of 23% versus 15% in the two groups and a progression-free survival of 14% versus 1%. Improved results were observed in patients with non-epithelioid tumors [172]. The results of this study led to the Food and Drug Administration (FDA) approval of this regimen and its inclusion in international guidelines as a first-line therapy for biphasic and sarcomatoid mesotheliomas and highlighted the importance of correct histological diagnosis of the tumors for choosing the right therapeutic plan [9, 133]. However, it is worth noting that patients with performance status zero or one were enrolled, which is a rare finding in mesothelioma, and that the rate of grade 3 side effects or higher was very high in the immunotherapy arm.

After the approval of nivolumab/ipilimumab, the potential use of other immunotherapy agents has been tested. In the phase II DREAM trial, the combination of durvalumab plus cisplatin-pemetrexed led to encouraging progression-free survival and objective response rates, without causing life-threatening adverse effects [173]. Durvalumab plus chemotherapy also showed promising results in the phase II PrE0505 trial, leading to a median survival of 20.4 months versus 12.1 in the control population. In this study, patients with germline mutations in BAP1 and DNA repair gene showed a significant survival benefit, highlighting the importance of genetic testing in the treatment decision-making process [174].

Following the successful use of immune checkpoint inhibitors as a first-line therapy, the phase III PROMISE-MESO randomized trial checked the efficacy of pembrolizumab as a second-line agent. The study included patients who had progressed while on standard chemotherapy, but it didn't reach the desired primary endpoints, which were progression-free or overall survival [175]. However, the phase III CONFIRM trial, comparing nivolumab with placebo in relapsed disease, showed significantly improved survival rates in the nivolumab group [176]. In the IFCT-1501 MAPS2 multicenter phase II trial, nivolumab was compared to the combination of nivolumab plus ipilimumab as a second-line therapy for relapsed mesothelioma. Although the combination treatment achieved better disease control in the 12-week endpoint, it was by higher rates of serious adverse events and treatment-related deaths [177].

In the search for effective mesothelioma therapies, the process of angiogenesis in tumors has been targeted, with heterogenic results between studies. The Mesothelioma Avastin Cisplatin

Pemetrexed Study (MAPS) phase III trial established the efficacy of antiangiogenic drugs for mesothelioma treatment. In this study, the addition of bevacizumab, a Vacular Endothelial Growth Factor (VEGF) inhibitor, to chemotherapy led to a significant, although modest, improvement in median survival of 17 months, thus similar to the ChekMate trial, but with no significant toxicities and no negative impact on the quality of life [178]. The addition of bevacizumab to standard chemotherapy as a frontline regimen can be considered in selected patients, with epithelioid tumors and good performance status. Contraindications for bevacizumab administration are old age, cardiovascular disease, hypertension, and bleeding or clotting risk [9, 133, 150].

The anti-VEGFR antibody nintedanib has been also tested in the LUME-Meso trial. In the phase II trial, the addition of nintedanib to standard chemotherapy in patients with non-sarcomatoid mesothelioma and good performance status showed improvement in progression-free survival with a manageable adverse effects profile. Despite these results, the phase III of this trial failed to reach the primary endpoint of progression-free survival in the intention-to-treat population, compared to the placebo group [179, 180].

When it comes to treatment plans targeting advanced disease, ramucirumab, an anti-VEGFR2 antibody, was used in combination with gemcitabine in the phase II RAMES study. The combination led to a significant survival advantage compared to chemotherapy alone [181].

These studies paved the way for ongoing clinical trials that are testing the effect of immunotherapy on mesothelioma. It should be noted, however, that these published studies that are showcasing survival benefits, can only prolong the survival for a few months. They often pose a high risk of adverse effects that may compromise the patient's quality of life, and also lead to significant dropout rates from the clinical studies, undermining their reporting strength. In a comparative study of 1,501 patients, the cost-effectiveness of the recommended therapies was assessed. The survival curve comparing CheckMate743 and MAPS trial failed to show a survival benefit with either of these treatments [182]. This study further raised concerns regarding the high rate of adverse events linked to immunotherapy and the high cost of this therapeutic plan, compared to anti-VEGF therapy, reinforcing the argument that more standardized studies need to be conducted in order to draw definitive conclusions on the success of each treatment. Confirming the concerns regarding the immunotherapeutic regimen, a study presented at the recent IASLC meeting in Singapore revealed that the real-world data differ significantly from the results of clinical trials. In this multicenter study, the patients who were treated with ipilimumab and nivolumab had a median survival of 14.5 months when they received a first-line treatment and 15.5 months when treated as a second-line scheme. Toxicity of grade 3–5 was reported in more than 22% of patients, while three treatment-related deaths were recorded [183].

10.6.4 Cell Therapies

Targeted therapies are being developed, and their safety and efficacy are being tested in mesothelioma. The development of Chimeric Antigen Receptor T-cell (CAR-T) therapies is aimed at the enhancement of the anti-tumor immune response by directing the T cells to specific tumor antigens. In mesothelioma, mesothelin was used as a target in multiple trials that used CAR-T-cell therapies, because of its high expression in mesothelioma, mostly of the epithelioid type, compared to its low expression in surrounding mesothelial cells and normal tissue [184]. It has been proven that high PD-1 expression in the tumor environment impairs CAR-T-cell efficacy, and PD-1 blockade by pembrolizumab can enhance their function. This observation led to a phase I trial evaluating the administration of a combination CAR-T-cell therapy and pembrolizumab in mesothelioma patients. In this trial, intrapleural administration of CAR-T cells was well tolerated, without significant adverse effects, and the T cells remained in adequate levels in the peripheral blood for a prolonged period. In the 18 patients from the cohort who also received pembrolizumab, the median overall survival was 23.9 months, with 8 patients exhibiting stable disease for 6 months and 2 of them having a complete metabolic response based on PET scan evaluation. This study highlighted the safety and the potential synergistic effect of the two therapeutic modalities in treating mesothelioma patients [147, 185, 186].

In the latest study targeting mesothelin, an anti-mesothelin antibody was integrated into a T-cell receptor fusion construct (TRuC), gavocabtagene autoleucel (gavo-cel). TRuCs can reprogram T-cell receptor (TCR) complexes to recognize tumor antigens, with high efficacy and lower cytokine release, and exhibit a more potent effect in solid tumor treatment than CAR-T cells. Mesothelin targeting TRuCs showed promising results in targeting mesothelin-expressing tumors, in in vitro and in vivo mouse xenograft models, showing higher intra-tumor accumulation and faster activation than CAR-T cells [187, 188]. In the phase I/II trial using gavo-cel, researchers evaluated the safety of the regimen and determined the recommended dose, in patients with chemoresistant, mesothelin-expressing tumors. Even though an overall response rate of 20% and a disease control rate of 77% were noted, the treatment caused grade 3 dose-limiting adverse effects in a high percentage of patients, with some of them exhibiting grade 4, and one of them having grade 5 bronchoalveolar hemorrhage. However, it is worth noting that a single gavo-cel injection was able to cause significant disease regression, and that the recommended dose was not accompanied by life-threatening adverse effects [189].

Another potential therapeutic target of precision therapies is the WT1 protein that is overexpressed and presented on the surface of mesothelioma tumor cells. In an attempt to enhance the immunogenic potential of WT1 and overcome the immune tolerance, a synthetic immunogenic peptide analog was designed. This peptide could cause cross-reactivity with native peptides and showcased improved stability, specific recognition of WT1, and enhanced reactivity of cytotoxic T cells against native WT1 [190]. In a recent phase II randomized trial, mesothelioma patients who had undergone surgery received synthetic WT1 analog peptide vaccination (galinpepimut-S) with GM-CSF and Montanide as immunologic adjuvants. The vaccination exhibited a favorable safety profile, with only mild and self-limited adverse effects reported. The median progression-free survival was 10.1 months in the patients who received vaccination, compared to 7.4 months in patients who only received GM-CSF and Montanide as control. Preliminary data on survival showed an overall survival of 22.8 months in the vaccine group, versus 18.3 months in the control group. The important limitation was, however, that the study was not powered for comparison between the two groups, and did not meet the recruitment goal in the patient groups, due to early closure. Even though definitive conclusions regarding overall survival cannot be derived from this study, the most important endpoint was the establishment of a safe profile that allows for further testing of the vaccine in future studies with higher statistical power [191].

An important part of the field of cell therapies deals with Dendritic Cell (DC)-based immunotherapy. DC therapies aim to boost the anti-tumor immune cell response, by increasing tumor cell antigen presentation to cytotoxic T cells. However, mesothelioma patients have a significantly reduced circulating number of dendritic cells that exhibit defects in their activation potential and their antigen processing capacity [192]. To overcome these limitations, DCs can be pulsed with tumor antigens ex vivo to ensure sufficient activation, and then be administered to patients. In murine mesothelioma models, mice received autologous DCs pulsed with autologous or allogeneic tumor lysate, and the survival and anti-tumor responses were assessed. Both lysates were able to induce adequate activation of DCs and the treatment led to significant survival advantages, compared to control animals. These results led to the application of this therapy to an in-human phase I clinical trial, where nine patients received DC vaccination with cells that were pulsed ex- vivo with lysate originating from five different mesothelioma cell lines. Although the study didn't reach an overall survival endpoint, no dose-limiting toxicities were observed and radiographic responses were evident [193].

10.6.5 Targeted Molecular Therapies

It is hoped that targeted therapy for mesothelioma will improve the clinical outcome [194]. The most recently discovered agents that are used for targeted therapies are presented in Figure 10.1. The characterization of BAP1 molecular interactions with BRCA complexes and its involvement in DNA repair through homologous recombination is clearly established. Mutations of BRCA-related genes have been proven to increase tumor sensitivity to PARP inhibitors, agents that cause accumulation of DNA single-strand breaks and contribute to synthetic lethality in DNA repair deficient tumors. This led to the investigation of the possible correlation of BAP1 status with the effect of PARP inhibitors in mesothelioma tumors. In a phase II trial using the PARP inhibitor olaparib, the response rate related to the mutation status of DNA repair genes was assessed. Patients with refractory mesothelioma received olaparib for 21 days or until disease progression or intolerable toxicity. The data regarding disease progression and survival did not show significant benefits after treatment, and the patient sample in this study is too small to create a generalizable result, however, germline BAP1 mutation was linked with relatively reduced survival (4.6 vs 9.6 months in control patients) and progression-free intervals (2.3 vs 4.1 months). Regarding the final endpoints of the study, treatment was safe and tolerable [195–198]. In a study on patient-derived mesothelioma cell lines treated with olaparib, talazoparib in combination with Temozolomide (TMZ), the sensitivity of cells to PARP inhibition was not dependent on BAP1 status, but was enhanced when a combination regimen was used [199]. This in vitro study did not show promising results regarding the importance of BAP1 status, and in a consequent clinical trial, the use of PARP inhibitors didn't lead to encouraging outcomes. In the phase IIa MiST1 trial, patients with progressing mesothelioma with BAP1 or BRCA1 mutations were treated with the PARP inhibitor rucaparib, and the disease control was monitored. Mutation status was not correlated with different responses to therapy. Rucaparib treatment was mostly linked to grades 1 and 2 adverse events, with 9% of patients developing grade 3 or 4 adverse events, mostly respiratory infections and anemia, and no treatment-related deaths were recorded. However, only 31% of patients completed all the therapy cycles, and 35% of them required a dose reduction. The study met its original endpoint with more than half the patients achieving disease control in 12 weeks (58%) and 23% maintaining disease control at 24 weeks [200].

In the search for an effective treatment for mesothelioma, more molecular targets were tested for their therapeutic effect. Focal Adhesion Kinase (FAK) is an important regulator of cancer cell proliferation and migration. Merlin (NF2) expression attenuates FAK phosphorylation and disrupts FAK downstream pathways. Its inactivation in mesothelioma is linked with FAK overexpression and increased invasiveness. Targeting of FAK with GSK2256098 showed improved progression-free survival in patients with Merlin-negative tumors. Based on the hypothesis that combined targeting of FAK and MEK, a component of the ERK pathway, a study evaluated the ideal dosage of combination MEK1/2 inhibitor trametinib and GSK2256098. This study evaluated the safety and pharmacokinetics of this regimen in mesothelioma and solid tumors. Preliminary data on the efficacy of the combination therapy showed progression-free survival of 11.8 weeks, in Merlin-negative tumors, versus 7.3 weeks in Merlin-positive tumors [201–203]. The activity of the Hippo-signaling pathway has been targeted through yes-associated protein (YAP), a downstream negative effector of this pathway that has been associated with the negative prognosis of mesothelioma. In vitro studies of mesothelioma cell lines showed decreased phosphorylated-YAP to YAP ratio in malignant cells compared to mesothelial cells and increased sensitivity of these cells to treatment with the YAP inhibitor verteporfin. Verteporfin significantly reduced the levels of YAP protein and mRNA of YAP downstream genes, and impaired invasion and sphere formation of malignant cells, showing the potential of this molecule for therapeutic targeting [204, 205]. One of the most commonly mutated genes in mesothelioma is CDKNA, on the chromosome 9p21.3 locus. Mutation of CDKNA leads to loss of the tumor suppressor p16ink4A, an inhibitory molecule that targets Cyclin-Dependent Kinase (CDK) 4 and CDK6, regulating cell cycle arrest. Small-molecule inhibitors of the p16ink4A targets have shown promising results in preclinical mesothelioma models [206, 207]. Combined treatment with CDK4/6 inhibitor palbociclib and PI3K/mTOR inhibitors showed a synergistic effect of these agents in inhibiting cell proliferation in vitro, in both normoxia and hypoxia, by reducing glucose uptake and consumption and mitochondrial respiration [208, 209]. Based on the promising effects of targeting CDKNA-related molecules in vitro and in mouse xenografts models, the phase II MiST2 trial evaluated the safety and efficacy of abemaciclib in p16ink4A negative mesothelioma patients with progressive disease. The study reached the primary endpoint of disease control in 12 weeks, in 54% of patients who enrolled, while 80% of patients also showed disease regression. However, an important drawback of this study was the high rate of adverse effects, with 27% of patients reporting grade 3 adverse effects and 12% of them reporting grade 4 or higher effects, while one patient died from treatment-related neutropenic sepsis [207].

In summary, the need to find an efficacious and safe targeted therapy that can improve the natural course of this malignancy still remains. Understanding the underlying mechanisms that drive mesothelioma pathogenesis and aggressive behavior is important for the development of effective therapies [210]. When reviewing the latest advances in the clinical setting, the heterogeneity between clinical trials remains a major problem. There is a need for standardization of patient selection and management between the studies to compare the results [122]. Also, the value of intermediate surrogate endpoints remains dubious, for example, patients do not care about "tumor-free survival", they care about survival. In addition, patients and physicians do not seem to agree on what is "tolerable toxicity" resulting in many patients dropping out of clinical trials because they find toxicity "intolerable".

10.6.6 Clinical Prognostic Scores

In order to select the right treatment plan for each patient and ensure the correct stratification of patients in clinical trials, so that beneficial effects can be reliably observed, certain clinical prognostic scores have been developed. The most widely used one was introduced by The European Organization for Research and Treatment of Cancer (EORTC). This scoring system takes into account the Eastern Cooperative Oncology Group (ECOG) performance status, histological subtype, sex, certainty of diagnosis, and WBC count [211]. EORTC score has been validated in clinical cohorts, with the latest one of them applying the score in a cohort of patients who underwent curative or palliative surgical treatment, where EORTC score showed an independent prognostic value in predicting patients' survival. In a study on mesothelioma patients who had overall survival that exceeded 5 years, assessment of patient clinical characteristics revealed significantly lower rates of reported asbestos exposure and lower lung fiber content compared to control patients. Other characteristics that contributed to these patients' improved survival were younger age, female gender, smaller tumor size, good performance status, and inclusion of both chemotherapy and surgery in the treatment plan [212].

A recently tested classification and regression tree system was developed based on a cohort of mesothelioma patients between 2005 and 2014. This system collected 29 clinical variables and evaluated patients' 18-month survival, taking into account the interactions of the independent variables. This method aimed to maximize sensitivity in determining the true at-risk patients and minimize misclassification, and stratified patients in distinct risk groups based on their clinical characteristics. The strongest predictor of worse survival was weight loss, followed by performance score and sarcomatoid histology. The group with the best survival had no weight loss, hemoglobin greater than 153 g/L, and serum albumin greater than 43 g/L. The predictive power of this model was validated in an external cohort [213].

The "Mesothelioma Risk Score" prediction system was developed with the purpose of establishing a reliable risk classification of surgical patients with mesothelioma. This model combined already established and newly obtained parameters, such as genomic signatures, molecular subtype, tumor volume, and Neutrophil-to-Lymphocyte Ratio (NLR), that were retrospectively collected from patients who underwent EPP or P/D. These parameters displayed an independent prognostic strength in patients with EPP, while the combination of molecular signatures and tumor volume was able to identify high-risk patients in the P/D group [214].

When it comes to histologic subtype identification and the effect on patient prognosis, a deep-learning tool, MesoNet, displayed high accuracy in predicting mesothelioma patients' survival based on histological characteristics from whole-slide images [215]. This model did not require pathologist annotations and performed significantly better when compared with current pathology models. The latest prediction model that was created, OncoCast-MPM, is a deep-learning tool that can stratify patients into low- and high-risk groups based on clinical characteristics, pathological features, and molecular profiling from standard next-generation sequencing testing. The advantage of this model is that it does not rely on subjective and fluctuating variables like performance score and laboratory values, and its performance was significantly more accurate in predicting patient survival compared to EORTC score and current stage and histology models. According to this model, features favoring survival were BAP1 and PBRM1 mutations, epithelioid histology, a history of smoking or tobacco use, and reported classic occupational asbestos exposure. Unfavorable features were male sex, mutations of CDKN2A/B, TP53, and TERT, older age, advanced-stage disease, and biphasic histology [216].

Overall these predictors of survival have a modest impact, because mesothelioma is a deadly disease, and differences in survival are measured in weeks to months. The only biomarker that distinguishes mesothelioma patients with significantly improved survival is the presence of germline mutations of BAP1 and of some other genes. These patients have a median survival of 6–7 years and over 20% of them are alive 10 years later, some survived 20 or more years and died of other causes [41].

10.6.7 Monitoring Disease Progression

Significant changes have been made in the protocols for monitoring disease and reporting treatment outcomes, in an attempt to standardize monitoring between studies and create comparable reports that minimize variability. European Respiratory Society (ERS) guidelines recommend regular and detailed clinical follow-up, with a CT scan every 3–4 months in the first year and adjustment according to the patient's profile after the first year [120, 217]. The latest modified Response Evaluation Criteria in Solid Tumors (RECIST1.1 criteria) aim to standardize the manner in which disease progression is assessed in CT scans and limit intra-observer variability. According to mRECIST1.1, complete response is the complete disappearance of imaging findings and needs to be confirmed 4 weeks after the first observation. Partial response is defined as a 30% or more reduction in the summed measured disease volume and progressive disease is an increase of 20% or more compared to all previous scans, and a 5mm or more increase compared to baseline scan. The minimum tumor thickness was defined as 5mm, as well as the ideal number of foci measured, to characterize lesions and disease extent. To ensure consistency between measurements, these criteria recommend that all scans have the same orientation, and a specific plane is used for defining the tumor longest diameter and thickness. The same observer should obtain all measurements, and the baseline measurements should always be used as reference [218]. The incorporation of immune-modified iRECIST criteria in clinical immunotherapy trials was based on RECIST criteria with some adjustments in defining and confirming disease progression and response, in order to ensure consistent data collection and report between trials [219].

10.7 CONCLUSIONS

In the past decade, major advances have been made in understanding the pathogenesis of mesothelioma and the molecular background in which it develops. The discovery of germline mutations that cause (BAP1) or predispose (BLM) to mesothelioma, and the characterization of the biological significance of some of these mutations, is helping in understanding the different biological behaviors of the disease and implement early detection strategies that benefit these patients. The significantly improved survival of patients carrying germline mutations of BAP1 and some other genes highlights the importance of genetic testing. The favorable outcome of patients diagnosed in the early stages emphasized the need for accurate and sensitive diagnostic procedures. The heterogeneity in reporting the incidence and survival data between countries remains an issue, originating from the different access of different medical centers to diagnostic measures and the different reporting systems. The development of nationwide registries that provide detailed information on asbestos exposure and most importantly combine standardized questionnaires with imaging supporting asbestos exposure and, when possible pathology showing the presence of ferruginous bodies in lung biopsies, and lung content analyses to identify the precise type of carcinogenic fibers responsible for the malignancy, would improve our ability to detect and reduce both occupational and environmental asbestos exposure worldwide. The role of surgery and immunotherapy in treating mesothelioma patients is being re-evaluated. It is hoped that randomized clinical trials will keep expanding the therapeutic landscape: hopefully, soon they will provide better options for mesothelioma patients. As more targeted therapies are being tested, standardization of clinical studies would increase their reporting strength and allow for more definitive conclusions to be drawn.

A very recent article reported that germline mutations of BARD1, the gene product of BARD1 binds BAP1, cause similar mechanistic alterations as BAP1 and similarly result in less aggressive minimally invasive mesotheliomas characterized by significantly improved survival. Some patients were cured. These findings underscore the difference between the aggressive sporadic and often asbestos-induced mesotheliomas versus those caused by genetics. The latter are a different disease, not only etiologically but also because for the most part they are much less aggressive, may remain indolent for years, if and when they grow and become invasive and visible on imaging, most patients respond to therapy, survive many years and some are cured [220].

REFERENCES

1. Sauter, J.L., et al., The 2021 WHO classification of tumors of the pleura: Advances since the 2015 classification. *Journal of Thoracic Oncology*, 2022. **17**(5): p. 608–622.
2. Marchevsky, A.M., et al., Localized malignant mesothelioma, an unusual and poorly characterized neoplasm of serosal origin: Best current evidence from the literature and the International Mesothelioma Panel. *Modern Pathology*, 2020. **33**(2): p. 281–296.
3. Meyerhoff, R.R., et al., Impact of mesothelioma histologic subtype on outcomes in the Surveillance, Epidemiology, and End Results database. *Journal of Surgical Research*, 2015. **196**(1): p. 23–32.
4. Verma, V., et al., Survival by histologic subtype of malignant pleural mesothelioma and the impact of surgical resection on overall survival. *Clinical Lung Cancer*, 2018. **19**(6): p. e901–e912.
5. Zhang, Y.Z., et al., Utility of nuclear grading system in epithelioid malignant pleural mesothelioma in biopsy-heavy setting: An external validation study of 563 cases. *American Journal of Surgical Pathology*, 2020. **44**(3): p. 347–356.
6. Rosen, L.E., et al., Nuclear grade and necrosis predict prognosis in malignant epithelioid pleural mesothelioma: A multi-institutional study. *Modern Pathology*, 2018. **31**(4): p. 598–606.
7. Nicholson, A.G., et al., EURACAN/IASLC proposals for updating the histologic classification of pleural mesothelioma: Towards a more multidisciplinary approach. *Journal of Thoracic Oncology*, 2020. **15**(1): p. 29–49.
8. Baas, P., et al., First-line nivolumab plus ipilimumab in unresectable malignant pleural mesothelioma (CheckMate 743): A multicentre, randomised, open-label, phase 3 trial. *The Lancet*, 2021. **397**(10272): p. 375–386.
9. NCCN, NCCN Clinical Practice Guidelines in Oncology (NCCN Guidelines®). Version 1.2023, 12/15/22 © 2022 National Comprehensive Cancer Network® (NCCN®).2022.
10. Carbone, M., Transitional mesothelioma and artificial intelligence: Do we need one more subtype? and do we need computers to identify them? *Journal of Thoracic Oncology*, 2020. **15**(6): p. 884–887.
11. Baumann, F., et al., Asbestos is not just asbestos: An unrecognised health hazard. *Lancet Oncology*, 2013. **14**(7): p. 576–578.
12. Larson, D., et al., Investigating palygorskite's role in the development of mesothelioma in southern Nevada: Insights into fiber-induced carcinogenicity. *Journal of Toxicology and Environmental Health. Part B Critical Reviews*, 2016. **19**(5–6): p. 213–230.
13. Dogan, A.U., et al., Genetic predisposition to fiber carcinogenesis causes a mesothelioma epidemic in Turkey. *Cancer Research*, 2006. **66**(10): p. 5063–5068.

14. Carbone, M., et al., Erionite exposure in North Dakota and Turkish villages with mesothelioma. *Proceedings of the National Academy of Sciences of the United States of America*, 2011. **108**(33): p. 13618–13623.
15. Jube, S., et al., Cancer cell secretion of the DAMP protein HMGB1 supports progression in malignant mesothelioma. *Cancer Research*, 2012. **72**(13): p. 3290–3301.
16. Qi, F., et al., Continuous exposure to chrysotile asbestos can cause transformation of human mesothelial cells via HMGB1 and TNF-alpha signaling. *American Journal of Pathology*, 2013. **183**(5): p. 1654–1666.
17. Xue, J., et al., Asbestos induces mesothelial cell transformation via HMGB1-driven autophagy. *Proceedings of the National Academy of Sciences of the United States of America*, 2020. **117**(41): p. 25543–25552.
18. Yang, H., et al., Programmed necrosis induced by asbestos in human mesothelial cells causes high-mobility group box 1 protein release and resultant inflammation. *Proceedings of the National Academy of Sciences of the United States of America*, 2010. **107**(28): p. 12611–12616.
19. Yang, H., et al., TNF-α inhibits asbestos-induced cytotoxicity via a NF-κB-dependent pathway, a possible mechanism for asbestos-induced oncogenesis. *Proceedings of the National Academy of Sciences of the United States of America*, 2006. **103**(27): p. 10397–10402.
20. Xue, J., et al., HMGB1 as a therapeutic target in disease. *Journal of Cellular Physiology*, 2021. **236**(5): p. 3406–3419.
21. Suarez, J, et al., HMGB1 released by mesothelial cells drives the development of asbestos-induced mesothelioma. *Proceedings of the National Academy of Sciences (PNAS)*, 2023. **120**(39): e2307999120.
22. Goparaju, C.M., et al., Onconase mediated NFKβ downregulation in malignant pleural mesothelioma. *Oncogene*, 2011. **30**(24): p. 2767–2777.
23. Nasu, M., et al., Ranpirnase interferes with NF– B pathway and MMP9 activity, inhibiting malignant mesothelioma cell invasiveness and xenograft growth. *Genes and Cancer*, 2011. **2**(5): p. 576–584.
24. Alpert, N., et al., Epidemiology of mesothelioma in the 21st century in Europe and the United States, 40 years after restricted/banned asbestos use. *Translational Lung Cancer Research*, 2020. **9**(S1): p. S28–S38.
25. Zhai, Z., et al., Assessment of global trends in the diagnosis of mesothelioma from 1990 to 2017. *JAMA Network Open*, 2021. **4**(8): p. e2120360.
26. Damiran, N. and A.L. Frank, Mongolia: Failure of total banning of asbestos. *Annals of Global Health*, 2023. **89**(1).
27. Carbone, M., et al., Mesothelioma: Scientific clues for prevention, diagnosis, and therapy. *CA: A Cancer Journal for Clinicians*, 2019. **69**(5): p. 402–429.
28. Liu, B., et al., Epidemiology of environmental exposure and malignant mesothelioma. *Journal of Thoracic Oncology*, 2017. **12**(7): p. 1031–1045.
29. Baumann, F., et al., The presence of asbestos in the natural environment is likely related to mesothelioma in Young individuals and women from Southern Nevada. *Journal of Thoracic Oncology*, 2015. **10**(5): p. 731–737.
30. BTS statement on malignant mesothelioma in the UK, 2007. *Thorax*, 2007. **62** (Suppl_2): p. ii1–ii19.
31. Attanoos, R.L., et al., Malignant mesothelioma and its non-asbestos causes. *Archives of Pathology and Laboratory Medicine*, 2018. **142**(6): p. 753–760.
32. Farioli, A., et al., Radiation-induced mesothelioma among long-term solid cancer survivors: A longitudinal analysis of SEER database. *Cancer Medicine*, 2016. **5**(5): p. 950–959.
33. Baiocco, G., et al., A matter of space: How the spatial heterogeneity in energy deposition determines the biological outcome of radiation exposure. *Radiation and Environmental Biophysics*, 2022. **61**(4): p. 545–559.
34. Chirieac, L.R., et al., Clinicopathologic characteristics of malignant mesotheliomas arising in patients with a history of radiation for Hodgkin and non-Hodgkin lymphoma. *Journal of Clinical Oncology: Official Journal of the American Society of Clinical Oncology*, 2013. **31**(36): p. 4544–4549.
35. Visci, G., et al., Relationship between exposure to ionizing radiation and mesothelioma risk: A systematic review of the scientific literature and meta-analysis. *Cancer Medicine*, 2022. **11**(3): p. 778–789.
36. De Bruin, M.L., et al., Malignant mesothelioma after radiation treatment for Hodgkin lymphoma. *Blood*, 2009. **113**(16): p. 3679–3681.
37. Mumma, M.T., et al., Mesothelioma mortality within two radiation monitored occupational cohorts. *International Journal of Radiation Biology*, 2022. **98**(4): p. 786–794.
38. Roushdy-Hammady, I., et al., Genetic-susceptibility factor and malignant mesothelioma in the Cappadocian region of Turkey. *The Lancet*, 2001. **357**(9254): p. 444–445.

39. Testa, J.R., et al., Germline BAP1 mutations predispose to malignant mesothelioma. *Nature Genetics*, 2011. **43**(10): p. 1022–1025.
40. Carbone, M., et al., Biological mechanisms and clinical significance of BAP1 mutations in human cancer. *Cancer Discovery*, 2020. **10**(8): p. 1103–1120.
41. Carbone, M., et al., Medical and surgical care of patients with mesothelioma and their relatives carrying germline BAP1 mutations. *Journal of Thoracic Oncology*, 2022. **17**(7): p. 873–889.
42. Carbone, M., et al., Combined Genetic and Genealogic Studies Uncover a Large BAP1 Cancer Syndrome Kindred Tracing Back Nine Generations to a Common Ancestor from the 1700s. *PLoS Genetics*, 2015. **11**(12): p. e1005633.
43. Carbone, M., et al., BAP1 cancer syndrome: Malignant mesothelioma, uveal and cutaneous melanoma, and MBAITs. *Journal of Translational Medicine*, 2012. **10**(1): p. 179.
44. Carbone, M., et al., Tumour predisposition and cancer syndromes as models to study gene–environment interactions. *Nature Reviews. Cancer*, 2020. **20**(9): p. 533–549.
45. Daou, S., et al., Monoubiquitination of ASXLs controls the deubiquitinase activity of the tumor suppressor BAP1. *Nature Communications*, 2018. **9**: p. 4385.
46. Masclef, L., et al., Roles and mechanisms of BAP1 deubiquitinase in tumor suppression. *Cell Death and Differentiation*, 2021. **28**(2): p. 606–625.
47. Bononi, A., et al., BAP1 regulates IP3R3-mediated Ca2+ flux to mitochondria suppressing cell transformation. *Nature*, 2017. **546**(7659): p. 549–553.
48. Bononi, A., et al., Germline BAP1 mutations induce a Warburg effect. *Cell Death and Differentiation*, 2017. **24**(10): p. 1694–1704.
49. Bononi, A., et al., BAP1 is a novel regulator of HIF-1α. *Proceedings of the National Academy of Sciences of the United States of America*, 2023. **120**(4): e2217840120.
50. Carbone, M., et al., Preventive and therapeutic opportunities: Targeting BAP1 and/or HMGB1 pathways to diminish the burden of mesothelioma. *Journal of Translational Medicine*, 2023. **21**(1): p. 749.
51. Novelli, F., et al., BAP1 forms a trimer with HMGB1 and HDAC1 that modulates gene × environment interaction with asbestos. *Proceedings of the National Academy of Sciences of the United States of America*, 2021. **118**(48): p. e2111946118.
52. Cicala, C.F.P. and M. Carbone, SV40 induces mesotheliomas in hamsters. *American Journal of Pathology*, 1993. **142**(5): p. 1524–1533.
53. Carbone, M., et al., Eighth international mesothelioma interest group. *Oncogene*, 2007. **26**(49): p. 6959–6967.
54. Bocchetta, M., et al., Human mesothelial cells are unusually susceptible to simian virus 40-mediated transformation and asbestos cocarcinogenicity. *Proceedings of the National Academy of Sciences of the United States of America*, 2000. **97**(18): p. 10214–10219.
55. Foddis, R., et al., SV40 infection induces telomerase activity in human mesothelial cells. *Oncogene*, 2002. **21**(9): p. 1434–1442.
56. Carbone, M., et al., New developments about the association of SV40 with human mesothelioma. *Oncogene*, 2003. **22**(33): p. 5173–5180.
57. Kroczynska, B., et al., Crocidolite asbestos and SV40 are cocarcinogens in human mesothelial cells and in causing mesothelioma in hamsters. *Proceedings of the National Academy of Sciences of the United States of America*, 2006. **103**(38): p. 14128–14133.
58. Cutrone, R., et al., Some oral poliovirus vaccines were contaminated with infectious SV40 after 1961. *Cancer Research*, 2005. **65**(22): p. 10273–10279.
59. Carbone, M.R.P., and H. Pass, Simian virus 40: the link with human malignant mesothelioma is well established. *Anticancer Research*, 2000. **20**(2A): p. 875–877.
60. Gazdar, A.F., et al., SV40 and human tumours: Myth, association or causality? *Nature Reviews. Cancer*, 2002. **2**(12): p. 957–964.
61. Rizzo, P.D.R.I., *et al.*, Unique strains of SV40 in commercial poliovaccines from 1955 not readily identifiable with current testing for SV40 infection. *Cancer Research*, 1999. **59**(24): p. 6103–6108.
62. Carbone, M., A. Gazdar, and J.S. Butel, SV40 and human mesothelioma. *Translational Lung Cancer Research*, 2020. **9**(S1): p. S47–S59.
63. Betti, M., et al., Germline mutations in DNA repair genes predispose asbestos-exposed patients to malignant pleural mesothelioma. *Cancer Letters*, 2017. **405**: p. 38–45.
64. Betti, M., et al., Sensitivity to asbestos is increased in patients with mesothelioma and pathogenic germline variants in BAP1 or other DNA repair genes. *Genes, Chromosomes and Cancer*, 2018. **57**(11): p. 573–583.

65. Napolitano, A., et al., Minimal asbestos exposure in germline BAP1 heterozygous mice is associated with deregulated inflammatory response and increased risk of mesothelioma. *Oncogene*, 2016. **35**(15): p. 1996–2002.
66. Luo, Y., et al., BRCA1 haploinsufficiency impairs iron metabolism to promote chrysotile-induced mesothelioma via ferroptosis resistance. *Cancer Science*, 2023. **114**(4): p. 1423–1436.
67. Oliveira, M.C., et al., Malignant epithelioid mesothelioma in senile Red Sindhi cows from Brazil. *Pesquisa Veterinária Brasileira*, 2023. **43:** e07279.
68. Guo, G., et al., Whole-exome sequencing reveals frequent genetic alterations in BAP1, NF2, CDKN2A, and CUL1 in malignant pleural mesothelioma, *Cancer Research*, 2015. **75**(2): p. 264–269.
69. Lo Iacono, M., et al., Targeted next-generation sequencing of cancer genes in advanced stage malignant pleural mesothelioma: A retrospective study. *Journal of Thoracic Oncology*, 2015. **10**(3): p. 492–499.
70. Carbone, M., et al., Recent insights emerging from malignant mesothelioma genome sequencing. *Journal of Thoracic Oncology*, 2015. **10**(3): p. 409–411.
71. Bueno, R., et al., Comprehensive genomic analysis of malignant pleural mesothelioma identifies recurrent mutations, gene fusions and splicing alterations. *Nature Genetics*, 2016. **48**(4): p. 407–416.
72. Hmeljak, J., et al., Integrative molecular characterization of malignant pleural mesothelioma. *Cancer Discovery*, 2018. **8**(12): p. 1548–1565.
73. Yoshikawa, Y., et al., Mesothelioma developing in carriers of inherited genetic mutations. *Translational Lung Cancer Research*, 2020. **9**(S1): p. S67–S76.
74. Sculco, M., et al., Malignant pleural mesothelioma: Germline variants in DNA repair genes may steer tailored treatment. *European Journal of Cancer*, 2022. **163**: p. 44–54.
75. Desmeules, P., et al., A subset of malignant mesotheliomas in Young adults are associated with recurrent EWSR1/FUS-ATF1 fusions. *American Journal of Surgical Pathology*, 2017. **41**(7): p. 980–988.
76. Pastorino, S., et al., A subset of mesotheliomas with improved survival occurring in carriers of BAP1 and other germline mutations. *Journal of Clinical Oncology*, 2018. **36**(35): p. 3485–3494.
77. Guo, R., et al., Novel germline mutations in DNA damage repair in patients with malignant pleural mesotheliomas. *Journal of Thoracic Oncology*, 2020. **15**(4): p. 655–660.
78. Bononi, A., et al., Heterozygous germline BLM mutations increase susceptibility to asbestos and mesothelioma. *Proceedings of the National Academy of Sciences of the United States of America*, 2020. **117**(52): p. 33466–33473.
79. Yoshikawa, Y., et al., High-density array-CGH with targeted NGS unmask multiple noncontiguous minute deletions on chromosome 3p21 in mesothelioma. *Proceedings of the National Academy of Sciences of the United States of America*, 2016. **113**(47): p. 13432–13437.
80. Oey, H., et al., Whole-genome sequencing of human malignant mesothelioma tumours and cell lines. *Carcinogenesis*, 2019. **40**(6): p. 724–734.
81. Mansfield, A.S., et al., Neoantigenic potential of complex chromosomal rearrangements in mesothelioma. *Journal of Thoracic Oncology*, 2019. **14**(2): p. 276–287.
82. Carbone, M., et al., Does chromothripsis make mesothelioma an immunogenic cancer? *Journal of Thoracic Oncology*, 2019. **14**(2): p. 157–159.
83. Lee, H.J., et al., The tumor suppressor BAP1 regulates the hippo pathway in pancreatic ductal adenocarcinoma. *Cancer Research*, 2020. **80**(8): p. 1656–1668.
84. Kakiuchi, T., et al., Modeling mesothelioma utilizing human mesothelial cells reveals involvement of phospholipase-C beta 4 in YAP-active mesothelioma cell proliferation. *Carcinogenesis*, 2016. **37**(11): p. 1098–1109.
85. Miyanaga, A., et al., Hippo pathway gene mutations in malignant mesothelioma: Revealed by RNA and targeted exon sequencing. *Journal of Thoracic Oncology*, 2015. **10**(5): p. 844–851.
86. Sato, T. and Y. Sekido, NF, NF2/merlin inactivation and potential therapeutic targets in mesothelioma. *International Journal of Molecular Sciences*, 2018. **19**(4): p. 988.
87. Sekido, Y. and T. Sato, NF2 alteration in mesothelioma. *Frontiers in Toxicology*, 2023. **5**: p. 1161995.
88. Baumann, F., et al., Mesothelioma patients with germline BAP1 mutations have 7-fold improved long-term survival. *Carcinogenesis*, 2015. **36**(1): p. 76–81.
89. Zauderer, M.G., et al., Prevalence and preliminary validation of screening criteria to identify carriers of germline BAP1 mutations. *Journal of Thoracic Oncology*, 2019. **14**(11): p. 1989–1994.
90. Walpole, S., et al., Microsimulation model for evaluating the cost-effectiveness of surveillance in BAP1 pathogenic variant carriers. *JCO Clinical Cancer Informatics*. **2021**(5): p. 143–154.
91. Hu, Z.I., et al., Meningiomas in patients with malignant pleural mesothelioma harboring germline BAP1 mutations. *Journal of Thoracic Oncology*, 2022. **17**(3): p. 461–466.

92. Parrotta, R., et al., A novel BRCA1-associated Protein-1 isoform affects response of mesothelioma cells to drugs impairing BRCA1-mediated DNA repair. *Journal of Thoracic Oncology*, 2017. **12**(8): p. 1309–1319.
93. Okonska A., et al., Functional genomic screen in mesothelioma reveals that loss of function of BRCA1-associated protein 1 induces chemoresistance to ribonucleotide reductase inhibition. *Molecular Cancer Therapeutics*, 2019.
94. Guazzelli, A., et al., BAP1 status determines the sensitivity of malignant mesothelioma cells to gemcitabine treatment. *International Journal of Molecular Sciences*, 2019. **20**(2): p. 429.
95. Oehl, K., et al., Alterations in BAP1 are associated with cisplatin resistance through inhibition of apoptosis in malignant pleural mesothelioma. *Clinical Cancer Research: An Official Journal of the American Association for Cancer Research*, 2021. **27**(8): p. 2277–2291.
96. Hassan, R., et al., Inherited predisposition to malignant mesothelioma and overall survival following platinum chemotherapy. *Proceedings of the National Academy of Sciences of the United States of America*, 2019. **116**(18): p. 9008–9013.
97. Ghafoor, A. and R. Hassan, Somatic BAP1 loss as a predictive biomarker of overall survival in patients with malignant pleural mesothelioma treated with chemotherapy. *Journal of Thoracic Oncology*, 2022. **17**(7): p. 862–864.
98. Louw, A., et al., BAP1 loss by immunohistochemistry predicts improved survival to first-line platinum and pemetrexed chemotherapy for patients with pleural mesothelioma: A validation study. *Journal of Thoracic Oncology*, 2022. **17**(7): p. 921–930.
99. Kim, K.H. and C.W.M. Roberts, Targeting EZH2 in cancer. *Nature Medicine*, 2016. **22**(2): p. 128–134.
100. Nair, N.U., et al., Genomic and transcriptomic analyses identify a prognostic gene signature and predict response to therapy in pleural and peritoneal mesothelioma. Cell. *Reproductive Medicine*, 2023. **4**(2): p. 100938.
101. Lee, J.S., et al., Synthetic lethality-mediated precision oncology via the tumor transcriptome. *Cell*, 2021. **184**(9): p. 2487-2502.e13.
102. Prevention, C.o.D.C.a., *Cancer Statistics at a Glance*. https://gis.cdc.gov/Cancer/USCS/#/AtAGlance/. 2020, .
103. Sahu, R.K., et al., Malignant mesothelioma tumours: Molecular pathogenesis, diagnosis, and therapies accompanying clinical studies. *Frontiers in Oncology*, 2023. **13**: p. 1204722.
104. Bou-Samra, P., et al., Epidemiological, therapeutic, and survival trends in malignant pleural mesothelioma: A review of the national cancer database. *Cancer Medicine*, 2023. **12**(11): p. 12208–12220.
105. Centers for Disease Control and Prevention. Incidence of Malignant Mesothelioma, 1999–2018. USCS Data Brief, no. 27. Atlanta, GA: Centers for Disease Control and Prevention, US Department of Health and Human Services. 2022.
106. Gerwen, M., et al., An overview of existing mesothelioma registries worldwide, and the need for a US Registry. *American Journal of Industrial Medicine*, 2019. **63**(2): p. 115–120.
107. Guo, Z., et al., Improving the accuracy of mesothelioma diagnosis in China. *Journal of Thoracic Oncology*, 2017. **12**(4): p. 714–723.
108. Mao, W., et al., Association of asbestos exposure with malignant mesothelioma incidence in Eastern China. *JAMA Oncology*, 2017. **3**(4): p. 562.
109. Mazurek, Jacek M.D.J.B., DrPH, and David N MD. Weissman, Malignant mesothelioma mortality in women — United States, 1999–2020. Morbidity and Mortality Weekly Report. *Center of Disease Control and Prevention*, 2022. **71**(19): p. 645–649.
110. Surveillance Research Program and N.C.I., SEER incidence data. *SEER Explorer: An Interactive* website for SEER cancer statistics, 2023.
111. Alpert, N., et al., Gender differences in outcomes of patients with mesothelioma. *American Journal of Clinical Oncology*, 2020. **43**(11): p. 792–797.
112. Barsky, A.R., et al., Gender-based disparities in receipt of care and survival in malignant pleural mesothelioma. *Clinical Lung Cancer*, 2020. **21**(6): p. e583–e591.
113. Woodard, G.A. and D.M. Jablons, Surgery for pleural mesothelioma, when it is indicated and why: Arguments against surgery for malignant pleural mesothelioma. *Translational Lung Cancer Research*, 2020. **9**(S1): p. S86–S91.
114. Huang, J., et al., Global incidence, risk factors, and temporal trends of mesothelioma: A population-based study. *Journal of Thoracic Oncology*, 2023. **18**(6): p. 792–802.
115. Zhu, W., et al., Global, regional, and national trends in mesothelioma burden from 1990 to 2019 and the predictions for the next two decades. *SSM – Population Health*, 2023. **23**: p. 101441.
116. Gao, Y., et al., Industry, occupation, and exposure history of mesothelioma patients in the U.S. National Mesothelioma Virtual Bank, 2006–2022. *Environmental Research*, 2023. **230**: p. 115085.

117. Gu, Y.F., et al., Epstein, How aging of the global population is changing oncology. *Ecancermedicalscience*, 2021. **15**: p. ed119.
118. Carbone, M., et al., Did the ban on asbestos reduce the incidence of mesothelioma? *Journal of Thoracic Oncology*, 2023. **18**(6): p. 694–697.
119. Sinha, S., et al., The role of imaging in malignant pleural mesothelioma: An update after the 2018 bts guidelines. *Clinical Radiology*, 2020. **75**(6): p. 423–432.
120. Martini, K. and T. Frauenfelder, Old borders and new horizons in multimodality imaging of malignant pleural mesothelioma. *The Thoracic and Cardiovascular Surgeon*, 2022. **70**(08): p. 677–683.
121. Armato, S.G., et al., Imaging in pleural mesothelioma: A review of the 14th International Conference of the International Mesothelioma Interest Group. *Lung Cancer*, 2019. **130**: p. 108–114.
122. Gill, R.R., et al., Radiologic considerations and standardization of malignant pleural mesothelioma imaging within clinical trials: Consensus statement from the NCI thoracic malignancy steering committee –. International Association for the Study of Lung Cancer – *Mesothelioma. Journal of Thoracic Oncology*, 2019. **14**(10): p. 1718–1731.
123. Tsim, S., et al., A comparison between MRI and CT in the assessment of primary tumour volume in mesothelioma. *Lung Cancer*, 2020. **150**: p. 12–20.
124. Blyth, K., et al., Fully automated volumetric measurement of malignant pleural mesothelioma from computed tomography images by deep learning: Preliminary results of an internal validation. Proceedings of the 13th International Joint Conference on Biomedical Engineering Systems and Technologies, 2020: p. 64–73.
125. Taralli, S., et al., The prognostic value of 18F-FDG PET imaging at staging in patients with malignant pleural mesothelioma: A literature review. *Journal of Clinical Medicine*, 2021. **11**(1): p. 33.
126. Pavic, M., et al., FDG PET versus CT radiomics to predict outcome in malignant pleural mesothelioma patients. *EJNMMI Research*, 2020. **10**(1): p. 81.
127. Ronneberger, O., P. Fischer, and T. Brox, U-net: Convolutional networks for biomedical image segmentation. In: *Lecture Notes in Computer Science*. Springer International Publishing, 2015: p. 234–241.
128. Berzenji, L., P.E. Van Schil, and L. Carp, The eighth TNM classification for malignant pleural mesothelioma. *Translational Lung Cancer Research*, 2018. **7**(5): p. 543–549.
129. Nowak, A.K., et al., The IASLC mesothelioma staging project: Proposals for revisions of the T descriptors in the forthcoming eighth edition of the TNM classification for pleural mesothelioma. *Journal of Thoracic Oncology*, 2016. **11**(12): p. 2089–2099.
130. Pairman, L., et al., Evaluation of pleural fluid cytology for the diagnosis of malignant pleural effusion: A retrospective cohort study. *Internal Medicine Journal*, 2022. **52**(7): p. 1154–1159.
131. Lynggard, L.A., et al., Diagnostic capacity of BAP1 and MTAP in cytology from effusions and biopsy in mesothelioma. *Journal of the American Society of Cytopathology*, 2022. **11**(6): p. 385–393.
132. Messina, G., et al., Diagnosis of malignant pleural disease: Ultrasound as "a detective probe". *Thoracic Cancer*, 2023. **14**(3): p. 223–230.
133. Popat, S., et al., Malignant pleural mesothelioma: ESMO clinical practice guidelines for diagnosis, treatment and follow-up☆up☆. *Annals of Oncology*, 2022. **33**(2): p. 129–142.
134. Carbone, M., et al., Positive nuclear BAP1 immunostaining helps differentiate non-small cell lung carcinomas from malignant mesothelioma. *Oncotarget*, 2016. **7**(37): p. 59314–59321.
135. Savic, I. and J. Myers, Update on diagnosing and reporting malignant pleural mesothelioma. *Acta Medica Academica*, 2021. **50**(1): p. 197.
136. Chapel, D.B., et al., Application of immunohistochemistry in diagnosis and management of malignant mesothelioma. *Translational Lung Cancer Research*, 2020. **9**(S1): p. S3–S27.
137. Chapel, D.B., et al., Clinical and molecular validation of BAP1, MTAP, P53, and Merlin immunohistochemistry in diagnosis of pleural mesothelioma. *Modern Pathology*, 2022. **35**(10): p. 1383–1397.
138. Husain, A.N., et al., Guidelines for pathologic diagnosis of malignant mesothelioma 2017 update of the consensus statement from the international mesothelioma interest group. *Archives of Pathology and Laboratory Medicine*, 2018. **142**(1): p. 89–108.
139. Patel, A., et al., Utility of Claudin-4 versus BerEP4 and B72.3 in pleural fluids with metastatic lung adenocarcinoma. *Journal of the American Society of Cytopathology*, 2020. **9**(3): p. 146–151.
140. Laury, A.R.M.H. et al., PAX8 reliably distinguishes ovarian serous tumors from malignant mesothelioma. *The American Journal of Surgical Pathology*, 2010. **34**(5): p. 627–635.
141. Terra, S.B.S.P., et al., Utility of immunohistochemistry for MUC4 and GATA3 to aid in the distinction of pleural sarcomatoid mesothelioma from pulmonary sarcomatoid carcinoma. *Archives of Pathology and Laboratory Medicine*, 2021. **145**(2): p. 208–213.
142. Prabhakaran, S., et al., The potential utility of GATA binding protein 3 for diagnosis of malignant pleural mesotheliomas. *Human Pathology*, 2020. **105**: p. 1–8.

143. Farkas, J.R., M. Sharobim, and J.J. Schulte, Updates on the pathologic diagnosis and classification of mesothelioma. *Journal of Cancer Metastasis and Treatment*, 2022. **8**.
144. Shaker, N., D. Wu, and A.M. Abid, Cytology of malignant pleural mesothelioma: Diagnostic criteria, WHO classification updates, and immunohistochemical staining markers diagnostic value. *Diagnostic Cytopathology*, 2022. **50**(11): p. 532–537.
145. Lenskaya, V. and C.A. Moran, Pleural mesothelioma: Current practice and approach. *Advances in Anatomic Pathology*, 2023. **30**(4): p. 243–252.
146. Chen, Z., et al., Diagnostic and prognostic biomarkers for malignant mesothelioma: An update. *Translational Lung Cancer Research*, 2017. **6**(3): p. 259–269.
147. Perera, N.D. and A.S. Mansfield, The evolving therapeutic landscape for malignant pleural mesothelioma. *Current Oncology Reports*, 2022. **24**(11): p. 1413–1423.
148. Bueno, R., I. Opitz, Surgery in malignant pleural mesothelioma. *Journal of Thoracic Oncology*, 2018. **13**(11): p. 1638–1654.
149. Friedberg, J.S., et al., A proposed system toward standardizing surgical-based treatments for malignant pleural mesothelioma, from the joint national cancer institute–international association for the study of lung cancer–mesothelioma applied research foundation taskforce. *Journal of Thoracic Oncology*, 2019. **14**(8): p. 1343–1353.
150. Kindler, H.L., et al., Treatment of malignant pleural mesothelioma: American society of clinical oncology clinical practice guideline. *Journal of Clinical Oncology*, 2018. **36**(13): p. 1343–1373.
151. Klotz, L.V., et al., Multimodal therapy of epithelioid pleural mesothelioma: Improved survival by changing the surgical treatment approach. *Translational Lung Cancer Research*, 2022. **11**(11): p. 2230–2242.
152. Aprile, V., et al., Hyperthermic intrathoracic chemotherapy for malignant pleural mesothelioma: The forefront of surgery-based multimodality treatment. *Journal of Clinical Medicine*, 2021. **10**(17): p. 3801.
153. Sugarbaker, D.J., et al., Hyperthermic intraoperative pleural cisplatin chemotherapy extends interval to recurrence and survival among low-risk patients with malignant pleural mesothelioma undergoing surgical macroscopic complete resection. *The Journal of Thoracic and Cardiovascular Surgery*, 2013. **145**(4): p. 955–963.
154. Ambrogi, M.C., et al., Diaphragm and lung–preserving surgery with hyperthermic chemotherapy for malignant pleural mesothelioma: A 10-year experience. *The Journal of Thoracic and Cardiovascular Surgery*, 2018. **155**(4): p. 1857–1866.e2.
155. Burt, B.M., et al., A Phase I trial of surgical resection and intraoperative hyperthermic cisplatin and gemcitabine for pleural mesothelioma. *Journal of Thoracic Oncology*, 2018. **13**(9): p. 1400–1409.
156. Opitz, I., et al., Intracavitary cisplatin-fibrin chemotherapy after surgery for malignant pleural mesothelioma: A phase I trial. *The Journal of Thoracic and Cardiovascular Surgery*, 2020. **159**(1): p. 330–340. e4.
157. Treasure, T.P., MD, et al., Extra-pleural pneumonectomy versus no extra-pleural pneumonectomy for patients with malignant pleural mesothelioma: Clinical outcomes of the Mesothelioma and Radical Surgery (MARS) randomised feasibility study. *Lancet Oncology*, 2011. **12**(8): p. 763–772.
158. Rintoul, R.C., et al., Efficacy and cost of video-assisted thoracoscopic partial pleurectomy versus talc pleurodesis in patients with malignant pleural mesothelioma (MesoVATS): An open-label, randomised, controlled trial. *Lancet*, 2014. **384**(9948): p. 1118–1127.
159. Thompson, A. B., et al., Addition of radiotherapy surgery and chemotherapy improves survival in localized malignant pleural mesothelioma. *Lung Cancer*, 2020. **146**: 120–126.
160. Nelson, D.B., et al., Defining the role of adjuvant radiotherapy for malignant pleural mesothelioma: A propensity-matched landmark analysis of the National Cancer Database. *Journal of Thoracic Disease*, 2019. **11**(4): p. 1269–1278.
161. Rimner, A., et al., Phase II study of hemithoracic intensity-modulated pleural radiation therapy (IMPRINT) as part of Lung-sparing multimodality therapy in patients with malignant pleural mesothelioma. *Journal of Clinical Oncology*, 2016. **34**(23): p. 2761–2768.
162. Foroudi, F., et al., High-dose palliative radiotherapy for malignant pleural mesothelioma. *Journal of Medical Imaging and Radiation Oncology*, 2017. **61**(6): p. 797–803.
163. Krayenbuehl, J., et al., Clinical outcome of postoperative highly conformal versus 3D conformal radiotherapy in patients with malignant pleural mesothelioma. *Radiation Oncology*, 2014. **9**(1): p. 32.
164. Simone, C.B. and K.A. Cengel, Photodynamic therapy for lung cancer and malignant pleural mesothelioma. *Seminars in Oncology*, 2014. **41**(6): p. 820–830.
165. Friedberg, J.S., et al., Photodynamic therapy and the evolution of a lung-sparing surgical treatment for mesothelioma. *The Annals of Thoracic Surgery*, 2011. **91**(6): p. 1738–1745.

166. Sun, H., et al., A real-time IR navigation system for pleural photodynamic therapy with a 3D surface acquisition system. *Proceedings of the SPIE - the International Society for Optical Engineering*, 2023. **12359**.
167. Rice, S.R., et al., A novel prospective study assessing the combination of photodynamic therapy and proton radiation therapy: Safety and outcomes when treating malignant pleural mesothelioma. *Photochemistry and Photobiology*, 2019. **95**(1): p. 411–418.
168. McCambridge, A.J., et al., Progress in the management of malignant pleural mesothelioma in 2017. *Journal of Thoracic Oncology*, 2018. **13**(5): p. 606–623.
169. Rondon, L., R. Fu, and M.R. Patel, Success of checkpoint blockade paves the way for novel immune therapy in malignant pleural mesothelioma. *Cancers*, 2023. **15**(11): p. 2940.
170. Ceresoli, G.L., et al., Tumour Treating Fields in combination with pemetrexed and cisplatin or carboplatin as first-line treatment for unresectable malignant pleural mesothelioma (STELLAR): A multicentre, single-arm phase 2 trial. *Lancet Oncology*, 2019. **20**(12): p. 1702–1709.
171. Okada, M., et al., Clinical Efficacy and Safety of Nivolumab: Results of a Multicenter, Open-label, Single-arm, Japanese Phase II study in Malignant Pleural mesothelioma (MERIT). *Clinical Cancer Research: An Official Journal of the American Association for Cancer Research*, 2019. **25**(18): p. 5485–5492.
172. Peters, S., et al., First-line nivolumab plus ipilimumab versus chemotherapy in patients with unresectable malignant pleural mesothelioma: 3-year outcomes from CheckMate 743. *Annals of Oncology: Official Journal of the European Society for Medical Oncology*, 2022. **33**(5): p. 488–499.
173. Nowak, A.K., et al., Durvalumab with first-line chemotherapy in previously untreated malignant pleural mesothelioma (DREAM): A multicentre, single-arm, phase 2 trial with a safety run-in. *The Lancet Oncology*, 2020. **21**(9): p. 1213–1223.
174. Forde, P.M., et al., Durvalumab with platinum-pemetrexed for unresectable pleural mesothelioma: Survival, genomic and immunologic analyses from the phase 2 PrE0505 trial. *Nature Medicine*, 2021. **27**(11): p. 1910–1920.
175. Popat, S., et al., A multicentre randomised phase III trial comparing pembrolizumab versus single-agent chemotherapy for advanced pre-treated malignant pleural mesothelioma: The European Thoracic Oncology Platform (ETOP 9–15) PROMISE-meso trial. *Annals of Oncology: Official Journal of the European Society for Medical Oncology*, 2020. **31**(12): p. 1734–1745.
176. Fennell, D.A., et al., Nivolumab versus placebo in patients with relapsed malignant mesothelioma (CONFIRM): A multicentre, double-blind, randomised, phase 3 trial. *The Lancet Oncology*, 2021. **22**(11): p. 1530–1540.
177. Scherpereel, A., et al., Nivolumab or nivolumab plus ipilimumab in patients with relapsed malignant pleural mesothelioma (IFCT-1501 MAPS2): A multicentre, open-label, randomised, non-comparative, phase 2 trial. *Lancet Oncology*, 2019. **20**(2): p. 239–253.
178. Zalcman, G., et al., Bevacizumab for newly diagnosed pleural mesothelioma in the mesothelioma Avastin cisplatin pemetrexed Study (MAPS): A randomised, controlled, open-label, phase 3 trial. *Lancet*, 2016. **387**(10026): p. 1405–1414.
179. Grosso, F., et al., Nintedanib plus pemetrexed/cisplatin in patients with malignant pleural mesothelioma: Phase II results from the randomized, placebo-controlled LUME-Meso trial. *Journal of Clinical Oncology: Official Journal of the American Society of Clinical Oncology*, 2017. **35**(31): p. 3591–3600.
180. Scagliotti, G., et al., Nintedanib in combination with pemetrexed and cisplatin for chemotherapy-naive patients with advanced malignant pleural mesothelioma (LUME-Meso): A double-blind, randomised, placebo-controlled phase 3 trial. *Lancet Respiratory Medicine*, 2019. **7**: p. 569–580.
181. Pinto, C., et al., Gemcitabine with or without ramucirumab as second-line treatment for malignant pleural mesothelioma (RAMES): A randomised, double-blind, placebo-controlled, phase 2 trial. *Lancet Oncology*, 2021. **22**: p. 1438–1447.
182. Meirson, T., et al., Comparison of 3 randomized clinical trials of frontline therapies for malignant pleural mesothelioma. *JAMA Network Open*, 2022. **5**(3): p. e221490.
183. McNamee, N., et al., Brief Report: Real-world toxicity and survival of combination immunotherapy in pleural mesothelioma - RIOMeso (article in press). *Journal of Thoracic Oncology*, 2024. **19**: p. 636–642.
184. Klampatsa, A., et al., Chimeric antigen receptor (CAR) T cell therapy for malignant pleural mesothelioma (MPM). *Cancers*, 2017. **9**(9): p. 115.
185. Adusumilli, P.S., et al., A Phase I trial of regional mesothelin-targeted CAR T-cell therapy in patients with malignant pleural disease, in combination with the anti-PD-1 agent pembrolizumab. *Cancer Discovery*, 2021. **11**(11): p. 2748–2763.

186. Cherkassky, L., et al., Human CAR T cells with cell-intrinsic PD-1 checkpoint blockade resist tumor-mediated inhibition. *Journal of Clinical Investigation*, 2016. **126**(8): p. 3130–3144.
187. Ding, J., et al., Mesothelin-targeting T cells bearing a novel T cell receptor fusion construct (TRuC) exhibit potent antitumor efficacy against solid tumors. *Oncoimmunology*, 2023. **12**(1): p. 2182058.
188. Baeuerle, P.A., et al., Synthetic TRuC receptors engaging the complete T cell receptor for potent anti-tumor response. *Nature Communications*, 2019. **10**(1): p. 2087.
189. Hassan, R., et al., Mesothelin-targeting T cell receptor fusion construct cell therapy in refractory solid tumors: Phase 1/2 trial interim results. *Nature Medicine*, 2023.
190. Pinilla-Ibarz, J., et al., Improved human T-cell responses against synthetic HLA-0201 analog peptides derived from the WT1 oncoprotein. *Leukemia*, 2006. **20**(11): p. 2025–2033.
191. Zauderer, M.G., et al., A randomized Phase II trial of adjuvant Galinpepimut-S, WT-1 analogue peptide vaccine, after multimodality therapy for patients with malignant pleural mesothelioma. *Clinical Cancer Research: An Official Journal of the American Association for Cancer Research*, 2017. **23**(24): p. 7483–7489.
192. Cornwall, S.M.J., et al., Human mesothelioma induces defects in dendritic cell numbers and antigen-processing function which predict survival outcomes. *OncoImmunology*, 2016. **5**(2): p. e1082028.
193. Aerts, J., et al., Autologous dendritic cells pulsed with allogeneic tumor cell lysate in mesothelioma: From mouse to human. *Clinical Cancer Research: An Official Journal of the American Association for Cancer Research*, 2018. **24**(4): p. 766–776.
194. Bononi, A., et al., Latest developments in our understanding of the pathogenesis of mesothelioma and the design of targeted therapies. *Expert Review of Respiratory Medicine*, 2015. **9**(5): p. 633–654.
195. Ghafoor, A., et al., Phase 2 study of olaparib in malignant mesothelioma and correlation of efficacy with germline or somatic mutations in BAP1 gene. *JTO Clinical and Research Reports*, 2021. **2**(10): p. 100231.
196. Ashworth, C.J.L.A., PARP inhibitors: Synthetic lethality in the clinic. *Science*, 2017. **355**(6330): p. 1152–1158.
197. Fong, P.C., et al., Inhibition of poly(ADP-ribose) polymerase in tumors from BRCA mutation carriers. *New England Journal of Medicine*, 2009. **361**(2): p. 123–134.
198. Jensen, D.E., et al., BAP1: A novel ubiquitin hydrolase which binds to the BRCA1 ring finger and enhances BRCA1-mediated cell growth suppression. *Oncogene*, 1998. **16**(9): p. 1097–1112.
199. Rathkey, D., et al., Sensitivity of mesothelioma cells to PARP inhibitors is not dependent on BAP1 but is enhanced by temozolomide in cells with high-schlafen 11 and low-O6-methylguanine-DNA methyltransferase expression. *Journal of Thoracic Oncology*, 2020. **15**(5): p. 843–859.
200. Fennell, D.A., et al., Rucaparib in patients with BAP1-deficient or BRCA1-deficient mesothelioma (MiST1): An open-label, single-arm, phase 2a clinical trial. *Lancet Respiratory Medicine*, 2021. **9**(6): p. 593–600.
201. Poulikakos, P.I., et al., Re-expression of the tumor suppressor NF2/merlin inhibits invasiveness in mesothelioma cells and negatively regulates FAK. *Oncogene*, 2006. **25**(44): p. 5960–5968.
202. Mak, G., et al., A phase Ib dose-finding, pharmacokinetic study of the focal adhesion kinase inhibitor GSK2256098 and trametinib in patients with advanced solid tumours. *British Journal of Cancer*, 2019. **120**(10): p. 975–981.
203. Soria, J.C., et al., A phase I, pharmacokinetic and pharmacodynamic study of GSK2256098, a focal adhesion kinase inhibitor, in patients with advanced solid tumors. *Annals of Oncology: Official Journal of the European Society for Medical Oncology*, 2016. **27**(12): p. 2268–2274.
204. Zhang, W.-Q., et al., Targeting YAP in malignant pleural mesothelioma. *Journal of Cellular and Molecular Medicine*, 2017. **21**(11): p. 2663–2676.
205. Dubois, F., et al., Molecular alterations in malignant pleural mesothelioma: A hope for effective treatment by targeting YAP. *Targeted Oncology*, 2022. **17**(4): p. 407–431.
206. Aliagas, E., et al., Efficacy of CDK4/6 inhibitors in preclinical models of malignant pleural mesothelioma. *British Journal of Cancer*, 2021. **125**(10): p. 1365–1376.
207. Fennell, D.A., et al., Abemaciclib in patients with p16ink4A-deficient mesothelioma (MiST2): A single-arm, open-label, phase 2 trial. *Lancet Oncology*, 2022. **23**(3): p. 374–381.
208. Bonelli, M.A., et al., Combined inhibition of CDK4/6 and PI3K/AKT/mTOR pathways induces a synergistic anti-tumor effect in malignant pleural mesothelioma cells. *Neoplasia*, 2017. **19**(8): p. 637–648.
209. Bonelli, M., et al., Dual inhibition of CDK4/6 and PI3K/AKT/mTOR signaling impairs energy metabolism in MPM cancer cells. *International Journal of Molecular Sciences*, 2020. **21**(14): p. 5165.

210. Carbone, M., M. Minaai, Y. Takinishi, I. Pagano, and H. Yang Preventive and therapeutic opportunities: Targeting BAP1 and/or HMGB1 pathways to diminish the burden of mesothelioma. *Journal of Translational Medicine*2023. **21**: p. 749.
211. Sandri, A., et al., Validation of EORTC and CALGB prognostic models in surgical patients submitted to diagnostic, palliative or curative surgery for malignant pleural mesothelioma. *Journal of Thoracic Disease*, 2016. **8**(8): p. 2121–2127.
212. Paajanen, J., et al., Clinical features in patients with malignant pleural mesothelioma with 5-year survival and evaluation of original diagnoses. *Clinical Lung Cancer*, 2020. **21**(6): p. e633–e639.
213. Brims, F.J.H., et al., A novel clinical prediction model for prognosis in malignant pleural mesothelioma using decision tree analysis. *Journal of Thoracic Oncology*, 2016. **11**(4): p. 573–582.
214. Yeap, B.Y., et al., Mesothelioma risk score: A new prognostic pretreatment, clinical-molecular algorithm for malignant pleural mesothelioma. *Journal of Thoracic Oncology*, 2021. **16**(11): p. 1925–1935.
215. Courtiol, P., et al., Deep learning-based classification of mesothelioma improves prediction of patient outcome. *Nature Medicine*, 2019. **25**(10): p. 1519–1525.
216. Zauderer, M.G., et al., The use of a next-generation sequencing-derived machine-learning risk-prediction model (OncoCast-MPM) for malignant pleural mesothelioma: A retrospective study. *Lancet Digit Health*, 2021. **3**(9): p. e565–e576.
217. Scherpereel, A., et al., ERS/ESTS/EACTS/ESTRO guidelines for the management of malignant pleural mesothelioma. *European Respiratory Journal*, 2020. **55**(6): p. 1900953.
218. Armato, S.G. and A.K. Nowak, Revised modified response evaluation criteria in solid tumors for assessment of response in malignant pleural mesothelioma (Version 1.1). *Journal of Thoracic Oncology*, 2018. **13**(7): p. 1012–1021.
219. Seymour, L., et al., iRECIST: Guidelines for response criteria for use in trials testing immunotherapeutics. *Lancet Oncology*, 2017. **18**(3): p. e143–e152.
220. Novelli, F., et al., Germline BARD1 variants predispose to mesothelioma by impairing DNA repair and Calcium signaling. *Proc Natl Acad Sci USA*, 2024. In press.

TABLE 10.1
Immunohistochemical Markers Commonly Used for the Differential Diagnosis of Malignant Mesothelioma.

Differential Diagnosis	Markers
Malignant mesothelioma	Pankeratin, CK7, Calretinin, WT1,* Cytokeratin 5 or 5/6 and HEG1,** Podoplanin (D2-40)***
Lung adenocarcinoma	Pankeratin, Claudin 4, TTF-1, Napsin A, MOC31
Lung squamous cell carcinoma	Pankeratin, Cytokeratin 5 or 5/6, p40, p63, Claudin 4,
Renal cell carcinoma	CK7, PAX8, CAIX9, CD10, RCC, Claudin 4
Breast/Ovarian/Endometrial	PAX8, WT1*, Estrogen receptor, Claudin 4, MOC31
Large cell lymphoma	CD45, CD20, CD3, CD30
Melanoma	S100, HMB-45, SOX-10, Melan-A
Angiosarcoma/Hemangioendothelioma	CD31, CD34, D2-40, ERG (or FLI-1)

Note: *WT1: often positive in ovarian and uterine malignancies.
**CK5, CK5/6, and HEG1 positive in epithelioid mesothelioma cells; HEG1 is also positive in ovarian carcinomas;
***D2-40: sensitive but not a specific marker.

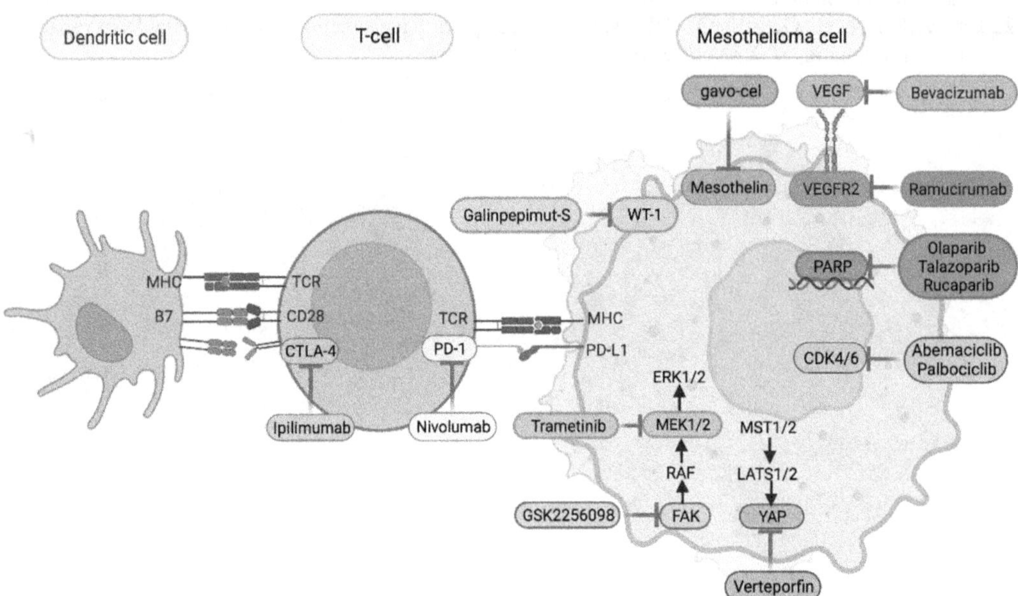

FIGURE 10.1 Latest therapeutic agents. The latest immunotherapeutic agents and targeted molecular therapies are presented. Ipilimumab and Nivolumab are the FDA approved drugs that target CTLA-4 and PD-1, respectively. Gavo-cel, an anti-mesothelin antibody integrated in a T-cell receptor construct effectively targets mesothelin, expressed on the surface of mesothelioma cells. The WT-1 analog peptide vaccine Galinpepimut-S targets WT-1 on the mesothelioma cell surface. In order to inhibit angiogenesis, Bevacizumab and Ramucirumab are used to target VEGF and VEGFR2, respectively. PARP inhibitors cause synthetic legality on BAP1 deficient cells that have defective double-strand break repair mechanisms. To induce cell cycle arrest and block the proliferation of cancer cells, CDK4/6 inhibitors are used. Targeting Hippo pathway through inhibition of its key regulator, YAP, can inhibit cell proliferation and slow cell growth. Trametinib and GSK2256098 are used to inhibit the function of MEK1/2 and FAK, both components of ERK pathway that regulates gene transcription and cell growth.

11 Pathologic Diagnosis of Mesothelioma

David B. Chapel, Aliya N. Husain, and Thomas Krausz

11.1 INTRODUCTION

Mesothelioma is a malignant neoplasm of the body's serosal surfaces. Approximately 85–90% arise in the pleura, 10–15% in the peritoneum, and ~1% each in the pericardium and tunica vaginalis.[1,2] Accurate diagnosis of mesothelial lesions (and their non-mesothelial mimics) is accomplished through integration of clinical, radiographic, morphological, immunophenotypic, and molecular data. Pathologic examination has four broad aims:

1) To distinguish mesothelial versus non-mesothelial (epithelial, mesenchymal, hematolymphoid, melanocytic) proliferations.
2) To distinguish benign versus malignant mesothelial proliferations.
3) To provide morphologic subclassification of mesotheliomas.
4) To provide clinically relevant immunohistochemical or molecular profiling.

This chapter is structured around these four aims, examining the role of histomorphology, immunohistochemistry, and molecular assays in routine diagnosis, classification, and grading of mesothelioma. Issues around epidemiology, radiology, molecular pathogenesis, and clinical management are addressed when relevant, but these are principally addressed in separate chapters. The pathologist should, whenever possible, review clinical and radiographic information prior to diagnosing mesothelioma (though the reported asbestos exposure history should not substantially influence the pathologist's evaluation). Collaboration between pathologists, pulmonologists, surgical and medical oncologists, and radiologists – ideally in the setting of a multidisciplinary tumor board – facilitates proper diagnosis and management.

Though mesotheliomas of the body's four serosal cavities are fundamentally similar, they show some differences in epidemiology, risk factors, histotype distribution, molecular pathogenesis, prognosis, and differential diagnosis. Where appropriate, diagnostically relevant differences between pleural and peritoneal mesothelioma are noted. Data on pericardial mesothelioma and mesothelioma of the tunica vaginalis are limited, particularly regarding modern diagnostic tests.

11.1.1 Terminology

In the most recent (5th) edition of the World Health Organization's *Classification of Thoracic Tumours*, "mesothelioma" is understood to be malignant, and the older term "malignant mesothelioma" is now simply "mesothelioma," and "well-differentiated papillary mesothelioma" and "multicystic mesothelioma" are replaced by "well-differentiated papillary mesothelial tumor" and "(multilocular) peritoneal inclusion cyst," respectively.

"Mesothelioma" without further specification is generally understood to refer to "diffuse mesothelioma," which shows multifocal or diffuse serosal involvement and accounts for 99% of mesotheliomas. Localized mesotheliomas, in contrast, account for just 1% of all mesotheliomas (see below).

DOI: 10.1201/9781003431909-11

11.2 GROSS PATHOLOGIC EXAMINATION

Serosal specimens received for pathologic examination include cytologic preparations, tissue biopsies, and resections. Cytology specimens almost entirely comprise effusion aspirates. Tissue biopsies include transcutaneous (blind or radiologically guided) core needle biopsies, open surgical biopsies, and video-assisted thoracoscopic (VATS) biopsies. VATS biopsies are increasingly preferred, as they permit detailed clinical evaluation and larger biopsies sampled from multiple serosal sites under direct examination, without the morbidity of open surgery. Gross evaluation of biopsies is generally not informative, but the aggregate three-dimensional tissue size and the size of the largest fragment(s) should be documented.

Resections for pleural mesothelioma include decortication and extrapleural pneumonectomy. Decortications are typically received as numerous unoriented fragments, which limits meaningful gross examination and obviates margin evaluation. At least 1 tissue block per cm of greatest aggregate dimension should be sampled, including areas of significant thickening or invasion of skeletal muscle or lung parenchyma.

Extrapleural pneumonectomy is increasingly rare. In these specimens, the tumor's relationship to parietal pleura, lung parenchyma, diaphragm, and pericardium should be documented. The bronchial margin may be received for frozen section. Comprehensive assessment of the final margin status is challenging, as virtually the entire parietal pleura represents a margin here.[3]

For peritoneal mesothelioma, cytoreduction surgery is roughly analogous to pleural decortication, albeit with frequent addition of abdominal viscera, including gynecologic organs, spleen, portions of liver, and segments of bowel. Gross invasion of serosa, omentum, diaphragm, and viscera should be sampled.

11.3 HISTOMORPHOLOGIC EXAMINATION

Morphology is the cornerstone of pathologic diagnosis. In evaluating serosal lesions, morphologic examination serves (1) to prompt recognition of mesothelial differentiation, (2) to distinguish benign mesothelial proliferations from mesothelioma (with immunohistochemical aid in challenging cases), and (3) to provide proper histologic subtyping. Morphologic evaluation is also central to the staging of pleural mesothelioma. There is currently no staging system in place for peritoneal, pericardial, or paratesticular mesotheliomas.

11.3.1 Morphologic Features of Mesothelium

Although immunohistochemistry plays a central role in the confirmation of mesothelial lineage, mesothelium has certain characteristic morphologic features that facilitate its recognition on H&E-stained slides. Normal quiescent mesothelium comprises a single layer of monomorphic cuboidal epithelioid cells, with scant-to-moderate eosinophilic cytoplasm and a bland, round nucleus, sometimes with a small nucleolus. As further detailed below, reactive mesothelium may proliferate to form multiple layers, simple surface papillae, and/or trabecular or retiform formations in a linear array parallel to the mesothelial surface. Mesothelial cell-cell adhesions leave a small space or "window" between adjacent cells, which may become more conspicuous in multilayered reactive mesothelium.

As detailed below, mesothelial tumors span a broad cytomorphologic and architectural spectrum, but some of the above-listed features – round monomorphic nuclei, eosinophilic cytoplasm, cell-cell "windows" – are often evident, particularly in well-differentiated low-grade tumors. The experienced pathologist's recognition of these features facilitates proper classification (though, outside of banal quiescent surface mesothelium or morphologically conventional reactive mesothelial hyperplasia, immunohistochemical confirmation of mesothelial lineage is almost always performed (see section 11.4.1, Distinguishing Mesothelial Versus Non-Mesothelial Proliferations.)

11.3.2 Distinguishing Mesothelioma from Reactive Mesothelial Proliferations

Here we detail the morphologic distinction between mesothelioma and reactive mesothelial proliferations. This differential presupposes that mesothelial lineage is confirmed, most often by immunohistochemistry, as detailed below (section 11.4.1). Mesothelioma's differential with benign indolent, predominantly peritoneal mesothelial tumors is discussed in a separate section below (section 11.8).

Reactive mesothelial proliferations can show epithelioid and/or spindled morphology, mimicking epithelioid, sarcomatoid, or biphasic mesothelioma. Accurate morphologic distinction relies on evaluation of mesothelial organization, tissue invasion, and mass-forming tumefactive growth. Good tissue orientation is essential, as tangential sectioning obscures tissue organization and can mimic sheet-like growth or invasion. Cytomorphologic features are often unhelpful, as reactive mesothelial hyperplasia can show nuclear atypia, mitoses, and necrosis (though frank pleomorphism and true coagulative necrosis are absent).[4]

At low magnification, reactive mesothelial hyperplasia generally has a regular or organized appearance, with mesothelial cords, trabeculae, and/or retiform spaces arranged in linear arrays parallel to the serosal surface (Figure 11.1). Reactive mesothelium with epithelioid cytomorphology can show surface multilayering or simple papillary projections. Mesothelial entrapment in granulation tissue or below a fibrous adhesion can mimic deep tissue invasion, but the mesothelial structures' orderly linear arrangement and parallel orientation to the overlying surface facilitate proper classification.

Reactive spindled mesothelial proliferations ("fibrous pleurisy") typically show fascicular (rather than storiform) growth. The reactive rind is typically of roughly uniform thickness, and there is zonation of cellularity, with hypercellularity toward the surface and lower cellularity in deeper layers ("maturation"). Capillary-sized vessels run perpendicular to the serosal surface at approximately even intervals (Figure 11.2). Storiform or haphazard growth, abrupt alterations between hypo- and hypercellular foci, and irregular expansile nodular growth are worrisome for sarcomatoid mesothelioma.

Invasion of extrapleural tissues is diagnostic of mesothelioma, but tissue invasion can be superficial and subtle, without desmoplasia or significant atypia. Cytokeratin immunostains may help confirm the extension of mesothelial nests into extrapleural tissues. Artifactual tissue spaces ("fake fat") within a reactive mesothelial proliferation can mimic adipose tissue, simulating invasion, and prompting overdiagnosis of mesothelioma.[5] "Fake fat" is recognized by the spaces' variable and irregular size and absence of adipocyte nuclei. Additionally, "fake fat" is negative for S100, collagen IV, and laminin, while true adipocytes are positive.

A gross tumor mass justifies the diagnosis of localized or diffuse mesothelioma, even in the absence of invasion.

Morphology may be insufficient for a definitive distinction of benign reactive versus malignant mesothelial proliferations, particularly in biopsies and florid lesions. Immunohistochemical surrogates for malignancy-defining molecular alterations, or direct molecular interrogation, are often helpful in such cases, as discussed below (section 11.4.2).

11.3.3 Morphologic Classification of Mesothelioma

Mesothelioma is classified into epithelioid, biphasic, and sarcomatoid types, which can then be further subcategorized by architectural, cytomorphologic, and stromal features. Among pleural mesothelioma, 60–70% are epithelioid, 15–30% biphasic, and 10–15% sarcomatoid.[6–9] Mesotheliomas of the tunica vaginalis are ~60% epithelioid and ~40% biphasic, with sarcomatoid tumors exceptionally rare.[10, 11] Non-epithelioid tumors are less common in the peritoneum, where 85–90% are epithelioid, 10–15% biphasic, and <5% sarcomatoid.[12–14] Histotype is strongly correlated with survival. Among pleural mesotheliomas, median survival is 15–16 months for epithelioid, 7–8 months for biphasic, and 4–6 months for sarcomatoid tumors.[6, 15–17]

Histotype should be reported in biopsies as well as resection specimens, as a significant proportion of mesotheliomas are not amenable to surgical resection. Concordance between histotype assigned on biopsy versus resection is 80%, but there is considerable variation: 90–98% of epithelioid mesotheliomas are accurately classified on biopsy, compared with just 45–55% of biphasic and sarcomatoid mesotheliomas.[18, 19]

Resections following chemotherapy do not typically show marked alterations in tumor morphology, though bizarre multinucleated tumors cells may be seen after radiation.[20] Patients with recurrent pleural effusion may be treated with pleurodesis, using talc or (less often) chemotherapeutic agents. This causes a diffuse foreign body giant cell reaction, often associated with superimposed reactive mesothelial hyperplasia.[20] Identification of residual tumor may require generous sampling. Immunohistochemical stains for mesothelioma-associated molecular alterations can be used to distinguish tumor from reactive epithelioid or spindled mesothelium in some cases (see section 11.4.2).

11.3.3.1 Epithelioid Mesothelioma

Epithelioid mesothelioma is characterized by cuboidal, columnar, or polyhedral cells, with usually moderate to voluminous cytoplasm. Nuclear atypia can be mild, moderate, or severe. Mitotic activity is most often low (median 3, range 0–64 mitoses per 10 high-power fields).[21] Necrosis is seen in 30–35%.[15, 16] Nuclear atypia, mitotic count, and necrosis are used to grade epithelioid mesothelioma, as detailed below.

Epithelioid mesotheliomas show a wide range of architectural patterns, and multiple patterns are frequently present in a single tumor. Some of these are prognostically significant, and architectural pattern(s) should be reported for both biopsies and resections. In resections, the percent contribution of each pattern is reported, estimated to the nearest 10%.[4, 22]

The most common patterns are tubulopapillary, trabecular, solid, adenomatoid, and micropapillary. *Tubulopapillary* architecture intuitively comprises variably dilated tubules with frequent intraluminal papillary projections (Figure 11.3). Occasional tumors show exclusively tubular or papillary growth, and some authors place cribriform or "adenoid cystic-like" architecture under the tubulopapillary umbrella.[23] *Trabecular* architecture comprises thin, sinuous, sometimes anastomosing cords (Figure 11.4). The *adenomatoid* pattern resembles adenomatoid tumor, with small tubules lined by cuboidal to attenuated mesothelium (Figure 11.5). Tubulopapillary, trabecular, and adenomatoid architecture are prognostically favorable.[22] Conversely, predominantly *solid* architecture, comprising cohesive tumor sheets or nests without other defining architectural features (Figure 11.6), is associated with a poorer prognosis.[16, 23] *Micropapillary* architecture, characterized by small cellular projections without fibrovascular stromal cores (Figure 11.7), is associated with a poorer prognosis and increased risk of lymph node metastases.[23, 24]

A number of "variant cytologic features" are defined for epithelioid mesothelioma, including rhabdoid, signet ring, small cell, clear cell, and deciduoid features.[22] Though data are limited, rhabdoid and small-cell morphologies appear to be prognostically adverse, while signet ring and clear-cell morphologies are prognostically neutral. Deciduoid mesothelioma may show low-grade or high-grade morphology, which corresponds to tumor behavior.[25] As these morphologies are regarded as variants of epithelioid mesothelioma, their co-occurrence with frankly sarcomatoid areas warrants diagnosis of biphasic mesothelioma.

- *Rhabdoid* morphology is marked by an eccentric nucleus, displaced by an eosinophilic cytoplasmic inclusion, positive for cytokeratin but negative for skeletal muscle markers (Figure 11.8). In mesotheliomas with "rhabdoid features," the rhabdoid cells account for 15–75% of tumor cells.[26] SWI/SNF protein deficiency is rare (<1%) in mesothelioma, but may sometimes be associated with rhabdoid morphology.[27, 28]
- *Signet ring* morphology is characterized by an eccentric, sometimes crescent-shaped nucleus, displaced by a clear or palely basophilic cytoplasmic vacuole (Figure 11.9). These vacuoles contain hyaluronic acid and are frequently accompanied by prominent

myxoid stroma. Signet ring cells account for 10–80% (median, 20–25%) of tumor cells in such cases. In some cases, signet ring formations coalesce into adenomatoid or nested structures.[29]

- *Small cell* morphology is characterized by scant cytoplasm and densely apposed nuclei. This may resemble small-cell lung cancer at low magnification, but mesothelioma with small-cell features, unlike small-cell lung cancer, shows slightly more abundant clear to eosinophilic cytoplasm, distinct cell borders, vesicular chromatin with small nucleoli, mitoses <5 per 10 high-power fields, and inconspicuous apoptoses (Figure 11.10). Small cells may predominate in biopsies, but they typically account for only 15–20% of tumor cells in resections.[30] Mesotheliomas with small cell features lack true neuroendocrine differentiation, and neuroendocrine and epithelial markers are negative while mesothelial markers are positive. The term "small cell mesothelioma" is discouraged to avoid conflation with true neuroendocrine neoplasia.[31]
- *Clear cell* morphology in mesothelioma[32] is a somewhat heterogeneous finding, characterized by optically clear or foamy cytoplasm, which can be caused by accumulation of glycogen and/or lipid, florid cytoplasmic vesicle or lumen formation, or mitochondrial swelling (Figure 11.11). Clear cells may be focal (20–40%) or diffuse. Solid growth often predominates, but tubulopapillary or papillary growth can also be present. Mesotheliomas with clear cell morphology may be enriched for *VHL* mutations and genomic near-haploidization.[33]
- *Deciduoid* mesothelioma refers to the typically solid growth of polygonal cells with abundant eosinophilic cytoplasm and distinct cell membranes, resembling decidualized endometrial stroma (Figure 11.12). Deciduoid cells may account for 10–100% of tumor cells in these cases. Contrary to initial reports, these tumors can occur in the pleura or peritoneum of both men and women, and they may show low- or high-grade morphology, which correlates with prognosis.[25]

Pleomorphic and lymphohistiocytoid mesothelioma are additional cytologic variants, but there is some debate as to whether these are best regarded as epithelioid or sarcomatoid morphologies.

Pleomorphic mesothelioma is defined by ≥10% of cells showing epithelioid or polygonal morphology, moderate to abundant cytoplasm, nuclear hyperchromasia and enlargement, anisonucleosis, and prominent nucleoli (Figure 11.13). Multinucleated tumor giant cells are often seen. Mitoses are usually brisk (>20 per 10 high-power fields), with frequent atypical mitoses. Survival in pleomorphic mesothelioma is comparable to sarcomatoid mesothelioma.[23, 34, 35] Some have proposed that their behavior warrants classification as a subtype of sarcomatoid mesothelioma,[23] while others counter that their ultrastructural features are more in line with epithelioid mesothelioma.[35] Median overall survival in pleomorphic mesothelioma (5 months) is significantly shorter than for high-grade epithelioid mesothelioma (9 months).[15] The most recent (5th edition) WHO classification acknowledges that pleomorphism may be encountered in epithelioid, biphasic, or sarcomatoid mesotheliomas and permits classification of pleomorphic mesotheliomas into any of these groups on the basis of individual cases' cytomorphology.[36]

In *lymphohistiocytoid* mesothelioma, >50% of the tumor comprises discohesive polygonal tumor cells resembling histiocytes, in a background of dense lymphoplasmacytic inflammation (Figure 11.14). These foci have an overall syncytial appearance. Adequate sampling almost always reveals areas of non-lymphohistiocytoid morphology, and the current recommendation is to histotype the tumor based on that latter component. The overall prognosis in lymphohistiocytoid mesothelioma most resembles epithelioid mesothelioma, and the rare (<1%) subset of sarcomatoid mesotheliomas with lymphohistiocytoid morphology appears to have a relatively favorable prognosis.[6, 37]

Note that dense inflammation alone does not warrant diagnosis of lymphohistiocytoid mesothelioma. Criteria have been proposed for routine reporting of tumor-infiltrating lymphocytes in mesothelioma,[38] though this is not currently standard practice, and there are conflicting data on the prognostic significance of tumor-infiltrating lymphocytes here.[39–42]

A subset of epithelioid mesotheliomas (~10% in one referral series[34]) have prominent myxoid stroma, which comprises >50% of the tumor volume (Figure 11.15). This finding is considered prognostically favorable,[34, 43] though data are conflicting.[23]

Grading: The most recent (5th edition) WHO classification endorses a two-tier grading system for all pleural epithelioid mesotheliomas, accounting for nuclear atypia, mitotic activity, and necrosis.[15, 22, 36] This represents a condensed version of a four-tier system[16] that evolved from a three-tier system proposed in 2012[21] (**Table 11.1**). Routine grading is not currently endorsed for biphasic or sarcomatoid mesotheliomas, or for peritoneal mesotheliomas. (Although the 2012 three-tier grading system is prognostic in peritoneal epithelioid mesothelioma, necrosis was not associated with survival in one large peritoneal cohort.[12])

By the 2012 three-tier system, 31–46% of pleural epithelioid mesotheliomas are grade I, 39–52% grade II, and 15–17% grade III. Overall survival is 25–28 months for grade I, 13–14 months for grade II, and 5–8 months for grade III.[15, 16, 21] Using the two-tier system, 53–65% are low-grade and 35–47% high-grade, with respective median survival of 18–19 and 9–11 months.[15, 44]

Although paired biopsy and resection specimens show only 75% concordance in grading,[19] the current two-tier system is highly prognostically significant in biopsy-heavy cohorts.[15] Due to morphologic heterogeneity, the prognostic significance of grading correlates with the number and size of biopsies. The minimum tissue required for meaningful grading is one intact, well-preserved biopsy measuring at least 10 mm. The optimal sample (i.e. the limit of marginal returns) is three biopsies from different sites, or a single biopsy measuring at least 20 mm. For any specimen with spatial heterogeneity of grade, the highest applicable grade should be reported.

Further modifications to these histomorphology-based grading systems have been proposed, including one applicable to sarcomatoid and biphasic as well as epithelioid mesothelioma.[44] These modifications are not yet widely accepted, but suggest that risk stratification models for mesothelioma will continue to evolve.

11.3.3.2 Sarcomatoid Mesothelioma

Sarcomatoid mesothelioma is defined by elongated spindled cells with fascicular, storiform, or haphazard architecture and invasion of extrapleural tissues (Figure 11.16). These tumors range from hypo- to hypercellular, and they can show mild, moderate, or marked nuclear atypia. Mitoses can be scarce or brisk, and atypical mitoses may be seen. Necrosis is common. Sarcomatoid mesothelioma carries a dismal prognosis, and there is no grading system in place for these tumors.

Heterologous osteosarcomatous, chondrosarcomatous, or rhabdomyosarcomatous differentiation is seen in ~2% of sarcomatoid mesotheliomas (Figure 11.17).[45] This finding does not appear to worsen prognosis. Ninety percent of such tumors are at least focally cytokeratin-positive, facilitating distinction from most primary or metastatic sarcomas. Ancillary testing for molecular alterations characteristic of mesothelioma or key sarcoma differentials may also be informative.

Desmoplastic mesothelioma is a sarcomatoid variant with a predominantly (>50%) hypocellular spindle cell population in collagenous to hyalinized stroma (Figure 11.18). So defined, desmoplastic mesothelioma accounts for ~20% of all sarcomatoid mesotheliomas, while an additional 35% of sarcomatoid mesotheliomas have "desmoplastic features" (i.e. 10–50% desmoplastic morphology).[6] The threshold between desmoplastic and conventional sarcomatoid mesothelioma is subjective, but this distinction is not prognostically or clinically significant. However, a high index of suspicion for desmoplastic mesothelioma will facilitate distinction from scar or fibrous pleurisy. Cytokeratin immunostains can be used to demonstrate areas of subtle extrapleural invasion.

Transitional mesothelioma shows features resembling a "transition" between epithelioid and sarcomatoid morphology: sheets of cohesive, elongated but plump, tapering cells with abundant cytoplasm, discrete cell borders, and large round nuclei with prominent nucleoli (Figure 11.19). Mitoses can be brisk, including atypical mitoses. "Frank sarcomatous features" are absent by definition, though this will be a subjective distinction in some cases. Though many were likely diagnosed as epithelioid mesothelioma historically, transitional mesothelioma is now classified as a variant of sarcomatoid mesothelioma due to its transcriptomic profile and dismal prognosis.[46] Interobserver reproducibility in diagnosis of transitional mesothelioma is moderate among pathologists with mesothelioma expertise,[46, 47] but it is likely lower among non-specialists. A reticulin stain may be helpful, revealing single-cell investment in transitional and sarcomatoid mesothelioma, versus a nested reticulin pattern in epithelioid mesothelioma.[46]

11.3.3.3 Biphasic Mesothelioma

Biphasic mesothelioma comprises distinct epithelioid and sarcomatoid components. The morphology of the individual elements is indistinguishable from that of pure epithelioid or sarcomatoid mesothelioma. In resections, diagnosis of biphasic mesothelioma requires that each component constitutes ≥10% of the tumor. In biopsies, by contrast, any amount of definitive epithelioid and sarcomatoid morphology is diagnosed as biphasic mesothelioma. A biopsy diagnosis of biphasic mesothelioma is confirmed on resection in 90% of cases, with the remainder roughly evenly split between epithelioid and sarcomatoid on resection.[19] Interobserver reproducibility in diagnosis of biphasic mesothelioma is fair to moderate among pathologists with mesothelioma expertise.[17, 48]

Biphasic mesotheliomas with predominantly (>50%) sarcomatoid morphology have a poorer prognosis than those with predominantly epithelioid morphology.[43, 49] Accordingly, the percent contribution of the epithelioid and sarcomatoid elements should be reported, estimated to the nearest 10%. This is best determined on a resection specimen, as an agreement is only fair (albeit greater than expected by chance alone) for distinguishing epithelioid-predominant versus sarcomatoid-predominant biphasic mesotheliomas in paired biopsies and resections.[19]

Epithelioid mesothelioma associated with a component of reactive spindled mesothelium is an important differential for biphasic mesothelioma. Frankly, malignant morphology in the spindled component is diagnostic of biphasic mesothelioma. In morphologically challenging cases, immunostains to detect malignancy-defining molecular alterations in the spindled component (often shared with the epithelioid component) can help establish the diagnosis (see below, section 11.4.2).

11.4 IMMUNOHISTOCHEMISTRY AND MOLECULAR ASSAYS IN DIAGNOSIS OF MESOTHELIOMA

Immunohistochemistry plays two principal roles in the diagnosis of mesothelioma: (1) distinguishing mesothelial versus non-mesothelial proliferations (i.e. establishing mesothelial lineage), and (2) distinguishing benign versus malignant mesothelial proliferations. One or the other of these functions may be more important in individual cases, depending on clinical, radiologic, and morphologic findings. By convention, ≥10% tumor cell staining is the threshold for "positive" staining in these differentials,[4] but this rather arbitrary threshold should not supersede the pathologist's judgment.[50]

Molecular assays – including fluorescence in situ hybridization (FISH), next-generation sequencing panels, and cytogenetics arrays – are also used to detect pathogenic molecular alterations and thus to distinguish benign from malignant mesothelial proliferations.

11.4.1 Distinguishing Mesothelial versus Non-mesothelial Proliferations

Immunohistochemistry plays a central role in the confirmation of mesothelial lineage, thus separating benign and malignant mesothelial proliferations from non-mesothelial mimics. The distinction between benign mesothelial and benign non-mesothelial lesions is often academic, but the accurate distinction between mesothelioma and non-mesothelial malignancies is of great clinical importance.

Mesothelioma's most common differential is carcinoma, with specific differentials depending on tumor morphology and site. Because both mesothelioma and carcinoma express broad-spectrum cytokeratins, more specific markers of mesothelial and epithelial lineage are indispensable. Suitable markers will show >80% sensitivity and >80% specificity. Because no marker is 100% sensitive or specific, they are applied as immunopanels. The initial immunopanel should include two epithelial and two mesothelial markers, followed by additional stains if initial results are ambiguous.

11.4.1.1 Cytokeratins

Broad-spectrum cytokeratins are positive in virtually 100% of epithelioid mesotheliomas and 90–95% of sarcomatoid mesotheliomas, particularly when multiple stains (e.g. cytokeratins 8/18, AE1/AE3, CAM 5.2, and MNF116) are used.[6] Staining is typically diffuse, even in sarcomatoid mesothelioma. The 5–10% of cytokeratin-negative sarcomatoid mesotheliomas are presumptively diagnosed as such in the context of supportive clinical and radiographic findings after other differentials have been reasonably excluded by ancillary studies. Detection of molecular alterations characteristic of mesothelioma is also supportive (Figure 11.20).

Mesothelioma is typically (~85%) CK 7-positive, and virtually all are CK 20-negative.[51–53]

11.4.1.2 Mesothelial Markers

The most common markers of mesothelial lineage are calretinin, WT1, D2-40, and cytokeratin (CK) 5/6. HEG-1 is a promising mesothelial marker not yet in widespread use (**Table 11.2**).

Calretinin is positive in 95% of epithelioid, 90% of biphasic, and 50% of sarcomatoid mesotheliomas.[9, 54] Only combined nuclear + cytoplasmic staining supports mesothelial lineage; other patterns are less specific. Calretinin is specific for mesothelioma in the differential with lung adenocarcinoma, high-grade serous carcinoma, and renal cell carcinoma, but it is positive in 40% of squamous cell carcinomas, 25% of sarcomatoid carcinomas, and 15–20% of breast cancers,[55–60] as well as in adrenal cortical carcinoma and sex cord-stromal tumors.

WT1 is a nuclear marker expressed in 90% of epithelioid, 60% of biphasic, and 40% of sarcomatoid mesotheliomas.[9, 54] Cytoplasmic-only staining is non-specific and should be regarded as negative. WT1 is specific for mesothelioma in most relevant differentials, but it is positive in virtually 100% of low-grade and high-grade serous ovarian carcinomas, as well as in metanephric adenoma, sex cord-stromal tumors, small-cell carcinoma of the ovary of hypercalcemic type, and CIC-DUX sarcoma.

D2-40 (podoplanin) is a membranous marker, positive in 95% of epithelioid, 80% of biphasic, and 50% of sarcomatoid mesotheliomas.[9, 54] Staining may be focal or patchy, and expression in entrapped lymphatics must be distinguished from true tumor cell positivity. D2-40 is specific for mesothelioma in the differential with lung adenocarcinoma and breast carcinoma, but it is positive in 60% of squamous cell carcinomas and 20% of sarcomatoid carcinomas and high-grade serous carcinomas.[55, 56, 61] D2-40 is also positive in seminoma/dysgerminoma, adrenal cortical carcinoma, and some angiosarcomas.

CK 5/6 is a cytoplasmic marker, positive in 90% of epithelioid, 75% of biphasic, and 25% of sarcomatoid mesotheliomas.[9, 54, 62] CK 5/6 is expressed in just 5% of lung adenocarcinomas, but it is positive in 98–100% of squamous cell carcinomas and 20–30% of sarcomatoid carcinomas, high-grade serous carcinomas, and breast carcinomas.[55, 56, 61, 63, 64] CK 5/6 is also positive in thymic and salivary tumors, basal cell carcinoma, two-thirds of urothelial carcinomas, and one-third of pancreatic adenocarcinomas.

HEG-1 is a recently described membranous marker, which has only recently become commercially available. HEG-1 is positive in 95% of epithelioid, 90% of biphasic, and 65% of sarcomatoid mesotheliomas,[65, 66] though staining in sarcomatoid tumors may be predominantly cytoplasmic and somewhat difficult to interpret. HEG-1 is highly specific for mesothelioma in most differentials, but it is positive in one-third to half of serous ovarian carcinomas and most thyroid carcinomas. HEG-1 is also positive in normal endothelial cells and in at least some vascular tumors.

Loss of BAP1 expression (see also below) is ~99% specific for mesothelioma in the differential with lung adenocarcinoma, squamous cell carcinoma, and high-grade serous ovarian carcinoma.[59, 67–72] However, outside of these specific differentials, BAP1 loss should not be regarded as specific for mesothelioma, as it is lost in 15% of clear cell renal cell carcinomas,[73] 10–30% of intrahepatic cholangiocarcinomas,[74] 10% of thymic carcinomas,[75] and 5–10% of uveal and cutaneous melanomas.[76–78] Loss of methylthioadenosine phosphorylase (MTAP) expression loss is not specific for mesothelioma in the differential with other malignancies,[79] and the specificity of Merlin loss has not yet been studied in this context.

11.4.1.3 Broad-Spectrum Epithelial Markers

The most common "broad-spectrum" epithelial markers (i.e. those expressed in most carcinomas) are claudin-4, MOC-31, and Ber-EP4. CEA, B72.3, and BG-8 also show acceptable sensitivity and specificity when properly validated (**Table 11.3**). Additional markers specific for particular types of carcinoma are also useful and are discussed below in the context of individual differentials.

Claudin-4 is a membranous marker expressed in 95% of squamous cell carcinomas and virtually 100% of lung adenocarcinomas, high-grade serous carcinomas, and breast carcinomas.[9, 54, 65] Claudin-4 is expressed in only 90% of renal cell carcinomas, including up to 100% of papillary and chromophobe but just 85% of clear cell renal cell carcinomas,[80, 81] perhaps reflecting the physiologic absence of claudin-4 from the proximal renal tubule.[82] Claudin-4 is also negative in normal liver and hepatocellular carcinoma[83, 84] and in adrenal cortical carcinoma.[85] Focal (<10%) membranous claudin-4 staining has been reported in 1% of epithelioid mesotheliomas, with most positive results coming from a single lab.[58, 86] Granular cytoplasmic claudin-4 is occasionally seen in mesothelioma and should be discounted.

Ber-EP4 and *MOC-31* are two clones targeting epithelial cell adhesion molecule (Ep-CAM). These are membranous markers, positive in 90–98% of lung adenocarcinoma, squamous cell carcinoma, and high-grade serous carcinoma. Like claudin-4, they have low sensitivity for renal cell carcinoma (~40%).[87] MOC-31 and Ber-EP4 are each positive (typically focal or patchy) in ~10–15% of epithelioid mesotheliomas,[54] with up to 35% staining in one recent tissue microarray-based study using modern immunohistochemical techniques.[88]

Sarcomatoid carcinomas lose epithelial differentiation and downregulate cell-cell adhesion molecules, resulting in diminished sensitivity of claudin-4 (35%), MOC-31 (35%), and Ber-EP4 (15–20%) for sarcomatoid carcinoma.[9, 54] These three markers are consistently negative in sarcomatoid mesothelioma.[88]

11.4.1.4 Epithelioid Mesothelioma: Important Differentials and Relevant Immunostains

The differential diagnosis for mesothelioma is dependent on tumor site and morphology, as well as clinical history and presentation. An exhaustive morphologic and immunophenotypic discussion of all primary and metastatic tumors that can be encountered in the serosa is beyond the scope of this chapter, but here we discuss key differentials and emphasize the findings most useful in their distinction from mesothelioma.

The most important differentials for epithelioid mesothelioma include lung adenocarcinoma, squamous cell carcinoma, low-grade and high-grade serous ovarian tumors, breast carcinoma, and renal cell carcinoma. Other notable differentials include gastrointestinal and pancreaticobiliary carcinomas, epithelioid angiosarcoma, and lymphoma. Melanoma can show epithelioid or sarcomatoid morphology.

Lung adenocarcinoma shows cytomorphologic and architectural features overlapping with epithelioid mesothelioma. Mesothelioma sometimes colonizes lung alveoli and mimics lepidic adenocarcinoma,[89] while rare (<5%) lung adenocarcinomas (or squamous cell carcinomas) show predominant "pseudomesotheliomatous" pleural involvement, which mimics mesothelioma clinically, radiographically, and grossly.[90, 91] Immunohistochemistry is indispensable, and all the broad-spectrum mesothelial and epithelial markers discussed above (see **Table 11.3**) are useful here. Additionally, TTF1 (particularly, clone 8G7G3/1) and Napsin A are both virtually 100% specific for lung adenocarcinoma,[6, 58, 92] and BAP1 loss is 99% specific for mesothelioma in this differential.[70] Occasional patients have both lung cancer and mesothelioma, and immunostaining of multiple blocks may be prudent in patients with pleural and parenchymal masses and/or multiple discrete morphologies suggesting multiple primaries.[93]

Well-differentiated *squamous cell carcinoma* is characterized by keratinization and cell-cell desmosomal bridges, which are extremely rare features in mesothelioma.[94] Poorly differentiated squamous cell carcinoma is a more challenging morphologic differential. WT1 (and, where available, HEG-1) are the best mesothelial markers in this differential.[9, 54, 66, 95] Broad-spectrum epithelial markers are sensitive for squamous cell carcinoma. p40 is more specific here than p63, positive in 5% and 17% of epithelioid mesotheliomas, respectively.[58, 67, 92]

Serous borderline tumor, low-grade serous carcinoma, and *high-grade serous carcinoma* can enter the differential for both pleural and peritoneal mesothelioma. Serous borderline tumor is non-invasive and shows hierarchical branching and polymorphous epithelium with ciliated cells, which are absent in mesothelioma. The nuclear pleomorphism and brisk mitoses of high-grade serous carcinoma are fairly uncommon in mesothelioma. Calretinin is the best mesothelial marker in the differential with high-grade serous carcinoma. Data on mesothelial markers in low-grade serous neoplasia are lacking. Broad-spectrum epithelial markers are sensitive for serous ovarian neoplasia. PAX8 is positive in virtually 100% of serous ovarian tumors, but it is also positive (often diffuse) in ~12–15% of peritoneal mesotheliomas, including 25% of peritoneal mesotheliomas in women.[96–98] Estrogen receptor (ER) and progesterone receptor (PR) are expressed in 7% and 2% of peritoneal mesothelioma.[98] PAX8, ER, and PR are likely expressed in lower percentages of pleural mesothelioma, though data are limited. BAP1 loss is specific for mesothelioma in this differential.[69] Approximately 15% of peritoneal mesotheliomas harbor *TP53* mutations, so mutant-pattern p53 is not specific for high-grade serous carcinoma in this differential.

Breast carcinoma may rarely present first with serosal spread, mimicking mesothelioma. Breast imaging is crucial in this context. Calretinin, WT-1, D2-40, and CK5/6 are each expressed in 10–20% of breast carcinomas.[9, 54, 57] Claudin-4 is expressed in 98% of breast cancer, versus 65% for MOC-31 and Ber-EP4. The breast marker GATA3 is positive in 40% of epithelioid and 70% of sarcomatoid mesotheliomas, but mammaglobin is negative,[57, 99–102] and ER and PR are only rarely expressed (see above).

Renal cell carcinoma more often enters the differential with peritoneal mesothelioma. Renal cell carcinoma is unlikely in the absence of a renal mass or history of renal cancer. Epithelioid mesothelioma with clear cell features can mimic clear cell renal cell carcinoma, though adequate sampling often reveals areas of more conventional mesothelioma morphology. As detailed above, claudin-4, MOC-31, and Ber-EP4 have limited sensitivity for renal cell carcinomas, particularly those of putative proximal tubule origin (e.g. clear cell renal cell carcinoma), and PAX8 is positive in a subset of peritoneal mesotheliomas. Given the diversity of renal cell carcinoma subtypes, immunopanels should be tailored to the specific morphologic differential. However, carbonic anhydrase IX is expressed in 90–100% of epithelioid mesotheliomas, CD10 in 50%, and RCC antigen in 10%.[80, 87, 103]

Gastrointestinal and pancreaticobiliary carcinomas may occasionally enter the differential with epithelioid mesothelioma, particularly in the peritoneum. A panel of mesothelial and epithelial markers should be diagnostic. Upper gastrointestinal and pancreaticobiliary carcinomas have a generally non-specific immunophenotype, but SMAD4 loss is not expected for mesothelioma. CK20, CDX2, and SATB2 are negative in mesothelioma.[104] Ten to 30% of intrahepatic cholangiocarcinomas lose BAP1.[74]

Epithelioid hemangioendothelioma (EHE) and *epithelioid angiosarcoma* rarely arise in the pleura. Cytoplasmic lumina with red blood cells are characteristic of EHE. Adequate sampling may reveal vasoformation and prominent hemorrhage in angiosarcoma. Epithelioid vascular tumors are negative for claudin-4, MOC-31, and Ber-EP4, and they may be positive for cytokeratins and HEG-1 – a treacherous pitfall. The vascular markers CD31, CD34, and ERG are specific in the differential with mesothelioma. EHE harbors diagnostic fusions in *CAMTA* or (less often) *TFE3*.

Lymphoma may rarely present in the serosa, particularly large-cell lymphomas such as diffuse large B cell lymphoma (DLBCL), anaplastic large-cell lymphoma (ALCL), and primary effusion lymphoma (PEL). DLBCL is negative for cytokeratin and positive for CD45 and CD20. ALCL is positive for ALK and CD30. PEL typically occurs in immunocompromized patients and is positive for CD30, HHV8, and EBV.

Melanoma can mimic epithelioid or sarcomatoid mesothelioma, particularly if a history of melanoma is unknown. Cytokeratins should be negative in melanoma, and melanoma markers – SOX10, S100, Melan-A, and HMB45 – are negative in mesothelioma. Five to 10% of uveal and cutaneous melanomas lose BAP1.[76–78]

11.4.1.5 Sarcomatoid Mesothelioma: Important Differentials and Relevant Immunostains

Important differentials for sarcomatoid mesothelioma include sarcomatoid carcinoma (most often sarcomatoid lung carcinoma, but also sarcomatoid renal cell carcinoma, metaplastic breast carcinoma, or other types) and solitary fibrous tumor. Synovial sarcoma can be biphasic or purely sarcomatous, and poorly differentiated or high-grade tumors with spindled growth (e.g. Mullerian carcinosarcoma) can mimic biphasic sarcoma.

Sarcomatoid carcinoma is positive for claudin-4, MOC-31, and Ber-EP4 in just 33%, 38%, and 23% of cases, respectively.[9, 54, 88] MUC4 is positive in ~60% of sarcomatoid carcinomas but <5% of sarcomatoid mesotheliomas.[50, 102, 105] Mesothelial markers show reduced sensitivity for sarcomatoid mesothelioma: ~50% for calretinin and D2-40, 30% for WT1, and 25% for CK 5/6. GATA3 is positive in 70% of sarcomatoid mesotheliomas, but also in ~10% of sarcomatoid carcinomas, including 50% of metaplastic breast carcinomas and 29% of sarcomatoid urothelial carcinomas.[101, 102, 106, 107] In the differential with sarcomatoid lung carcinoma, BAP1 loss supports sarcomatoid mesothelioma, but it is only ~20% sensitive. Conversely, expression of TTF1, Napsin A, or p40 supports diagnosis of sarcomatoid lung carcinoma, though each is only ~15–20% sensitive.[50] PAX8 is positive in 45–70% of sarcomatoid renal cell carcinoma but typically negative in sarcomatoid mesothelioma.[108] Sarcomatoid renal cell carcinoma can show BAP1 loss.[109] Clearly, this is a challenging differential, and in many cases clinical and radiographic findings will be more diagnostically informative than even a wide-ranging immunopanel.[50]

Solitary fibrous tumor (SFT) is usually a solitary mass, raising consideration of localized mesothelioma. SFT shows a haphazard arrangement of short spindle cells with staghorn vessels, ropy stromal collagen bands, and alternating hypo- and hypercellular foci. SFT can be positive for cytokeratins and D2-40, but other mesothelial markers are negative, while CD34 and STAT6 are positive.

Synovial sarcoma may be primary to the pleura,[110] often forming a solitary mass. Monophasic synovial sarcoma shows cellular fascicular growth of plump spindle cells with overlapping nuclei. Biphasic synovial sarcoma harbors an additional component of epithelial nests or tubules. Synovial sarcoma is typically positive for cytokeratins and Ber-EP4, and a subset expresses claudin-4.[111] (These markers are all typically more diffusely expressed in the epithelial component of biphasic synovial sarcoma.) Calretinin is at least focally positive in ~60% of synovial sarcomas, most often in sarcomatous foci, but WT1 is negative.[111] TLE1 is non-specific.[112] Detection of the *SS18-SSX* fusion is diagnostic, either by molecular testing or by the translocation-specific immunostain.[113, 114]

Among other spindle cell sarcomas, 10-15% of malignant peripheral nerve sheath tumors express calretinin, while epithelioid sarcoma, leiomyosarcoma, GIST, and angiosarcoma are calretinin-negative.[111]

11.4.2 Distinguishing Mesothelioma from Benign Mesothelial Proliferations

Recent advances in our understanding of mesothelioma biology have revolutionized the approach to mesothelioma diagnosis, particularly in biopsies. Immunohistochemical stains for BAP1, MTAP, Merlin, and p53 are surrogates for underlying alterations in *BAP1, CDKN2A, NF2,* and *TP53*, which are pathognomonic for malignancy, provided mesothelial lineage has been established (see above). Molecular assays are also used to detect pathogenic alterations in these and other genes, as well as cytogenetic alterations. *CDKN2A* FISH is well established in mesothelioma diagnosis, and next-generation sequencing panels and cytogenetics arrays have more recently come into use in this context, particularly in large referral centers.

Alterations in *BAP1, CDKN2A, NF2*, and *TP53* are reported in all three mesothelioma histotypes and all four serosal sites (though data on tumors of the pericardium and tunica vaginalis are rare[10, 115]). However, no single gene is altered in all mesotheliomas, and the sensitivity of our diagnostic assays varies by tumor morphology and site (**Table 11.4**). Alterations in *BAP1, CDKN2A, NF2*, and *TP53* are largely independent events,[116] so immunohistochemical panels can achieve sensitivity >90%.[117]

GLUT1, IMP3, EMA, and desmin immunostains were previously advocated to distinguish mesothelioma from benign mesothelial proliferations, but these lack sensitivity and/or specificity and should be discarded in this context.[118]

11.4.2.1 BAP1

BAP1 alterations in mesothelioma include missense, nonsense, frameshift, and splice site mutations; small insertion and deletion events, whole-gene deletion, and truncating rearrangements.[119] Pathogenic *BAP1* alterations are considered impermissible in benign mesothelium (see section on mesothelioma in situ below). Genetic sequencing can detect *BAP1* alterations directly, or (more often) loss of nuclear BAP1 by immunohistochemistry provides an accurate surrogate for pathogenic *BAP1* alteration.[117, 120]

BAP1 loss is detected in 50-60% of pleural mesotheliomas, including 60-70% of epithelioid, 50% of biphasic, and 20% of sarcomatoid tumors.[9, 54, 117] BAP1 loss is detected in ~60% of peritoneal mesotheliomas,[98, 120–123] which are predominantly epithelioid. As noted above, BAP1 loss is specific for mesothelioma in the differential with lung adenocarcinoma and high-grade serous ovarian carcinoma.

Interpretation of BAP1 is contingent on an appropriate positive internal control, typically inflammatory, stromal, or endothelial cells. Only nuclear BAP1 is regarded as retained expression. The significance (if any) of cytoplasmic BAP1 localization remains unclear,[117, 124–126] but cytoplasmic BAP1 should not be interpreted as abnormal if nuclear staining is retained.

BAP1 expression patterns can help distinguish biphasic mesothelioma from epithelioid mesothelioma associated with reactive spindled mesothelium. BAP1 loss in both the epithelioid and spindled components strongly supports diagnosis of biphasic mesothelioma, whereas BAP1 loss in the epithelioid component only would favor epithelioid mesothelioma associated with reactive spindled mesothelium. Because data on this application are conflicting,[17, 124, 125, 127, 128] discordant BAP1 staining should not preclude a diagnosis of biphasic mesothelioma if there is frankly malignant biphasic morphology. BAP1 loss confined to the spindled component would be unusual,[17] but this could prompt consideration of a sarcomatoid mesothelioma associated with reactive mesothelial hyperplasia, particularly if the epithelioid component is at or near the serosal surface.

11.4.2.2 CDKN2A / MTAP

CDKN2A alterations in mesothelioma are essentially restricted to whole-gene deletions, and either heterozygous or homozygous *CDKN2A* deletion is specific for mesothelioma in the differential with reactive mesothelium. *CDKN2A* deletion is found in 65–70% of pleural mesotheliomas, including 60% of epithelioid, 75% of biphasic, and 90–95% of sarcomatoid tumors,[9, 54, 128–131] but in just 25–30% of peritoneal mesotheliomas.[116, 132]

Historically, *CDKN2A* deletion was detected by FISH, as immunohistochemical studies for its gene product, p16, are a poor surrogate.[130] However, FISH is more technically challenging and less widely available than immunohistochemistry. *MTAP*, located ~ 100 kb telomeric of *CDKN2A* on chromosome 9p21, encodes methylthioadenosine phosphorylase, a housekeeping gene involved in purine salvage. MTAP immunohistochemistry is a valuable surrogate for *CDKN2A* deletion because (1) *MTAP* is deleted in 75–90% of mesotheliomas with *CDKN2A* deletion,[117, 133, 134] and

(2) MTAP immunohistochemistry accurately reflects *MTAP* deletion.[117, 133] (One exception: MTAP immunohistochemistry is frequently uninterpretable in desmoplastic mesothelioma, due to scant tumor cell cytoplasm and poor positive internal control; in this scenario, *CDKN2A* FISH may be necessary.[135]) As for *CDKN2A, MTAP* alterations in mesothelioma are almost exclusively deletions, and *MTAP* deletion without *CDKN2A* deletion appears to be exceedingly rare.

MTAP loss – defined by absent cytoplasmic expression – is reported in ~50% of pleural mesotheliomas, including 40% of epithelioid and biphasic tumors and 75% of sarcomatoid tumors.[54, 117] Nuclear MTAP lose is a less reliable surrogate for *MTAP* deletion.[136, 137] Like BAP1, interpretation of MTAP depends on an appropriate positive internal control. In some cases, particularly sarcomatoid or lymphohistiocytoid mesotheliomas, admixed inflammatory cells can be so prominent that MTAP expression appears retained at low magnification, so examination at high magnification and correlation with morphology is necessary.

Like BAP1, MTAP can help distinguish biphasic mesothelioma from epithelioid mesothelioma associated with reactive spindled mesothelium (Figure 11.21). MTAP loss in both the epithelioid and spindled components supports the diagnosis of biphasic mesothelioma, while MTAP loss in the epithelioid component only supports the diagnosis of epithelioid mesothelioma associated with reactive spindled mesothelium. A subset of clear-cut biphasic mesotheliomas shows MTAP loss in the sarcomatoid component only, suggesting that deletion of chr 9p21 can sometimes play a role in the evolution of sarcomatoid morphology.[133]

Some mesotheliomas show subclonal MTAP loss, affecting 1-80% of immunostained tumor cells, which appears to correlate with subclonal *MTAP* and *CDKN2A* deletion.[133] This subclonal MTAP immunostaining pattern is not seen in reactive mesothelial hyperplasia.[117] Thus, although early studies required MTAP loss in ≥50% of tumor cells for a binary designation of "MTAP loss," recent evidence suggests that focal but convincing subclonal loss of MTAP immunostaining supports *MTAP/CDKN2A* deletion and thus a diagnosis of malignancy.

11.4.2.3 Merlin (NF2)

NF2 alterations – including missense, nonsense, and frameshift mutations, small insertions and deletions, whole-gene deletions, and truncating rearrangements are present in 33–74% of pleural and 27% of peritoneal mesotheliomas and are specific for mesothelioma in the differential with reactive mesothelial proliferations.[116, 117, 138, 139] FISH to detect hemizygous *NF2* deletion is reportedly 55% sensitive and 100% specific for pleural mesothelioma in the differential with reactive mesothelial hyperplasia, but this assay is not in widespread use.[140–142] However, immunohistochemistry for the *NF2* protein product, Merlin, was recently shown to be reliable for mesothelioma diagnosis. Immunohistochemical loss of Merlin is detected in 45% of pleural mesotheliomas (40% of epithelioid and 55% of biphasic and sarcomatoid tumors) but not in reactive mesothelium.[117, 143]

In reactive mesothelium, Merlin shows linear or granular staining of the apicolateral cell membrane, sometimes with faint cytoplasmic staining. Similar apicolateral membranous staining is seen in epithelioid mesotheliomas with tubulopapillary, micropapillary, or acinar growth and retained Merlin, while those with solid growth can show circumferential membranous or cytoplasmic staining. In sarcomatoid mesothelioma, Merlin expression is cytoplasmic. The basis for these different Merlin localization patterns is unclear, but all appear to signify wildtype *NF2*. At present, only complete loss of Merlin in a well-validated immunostain supports diagnosis of mesothelioma. Data are limited, but convincing subclonal Merlin loss likely reflects underlying *NF2* alteration, as *NF2* alteration is a late event in mesothelioma pathogenesis.[144]

11.4.2.4 p53 (TP53)

TP53 alterations are detected in ~15% of pleural and peritoneal mesotheliomas,[116, 117, 121] and pattern-based interpretation of p53 immunohistochemistry (borrowed from experience in serous ovarian carcinomas) is a reliable surrogate for *TP53* mutation. Strong p53 staining in ≥80% of tumor cells corresponds to underlying *TP53* mutation and is found in ~10% of pleural mesothelioma, but not in reactive mesothelium.[117, 145] Data on the specificity of a "null" mutant p53 pattern in mesothelioma are conflicting, so caution is warranted in interpreting this pattern until additional data are available.

11.4.2.5 Immunohistochemical Panels

Because molecular alterations in *BAP1*, *CDKN2A/MTAP*, *NF2*, and *TP53* are generally independent of one another, an immunopanel including BAP1, MTAP, Merlin, and p53 attains 93% sensitivity for pleural mesothelioma.[117] Although mutant-pattern p53 is seen in <10% of pleural mesotheliomas, *TP53* mutations are enriched in mesotheliomas with genomic near-haploidization, which lack *BAP1*, *CDKN2A*, and *NF2* alterations.[116, 117, 138] As a result, aberrant p53 is observed in a subset of mesotheliomas with normal BAP1, MTAP, and Merlin expression.

In routine diagnostic practice, it is reasonable to use BAP1 and MTAP (combined sensitivity, ~80%[117, 146]) as first-line immunostains for the evaluation of malignancy in a mesothelial proliferation. Merlin is not yet in widespread use, but it could be reasonably regarded as a first-line or second-line study, pending additional data. Given its low sensitivity, p53 is likely best reserved for challenging cases with retained BAP1 and MTAP (and, where available, Merlin).

11.4.2.6 Molecular Assays in Mesothelioma Diagnosis

As noted above, *CDKN2A* FISH is in widespread diagnostic use, and *NF2* FISH is also used in some institutions. Additional molecular assays used in mesothelioma diagnosis include array comparative genomic hybridization, next-generation sequencing panels, and fusion assays.

Array comparative genomic hybridization (aCGH) can detect copy number alterations characteristic of mesothelioma, including deletions of *BAP1* (chr 3p21.1), *CDKN2A* (chr 9p21), and *NF2* (chr 22q12). This assay can also detect loss of heterozygosity at individual loci, as well as genomic near-haploidization, a recently described molecular subcategory comprising ~5% of mesothelioma. Genomic near-haploidization in mesothelioma is associated with mutant *TP53* and wildtype *BAP1*, *CDKN2A*, and *NF2* (see above).

The diagnostic capacity of next-generation sequencing panels depends on panel size and composition as well as the sophistication of the bioinformatics analysis pipeline. Large panels include hundreds of genes and are capable of detecting copy number alterations, loss of heterozygosity, microsatellite instability, and at least some fusions or translocations. Such panels provide functionalities comparable to aCGH, in addition to direct detection of pathogenic point mutations and small insertion or deletion events in targeted genes. A next-generation sequencing panel including these functionalities will detect a pathogenic alteration in *BAP1*, *CDKN2A/MTAP*, *NF2*, or *TP53* in 91–95% of all pleural mesotheliomas.[117, 147]

Recurrent fusions are found in minor subsets of peritoneal mesotheliomas, and targeted fusion assays (including FISH and next-generation sequencing-based fusion panels) may be applied to detect these rare cases. *ALK* rearrangements and *EWSR1::ATF1* or *EWSR1::CREB* fusions occur in peritoneal mesotheliomas in children and young adults, while *EWSR1::YY1* fusions are found in peritoneal mesotheliomas in middle age or older adults.[139, 148–152] Recurrent *NR4A3* fusions are reported in diffuse or localized peritoneal mesotheliomas with pure adenomatoid/microcystic morphology and possibly indolent behavior.[153] These various arrangements appear to define a unique molecular subset, which lack alterations in genes commonly mutated in mesothelioma. *ALK* rearrangement is a targetable alteration, as discussed below.

11.4.2.7 Prognostic and Predictive Immunostains and Molecular Assays

ALK rearrangement is a targetable alteration, and targeted therapy can produce a dramatic treatment response. Although guidelines are lacking, it is reasonable to perform ALK immunohistochemistry on peritoneal mesotheliomas and mesotheliomas from young patients, particularly if they show normal BAP1, MTAP, Merlin, and p53 expression. Molecular confirmation of *ALK* rearrangement should be performed for any tumor with a positive ALK immunostain.

Mismatch repair deficiency is reportedly rare in mesothelioma,[154–156] though next-generation sequencing panels have detected microsatellite instability in 2–4% of mesotheliomas.[157, 158] As these patients may benefit from immune checkpoint inhibitor therapy, testing for mismatch repair deficiency or microsatellite instability can be considered in individual cases.

Programmed death 1-ligand 1 (PD-L1) is positive (>1% tumor cell staining) in variable proportions of epithelioid (10–49%), biphasic (9–67%), and sarcomatoid (22–100%) mesothelioma, depending on antibody clone and staining conditions.[159–163] However, routine PD-L1 immunohistochemistry is not recommended in mesothelioma. The FDA has approved first-line ipilimumab and nivolumab for the treatment of unresectable diffuse pleural mesothelioma, which shows clinical benefit compared to chemotherapy, regardless of histotype or PD-L1 status.[164–166]

11.5 MESOTHELIOMA IN SITU

Mesothelioma in situ is defined by (1) surface-confined (i.e. noninvasive) mesothelium with flat or papillary architecture, (2) lined by a single layer of cuboidal mesothelial cells with usually minimal nuclear atypia, (3) harboring a mesothelioma-defining alteration in *BAP1* (almost all) or *CDKN2A* (rare cases), (4) in the absence of a serosal mass on clinical and radiographic exam (Figure 11.22). A sarcomatoid variant of mesothelioma in situ is not described, though one case of stereotypical mesothelioma in situ apparently progressed to sarcomatoid mesothelioma.[167] Mesothelioma in situ can occur in the pleura or, slightly less often, the peritoneum. Cases in the pericardium or tunica vaginalis are not well attested. Patients with germline *BAP1* mutation may have multicavity involvement.[168]

Mesothelioma in situ has a progression rate of at least 70% to invasive mesothelioma over a median interval of 60 months.[169] *CDKN2A* deletion may confer a more aggressive course, with shorter time to progression, though data are limited.[167] Few studies have indicated that mesothelioma in situ can be associated with microscopic foci of invasion (i.e. in the absence of any clinical or radiographic mass lesion). These "minimally invasive" mesotheliomas associated with a predominantly in situ lesions appear to have a significantly better prognosis than mesotheliomas presenting with diffuse gross clinical disease.[170, 171] Optimal management of mesothelioma in situ (with or without associated microscopic invasion) remains unclear, but at least some patients are treated aggressively, with surgical decortication and, in the peritoneum, hyperthermic intraperitoneal chemotherapy.

Mesothelioma in situ is diagnosed most often in the context of an unexplained, non-resolving effusion, but it may rarely be an incidental finding in specimens obtained for another indication.[169] Patients with unexplained, unresolving effusion warrant careful examination and consideration of serosal biopsy.[172] Diagnosis of mesothelioma in situ also requires the absence of any clinical or radiographic evidence of a serosal mass. If mesothelioma in situ morphology is encountered in a serosal biopsy from a patient with a gross serosal mass, then the biopsy likely represents undersampling of a more significant lesion.

Particularly in the peritoneum, mesothelioma in situ may show long, slender papillae lined by a single layer of bland cuboidal epithelium, morphologically indistinguishable from well-differentiated papillary mesothelial tumor (WDPMT). However, these so-called "mesotheliomas in situ with WDPMT -like morphology" are frequently associated with recurrent effusion or ascites and show extensive or diffuse carcinomatosis-like serosal involvement – both features that would be unusual in banal WDPMT.[171]

It is impractical to perform immunohistochemical studies on all serosal biopsies. The current literature consensus advocates BAP1 (and, where feasible, MTAP) immunohistochemistry on any serosal biopsy from a patient with an unexplained, non-resolving effusion. These stains are also recommended at least for apparent WDPMT with "invasive foci" (see below), with multifocal or confluent growth, or with associated ascites, though some authors advocate ancillary studies even in solitary, incidental WDPMT.[171] In these scenarios, *CDKN2A* FISH should be considered if BAP1 and MTAP are retained and clinical or pathologic suspicion is high.

The WHO classification regards mesothelioma in situ as a diagnosis for surgical specimens, but some authors have also advocated that these ancillary studies be performed on cell block preparations from patients with unexplained, non-resolving effusion and no clinical or radiographic serosal mass, as this may permit earlier detection of mesothelioma, with the hope for improved outcomes.[173–175] Because invasive versus noninvasive growth cannot be determined in exfoliative effusion cytology, some have proposed descriptive terminology such as "at least mesothelioma in situ, cannot exclude invasive mesothelioma," in this situation.[176]

NF2 alterations have not been detected in mesothelioma in situ, though data thus far are limited to just two cases.[177] Molecular evidence suggests that *NF2* mutations are typically late events in mesothelioma tumorigenesis, so they may indeed be rare or absent at the in situ stage. The possibility of mutant-pattern p53 immunostaining in mesothelioma in situ remains unexplored.

11.6 CYTOPATHOLOGIC DIAGNOSIS OF MESOTHELIOMA

Although 90% of mesotheliomas are accompanied by effusion, cytopathologic diagnosis of mesothelioma remains challenging and controversial. As for tissue diagnosis, cytologic diagnosis of mesotheliomas has been revolutionized by widely available ancillary studies for malignancy-defining molecular alterations. In one survey of pathologists with mesotheliomas expertise, 35% felt comfortable diagnosing mesothelioma in a cytology specimen by atypical morphology alone; 53% by atypical morphology and loss of BAP or MTAP or CDKN2A deletion; and 65% by these two findings plus abnormal radiology.[173]

Aspirated effusion fluid containing exfoliated mesothelial cells is by far the most common cytology specimen received for evaluation of mesothelioma, and this may be the only diagnostic specimen obtainable in patients with poor performance status. Diagnosis of mesothelioma in sputum cytology, bronchial lavage or brushing, or transbronchial fine needle aspiration, though possible, is exceptionally rare.

Nonetheless, cytology has certain disadvantages, compared to biopsies or resections. First, only epithelioid mesothelioma sheds into effusion, so sarcomatoid and biphasic mesothelioma cannot generally be diagnosed by effusion cytology. (Transbronchial fine needle aspiration may sample sarcomatoid mesothelioma, though this is rare.) Second, sensitivity for mesothelioma is just 30–75% (though a low threshold for application of ancillary studies will likely increase detection[174]). Third, as discussed above, mesothelioma in situ cannot be definitively distinguished from invasive mesothelioma by cytology. Fourth, grading and architectural subtyping are not readily performed in cytology preparations.

Effusions range from hypocellular (particularly early in tumorigenesis) to hypercellular.[175] Mesothelioma effusions range from single cells and cell clusters with only mild atypia (overlapping morphologically with reactive mesothelium) to abundant large tumor fragments and clusters with overt nuclear atypia. Morphologic features consistent with mesothelioma include cell-in-cell arrangement, mesothelial cells with a peripheral "hump," orangeophilic cytoplasm, multinucleated cells, and papillary clusters with basement membrane cores.

As for tissue diagnosis, cytopathologic diagnosis of mesothelioma requires both (1) confirmation of mesothelial lineage, and (2) confirmation of malignancy. The ancillary studies applied in tissue diagnosis can also be applied to effusion cell blocks (or, less often, smears), though these studies must be specifically validated for this application, given differences in fixation.[178] In cytologic preparations, *CDKN2A* deletion by FISH in mesothelial cells is 100% specific for mesothelioma, while BAP1 loss and MTAP loss are each 99% specific. A panel of BAP1 immunohistochemistry and *CDKN2A* FISH offered 83% sensitivity for diagnosis of mesothelioma in cytologic preparations.[179] The role of Merlin and p53 immunostains in cytopathologic diagnosis of mesothelioma remains unexamined.

11.7 LOCALIZED MESOTHELIOMA

Localized mesotheliomas account for ~1% of all mesotheliomas. These are solitary, circumscribed pleural (80–90%) or peritoneal tumors, ranging from 0.5 cm to 20 cm. Fifty-five to 70% are epithelioid, 20–25% biphasic, and 10–18% sarcomatoid.[180, 181] They are microscopically indistinguishable from diffuse mesothelioma, so clinical and radiographic correlation is essential. An effusion may be present, but a malignant effusion precludes diagnosis of localized mesothelioma. Multifocal or diffuse microscopic involvement in biopsies taken from clinically normal background serosa would also preclude this diagnosis, though there is no agreed-upon standard for biopsy of grossly uninvolved serosa. The precise relationship of localized mesothelioma to mesothelioma in situ and diffuse mesothelioma remains unclear. Some localized mesotheliomas are biologically similar to diffuse mesothelioma, with pathogenic alterations in *BAP1*, *CDKN2A*, and *NF2* or genomic near-haploidization. However, some localized mesotheliomas harbor *TRAF7* mutation and may be more closely related to benign or indolent peritoneal mesothelial tumors.[182] Perhaps reflecting this molecular heterogeneity, median survival in localized mesothelioma is 134 months, significantly longer than for diffuse mesothelioma.[181]

11.8 NONMALIGNANT MESOTHELIAL TUMORS

The nonmalignant mesothelial tumors discussed in this section are often easily distinguished from mesothelioma by morphology alone, but diagnostic immunostains may be used to confirm mesothelial lineage or to help rule out a subtle malignant lesion. The tumors detailed here are predominantly encountered in the peritoneum, and their occurrence in the pleura should be carefully scrutinized to exclude mesothelioma or mesothelioma in situ.

These lesions are typically uni- or oligofocal, though rare examples show multifocal or (in the case of peritoneal inclusion cysts) diffuse growth. Available molecular data show that these lesions are biologically distinct from mesothelioma, with no alterations in *BAP1*, *CDKN2A*, and *NF2*.[183, 184] Their benign or at most indolent clinical behavior also separates them from mesothelioma.

11.8.1 Well-differentiated Papillary Mesothelial Tumor

Well-differentiated papillary mesothelial tumor (WDPMT) is characterized by slender papillae with myxoid, fibromyxoid, or collagenous stromal cores lined by a single layer of bland cuboidal or flattened mesothelium.[185–187] Sixty to 95% are PAX8-positive.[97, 186]

Rare WDPMT show florid confluent papillary growth and/or nests or cords of mesothelium within the papillary cores – both of these patterns have been termed "WDPMT with invasive foci."[188] Despite this potentially confusing name, the "invasive foci" here are confined to the stromal cores of the WDPMT, and infiltration of underlying subserosal tissues should be absent. Because this variant was described before the modern concept of mesothelioma in situ was formulated, the relationship between these two remains unclear.

11.8.2 Adenomatoid Tumor

Adenomatoid tumor is encountered most often in the paratesticular region in men and in the uterine corpus or fallopian tube in women.[189] Rare cases can occur in the pelvic peritoneum or colonic serosa.[190] They are typically small (<2 cm). Microscopically, adenomatoid tumor comprises small tubules lined by bland cuboidal to flattened mesothelium, as well as small solid nests and signet ring cells. Thin mucoid strands characteristically bridge the tubular lumina. Adenomatoid tumor may be circumscribed or infiltrate around background structures, but destructive infiltration is absent.

11.8.3 Peritoneal Inclusion Cysts

"Peritoneal inclusion cyst" refers to a broad spectrum of lesions, ranging from incidental minute unilocular inclusions to large multiloculated lesions presenting with mass effect. In either case, the cysts are lined by bland, cuboidal to flattened mesothelium, which is occasionally partly or diffusely squamatized. Minor adenomatoid proliferations can be present in the cyst walls, and when large enough these may be considered hybrids of peritoneal inclusion cyst and adenomatoid tumor. Peritoneal inclusion cysts differ somewhat from the other lesions in this section, insofar as they may be massive (up to 30 cm) and multifocal or diffuse, with recurrence rates up to 50% in such florid cases.[191–193] However, more recent series better reflecting the full morphologic spectrum of peritoneal inclusion cysts (i.e. including a higher proportion of small, unicystic, incidental lesions) indicates a recurrence rate of just 3%.[194]

Morphologically identical "mesothelial inclusion cysts" are rarely encountered in the pericardium, but these are exceptionally rare in the pleura.

11.8.4 Other Lesions

Occasional incidental, bland, circumscribed, uni- or oligofocal peritoneal mesothelial proliferations defy easy classification. One such group was recently codified as "solid papillary mesothelial tumor," characterized by predominantly solid and focally (pseudo)papillary growth of epithelioid cells with moderate eosinophilic cytoplasm, sharp cell membranes, and bland nuclei with frequent nuclear grooves.[195]

It is reasonable to exclude mesothelioma in situ or localized mesothelioma in any unclassifiable mesothelial tumor. Otherwise, these may be diagnosed descriptively. Clinical follow-up is prudent in these cases, given the likely heterogeneity of these unclassifiable lesions and limited data on their behavior.

11.9 CONCLUSION

Diagnosis of mesothelioma remains a challenge for surgical pathologists in both general and subspecialized practice. Morphology is the cornerstone of pathologic diagnosis. However, the development and refinement of robust immunohistochemical stains to confirm mesothelial lineage and, more significantly, to detect malignancy-defining pathogenic molecular alterations in *BAP1*, *CDKN2A*, *NF2*, and *TP53* have significantly altered diagnostic practice, permitting more confident diagnosis in morphologically challenging cases, including small biopsies and effusion cytology preparations. These powerful tools have also revivified the concept of mesothelioma in situ, raising the hope for earlier diagnosis and meaningful early interventions. More robust molecular techniques, including next-generation sequencing panels, are already in routine diagnostic use in some institutions. This growing arsenal must be applied in the context of a differential diagnosis generated through rigorous morphologic evaluation, and the composite pathologic results should be interpreted alongside clinical and radiographic data, ideally in the form of a multidisciplinary tumor board. Given the substantial clinical implications of a mesothelioma diagnosis, evaluation by a pathologist with mesothelioma expertise is prudent for challenging or unusual cases.

REFERENCES

1. Beebe-Dimmer, J. L. *et al.* Mesothelioma in the United States: A Surveillance, Epidemiology, and End Results (SEER)-Medicare investigation of treatment patterns and overall survival. *Clin. Epidemiol.* **8**, 743–750 (2016).
2. Bray, F. *et al.* Global cancer statistics 2018: GLOBOCAN estimates of incidence and mortality worldwide for 36 cancers in 185 countries. *CA Cancer J. Clin.* **68**(6), 394–424 (2018).

3. Churg, A. *et al.* Dataset for reporting of malignant mesothelioma of the pleura or peritoneum: Recommendations from the international collaboration on cancer reporting (ICCR). *Arch. Pathol. Lab. Med.* **140**(10), 1104–1110 (2016).
4. Husain, A. N. *et al.* Guidelines for pathologic diagnosis of malignant mesothelioma 2017 update of the consensus statement from the international mesothelioma interest group. *Arch. Pathol. Lab. Med.* **142**(1), 89–108 (2018).
5. Churg, A. *et al.* The fake fat phenomenon in organizing pleuritis: A source of confusion with desmoplastic malignant mesotheliomas. *Am. J. Surg. Pathol.* **35**(12), 1823–1829 (2011).
6. Klebe, S. *et al.* Sarcomatoid mesothelioma: A clinical-pathologic correlation of 326 cases. *Mod. Pathol. Off. J. US Can. Acad. Pathol. Inc.* **23**(3), 470–479 (2010).
7. Verma, V. *et al.* Survival by histologic subtype of malignant pleural mesothelioma and the impact of surgical resection on overall survival. *Clin. Lung Cancer* **19**(6), e901–e912 (2018).
8. Chirieac, L. R. *et al.* Diagnostic value of biopsy sampling in predicting histology in patients with diffuse malignant pleural mesothelioma. *Cancer* **125**(23), 4164–4171 (2019).
9. Chapel, D. B., VIvero, M. & Sholl, L. M. Mesothelioma. In: *Practical Pulmonary Pathology.*
10. Anderson, W. J. *et al.* Molecular and immunohistochemical characterisation of mesothelioma of the tunica vaginalis. *Histopathology* **81**(1), 65–76 (2022).
11. Butnor, K. J., Pavlisko, E. N., Sporn, T. A. & Roggli, V. L. Mesothelioma of the tunica vaginalis testis. *Hum. Pathol.* **92**, 48–58 (2019).
12. Chapel, D. B. *et al.* Malignant peritoneal mesothelioma: Prognostic significance of clinical and pathologic parameters and validation of a nuclear-grading system in a multi-institutional series of 225 cases. *Mod. Pathol. Off. J. US Can. Acad. Pathol. Inc.* **34**(2), 380–395 (2021).
13. Malpica, A. *et al.* Malignant mesothelioma of the peritoneum in women: A clinicopathologic study of 164 cases. *Am. J. Surg. Pathol.* **45**(1), 45–58 (2021).
14. Pavlisko, E. N. & Roggli, V. L. Sarcomatoid peritoneal mesothelioma: Clinicopathologic correlation of 13 cases. *Am. J. Surg. Pathol.* **39**(11), 1568–1575 (2015).
15. Zhang, Y. Z. *et al.* Utility of nuclear grading system in epithelioid malignant pleural mesothelioma in biopsy-heavy setting: An external validation study of 563 cases. *Am. J. Surg. Pathol.* **44**(3), 347–356 (2020).
16. Rosen, L. E. *et al.* Nuclear grade and necrosis predict prognosis in malignant epithelioid pleural mesothelioma: A multi-institutional study. *Mod. Pathol. Off. J. US Can. Acad. Pathol. Inc.* **31**(4), 598–606 (2018).
17. Galateau Salle, F. *et al.* New insights on diagnostic reproducibility of biphasic mesotheliomas: A multi-institutional evaluation by the international mesothelioma panel from the MESOPATH reference center. *J. Thorac. Oncol. Off. Publ. Int. Assoc. Study Lung Cancer* **13**(8), 1189–1203 (2018).
18. Bueno, R. *et al.* Pleural biopsy: A reliable method for determining the diagnosis but not subtype in mesothelioma. *Ann. Thorac. Surg.* **78**(5), 1774–1776 (2004).
19. Schulte, J. J. *et al.* Comparison of nuclear grade, necrosis, and histologic subtype between biopsy and resection in pleural malignant mesothelioma: An international multi-institutional analysis. *Am. J. Clin. Pathol.* **156**(6), 989–999 (2021).
20. Attanoos, R. L. & Gibbs, A. R. The pathology associated with therapeutic procedures in malignant mesothelioma. *Histopathology* **45**(4), 393–397 (2004).
21. Kadota, K. *et al.* A nuclear grading system is a strong predictor of survival in epitheloid diffuse malignant pleural mesothelioma. *Mod. Pathol. Off. J. US Can. Acad. Pathol. Inc.* **25**(2), 260–271 (2012).
22. Nicholson, A. G. *et al.* EURACAN/IASLC proposals for updating the histologic classification of pleural mesothelioma: Towards a more multidisciplinary approach. *J. Thorac. Oncol. Off. Publ. Int. Assoc. Study Lung Cancer* **15**(1), 29–49 (2020).
23. Kadota, K. *et al.* Pleomorphic epithelioid diffuse malignant pleural mesothelioma: A clinicopathological review and conceptual proposal to reclassify as biphasic or sarcomatoid mesothelioma. *J. Thorac. Oncol. Off. Publ. Int. Assoc. Study Lung Cancer* **6**(5), 896–904 (2011).
24. Mogi, A. *et al.* Pleural malignant mesothelioma with invasive micropapillary component and its association with pulmonary metastasis. *Pathol. Int.* **59**(12), 874–879 (2009).
25. Ordóñez, N. G. Deciduoid mesothelioma: Report of 21 cases with review of the literature. *Mod. Pathol. Off. J. US Can. Acad. Pathol. Inc.* **25**(11), 1481–1495 (2012).
26. Ordóñez, N. G. Mesothelioma with rhabdoid features: An ultrastructural and immunohistochemical study of 10 cases. *Mod. Pathol. Off. J. US Can. Acad. Pathol. Inc.* **19**(3), 373–383 (2006).
27. Kimura, N., Hasegawa, M. & Hiroshima, K. SMARCB1/INI1/BAF47- deficient pleural malignant mesothelioma with rhabdoid features. *Pathol. Int.* **68**(2), 128–132 (2018).

28. Ahadi, M. S. & Gill, A. J. SMARCA4 loss is very rare in thoracic mesothelioma. *Am. J. Surg. Pathol.* **43**(8), 1154–1155 (2019).
29. Ordóñez, N. G. Mesothelioma with signet-ring cell features: Report of 23 cases. *Mod. Pathol. Off. J. US Can. Acad. Pathol. Inc.* **26**(3), 370–384 (2013).
30. Ordóñez, N. G. Mesotheliomas with small cell features: Report of eight cases. *Mod. Pathol. Off. J. US Can. Acad. Pathol. Inc.* **25**(5), 689–698 (2012).
31. Sauter, J. L. *et al.* The 2021 WHO classification of tumors of the pleura: Advances since the 2015 classification. *J. Thorac. Oncol. Off. Publ. Int. Assoc. Study Lung Cancer* **17**(5), 608–622 (2022).
32. Ordóñez, N. G. Mesothelioma with clear cell features: An ultrastructural and immunohistochemical study of 20 cases. *Hum. Pathol.* **36**(5), 465–473 (2005).
33. Michal, M. *et al.* Clear cell mesotheliomas with inactivating VHL mutations and near-haploid genomic features. *Genes Chromosomes Cancer* **62**(5), 267–274 (2023).
34. Shia, J. *et al.* Malignant mesothelioma with a pronounced myxoid stroma: A clinical and pathological evaluation of 19 cases. *Virchows Arch. Int. J. Pathol.* **447**(5), 828–834 (2005).
35. Ordóñez, N. G. Pleomorphic mesothelioma: Report of 10 cases. *Mod. Pathol. Off. J. US Can. Acad. Pathol. Inc.* **25**(7), 1011–1022 (2012).
36. Sauter, J. L. *et al.* Diffuse pleural mesothelioma. In: *Thoracic Tumours 204–219* (International Agency for Research on Cancer, 2021).
37. Galateau-Sallé, F. *et al.* Lymphohistiocytoid variant of malignant mesothelioma of the pleura: A series of 22 cases. *Am. J. Surg. Pathol.* **31**(5), 711–716 (2007).
38. Hendry, S. *et al.* Assessing tumor-infiltrating lymphocytes in solid tumors: A practical review for pathologists and proposal for a standardized method from the international immuno-oncology biomarkers working group: Part 2: TILs in melanoma, gastrointestinal tract carcinomas, non-small cell lung carcinoma and mesothelioma, endometrial and ovarian carcinomas, squamous cell carcinoma of the head and neck, genitourinary carcinomas, and primary brain tumors. *Adv. Anat. Pathol.* **24**(6), 311–335 (2017).
39. Anraku, M. *et al.* Impact of tumor-infiltrating T cells on survival in patients with malignant pleural mesothelioma. *J. Thorac. Cardiovasc. Surg.* **135**(4), 823–829 (2008).
40. Fuchs, T. L., Chou, A., Sioson, L., Sheen, A. & Gill, A. J. Stromal tumour-infiltrating lymphocytes (TILs) assessed using the ITWG system do not predict overall survival in a cohort of 337 cases of mesothelioma. *Histopathology* **76**(7), 1095–1101 (2020).
41. Yamada, N. *et al.* CD8+ tumor-infiltrating lymphocytes predict favorable prognosis in malignant pleural mesothelioma after resection. *Cancer Immunol. Immunother. CII* **59**(10), 1543–1549 (2010).
42. Fusco, N. *et al.* Characterization of the immune microenvironment in malignant pleural mesothelioma reveals prognostic subgroups of patients. *Lung Cancer, (Amst., Neth.)* **150**, 53–61 (2020).
43. Alchami, F. S., Attanoos, R. L. & Bamber, A. R. Myxoid variant epithelioid pleural mesothelioma defines a favourable prognosis group: An analysis of 191 patients with pleural malignant mesothelioma. *J. Clin. Pathol.* **70**(2), 179–182 (2017).
44. Fuchs, T. L. *et al.* A critical assessment of current grading schemes for diffuse pleural mesothelioma with a proposal for a novel mesothelioma weighted grading scheme (MWGS). *Am. J. Surg. Pathol.* **46**(6), 774–785 (2022).
45. Klebe, S., Mahar, A., Henderson, D. W. & Roggli, V. L. Malignant mesothelioma with heterologous elements: Clinicopathological correlation of 27 cases and literature review. *Mod. Pathol. Off. J. US Can. Acad. Pathol. Inc.* **21**(9), 1084–1094 (2008).
46. Galateau Salle, F. *et al.* Comprehensive molecular and pathologic evaluation of transitional mesothelioma assisted by deep learning approach: A multi-institutional study of the international mesothelioma panel from the MESOPATH reference center. *J. Thorac. Oncol. Off. Publ. Int. Assoc. Study Lung Cancer* **15**(6), 1037–1053 (2020).
47. Dacic, S. *et al.* Interobserver variation in the assessment of the sarcomatoid and transitional components in biphasic mesotheliomas. *Mod. Pathol. Off. J. US Can. Acad. Pathol. Inc.* **33**(2), 255–262 (2020).
48. Brcic, L., Vlacic, G., Quehenberger, F. & Kern, I. Reproducibility of malignant pleural mesothelioma histopathologic subtyping. *Arch. Pathol. Lab. Med.* **142**(6), 747–752 (2018).
49. Vigneswaran, W. T. *et al.* Amount of epithelioid differentiation is a predictor of survival in malignant pleural mesothelioma. *Ann. Thorac. Surg.* **103**(3), 962–966 (2017).
50. Marchevsky, A. M. *et al.* The differential diagnosis between pleural sarcomatoid mesothelioma and spindle cell/pleomorphic (sarcomatoid) carcinomas of the lung: Evidence-based guidelines from the International Mesothelioma Panel and the MESOPATH National Reference Center. *Hum. Pathol.* **67**, 160–168 (2017).

51. Tot, T. The value of cytokeratins 20 and 7 in discriminating metastatic adenocarcinomas from pleural mesotheliomas. *Cancer* **92**(10), 2727–2732 (2001).
52. Winstanley, A. M. *et al.* The immunohistochemical profile of malignant mesotheliomas of the tunica vaginalis: A study of 20 cases. *Am. J. Surg. Pathol.* **30**(1), 1–6 (2006).
53. Chu, P., Wu, E. & Weiss, L. M. Cytokeratin 7 and cytokeratin 20 expression in epithelial neoplasms: A survey of 435 cases. *Mod. Pathol. Off. J. US Can. Acad. Pathol. Inc.* **13**(9), 962–972 (2000).
54. Chapel, D. B., Schulte, J. J., Husain, A. N. & Krausz, T. Application of immunohistochemistry in diagnosis and management of malignant mesothelioma. *Transl. Lung Cancer Res.* **9**(Supplement 1), S3–S27 (2020).
55. Ordóñez, N. G. The diagnostic utility of immunohistochemistry in distinguishing between epithelioid mesotheliomas and squamous carcinomas of the lung: A comparative study. *Mod. Pathol. Off. J. US Can. Acad. Pathol. Inc.* **19**(3), 417–428 (2006).
56. Ordóñez, N. G. Value of immunohistochemistry in distinguishing peritoneal mesothelioma from serous carcinoma of the ovary and peritoneum: A review and update. *Adv. Anat. Pathol.* **13**(1), 16–25 (2006).
57. Ordóñez, N. G. & Sahin, A. A. Diagnostic utility of immunohistochemistry in distinguishing between epithelioid pleural mesotheliomas and breast carcinomas: A comparative study. *Hum. Pathol.* **45**(7), 1529–1540 (2014).
58. Kushitani, K. *et al.* Utility and pitfalls of immunohistochemistry in the differential diagnosis between epithelioid mesothelioma and poorly differentiated lung squamous cell carcinoma. *Histopathology* **70**(3), 375–384 (2017).
59. Le Stang, N. *et al.* Differential diagnosis of epithelioid malignant mesothelioma with lung and breast pleural metastasis: A systematic review compared with a standardized panel of antibodies-A new proposal that may influence pathologic practice. *Arch. Pathol. Lab. Med.* **144**(4), 446–456 (2020).
60. Padgett, D. M., Cathro, H. P., Wick, M. R. & Mills, S. E. Podoplanin is a better immunohistochemical marker for sarcomatoid mesothelioma than calretinin. *Am. J. Surg. Pathol.* **32**(1), 123–127 (2008).
61. Ordóñez, N. G. The diagnostic utility of immunohistochemistry and electron microscopy in distinguishing between peritoneal mesotheliomas and serous carcinomas: A comparative study. *Mod. Pathol. Off. J. US Can. Acad. Pathol. Inc.* **19**(1), 34–48 (2006).
62. Chu, P. G. & Weiss, L. M. Expression of cytokeratin 5/6 in epithelial neoplasms: An immunohistochemical study of 509 cases. *Mod. Pathol. Off. J. US Can. Acad. Pathol. Inc.* **15**(1), 6–10 (2002).
63. Attanoos, R. L., Webb, R., Dojcinov, S. D. & Gibbs, A. R. Value of mesothelial and epithelial antibodies in distinguishing diffuse peritoneal mesothelioma in females from serous papillary carcinoma of the ovary and peritoneum. *Histopathology* **40**(3), 237–244 (2002).
64. Comin, C. E. *et al.* Expression of thrombomodulin, calretinin, cytokeratin 5/6, D2-40 and WT-1 in a series of primary carcinomas of the lung: An immunohistochemical study in comparison with epithelioid pleural mesothelioma. *Tumori* **100**(5), 559–567 (2014).
65. Churg, A. & Naso, J. R. Hypothesis: HEG1 and claudin-4 staining will allow a diagnosis of epithelioid and biphasic mesothelioma versus non-small-cell lung carcinoma with only two stains in most cases. *Histopathology* **82**(3), 385–392 (2023).
66. Naso, J. R., Tsuji, S. & Churg, A. HEG1 is a highly specific and sensitive marker of epithelioid malignant mesothelioma. *Am. J. Surg. Pathol.* **44**(8), 1143–1148 (2020).
67. Carbone, M. *et al.* Positive nuclear BAP1 immunostaining helps differentiate non-small cell lung carcinomas from malignant mesothelioma. *Oncotarget* **7**(37), 59314–59321 (2016).
68. Yoshimura, M. *et al.* Diagnostic application of BAP1 immunohistochemistry to differentiate pleural mesothelioma from metastatic pleural tumours. *Histopathology* **71**(6), 1011–1014 (2017).
69. Andrici, J. *et al.* Loss of BAP1 expression is very rare in peritoneal and gynecologic serous adenocarcinomas and can be useful in the differential diagnosis with abdominal mesothelioma. *Hum. Pathol.* **51**, 9–15 (2016).
70. Andrici, J. *et al.* Loss of expression of BAP1 is very rare in non-small cell lung carcinoma. *Pathology (Phila.)* **48**(4), 336–340 (2016).
71. Owen, D., Sheffield, B. S., Ionescu, D. & Churg, A. Loss of BRCA1-associated protein 1 (BAP1) expression is rare in non-small cell lung cancer. *Hum. Pathol.* **60**, 82–85 (2017).
72. Sun, T. *et al.* Somatic mutation of BAP1 can lead to expression loss in non-small cell lung carcinoma: Next generation sequencing and IHC analysis in A large single institute cohort. *Int. J. Surg. Pathol.* **30**(5), 512–519 (2022).
73. Ricketts, C. J. *et al.* The cancer genome atlas comprehensive molecular characterization of renal cell carcinoma. *Cell Rep.* **23**, 313–326.e5 (2018).

74. Lowery, M. A. *et al.* Comprehensive molecular profiling of intrahepatic and extrahepatic cholangiocarcinomas: Potential targets for intervention. *Clin. Cancer Res. Off. J. Am. Assoc. Cancer Res.* **24**(17), 4154–4161 (2018).
75. Wang, Y. *et al.* Mutations of epigenetic regulatory genes are common in thymic carcinomas. *Sci. Rep.* **4**, 7336 (2014).
76. Murali, R. *et al.* BAP1 expression in cutaneous melanoma: A pilot study. *Pathology (Phila.)* **45**(6), 606–609 (2013).
77. Di Nunno, V. *et al.* BAP1 in solid tumors. *Future Oncol., (Lond.) Engl.* **15**(18), 2151–2162 (2019).
78. Laitman, Y., Newberg, J., Molho, R. B., Jin, D. X. & Friedman, E. The spectrum of tumors harboring BAP1 gene alterations. *Cancer Genet.* **256–257**, 31–35 (2021).
79. Terra, S., Roden, A. C., Yi, E. S., Aubry, M. C. & Boland, J. M. Loss of methylthioadenosine phosphorylase by immunohistochemistry is common in pulmonary sarcomatoid carcinoma and sarcomatoid mesothelioma. *Am. J. Clin. Pathol.* **157**(1), 33–39 (2022).
80. Ordóñez, N. G. Value of PAX8, PAX2, napsin A, carbonic anhydrase IX, and claudin-4 immunostaining in distinguishing pleural epithelioid mesothelioma from metastatic renal cell carcinoma. *Mod. Pathol. Off. J. US Can. Acad. Pathol. Inc.* **26**(8), 1132–1143 (2013).
81. Ordóñez, N. G. Value of claudin-4 immunostaining in the diagnosis of mesothelioma. *Am. J. Clin. Pathol.* **139**(5), 611–619 (2013).
82. Lechpammer, M. *et al.* The diagnostic and prognostic utility of claudin expression in renal cell neoplasms. *Mod. Pathol. Off. J. US Can. Acad. Pathol. Inc.* **21**(11), 1320–1329 (2008).
83. Ono, Y. *et al.* Claudins-4 and –7 might be valuable markers to distinguish hepatocellular carcinoma from cholangiocarcinoma. *Virchows Arch. Int. J. Pathol.* **469**(4), 417–426 (2016).
84. Lódi, C. *et al.* Claudin-4 differentiates biliary tract cancers from hepatocellular carcinomas. *Mod. Pathol. Off. J. US Can. Acad. Pathol. Inc.* **19**(3), 460–469 (2006).
85. Facchetti, F. *et al.* Claudin 4 identifies a wide spectrum of epithelial neoplasms and represents a very useful marker for carcinoma versus mesothelioma diagnosis in pleural and peritoneal biopsies and effusions. *Virchows Arch. Int. J. Pathol.* **451**(3), 669–680 (2007).
86. Kai, Y. *et al.* Mucin 21 is a novel, negative immunohistochemical marker for epithelioid mesothelioma for its differentiation from lung adenocarcinoma. *Histopathology* **74**(4), 545–554 (2019).
87. Ordóñez, N. G. The diagnostic utility of immunohistochemistry in distinguishing between mesothelioma and renal cell carcinoma: A comparative study. *Hum. Pathol.* **35**(6), 697–710 (2004).
88. Naso, J. R. & Churg, A. Claudin-4 shows superior specificity for mesothelioma vs non-small-cell lung carcinoma compared with MOC-31 and Ber-EP4. *Hum. Pathol.* **100**, 10–14 (2020).
89. Rossi, G., Caroli, G., Caruso, D., Stella, F. & Davoli, F. Pseudocarcinomatous mesothelioma: A Hitherto Unreported Presentation closely simulating primary lung cancer. *Int. J. Surg. Pathol.* **29**(7), 775–779 (2021).
90. Harwood, T. R., Gracey, D. R. & Yokoo, H. Pseudomesotheliomatous carcinoma of the lung. A variant of peripheral lung cancer. *Am. J. Clin. Pathol.* **65**(2), 159–167 (1976).
91. Attanoos, R. L. & Gibbs, A. R. 'Pseudomesotheliomatous' carcinomas of the pleura: A 10-year analysis of cases from the environmental lung disease research group, Cardiff. *Histopathology* **43**(5), 444–452 (2003).
92. Mawas, A. S. *et al.* MUC4 immunohistochemistry is useful in distinguishing epithelioid mesothelioma from adenocarcinoma and squamous cell carcinoma of the lung. *Sci. Rep.* **8**(1), 134 (2018).
93. Butnor, K. J. *et al.* Diffuse malignant mesothelioma and synchronous lung cancer: A clinicopathological study of 18 cases. *Lung Cancer, (Amst., Neth.)* **95**, 1–7 (2016).
94. Tanaka, H. *et al.* Malignant mesothelioma with squamous differentiation. *Histopathology* **72**(7), 1216–1220 (2018).
95. Hiroshima, K. *et al.* Membranous HEG1 expression is a useful marker in the differential diagnosis of epithelioid and biphasic malignant mesothelioma versus carcinomas. *Pathol. Int.* **71**(9), 604–613 (2021).
96. Chapel, D. B., Husain, A. N., Krausz, T. & McGregor, S. M. PAX8 Expression in a subset of malignant peritoneal mesotheliomas and benign mesothelium has diagnostic implications in the differential diagnosis of ovarian serous carcinoma. *Am. J. Surg. Pathol.* **41**(12), 1675–1682 (2017).
97. Xing, D. *et al.* Aberrant Pax-8 expression in well-differentiated papillary mesothelioma and malignant mesothelioma of the peritoneum: A clinicopathologic study. *Hum. Pathol.* **72**, 160–166 (2018).
98. Tandon, R. T., Jimenez-Cortez, Y., Taub, R. & Borczuk, A. C. Immunohistochemistry in peritoneal mesothelioma: A single-center experience of 244 cases. *Arch. Pathol. Lab. Med.* **142**(2), 236–242 (2018).

99. Piao, Z. H., Zhou, X. C. & Chen, J. Y. GATA3 is a useful immunohistochemical marker for distinguishing sarcomatoid malignant mesothelioma from lung sarcomatoid carcinoma and organizing pleuritis. *Virchows Arch. Int. J. Pathol.* **479**(2), 257–263 (2021).
100. Miettinen, M. *et al.* GATA3: A multispecific but potentially useful marker in surgical pathology: A systematic analysis of 2500 epithelial and nonepithelial tumors. *Am. J. Surg. Pathol.* **38**(1), 13–22 (2014).
101. Berg, K. B. & Churg, A. GATA3 immunohistochemistry for distinguishing sarcomatoid and desmoplastic mesothelioma from sarcomatoid carcinoma of the lung. *Am. J. Surg. Pathol.* **41**(9), 1221–1225 (2017).
102. Terra, S. B. S. P., Roden, A. C., Aubry, M. C., Yi, E. S. J. & Boland, J. M. Utility of immunohistochemistry for MUC4 and GATA3 to aid in the distinction of pleural sarcomatoid mesothelioma from pulmonary sarcomatoid carcinoma. *Arch. Pathol. Lab. Med.* **145**(2), 208–213 (2021).
103. Ananthanarayanan, V., Tretiakova, M., Husain, A. N., Krausz, T. & Antic, T. Carbonic anhydrase IX (CAIX) does not differentiate between benign and malignant mesothelium. *Am. J. Clin. Pathol.* **142**(1), 82–87 (2014).
104. Lin, F. *et al.* Cadherin-17 and SATB2 are sensitive and specific immunomarkers for medullary carcinoma of the large intestine. *Arch. Pathol. Lab. Med.* **138**(8), 1015–1026 (2014).
105. Amatya, V. J. *et al.* MUC4, a novel immunohistochemical marker identified by gene expression profiling, differentiates pleural sarcomatoid mesothelioma from lung sarcomatoid carcinoma. *Mod. Pathol. Off. J. US Can. Acad. Pathol. Inc.* **30**(5), 672–681 (2017).
106. Yoon, E. C. *et al.* TRPS1, GATA3, and SOX10 expression in triple-negative breast carcinoma. *Hum. Pathol.* **125**, 97–107 (2022).
107. Prabhakaran, S., Hocking, A., Kim, C., Hussey, M. & Klebe, S. The potential utility of GATA binding protein 3 for diagnosis of malignant pleural mesotheliomas. *Hum. Pathol.* **105**, 1–8 (2020).
108. Chang, A., Brimo, F., Montgomery, E. A. & Epstein, J. I. Use of PAX8 and GATA3 in diagnosing sarcomatoid renal cell carcinoma and sarcomatoid urothelial carcinoma. *Hum. Pathol.* **44**(8), 1563–1568 (2013).
109. Gallan, A. J., Parilla, M., Segal, J., Ritterhouse, L. & Antic, T. BAP1-mutated clear cell renal cell carcinoma. *Am. J. Clin. Pathol.* **155**(5), 718–728 (2021).
110. Klebe, S. *et al.* Pleural malignant mesothelioma versus pleuropulmonary synovial sarcoma: A clinicopathological study of 22 cases with molecular analysis and survival data. *Pathology (Phila.)* **50**(6), 629–634 (2018).
111. Miettinen, M., Limon, J., Niezabitowski, A. & Lasota, J. Calretinin and other mesothelioma markers in synovial sarcoma: Analysis of antigenic similarities and differences with malignant mesothelioma. *Am. J. Surg. Pathol.* **25**(5), 610–617 (2001).
112. Matsuyama, A. *et al.* TLE1 expression in malignant mesothelioma. *Virchows Arch. Int. J. Pathol.* **457**(5), 577–583 (2010).
113. Baranov, E. *et al.* A novel SS18-SSX fusion-specific antibody for the diagnosis of synovial sarcoma. *Am. J. Surg. Pathol.* **44**(7), 922–933 (2020).
114. Weinbreck, N. *et al.* SYT-SSX fusion is absent in sarcomatoid mesothelioma allowing its distinction from synovial sarcoma of the pleura. *Mod. Pathol. Off. J. US Can. Acad. Pathol. Inc.* **20**(6), 617–621 (2007).
115. Schaefer, I.-M., Mariño-Enríquez, A., Hammer, M. M., Padera, R. F. & Sholl, L. M. Recurrent tumor suppressor alterations in primary pericardial mesothelioma. *Mod. Pathol. Off. J. US Can. Acad. Pathol. Inc.* **36**(9), 100237 (2023). doi:10.1016/j.modpat.2023.100237.
116. Hiltbrunner, S. *et al.* Tumor immune microenvironment and genetic alterations in mesothelioma. *Front. Oncol.* **11**, 660039 (2021).
117. Chapel, D. B., Hornick, J. L., Barlow, J., Bueno, R. & Sholl, L. M. Clinical and molecular validation of BAP1, MTAP, P53, and Merlin immunohistochemistry in diagnosis of pleural mesothelioma. *Mod. Pathol. Off. J. US Can. Acad. Pathol. Inc.* **35**(10), 1383–1397 (2022).
118. Churg, A., Sheffield, B. S. & Galateau-Salle, F. New markers for separating benign from malignant mesothelial proliferations: Are we there yet? *Arch. Pathol. Lab. Med.* **140**(4), 318–321 (2016).
119. Jama, M. *et al.* Gene fusions during the early evolution of mesothelioma correlate with impaired DNA repair and Hippo pathways. *Genes Chromosomes Cancer* (2023). doi:10.1002/gcc.23189.
120. Leblay, N. *et al.* BAP1 is altered by copy number loss, mutation, and/or loss of protein expression in more than 70% of malignant peritoneal mesotheliomas. *J. Thorac. Oncol. Off. Publ. Int. Assoc. Study Lung Cancer* **12**(4), 724–733 (2017).
121. Offin, M. *et al.* Molecular characterization of peritoneal mesotheliomas. *J. Thorac. Oncol. Off. Publ. Int. Assoc. Study Lung Cancer* **17**(3), 455–460 (2022).

122. Singhi, A. D. *et al.* The prognostic significance of BAP1, NF2, and CDKN2A in malignant peritoneal mesothelioma. *Mod. Pathol. Off. J. US Can. Acad. Pathol. Inc.* **29**(1), 14–24 (2016).
123. Devins, K. M., Zukerberg, L., Watkins, J. C., Hung, Y. P. & Oliva, E. BAP1 and Claudin-4, but not MTAP, reliably distinguish borderline and low-grade serous ovarian tumors from peritoneal mesothelioma. *Int. J. Gynecol. Pathol. Off. J. Int. Soc. Gynecol. Pathol.* (2022). doi:10.1097/PGP.0000000000000877.
124. Righi, L. *et al.* BRCA1-associated protein 1 (BAP1) immunohistochemical expression as a diagnostic tool in malignant pleural mesothelioma classification: A large retrospective study. *J. Thorac. Oncol. Off. Publ. Int. Assoc. Study Lung Cancer* **11**(11), 2006–2017 (2016).
125. De Rienzo, A. *et al.* Large-scale analysis of BAP1 expression reveals novel associations with clinical and molecular features of malignant pleural mesothelioma. *J. Pathol.* **253**(1), 68–79 (2021).
126. Bononi, A. *et al.* BAP1 regulates IP3R3-mediated Ca2+ flux to mitochondria suppressing cell transformation. *Nature* **546**(7659), 549–553 (2017).
127. McGregor, S. M. *et al.* BAP1 facilitates diagnostic objectivity, classification, and prognostication in malignant pleural mesothelioma. *Hum. Pathol.* **46**(11), 1670–1678 (2015).
128. Wu, D. *et al.* Usefulness of p16/CDKN2A fluorescence in situ hybridization and BAP1 immunohistochemistry for the diagnosis of biphasic mesothelioma. *Ann. Diagn. Pathol.* **26**, 31–37 (2017).
129. Hwang, H. C. *et al.* Utility of BAP1 immunohistochemistry and p16 (CDKN2A) FISH in the diagnosis of malignant mesothelioma in effusion cytology specimens. *Am. J. Surg. Pathol.* **40**(1), 120–126 (2016).
130. Hida, T. *et al.* Immunohistochemical detection of MTAP and BAP1 protein loss for mesothelioma diagnosis: Comparison with 9p21 FISH and BAP1 immunohistochemistry. *Lung Cancer, (Amst., Neth.)* **104**, 98–105 (2017).
131. Wu, D. *et al.* Diagnostic usefulness of p16/CDKN2A FISH in distinguishing between sarcomatoid mesothelioma and fibrous pleuritis. *Am. J. Clin. Pathol.* **139**(1), 39–46 (2013).
132. Hung, Y. P. *et al.* Molecular characterization of diffuse malignant peritoneal mesothelioma. *Mod. Pathol. Off. J. US Can. Acad. Pathol. Inc.* (2020). doi:10.1038/s41379-020-0588-y.
133. Chapel, D. B., Dubuc, A. M., Hornick, J. L. & Sholl, L. M. Correlation of methylthioadenosine phosphorylase (MTAP) protein expression with MTAP and CDKN2A copy number in malignant pleural mesothelioma. *Histopathology* **78**(7), 1032–1042 (2021).
134. Illei, P. B., Rusch, V. W., Zakowski, M. F. & Ladanyi, M. Homozygous deletion of CDKN2A and codeletion of the methylthioadenosine phosphorylase gene in the majority of pleural mesotheliomas. *Clin. Cancer Res. Off. J. Am. Assoc. Cancer Res.* **9**(6), 2108–2113 (2003).
135. Sa-Ngiamwibool, P. *et al.* Challenges and limitation of MTAP immunohistochemistry in diagnosing desmoplastic mesothelioma/sarcomatoid pleural mesothelioma with desmoplastic features. *Ann. Diagn. Pathol.* **60**, 152004 (2022).
136. Chapel, D. B. *et al.* MTAP immunohistochemistry is an accurate and reproducible surrogate for CDKN2A fluorescence in situ hybridization in diagnosis of malignant pleural mesothelioma. *Mod. Pathol. Off. J. US Can. Acad. Pathol. Inc.* **33**(2), 245–254 (2020).
137. Berg, K. B., Dacic, S., Miller, C., Cheung, S. & Churg, A. Utility of methylthioadenosine phosphorylase compared with BAP1 immunohistochemistry, and CDKN2A and NF2 fluorescence in situ hybridization in separating reactive mesothelial proliferations from epithelioid malignant mesotheliomas. *Arch. Pathol. Lab. Med.* **142**(12), 1549–1553 (2018).
138. Hmeljak, J. *et al.* Integrative molecular characterization of malignant pleural mesothelioma. *Cancer Discov.* **8**(12), 1548–1565 (2018).
139. Dagogo-Jack, I. *et al.* Molecular characterization of mesothelioma: Impact of histologic type and site of origin on molecular landscape. *JCO Precis. Oncol.* **6**, e2100422 (2022).
140. Kinoshita, Y. *et al.* Hemizygous loss of NF2 detected by fluorescence in situ hybridization is useful for the diagnosis of malignant pleural mesothelioma. *Mod. Pathol. Off. J. US Can. Acad. Pathol. Inc.* **33**(2), 235–244 (2020).
141. Sa-Ngiamwibool, P. *et al.* Usefulness of NF2 hemizygous loss detected by fluorescence in situ hybridization in diagnosing pleural mesothelioma in tissue and cytology material: A multi-institutional study. *Lung Cancer, (Amst., Neth.)* **175**, 27–35 (2022).
142. Sa-Ngiamwibool, P. *et al.* Usefulness of NF2 hemizygous loss detected by fluorescence in situ hybridization in diagnosing pleural mesothelioma in tissue and cytology material: A multi-institutional study. *Lung Cancer, (Amst., Neth.)* **175**, 27–35 (2023).
143. Martin, S. D., Cheung, S. & Churg, A. Immunohistochemical demonstration of Merlin/NF2 loss in mesothelioma. *Mod. Pathol. Off. J. US Can. Acad. Pathol. Inc.* **36**. doi:10.1016/j.modpat.2022.100036.
144. Meiller, C. *et al.* Multi-site tumor sampling highlights molecular intra-tumor heterogeneity in malignant pleural mesothelioma. *Genome Med.* **13**(1), 113 (2021).

145. Naso, J. R., Tessier-Cloutier, B., Senz, J., Huntsman, D. G. & Churg, A. Significance of p53 immunostaining in mesothelial proliferations and correlation with TP53 mutation status. *Mod. Pathol. Off. J. US Can. Acad. Pathol. Inc.* (2021). doi:10.1038/s41379-021-00920-9.
146. Lynggård, L. A., Panou, V., Szejniuk, W., Røe, O. D. & Meristoudis, C. Diagnostic capacity of BAP1 and MTAP in cytology from effusions and biopsy in mesothelioma. *J. Am. Soc. Cytopathol.* **11**(6), 385–393 (2022).
147. Chen-Yost, H. I.-H. *et al.* Characterizing the distribution of alterations in mesothelioma and their correlation to morphology. *Am. J. Clin. Pathol*, aqad041 (2023). doi:10.1093/ajcp/aqad041.
148. Hung, Y. P. *et al.* Identification of ALK rearrangements in malignant peritoneal mesothelioma. *JAMA Oncol.* **4**(2), 235–238 (2018).
149. Argani, P. *et al.* Pediatric mesothelioma with ALK fusions: A molecular and pathologic study of 5 cases. *Am. J. Surg. Pathol.* **45**(5), 653–661 (2021).
150. Ren, H. *et al.* Malignant mesothelioma with EWSR1-ATF1 fusion in two adolescent male patients. *Pediatr. Dev. Pathol. Off. J. Soc. Pediatr. Pathol. Paediatr. Pathol. Soc.* **24**(6), 570–574 (2021).
151. Ke, H. *et al.* Malignant peritoneal mesothelioma with EWSR1-ATF1 fusion: A case report. *JTO Clin. Res. Rep.* **2** (2021). doi:10.1016/j.jtocrr.2021.100236.
152. Dermawan, J. K. *et al.* EWSR1::YY1 fusion positive peritoneal epithelioid mesothelioma harbors mesothelioma epigenetic signature: Report of 3 cases in support of an emerging entity. *Genes Chromosomes Cancer* **61**(10), 592–602 (2022).
153. Agaimy, A. *et al.* NR4A3 fusions characterize a distinctive peritoneal mesothelial neoplasm of uncertain biological potential with pure adenomatoid/microcystic morphology. *Genes Chromosomes Cancer* **62**(5), 256–266 (2023).
154. Arulananda, S. *et al.* Mismatch repair protein defects and microsatellite instability in malignant pleural mesothelioma. *J. Thorac. Oncol. Off. Publ. Int. Assoc. Study Lung Cancer* **13**(10), 1588–1594 (2018).
155. Cedrés, S. *et al.* Analysis of mismatch repair (MMR) proteins expression in a series of malignant pleural mesothelioma (MPM) patients. *Clin. Transl. Oncol.* **22**(8), 1390–1398 (2020).
156. Losi, L. *et al.* Role of evaluating tumorinfiltrating lymphocytes, programmed death1 ligand 1 and mismatch repair proteins expression in malignant mesothelioma. *Int. J. Oncol.* **55**(5), 1157–1164 (2019).
157. Bonneville, R. *et al.* Landscape of microsatellite instability across 39 cancer types. *JCO Precis. Oncol.* (2017). doi:10.1200/PO.17.00073.
158. Latham, A. *et al.* Microsatellite instability is associated with the presence of Lynch syndrome pan-cancer. *J. Clin. Oncol. Off. J. Am. Soc. Clin. Oncol.* **37**(4), 286–295 (2019).
159. Combaz-Lair, C. *et al.* Immune biomarkers PD-1/PD-L1 and TLR3 in malignant pleural mesotheliomas. *Hum. Pathol.* **52**, 9–18 (2016).
160. Chapel, D. B. *et al.* Tumor PD-L1 expression in malignant pleural and peritoneal mesothelioma by Dako PD-L1 22C3 pharmDx and Dako PD-L1 28–8 pharmDx assays. *Hum. Pathol.* **87**, 11–17 (2019).
161. Nguyen, B. H., Montgomery, R., Fadia, M., Wang, J. & Ali, S. PD-L1 expression associated with worse survival outcome in malignant pleural mesothelioma. *Asia Pac. J. Clin. Oncol.* **14**(1), 69–73 (2018).
162. Forest, F. *et al.* Nuclear grading, BAP1, mesothelin and PD-L1 expression in malignant pleural mesothelioma: Prognostic implications. *Pathology (Phila.)* **50**(6), 635–641 (2018).
163. Cedrés, S. *et al.* Analysis of expression of programmed cell death 1 ligand 1 (PD-L1) in malignant pleural mesothelioma (MPM). *PLOS One* **10**(3), e0121071 (2015).
164. Baas, P. *et al.* First-line nivolumab plus ipilimumab in unresectable malignant pleural mesothelioma (CheckMate 743): A multicentre, randomised, open-label, phase 3 trial. *Lancet* **397**(10272), 375–386 (2021).
165. Peters, S. *et al.* First-line nivolumab plus ipilimumab versus chemotherapy in patients with unresectable malignant pleural mesothelioma: 3-year outcomes from CheckMate 743. *Ann. Oncol. Off. J. Eur. Soc. Med. Oncol.* **33**(5), 488–499 (2022).
166. Scherpereel, A. *et al.* First-line nivolumab plus ipilimumab versus chemotherapy for the treatment of unresectable malignant pleural mesothelioma: Patient-reported outcomes in CheckMate 743. *Lung Cancer, (Amst., Neth.)* **167**, 8–16 (2022).
167. Nishikubo, M. *et al.* Sarcomatoid mesothelioma originating from mesothelioma in situ: Are methylthioadenosine phosphorylase loss and CDKN2A homozygous deletion poor prognostic factors for preinvasive mesothelioma? *Virchows Arch. Int. J. Pathol.* **481**(2), 307–312 (2022).
168. MacLean, A., Churg, A. & Johnson, S. T. Bilateral pleural mesothelioma in situ and peritoneal mesothelioma in situ associated with BAP1 germline mutation: A case report. *JTO Clin. Res. Rep.* **3** (2022). doi:10.1016/j.jtocrr.2022.100356.

169. Churg, A. *et al.* Malignant mesothelioma in situ: Morphologic features and clinical outcome. *Mod. Pathol. Off. J. US Can. Acad. Pathol. Inc.* **33**(2), 297–302 (2020).
170. Pulford, E., Henderson, D. W. & Klebe, S. Malignant mesothelioma in situ: Diagnostic and clinical considerations. *Pathology (Phila.)* **52**(6), 635–642 (2020).
171. Galateau-Salle, F. *et al.* Mesothelioma in situ mimicking well-differentiated papillary mesothelial tumor. *Am. J. Surg. Pathol.* **47**(5), 611–617 (2023).
172. Churg, A., Dacic, S., Galateau-Salle, F., Attanoos, R. & de Perrot, M. Malignant mesothelioma in situ: Clinical and pathologic implications. *J. Thorac. Oncol.* **15**(6), 899–901 (2020).
173. Klebe, S. *et al.* The concept of mesothelioma in situ, with consideration of its potential impact on cytology diagnosis. *Pathology (Phila.)* **53**(4), 446–453 (2021).
174. Louw, A. *et al.* Analysis of early pleural fluid samples in patients with mesothelioma: A case series exploration of morphology, BAP1, and CDKN2A status with implications for the concept of mesothelioma in situ in cytology. *Cancer Cytopathol.* **130**(5), 352–362 (2022).
175. Michael, C. W., Bedrossian, C. C. W. M., Sadri, N. & Klebe, S. The cytological features of effusions with mesothelioma in situ: A report of 9 cases. *Diagn. Cytopathol.* **51**(6), 374–388 (2023).
176. Churg, A., Galateau-Salle, F., Tan, L. & Qing, G. Cytological diagnosis of mesothelioma in situ versus invasive mesothelioma. *Pathology (Phila.)* **54**(1), 133–136 (2022).
177. Churg, A. *et al.* Malignant mesothelioma in situ. *Histopathology* **72**(6), 1033–1038 (2018).
178. Sauter, J. L. *et al.* Young investigator challenge: Validation and optimization of immunohistochemistry protocols for use on cellient cell block specimens. *Cancer Cytopathol.* **124**(2), 89–100 (2016).
179. Girolami, I. *et al.* Evidence-based diagnostic performance of novel biomarkers for the diagnosis of malignant mesothelioma in effusion cytology. *Cancer Cytopathol.* **130**(2), 96–109 (2022).
180. Allen, T. C. *et al.* Localized malignant mesothelioma. *Am. J. Surg. Pathol.* **29**(7), 866–873 (2005).
181. Marchevsky, A. M. *et al.* Localized malignant mesothelioma, an unusual and poorly characterized neoplasm of serosal origin: Best current evidence from the literature and the International Mesothelioma Panel. *Mod. Pathol. Off. J. US Can. Acad. Pathol. Inc.* **33**(2), 281–296 (2020).
182. Hung, Y. P. *et al.* Molecular characterization of localized pleural mesothelioma. *Mod. Pathol. Off. J. US Can. Acad. Pathol. Inc.* **33**(2), 271–280 (2020).
183. Shrestha, R. *et al.* Well-differentiated papillary mesothelioma of the peritoneum is genetically distinct from malignant mesothelioma. *Cancers* **12**(6) (2020). doi:10.3390/cancers12061568.
184. Stevers, M. *et al.* Well-differentiated papillary mesothelioma of the peritoneum is genetically defined by mutually exclusive mutations in TRAF7 and CDC42. *Mod. Pathol. Off. J. US Can. Acad. Pathol. Inc.* **32**(1), 88–99 (2019).
185. Malpica, A., Sant'Ambrogio, S., Deavers, M. T. & Silva, E. G. Well-differentiated papillary mesothelioma of the female peritoneum: A clinicopathologic study of 26 cases. *Am. J. Surg. Pathol.* **36**(1), 117–127 (2012).
186. Sun, M., Zhao, L., Weng Lao, I., Yu, L. & Wang, J. Well-differentiated papillary mesothelioma: A 17-year single institution experience with a series of 75 cases. *Ann. Diagn. Pathol.* **38**, 43–50 (2019).
187. Butnor, K. J., Sporn, T. A., Hammar, S. P. & Roggli, V. L. Well-differentiated papillary mesothelioma. *Am. J. Surg. Pathol.* **25**(10), 1304–1309 (2001).
188. Churg, A. *et al.* Well-differentiated papillary mesothelioma with invasive foci. *Am. J. Surg. Pathol.* **38**(7), 990–998 (2014).
189. Karpathiou, G., Hiroshima, K. & Peoc'h, M. Adenomatoid tumor: A review of pathology with focus on unusual presentations and sites, histogenesis, differential diagnosis, and molecular and clinical aspects with a historic overview of its description. *Adv. Anat. Pathol.* **27**(6), 394–407 (2020).
190. Hissong, E. *et al.* Adenomatoid tumours of the gastrointestinal tract - A case-series and review of the literature. *Histopathology* **80**(2), 348–359 (2022).
191. Ross, M. J., Welch, W. R. & Scully, R. E. Multilocular peritoneal inclusion cysts (so-called cystic mesotheliomas). *Cancer* **64**(6), 1336–1346 (1989).
192. Weiss, S. W. & Tavassoli, F. A. Multicystic mesothelioma. An analysis of pathologic findings and biologic behavior in 37 cases. *Am. J. Surg. Pathol.* **12**(10), 737–746 (1988).
193. Nizri, E. *et al.* Multicystic mesothelioma: Operative and long-term outcomes with cytoreductive surgery and hyperthermic intra peritoneal chemotherapy. *Eur. J. Surg. Oncol. J. Eur. Soc. Surg. Oncol. Br. Assoc. Surg. Oncol.* **44**(7), 1100–1104 (2018).
194. Karpathiou, G., Casteillo, F., Dridi, M. & Peoc'h, M. Mesothelial cysts. *Am. J. Clin. Pathol.* **155**(6), 853–862 (2021).
195. Churg, A. *et al.* Solid papillary mesothelial tumor. *Mod. Pathol. Off. J. US Can. Acad. Pathol. Inc.* **35**(1), 69–76 (2022).

TABLE 11.1
Established Grading Systems for Pleural Epithelioid Mesothelioma

MSKCC Grading System for Pleural Epithelioid Mesothelioma (Kadota, et al., 2012)

Nuclear atypia	Mild (uniform nuclear size and shape)	1	
	Moderate (intermediate-sized nuclei with slight irregularity of shape)	2	
	Severe (bizarre, enlarged, variably sized nuclei; at least 2:1 variation in nuclear size)	3	
Mitotic index (per 10 high-power fields (40x objective, 0.237 mm^2 field of view))	0-1	1	
	2–4	2	
	≥5	3	
			Composite MSKCC Nuclear Grade
Combined atypia and mitosis scores		2–3	I
		4–5	II
		6	III

Modified Two- and Four-Tier Grading Systems for Pleural Epithelioid Mesothelioma

	Four-Tier (Rosen, et al, 2018)		WHO Two-Tier (Nicholson, et al, 2020)	
Morphologic Criteria	Grade	Median Survival (Rosen, et al, 2018)	Grade	Median Survival (Zhang, et al., 2020; Fuchs, et al., 2022)
MSKCC Grade I, no tumor necrosis	1	29 mo.	Low Grade	18-19 mo.
MSKCC Grade I, with tumor necrosis, *OR* MSKCC Grade II, no tumor necrosis	2	16 mo.		
MSKCC Grade II, with tumor necrosis	3	10 mo.	High Grade	9-11 mo
MSKCC Grade III	4	8 mo.		

TABLE 11.2
Mesothelial Markers.

	Mesothelial Markers Median Percent Positivity (Interquartile Range)								
	Calretinin (number of studies = 49)	WT-1 (n = 25)	D2-40 (n = 15)	CK 5/6 N = 29	HEG1 (n = 6)	Mesothelin (n = 9)	HBME-1 (n = 18)	Thrombomodulin (n = 24)	Vimentin (n = 15)
EMM	95 (88–100)	88 (77–93)	93 (88–96)	91 (75–100)	94 (93–98)	89 (77–100)	88 (80–90)	78 (68–91)	65 (33–81)
BMM	90 (84–90)	60 (60–73)	81 (74–82)	76 (67–79)	90 (86–95)	.	.	90	0
SMM	49 (33–66)	42 (13–45)	50 (38–74)	25 (21–29)	64 (54–72)	0	.	45 (26–60)	90 (88–91)
LUAD	8 (5–24)	0 (0–18)	3 (2–8)	6 (5–19)	0	38 (28–69)	68 (64–75)	14 (6–20)	17 (5–38)
SqCC	40 (23–40)	2 (0–3)	61 (42–61)	98 (97–100)	0	37	.	71	.
SARC	24 (8–52)	7 (0–31)	19 (8–26)	20 (7–28)	.	.	.	40 (25–42)	56
HGSC	5 (0–20)	100	20 (13–27)	28 (25–52)	37 (14–58)	.	3 (1–17)	96 (89–100)	33
RCC	0	0	.	0	.	.	.	2	.
BRCA	17 (13–21)	10 (4–15)	0	19 (5–33)	0	29 (3–55)	.	13	.

The “n” statistic over each column represents the total number of studies of a given marker represented in the column, and not all tumor types are represented in all studies. The HEG1 sensitivity figure for epithelioid and biphasic mesothelioma includes membranous staining only, while the figure for sarcomatoid mesothelioma includes cytoplasmic staining. BMM, biphasic mesothelioma; BRCA, breast carcinoma; EMM, epithelioid mesothelioma; HGSC, high-grade serous carcinoma; LUAD, lung adenocarcinoma; RCC, renal cell carcinoma; SARC, sarcomatoid carcinoma; SMM, sarcomatoid mesothelioma; SqCC, squamous cell carcinoma.

TABLE 11.3
Epithelial Markers and Carcinoma Subtyping Markers.

	Epithelial Markers Median Percent Positivity (Interquartile Range)													
	Claudin-4 (number of studies = 10)	MOC-31 (n = 17)	Ber-EP4 (n = 39)	BG-8 (n = 11)	CEA (n = 48)	CD15 (n = 41)	B72.3 (n = 26)	MUC4 (n = 4)	TTF-1 (n = 10)	Napsin A (n = 4)	GATA3 (n = 3)	PAX8 (n = 5)	p63 (n = 3)	p40 (n = 2)
EMM	0 (0–2)	8 (5–17)	14 (5–18)	7 (6–17)	0 (0–8)	0 (0–7)	2 (0–5)	0	0	0	40 (32–49)	12 (6–18)**	17 (7–23)	5–6
BMM	0	0	.	.	.	.	.	.	0	.	50	.	.	.
SMM	0	0	0	0	0 (0–1)	0	0	2 (0–3)	0	0	72 (70–78)	.	1	0–7
LUAD	99 (96–100)	92 (90–100)	96 (91–100)	96 (94–98)	84 (75–96)	77 (70–82)	84 (81–90)	80 (78–81)	82 (73–91)	83 (82–90)	8	0	30 (9–53)	10
SqCC	95 (92–98)	91 (87–97)	87	80	92 (77–100)	30	40	89	9 (4–11)	6 (3–8)	12	33	99 (97–100)	95–98
SARC	33 (20–45)	34 (15–38)	17 (10–24)	.	15 (6–22)	.	.	60 (38–72)	15 (14–17)	20	9 (0–17)	.	73	21–33
HGSC	98 (96–100)	98 (73–98)	100 (98–100)	73	10 (0–16)	58 (35–62)	80 (73–87)	.	0	0–6	6	99–100	.	.
RCC	90 (86–92)	39 (27–50)	42	8	0	63	0	.	.	52	2–51	90	0	0
BRCA	100 (98–100)	.	63 (55–71)	.	49 (18–79)	.	.	.	15	3	99 (98–100)	0	6–30	2–12

The "n" statistic over each column represents the total number of studies of a given marker represented in the column, and not all tumor types are represented in all studies. ** The PAX8 sensitivity figure for epithelioid mesothelioma represents peritoneal tumors; PAX8 expression in pleural mesothelioma is rare. BMM, biphasic mesothelioma; BRCA, breast carcinoma; EMM, epithelioid mesothelioma; HGSC, high-grade serous carcinoma; LUAD, lung adenocarcinoma; RCC, renal cell carcinoma; SARC, sarcomatoid carcinoma; SMM, sarcomatoid mesothelioma; SqCC, squamous cell carcinoma.

TABLE 11.4
Markers of Mesothelial Malignancy.

	Markers of Mesothelial Malignancy Median Percent Positivity (Interquartile Range)				
	BAP1 loss (n = 36)	CDKN2A deletion (n = 24)	MTAP loss (n = 16)	Merlin loss (n = 2)	p53 aberrant (n = 2)
All MM	56 (60–61)	67 (69–73)	52 (46–59)	44 (40–48)	10 (9–12)
EMM	67 (60–72)	60 (57–69)	41 (37–55)	38 (37–40)	11 (10–11)
BMM	50 (39–56)	74 (69–90)	40 (37–56)	70	17
SMM	22 (10–33)	93 (80–100)	75 (51–90)	53 (46–60)	.
LUAD	0 (0–1)	3	14	.	.
SCC	0	29	.	.	.
RCC	22 (18–25)	32	.	.	.
BRCA	6 (3–9)	15	.	.	.
HGSC	0.15 (0–0.3)	6	8	.	.
RMH	0	0	0	0	0

Note that these figures represent primarily pleural mesothelioma, with *CDKN2A* deletion and MTAP loss being somewhat less common in peritoneal mesothelioma (see text). The "n" statistic over each column represents the total number of studies of a given marker represented in the column, and not all tumor types are represented in all studies. BMM, biphasic mesothelioma; BRCA, breast carcinoma; EMM, epithelioid mesothelioma; HGSC, high-grade serous carcinoma; LUAD, lung adenocarcinoma; RCC, renal cell carcinoma; RMH, reactive mesothelial hyperplasia; SARC, sarcomatoid carcinoma; SMM, sarcomatoid mesothelioma; SqCC, squamous cell carcinoma.

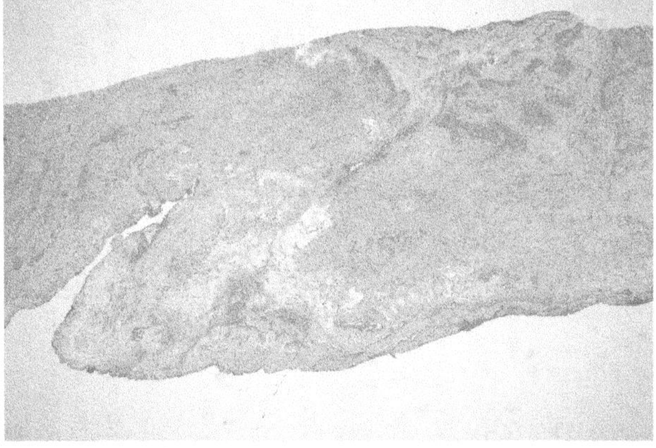

FIGURE 11.1 Reactive mesothelial hyperplasia. Retiform mesothelial arrays run parallel to the serosal surface (bottom right). Tissue twisting and tangential sectioning simulate more expansile growth (running bottom left to top right), mimicking mesothelioma. BAP1, MTAP, and Merlin were retained (not shown).

FIGURE 11.2 Fibrous pleuritis. Reactive spindled mesothelium shows a generally organized arrangement of short fascicles, with a rather hypercellular surface "maturing" toward deeper, uniformly hypocellular layers. Capillary vessels run perpendicular to the serosal surface at generally regular intervals.

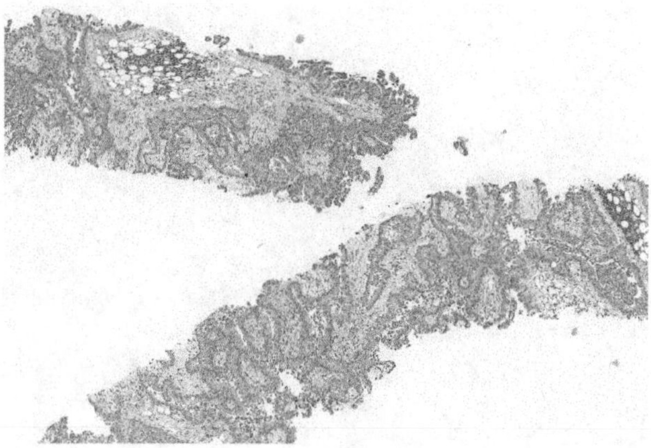

FIGURE 11.3 Epithelioid mesothelioma with tubulopapillary architecture, core biopsies. The tumor is formed of broad papillary fronds, projecting into variably dilated tubular spaces, imparting an overall "puzzle-like" appearance.

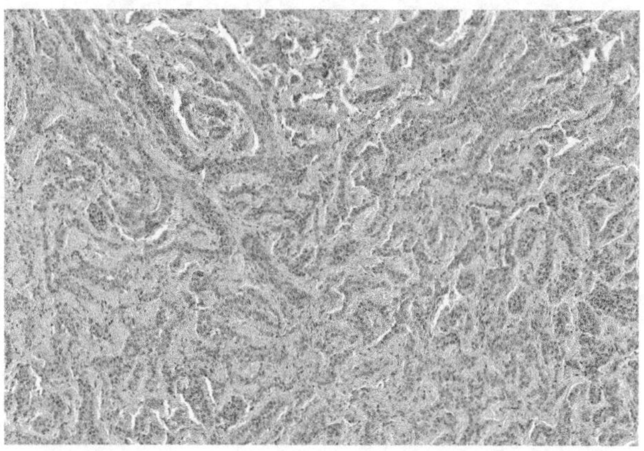

FIGURE 11.4 Epithelioid mesothelioma with trabecular architecture. The tumor comprises a dense arrangement of sinuous, variably anastomosing cords, roughly 2–4 cells wide, separated by fibrous stroma.

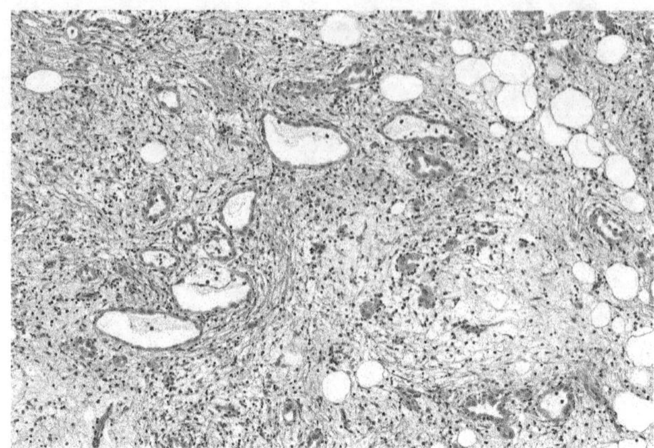

FIGURE 11.5 Epithelioid mesothelioma with adenomatoid (microcystic) architecture. This tumor comprises simple, rounded to angulated tubules, which resemble the tubules of an adenomatoid tumor. However, infiltration of adipose tissue is diagnostic of mesothelioma.

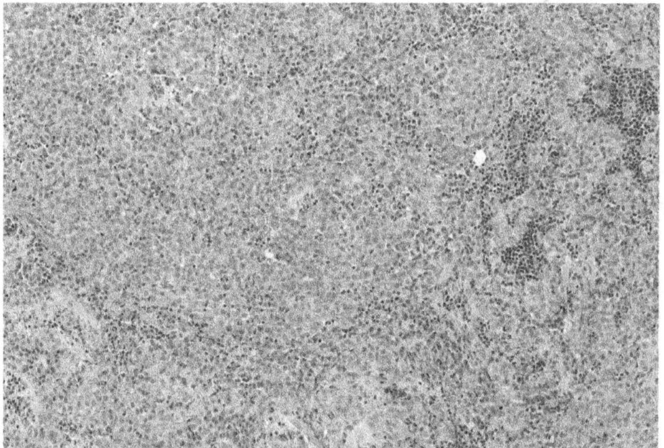

FIGURE 11.6 Epithelioid mesothelioma with solid architecture. This tumor grows as sheets of epithelioid cells, with no other discernible architectural pattern.

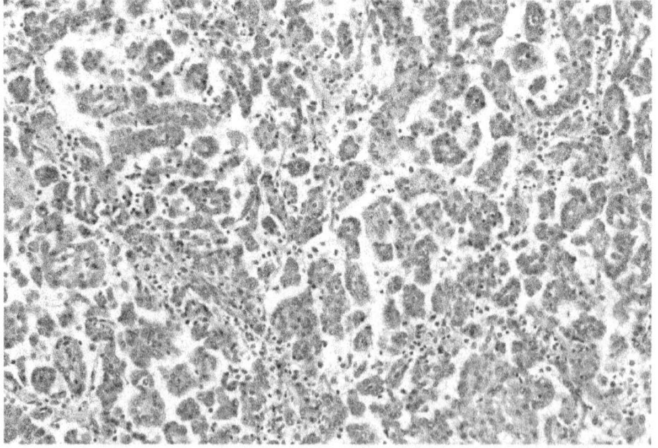

FIGURE 11.7 Epithelioid mesothelioma with micropapillary architecture. This tumor comprises sheets of slender "floating" papillae, lacking fibrovascular stromal cores.

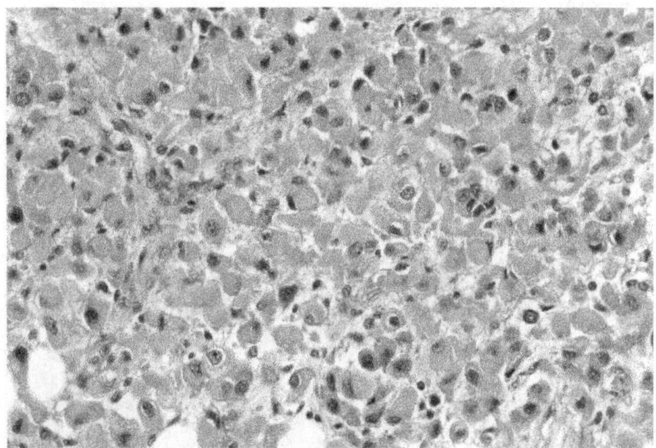

FIGURE 11.8 Epithelioid mesothelioma with rhabdoid features. This tumor grows as solid sheets of epithelioid cells with eccentric nuclei and brightly eosinophilic cytoplasmic inclusions, imparting a rhabdoid appearance.

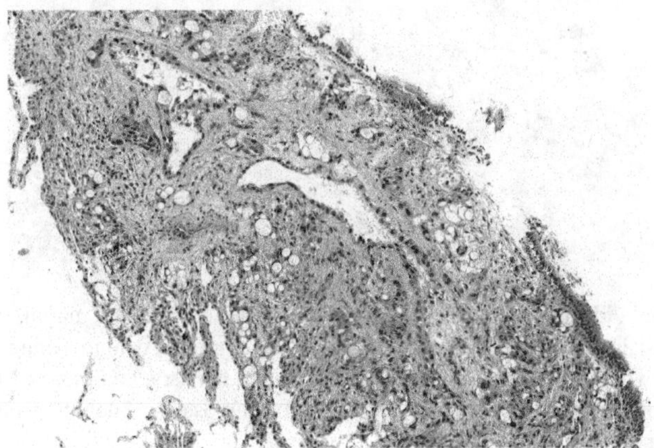

FIGURE 11.9 Epithelioid mesothelioma with signet ring features, core biopsy. This tumor shows predominantly signet ring cell morphology, present as single cells in stroma, small confluent signet ring nests, and scattered signet ring-type vacuoles in tumor tubules. The vacuoles contain flocculent basophilic material, consistent with hyaluronic acid.

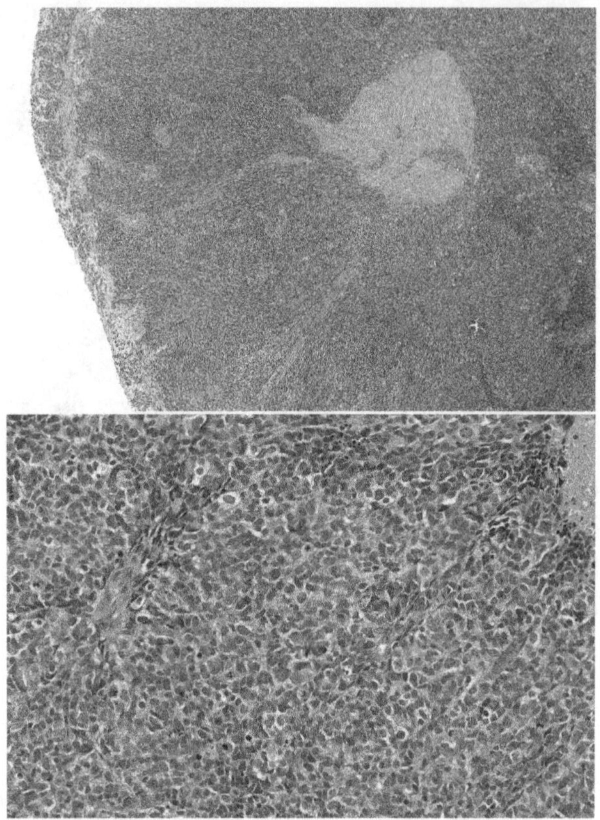

FIGURE 11.10 Epithelioid mesothelioma with small cell features. At low magnification (top), this tumor is deeply basophilic, raising consideration of a small-cell carcinoma. At higher magnification (bottom), the tumor cells show somewhat more cytoplasm, more distinct cell borders, and more conspicuous nucleoli than small-cell lung carcinoma. Nuclear molding is not seen. Immunostains (including negative neuroendocrine markers) were confirmatory (not shown).

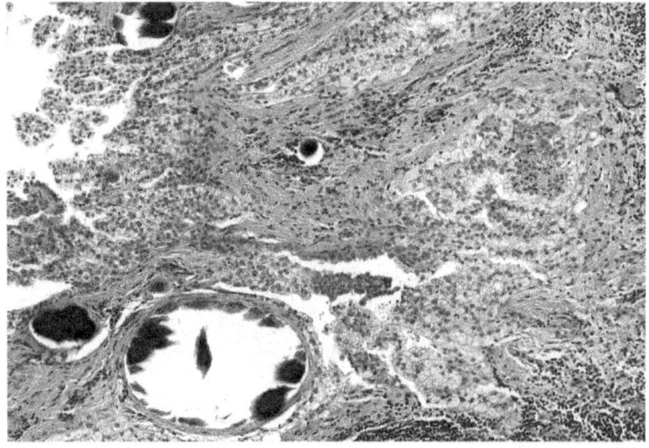

FIGURE 11.11 Epithelioid mesothelioma with clear cell features. This tumor shows tubulopapillary architecture and clear cell cytomorphology, characterized by flocculent, foamy cytoplasm.

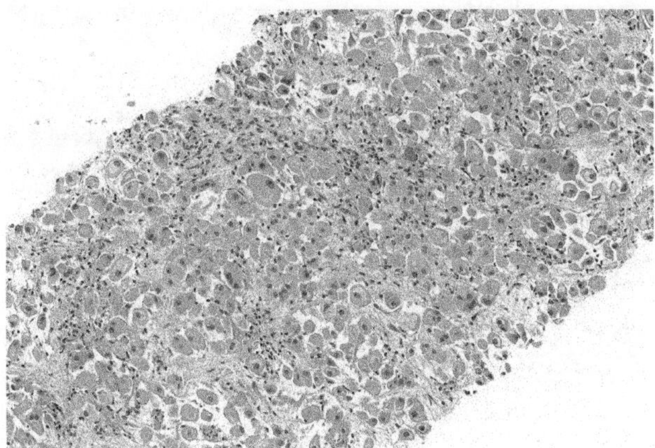

FIGURE 11.12 Epithelioid mesothelioma with deciduoid features. This tumor shows sheet-like growth of large, polyhedral cells with abundant eosinophilic to foamy cytoplasm. This imparts a passing appearance to decidualized endometrium.

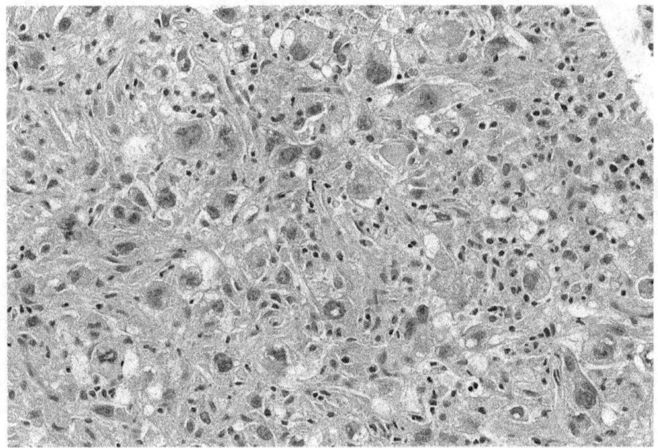

FIGURE 11.13 Pleomorphic mesothelioma. This tumor comprises large, epithelioid to polyhedral cells with abundant eosinophilic cytoplasm and markedly atypical nuclei, with prominent nucleoli and occasional multinucleated tumor cells.

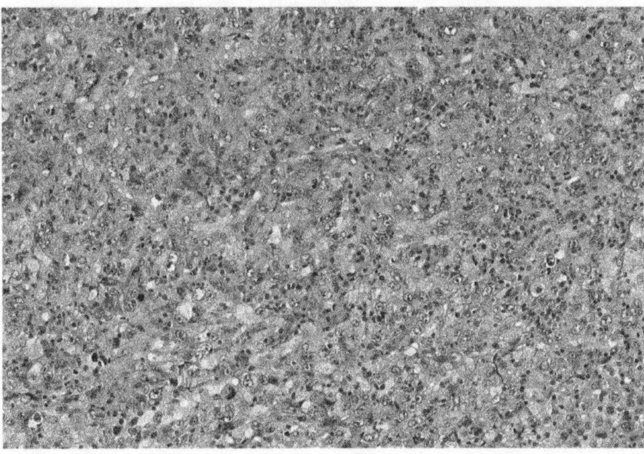

FIGURE 11.14 Lymphohistiocytoid mesothelioma. This tumor comprises sheets of elongated epithelioid cells with pale, flocculent cytoplasm and atypical nuclei, resembling histiocytes. Tumor cells are interposed in a predominantly lymphocytic infiltrate. Individual tumor cells are difficult to pick out, and tumor architectural formations are lacking.

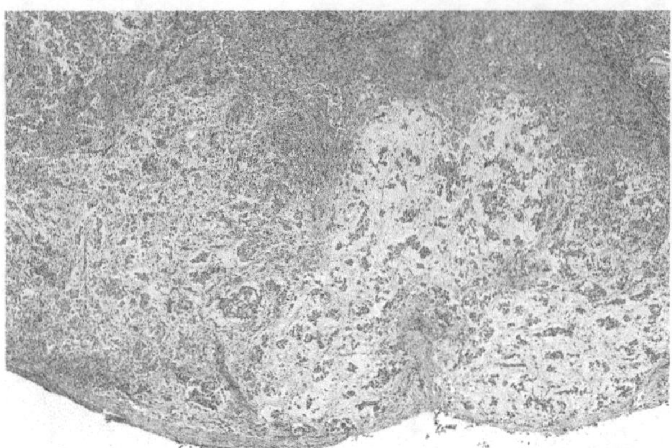

FIGURE 11.15 Mesothelioma with prominent myxoid stroma. This epithelioid mesothelioma shows prominent myxoid stroma, composing >50% of the tumor volume. Such prominent myxoid stroma is reportedly a favorable prognostic finding.

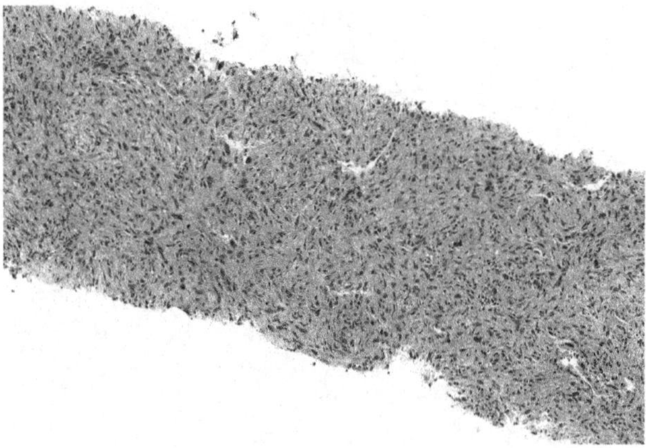

FIGURE 11.16 Sarcomatoid mesothelioma, core biopsy. This tumor is characterized by a haphazard arrangement of short spindled cells with nuclear atypia.

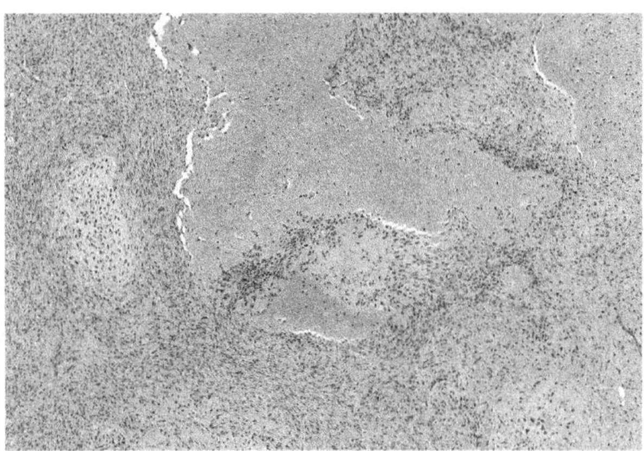

FIGURE 11.17 Sarcomatoid mesothelioma with heterologous differentiation. This tumor shows osseus and cartilaginous differentiation. The spindled proliferation was cytokeratin-positive (not shown), supporting the diagnosis.

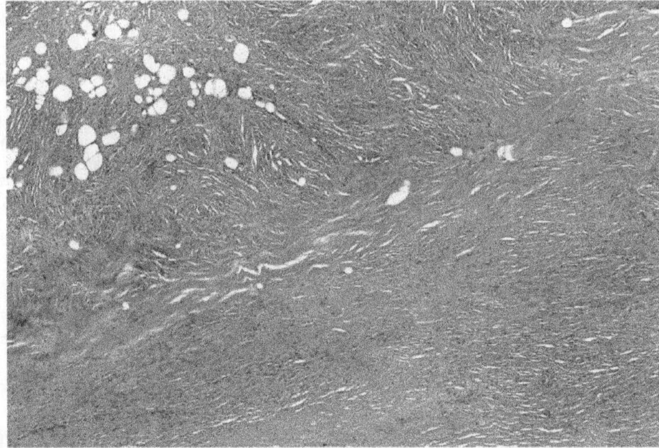

FIGURE 11.18 Desmoplastic mesothelioma. This tumor comprises a haphazard to storiform arrangement of hypocellular fascicles with densely hyalinized, cracked stroma and infiltration of adipose tissue (upper left).

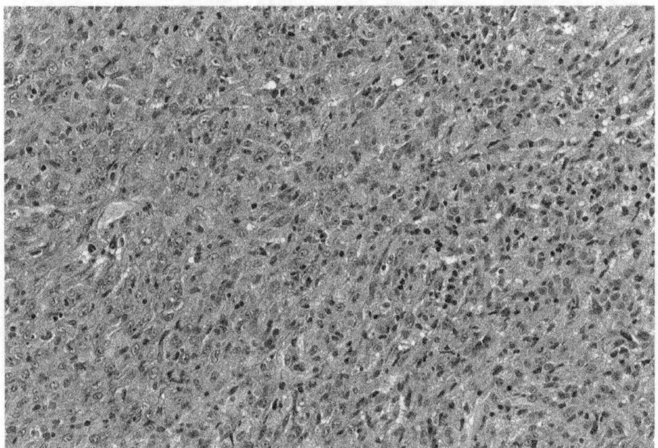

FIGURE 11.19 Transitional mesothelioma. This tumor comprises cohesive sheets of elongated but plump, tapering cells with abundant cytoplasm, discrete cell borders, and large round nuclei with prominent nucleoli, resembling overall a "transition" between epithelioid and sarcomatoid morphology.

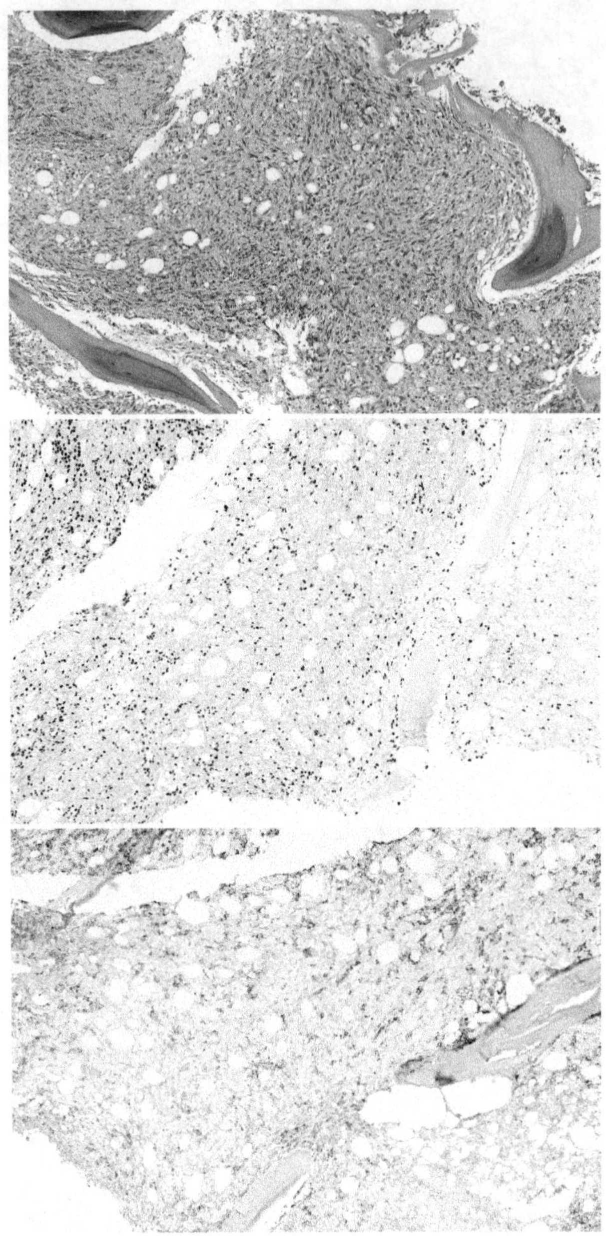

FIGURE 11.20 Metastatic sarcomatoid mesothelioma, core biopsy. This high-grade sarcomatoid malignant neoplasm (top) was positive for cytokeratin and calretinin (not shown) and showed loss of BAP1 (middle) and Merlin (bottom). (Note positive staining in interspersed inflammatory cells, requiring close attention to tumor cell contours.) Based on this immunophenotype, a diagnosis of metastatic sarcomatoid mesothelioma was favored.

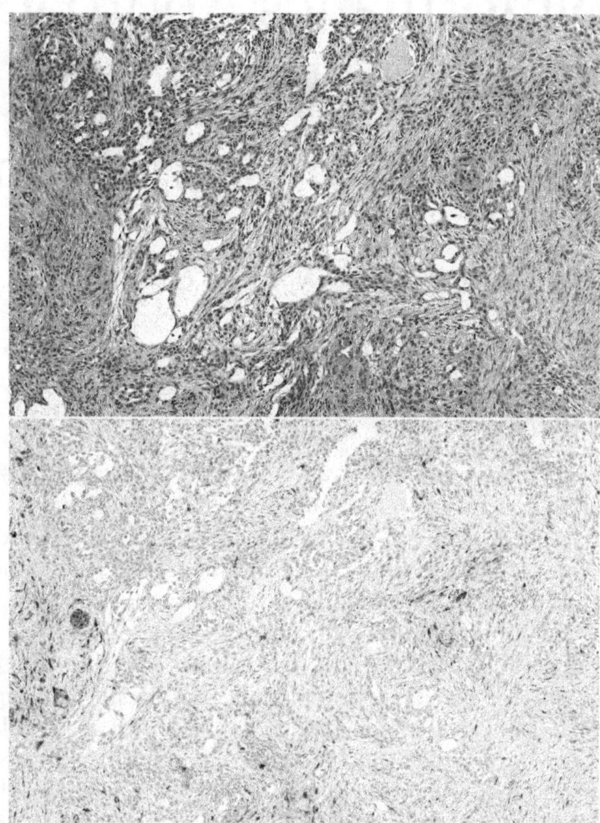

FIGURE 11.21 Biphasic mesothelioma. This diagnostically challenging case shows (top) an epithelioid mesothelioma (upper left) admixed with a morphologically bland spindle cell proliferation (right). By immunohistochemistry (bottom), both components show loss of MTAP expression, supporting a diagnosis of biphasic mesothelioma.

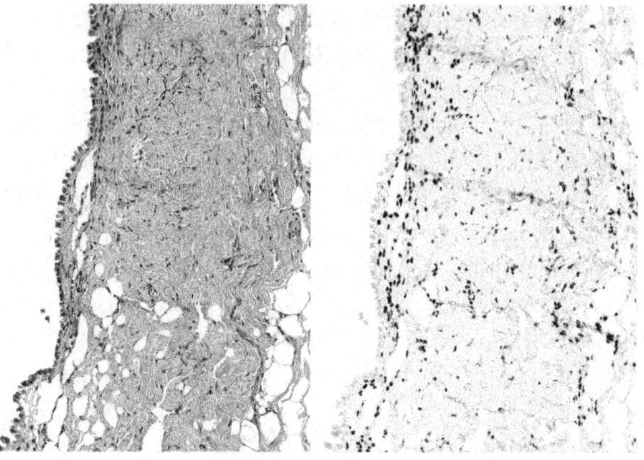

FIGURE 11.22 Mesothelioma in situ. A single, flat layer of cytologically banal mesothelium (left), with loss of BAP1 expression by immunohistochemistry (right). This patient presented with recurrent, unexplained effusion.

12 Bioinformatics Approaches to Studying Diffuse Malignant Mesothelioma

Alicia A. Zolondick and Michele C. Carbone

12.1 INTRODUCTION

Malignant pleural mesothelioma (MPM) is an aggressive cancer typically caused by chronic exposure to carcinogenic mineral fibers, such as asbestos, in the workplace or naturally present in the environment. Each year, there are about 3,200 new cases of MPM and about 3,000 deaths in the US and this incidence rate has remained stable since 2000 [1, 2]. Once inhaled, asbestos fibers are never properly cleared from the body and remain *in situ* in the pleura. Mesothelial cells unsuccessfully attempt to phagocytize the fibers, leading to necrotic cell death and initiating a chronic inflammatory response. Additionally, asbestos-exposed mesothelial cells accumulate DNA damage and undergo cellular transformation. Mesothelial cell transformation coupled with the localized inflammatory environment promotes mesothelioma development and growth. MPM is resistant to current therapies with a median survival of about one year, and less than 30% of patients respond to first-line therapies that may extend median survival to two years [3]. Developing countries lack asbestos regulations; thus, the global MPM incidence is expected to increase worldwide [1].

In Turkey, there was an MPM epidemic with more than 50% incidence [4]. The homes in these villages were made out of and built into the hillsides comprising of erionite, another carcinogenic mineral fiber. Initially, it was believed that the incredibly high incidence of MPM in this region must be due to an increased carcinogenicity of erionite compared to asbestos. However, it was later discovered in 2001 that many families in this region have a genetic predisposition to MPM that increases susceptibility to environmental carcinogenesis [5]. In the following years, genetic and genealogic studies revealed a familial cancer syndrome tracing back to a common ancestor from the 1700s [6]. BRCA1-associated protein 1 (BAP1) is a powerful deubiquitylating tumor suppressor that regulates several essential cellular functions such as transcription, DNA repair, inflammation, metabolism, and cell death [7–12]. The BAP1 cancer syndrome is caused by inherited heterozygous *BAP1* (*BAP1*$^{+/-}$) mutations and carriers are very susceptible to developing MPM, uveal melanoma (UVM), and renal cell carcinoma (RCC), and, less commonly, almost any other cancer type [13]. Patients affected by the BAP1 cancer syndrome show high cancer incidence approaching 100%, and about a third of them develop multiple cancers [4, 14, 15]. Since then, multiple reports elucidated the mechanisms of BAP1 activities and how germline *BAP1*$^{+/-}$ mutations promote cancer growth [7–12]. Irrespective of germline *BAP1*$^{+/-}$ mutation status, genetic analyses of MPM show frequent genetic alterations in several tumor suppressor genes [16]. Furthermore, sequencing of MPM reveals that more than 60% of sporadic MPM and all MPM developing in carriers of germline *BAP1*$^{+/-}$ mutations acquired biallelic inactivation (*BAP1*$^{-/-}$) [17].

Despite the fact that carriers of germline *BAP1*$^{+/-}$ mutations are more likely to develop MPM, these patients have a sevenfold improved survival of 5–10 years, and their tumors are less aggressive and invasive compared to *BAP1*^{WT} MPM patients [18–21]. This paradox is poorly understood:

DOI: 10.1201/9781003431909-12

how can germline $BAP1^{+/-}$ mutations both favor the development of cancer but impede its progression? The cause of the prolonged survival of MPM patients carrying germline $BAP1^{+/-}$ mutations is unknown. It does not appear to be related exclusively to the biallelic *BAP1* inactivation ($BAP1^{-/-}$) of MPM cells because more than 60% of MPM acquire somatic $BAP1^{-/-}$ and only show a modest, if any, survival improvement [17]. Understanding the mechanisms behind this paradox should help all MPM patients, and possibly the entire field of cancer therapeutics.

These various factors that may lead to MPM development and progression attest to its complexity to manage, treat, and characterize. Germline $BAP1^{WT}$ MPM patients exposed to carcinogenic mineral fibers over many years often do not present symptoms until the advanced stage at the time of diagnosis. Families carrying germline $BAP1^{+/-}$ mutations are particularly susceptible to environmental carcinogenesis and have an increased risk of developing MPM and other cancers, yet MPM patients carrying germline $BAP1^{+/-}$ mutations have a significantly improved prognosis and respond better to treatment compared to $BAP1^{WT}$ MPM patients [17]. Bioinformatics approaches to studying MPM have only recently made noteworthy advancements. Moreover, there is still a considerable need to improve molecular profiling of all MPM as there are significant clinical variations between individuals, intratumor heterogeneity, and patients carrying germline $BAP1^{+/-}$ mutations are largely excluded from MPM patient cohorts. The purpose of this review is to highlight the key findings and current advancements in bioinformatics approaches to studying MPM, as well as emphasize the need for MPM databases to include data from MPM patients carrying germline $BAP1^{+/-}$ mutations which will strengthen our knowledge of both asbestos-induced MPM and germline $BAP1^{+/-}$ MPM.

12.2 INITIAL INVESTIGATIONS OF GENETIC LANDSCAPE OF MALIGNANT PLEURAL MESOTHELIOMA

Over the last 30 years, significant advancements in bioinformatics approaches to studying MPM have been developed. MPM impacts various populations worldwide, as asbestos is naturally present in the environment, still mined and used commercially, and there are families living all over the world with a genetic predisposition to MPM. Although numerous studies have characterized the key players involved in asbestos carcinogenesis, current standard-of-care methods are ineffective in improving patient prognosis. Thus, several studies have documented the genomic landscape of MPM in order to identify possible driver genes and novel therapeutic targets.

In the late 1990s, initial studies reported the identification of extensive chromosomal copy-number variations observed in most MPM utilizing karyotyping, comparative genomic hybridization (CGH), and array methods. In CGH analysis of 24 MPM cell lines, significant genomic imbalances were reported and demonstrated that chromosomal losses were more frequent than gains [22]. Furthermore, recurrent somatic mutations in multiple tumor suppressor genes were shown, which supported the observed frequent chromosomal losses—the most frequent are *CDKN2A*, *BAP1*, and *NF2[23]*. These initial findings have been confirmed by countless studies with different sequencing methods over the years in various cohorts of MPM patient biopsies and cell lines [24–27].

12.3 NEXT-GENERATION SEQUENCING OF MALIGNANT PLEURAL MESOTHELIOMA

In recent years, the utilization of massively parallel sequencing (MPS) techniques has become increasingly common in the identification of driver genetic alterations that contribute to disease. MPS, commonly known as next-generation sequencing, refers to high-throughput DNA sequencing methods such as whole-genome sequencing, whole transcriptome sequencing, and targeted sequencing; these methods are capable of simultaneous production of millions of sequence reads.

TABLE 12.1
Overview of Major Studies Using MPS in MPM.

Study	Sequencing Type	Platform
Sugarbarker et al. (2008)[28]; Dong et al. (2009)[29]	Transcriptome	Roche/454-pyrosequencing
Bueno et al. (2010)[30]	Genome	Illumnia Genome Analays=zer 2, Roche/454-pyrosequencing
Guo et al. (2015)[31]	Exome	Illumnia Hiseq
Lo lacono et al. (2015)[32]	Targeted	Ion Torrent Personal Genome Machine
Maki-Nevala et al. (2016)[33]	Exome	Illumnia Hiseq
Kang et al. (2016)[34]	Exome and Targeted	SOLiD 5500 and Ion Torrent Personal Genome Machine
Bueno et al. (2016)[35]	Transcriptome, Exome and Targeted	Illumina HiSeq2500
Hmeljak et al. (2018)[36]	Transcriptome, Exome and Tageted	Illumina HiSeq2500
Mangiante et al. (2021)[37]	Transcriptome and Genome	Illumina Novaseq6000, Illumina HiseqX5

MPS, massively parallel sequencing; MPM, malignant pleural mesothelioma. *Created with Biorender.com*

The complete determination of the human DNA sequence is made possible by whole-genome sequencing, rendering it an indispensable resource for identifying a spectrum of genetic variations. Meanwhile, transcriptome sequencing allows for the examination of RNA transcript presence and abundance in a specific tissue at a particular point in time, thereby facilitating the detection of variations in gene expression and alternative splicing events. Furthermore, targeted sequencing permits the sequencing of specific genomic segments, such as the exome, or specific sets of genes. An overview of the studies utilizing MPS of large cohorts of MPM patients that have had a major impact on our understanding of the genomic landscape of MPM are summarized in Table 12.1 [28–37].

Applying these next-generation sequencing methods to studying MPM has allowed us to report genetic variations seen in MPM, analyze differentially expressed genes and affected pathways in MPM, and correlate these biological subtypes with patient prognosis. In 2016, several reports using MPS techniques to study molecular alterations in MPM were comprehensively reviewed [16], summarizing the genes reported in these studies that exhibit molecular alterations in MPM, the genetic variants linked to MPM, and the main pathways that the reported mutations are involved in [16]. Notably, Guo et al. were the pioneers in performing whole-exome sequencing on 22 MPMs and paired blood samples utilizing the Illumina HiSeq platform and confirmed frequent genetic alterations in *BAP1*, *NF2*, *CDKN2A*, and *CUL1* in MPM [31]. Pathway enrichment analysis was performed using the WebGestalt (Web-based Gene Analysis Toolkit) [38] to compare their findings with the genes reported to have frequent somatic mutations of copy-number changes in the KEGG database[39] and identified the cell cycle, MAPK, and Wnt signaling pathways to be significantly altered in MPM [31].

12.4 INTEGRATIVE ANALYSES OF MALIGNANT PLEURAL MESOTHELIOMA

Due to its rarity, genomic investigations into MPM are constrained, ineffective at identifying clear molecular targets, and often include only a limited number of samples. Therefore, recent studies have included a larger number of samples and applied integrative analyses on MPS data to identify molecular pathways, characterize MPM histotypes, and correlate these findings with clinical outcomes utilizing novel computational algorithms.

A comprehensive genomic analysis including 211 transcriptomes, 99 whole exomes, and 103 targeted exomes from 216 MPM tumors made a notable impact on the field of MPM and identified new recurrent mutations, gene fusions, and splicing alterations, as well as determined clusters of distinct MPM histotypes based on expression [35]. Bueno et al. sequenced the libraries on Illumina HiSeq2500 and analyzed the impact of nonsynonymous variants on gene function using the tools: PolyPhen, SIFT, and Condel and found that 52% of variants have a functional impact [35]. Mesotheliomas are sorted into epithelioid, biphasic, or sarcomatoid categories based on histological features, and exhibit heterogeneity with varying ratios of epithelioid and sarcomatoid characteristics [40]. RNA-sequencing data from this cohort was used in unsupervised consensus clustering and identified differentially expressed genes present in four clusters: sarcomatoid, epithelioid, biphasic-sarcomatoid, and biphasic-epithelioid, and correlated these distinct clusters with patient survival data [35]. It was reported that the MPM biopsies of the epithelioid histotype had the longest patient survival when compared to all other subtypes grouped together or when compared with the clustered subtypes individually [35]. The diagnosis of MPM requires histological evaluation, and historically, classification of histological subtypes has been an arguably reliable prognostic marker [1]. However, it was reported that 16% of histo-type classifications have discrepancies and clinicians rely on histological classification for determining therapeutic intervention [1, 41]. Therefore, the clustering of expression-based MPM subtypes in this large cohort provides key insights into the mutation signatures of each subtype, which may provide novel alternative prognostic markers [35].

In 2018, a comprehensive, multiplatform, genomic study of MPM was published [36]. This report was a part of The Cancer Genome Atlas (TCGA) study and aimed to characterize the molecular landscapes of MPM that may contribute to distinct survival clusters of MPM patients in addition to the clustered histo-types in the previous report by Bueno et al. [35, 36], as within each subtype there are still clinical variations observed between patients in survival. In this cohort of 74 MPM patients, a comprehensive molecular profiling study including copy-number arrays, mRNA sequencing, exome sequencing, reverse-phase protein arrays, noncoding RNA profiling, and DNA methylation were performed and clustered using iCluster and PARADIGM [36]. The results demonstrated four different clusters of histological subtypes correlated with survival markedly similar to the observations reported in the Bueno et al. cohort [35, 36].

Epithelioid MPM seems to be the subtype that has the most variability between patient outcomes. Thus, the authors aimed to identify key molecular differences between patients within the epithelioid cluster. The clustering of epithelioid MPM alone was compared to the clustering of all 74 MPM; the integrative clustering analysis revealed a close resemblance between these results. This suggests that the clustering of all 74 MPM was not based on histological subtype as many of the key features of the epithelioid MPM clusters were also seen in all 74 MPM clustering [36], including survival analysis [36]. To define possible pathways in the epithelioid MPM clustering that may contribute to poor prognosis, PATHMARK analysis was performed [36]. In addition, the TCGA study confirmed their comprehensive molecular profiling of epithelioid MPM would demonstrate similar observations in other cohorts by applying these integrative clustering analyses to 141 epithelioid MPM from the Bueno et al. cohort and confirmed the reproducibility of their clustering model [35, 36].

Although the TCGA study performed extensive integrative analysis and characterized molecular features that are associated with patient prognosis, an obvious limitation of this study is that none of the individuals included in this cohort carried germline *BAP1*$^{+/-}$ mutations. The study included integrative analyses of BAP1 status in this cohort and 57% demonstrated BAP1 alterations [36], yet all were somatic variants, and the molecular differences reported between *BAP1*-inactivated samples and *BAP1*^{WT} seemed less impactful than expected for such a high frequency of BAP1 alterations in this cohort, and observed in MPM patients in general. A clearly stated goal of their study was to define the subsets of MPM in a comprehensive genomic study using integrative analyses that reveal molecular profiles associated with prognosis, however, none of the MPM patients reported to have the best prognosis (patients carrying germline *BAP1*$^{+/-}$ mutations) was included in this cohort and thus the most publicly available data set of MPM is lacking key information that may reveal novel targets in MPM and the BAP1 Cancer Syndrome.

12.5 NOVEL ADVANCES IN ANALYSES OF MALIGNANT PLEURAL MESOTHELIOMA

In the last five years, unprecedented advances in bioinformatics approaches to studying MPM have been developed. In 2019, MesoNet, a deep learning framework for classifying MPM and predicting patient prognosis based on histological slides, was developed and was shown to be more accurate in predicting patient clinical outcomes than any model to date [42]. MesoNet was generated based on algorithms designed to classify and identify disease on histological slides using global data labels [43] from whole slide images (WSIs) of slides from 2,981 patients in the French MESOPATH/MESOBANK database [42]. The WSIs were sectioned into small tiles, selected for regions of interest that were predictive of survival, and given a survival score by a computational learning model employing fivefold cross-validation [42]. Two thousand and three hundred of the 2,981 slides were chosen randomly to be the training set, and the remaining 681 were used as the testing set to evaluate the model [42]. The model was then validated using 56 slides from the TCGA cohort [36, 42]. MesoNet can identify histological subtypes of MPM and has accurately reclassified patients as sarcomatoid MPM instead of the previously determined epithelioid MPM subtype and changed the course of clinical intervention [42]. MesoNet described the tumor stroma to be a crucial region in MPM that predicts patient prognosis and therapeutic response—a key finding to pivot the way researchers investigate and clinicians treat ~~and treat~~ MPM [42]. This tool effectively predicts patient outcomes with either WSIs from large biopsies or as small as a needle size can be a useful and minimally invasive tool to observe MPM patient response to treatment during active clinical trials. In summary, MesoNet made leaps forward in the future of MPM diagnostic methodologies and guides MPM research in a new direction to future studies of the effects of the tumor microenvironment on MPM progression and prognosis.

Following the development of MesoNet, the same research group has become the pioneers of multi-omic factor analyses (MOFA) analyses of MPM and included the MESOBANK [42], TCGA [36], and Bueno et al. [35] cohorts, as well as developed the MESOMICS study [37, 44]. The MESOMICS study was established with the goal of characterizing the heterogeneity of MPM tumors, unraveling the primary sources of molecular variation, and determining their underlying biological functions [37, 44]. The MESOMICS study included the addition of a MESOMICS cohort with whole-genome sequencing data from 115 tumors, along with 109 transcriptomes, 119 epigenomes, and 13 multi-region samples, and extensively maps the genomic landscape of 120 MPM revealing implications for the molecular profiles [37, 44].

The MESOMICS study found that MPM heterogeneity stems from four distinct sources of variation: tumor cell morphology, ploidy, adaptive immune response, and CpG island methylator phenotype [44]. While earlier genomic analyses described tumor cell morphology as a key factor influencing variation, the MESOMICS study identified and extensively characterized the presence of the remaining three sources across all publicly accessible cohorts, demonstrating how these variations alter the behavior of cancer cells and how genomic events influence the molecular profiles observed in MPM [35–37, 44]. In addition, the MESOMICS study demonstrated how these newly identified sources of variation explain the heterogeneity in the clinical outcome of MPM. These discoveries revealed the relationship between functional biology and the genomic lineage of MPM, providing crucial insights for histological classification, prognostic prediction, and therapeutic models.

The MESOMICS study integrated their findings with previously published multi-omic MPM datasets mentioned above (a total of n = 374) and produced a comprehensive molecular phenotype map of MPM [44, 45]. This map is publicly available on the UCSC TumorMap portal (https://tumormap.ucsc.edu/?p=RCG_MESOMICS/MPM_Archetypes) [46]. This newly established, high-quality MPM multi-omics dataset, in conjunction with cutting-edge bioinformatics and user-friendly visualization tools, will aid in advancing therapeutic development in MPM.

12.6 DISCUSSION

The extensive genomic studies, multi-omic analyses, and cutting-edge bioinformatics approaches to studying MPM have led to considerable advancements in our understanding of the molecular complexities and genetic variations that shape MPM development, progression, and patient prognosis. Integrative analyses have revealed the crucial driver genes, key pathways, and characteristics of histological class that contribute to clinical outcomes. Breakthroughs in accurate diagnosis and prediction of MPM patient survival are now possible through deep learning frameworks, which implicate the tumor microenvironment plays an essential role in MPM development. It is hoped that these novel tools will aid in developing effective therapeutic approaches and ultimately improve the lives of patients living with MPM. Although the recent findings of the MESOMICs study and the phenotypic map of MPM paved the way for the identification of genomic events that influence molecular profiles in MPM, the continued collaboration between computational biologists, molecular biologists, and clinicians is essential to identify the mechanisms behind MPM progression so that we may develop targeted therapies. Furthermore, future studies would benefit significantly by including MPM patients carrying germline $BAP1^{+/-}$ mutations and $BARD1^{+/-}$ mutations [17,47] to identify a biological explanation for their significantly improved prognosis and less aggressive tumor phenotype. In conclusion, bioinformatics tools to study MPM have made leaps forward in recent years which will aid in directing future studies in MPM, but the work has just begun.

REFERENCES

1. Carbone, M., et al., Mesothelioma: Scientific clues for prevention, diagnosis, and therapy. *CA Cancer J Clin*, 2019. **69**(5): p. 402–29.
2. Carbone, M., et al., Malignant mesothelioma: Facts, myths, and hypotheses. *J Cell Physiol*, 2012. **227**(1): p. 44–58.
3. Cedres, S., et al., Efficacy of chemotherapy for malignant pleural mesothelioma according to histology in a real-world cohort. *Sci Rep*, 2021. **11**(1): p. 21357.
4. Testa, J.R., et al., Germline BAP1 mutations predispose to malignant mesothelioma. *Nat Genet*, 2011. **43**(10): p. 1022–5.
5. Roushdy-Hammady, I., et al., Genetic-susceptibility factor and malignant mesothelioma in the Cappadocian region of Turkey. *Lancet*, 2001. **357**(9254): p. 444–5.
6. Carbone, M., et al., Combined genetic and genealogic studies uncover a large BAP1 cancer syndrome kindred tracing back nine generations to a common ancestor from the 1700s. *PLOS Genet*, 2015. **11**(12): p. e1005633.
7. Affar, E.B. and M. Carbone, BAP1 regulates different mechanisms of cell death. *Cell Death Dis*, 2018. **9**(12): p. 1151.
8. Han, A., T.J. Purwin, and A.E. Aplin, Roles of the BAP1 tumor suppressor in cell metabolism. *Cancer Res*, 2021. **81**(11): p. 2807–14.
9. Bononi, A., et al., BAP1 regulates IP3R3-mediated Ca(2+) flux to mitochondria suppressing cell transformation. *Nature*, 2017. **546**(7659): p. 549–53.
10. Novelli, F., et al., BAP1 forms a trimer with HMGB1 and HDAC1 that modulates gene x environment interaction with asbestos. *Proc Natl Acad Sci U S A*, 2021. **118**(48): p. e2111946118.
11. Bononi, A., et al., Germline BAP1 mutations induce a Warburg effect. *Cell Death Differ*, 2017. **24**(10): p. 1694–704.
12. Zhang, Y., et al., BAP1 links metabolic regulation of ferroptosis to tumour suppression. *Nat Cell Biol*, 2018. **20**(10): p. 1181–92.
13. Carbone, M., et al., BAP1 cancer syndrome: Malignant mesothelioma, uveal and cutaneous melanoma, and MBAITs. *J Transl Med*, 2012. **10**: p. 179.
14. Carbone, M., et al., BAP1 and cancer. *Nat Rev Cancer*, 2013. **13**(3): p. 153–9.
15. Cebulla, C.M., et al., Analysis of BAP1 germline gene mutation in young uveal melanoma patients. *Ophthal Genet*, 2015. **36**(2): p. 126–31.
16. Hylebos, M., et al., The genetic landscape of malignant pleural mesothelioma: Results from massively parallel sequencing. *J Thorac Oncol*, 2016. **11**(10): p. 1615–26.

17. Carbone, M., et al., Medical and surgical care of patients with mesothelioma and their relatives carrying germline BAP1 mutations. *J Thorac Oncol*, 2022. **17**(7): p. 873–89.
18. Pastorino, S., et al., A subset of mesotheliomas with improved survival occurring in carriers of BAP1 and other germline mutations. *J Clin Oncol*, 2018. **36**(35): p. JCO2018790352.
19. Baumann, F., et al., Mesothelioma patients with germline BAP1 mutations have 7-fold improved long-term survival. *Carcinogenesis*, 2015. **36**(1): p. 76–81.
20. Hassan, R., et al., Inherited predisposition to malignant mesothelioma and overall survival following platinum chemotherapy. *Proc Natl Acad Sci U S A*, 2019. **116**(18): p. 9008–13.
21. Panou, V., et al., Frequency of germline mutations in cancer susceptibility genes in malignant mesothelioma. *J Clin Oncol*, 2018. **36**(28): p. 2863–71.
22. Balsara, B.R., et al., Comparative genomic hybridization and loss of heterozygosity analyses identify a common region of deletion at 15q11.1-15 in human malignant mesothelioma. *Cancer Res*, 1999. **59**(2): p. 450–4.
23. Hiltbrunner, S., et al., Genomic landscape of pleural and peritoneal mesothelioma tumours. *Br J Cancer*, 2022. **127**(11): p. 1997–2005.
24. Nasu, M., et al., High incidence of somatic BAP1 alterations in sporadic malignant mesothelioma. *J Thorac Oncol*, 2015. **10**(4): p. 565–76.
25. Prins, J.B., et al., The gene for the cyclin-dependent-kinase-4 inhibitor, CDKN2A, is preferentially deleted in malignant mesothelioma. *Int J Cancer*, 1998. **75**(4): p. 649–53.
26. Sekido, Y., et al., Neurofibromatosis type 2 (NF2) gene is somatically mutated in mesothelioma but not in lung cancer. *Cancer Res*, 1995. **55**(6): p. 1227–31.
27. Bott, M., et al., The nuclear deubiquitinase BAP1 is commonly inactivated by somatic mutations and 3p21.1 losses in malignant pleural mesothelioma. *Nat Genet*, 2011. **43**(7): p. 668–72.
28. Sugarbaker, D.J., et al., Transcriptome sequencing of malignant pleural mesothelioma tumors. *Proc Natl Acad Sci U S A*, 2008. **105**(9): p. 3521–6.
29. Dong, L., et al., Differentially expressed alternatively spliced genes in malignant pleural mesothelioma identified using massively parallel transcriptome sequencing. *BMC Med Genet*, 2009. **10**: p. 149.
30. Bueno, R., et al., Second generation sequencing of the mesothelioma tumor genome. *PLOS ONE*, 2010. **5**(5): p. e10612.
31. Guo, G., et al., Whole-exome sequencing reveals frequent genetic alterations in BAP1, NF2, CDKN2A, and CUL1 in malignant pleural mesothelioma. *Cancer Res*, 2015. **75**(2): p. 264–9.
32. Lo Iacono, M., et al., Targeted next-generation sequencing of cancer genes in advanced stage malignant pleural mesothelioma: A retrospective study. *J Thorac Oncol*, 2015. **10**(3): p. 492–9.
33. Maki-Nevala, S., et al., Driver gene and novel mutations in asbestos-exposed lung adenocarcinoma and malignant mesothelioma detected by exome sequencing. *Lung*, 2016. **194**(1): p. 125–35.
34. Kang, H.C., et al., Whole exome and targeted deep sequencing identify genome-wide allelic loss and frequent SETDB1 mutations in malignant pleural mesotheliomas. *Oncotarget*, 2016. **7**(7): p. 8321–31.
35. Bueno, R., et al., Comprehensive genomic analysis of malignant pleural mesothelioma identifies recurrent mutations, gene fusions and splicing alterations. *Nat Genet*, 2016. **48**(4): p. 407–16.
36. Hmeljak, J., et al., Integrative molecular characterization of malignant pleural mesothelioma. *Cancer Discov*, 2018. **8**(12): p. 1548–65.
37. Mangiante, L., et al., Disentangling heterogeneity of Malignant Pleural mesothelioma through deep integrative omics analyses. *bioRxiv*, 2021: p.09.27.461908.
38. Zhang, B., S. Kirov, and J. Snoddy, WebGestalt: An integrated system for exploring gene sets in various biological contexts. *Nucleic Acids Res*, 2005. **33**(Web Server issue): p. W741–8.
39. Tanabe, M. and M. Kanehisa, Using the KEGG database resource. *Curr Protoc Bioinformatics*, 2012. **1**: p. 1 12 1–1 12 43.
40. Travis, W.D., et al., The 2015 World Health Organization classification of lung tumors: Impact of genetic, clinical and radiologic advances since the 2004 classification. *J Thorac Oncol*, 2015. **10**(9): p. 1243–60.
41. Galateau Salle, F., et al., New insights on diagnostic reproducibility of biphasic mesotheliomas: A multi-institutional evaluation by the international mesothelioma panel from the MESOPATH reference center. *J Thorac Oncol*, 2018. **13**(8): p. 1189–203.
42. Courtiol, P., et al., Deep learning-based classification of mesothelioma improves prediction of patient outcome. *Nat Med*, 2019. **25**(10): p. 1519–25.
43. Courtiol, P., E.W. Tramel, M. Sanselme, and G. Wainrib, Classification and disease localization in histopathology using only global labels: A weakly-supervised approach, 2018. https://arxiv.org/abs/1802.02212.

44. Mangiante, L., et al., Multiomic analysis of malignant pleural mesothelioma identifies molecular axes and specialized tumor profiles driving intertumor heterogeneity. *Nat Genet*, 2023. **55**(4): p. 607–18.
45. Di Genova, A., et al., A molecular phenotypic map of malignant pleural mesothelioma. *GigaScience*, 2022. **12**.
46. Alex Di Genova, L.M., A. Sexton-Oates, C. Voegele, L. Fernandez-Cuesta, N. Alcala, and M. Foll, MESOMICS, 2023. https://github.com/IARCbioinfo/MESOMICS_data.
47. Novelli, F., et al., Germline BARD1 variants predispose to mesothelioma by impairing DNA repair and Calcium signaling. *Proc Natl Acad Sci USA*, 2024, In press.

13 OncoTherapy in Mesothelioma

Steven G. Gray, Tomer Meirson, and Luciano Mutti

13.1 INTRODUCTION

Pleural mesothelioma (PM) is a rare aggressive inflammatory cancer arising from mesothelial lining of the pleura [1], and a recent estimate suggests that 29,300 people worldwide die each year from PM [2]. Classified as an orphan disease, PM is traditionally associated with previous exposure to asbestos fibers, and while over 400 fibrous minerals have been identified only six are considered carcinogenic [3]. As PM is considered to be predominantly associated with environmental and occupational exposure to asbestos it is considered to be an avoidable cancer, and a recent study found that lung, colorectal, and female breast cancer contributed to having the largest avoidable cancer burden, this was followed by PM as a major contributor [4]. The avoidable proportion in PM was found to be 88.6% in the male populace [4], and reflects the emergence of a subset of PM which have heritable components [5–7], often called BAP1 cancer syndrome [8, 9].

Given that the use of asbestos has been banned in many countries, it was expected that levels of PM would decrease, but many countries including the USA continue to allow its use [10–12]. And while the incidence of PM has apparently remained stable over time with world standardized incidence rates (WSIR) for males and females (per 100,000), respectively, of 0.9 and 0.3 in the United States and 1.7 and 0.4 for Europe [1, 10, 13], overall the global burden of PM has declined over the past 30 years [14]. Despite this drop in overall global burden deaths attributed to PM continue to rise [1].

Due to the long latency associated with the development of PM, the age at diagnosis often lies within an estimated range with means between 50 and 80 years [13, 15–17]. The vast majority of patients are predominantly male with an approximate split between 75–80%: 25–20% (male: female) [13, 16, 17]. Historically, female patients have a better overall survival (OS) than males [16–18], with a threefold better 5-year OS rate than men [18], although a recent study modeling prognostic factors in PM did not find an apparent association [19]. Other prognostic variables associated with prognosis or survival include histological subtype [13, 16], clinical staging [16], germline BAP1 mutational status [1], anemia and serum mesothelin levels [19].

The vast majority of patients presenting with PM are often unable to avail of surgical treatment [1, 20–22], and the role of surgery and multimodality therapy is controversial [23]. As such patients are subsequently offered chemotherapy and more recently immunotherapy. The following sections describe the current status of such therapies in the treatment of PM.

13.2 CHEMOTHERAPY IN THE FIRST-LINE SETTING

Cisplatin entered the clinic for anti-cancer use in 1978 [24], and platinum-based compounds mainly elicit their effects by impairing normal DNA functions and rely on cancer cells having aberrant repair responses [24] such as those seen in PM [25]. It's approval for use in PM as a combination therapy with Pemetrexed/Raltitrexed emerged from two important Phase III studies [26–28], and it has been the established first-line chemotherapy option to date [15, 29–33]. Treatment with this regimen is effectively non-curative and results in only response rates of approximately 40%.

In the 20 years since, only one potential advance has been found in first-line chemotherapy for PM, which was the addition of Bevacizumab (an anti-angiogenic targeting agent) to the Cisplatin/

DOI: 10.1201/9781003431909-13

Pemetrexed regimen. This combination is based on a solid preclinical background [34], and results in an increased OS benefit of just over 2 months (18·8 vs 16.1 months)[35], nevertheless uptake of this combination is arguable due to the lack of efficacy of other anti-angiogenic combinations such as Cediranib [36].

As a consequence, many different therapies with similar strong rationales such as targeted therapies have been tested in the clinic to see if this regimen can be improved upon [37], but at the present moment none has had any significant effect on patient outcome. One of these early combinatorial strategies involved the use of Vinorelbine and while this chemotherapy was not able to improve on the existing combination in the first-line setting [38, 39], it has been recommended for use in the second- or third-line setting [15, 29–32, 40, 41], and is discussed in more detail in the next section.

13.3 CHEMOTHERAPEUTIC OPTIONS IN THE SECOND-LINE SETTING

13.3.1 Vinorelbine

Vinorelbine belongs to a family of drugs called the vinca alkaloids [42] and is a commonly used chemotherapeutic for various cancers. The original trials of Vinorelbine in both first-line and second-line settings have been well summarized by Ceresoli and Zucali [43], but in the current guidelines for the treatment of PM, Vinorelbine is suggested as a therapeutic option to be used in the second-line setting [15, 22, 30, 31], although some single institution analyses suggest that while a high rate of stable disease is observed, actual patient responses to Vinorelbine even at second- or third-line settings are rare [39]. Nevertheless, the OS benefit obtained in patients from these initial trials of Vinorelbine in the second-line setting is within the range of 2.5–11.2 months [43].

A more recent trial attempted to assess the efficacy of Vinorelbine in a randomized setting. This Phase II trial (the VIM Trial) randomized patients (1:2) to receive either active symptom control (ASC) (which is all supportive care deemed necessary for pain management excluding disease-modifying treatment) or ASC with Vinorelbine [44]. The results of this trial were positive meeting its primary endpoint of PFS with the ASC plus Vinorelbine arm versus ASC alone (4.2 months vs 2.8 months) [44].

In a separate randomized Phase II trial the ARCS-M Trial, patients were randomized (2:1) to receive either Anetumab ravtansine (BAY94-9343) a human anti-mesothelin antibody conjugated to a tubulin versus Vinorelbine. This trial did not meet its primary endpoint (PFS) with Anetumab ravtansine not providing any superiority to Vinorelbine (median PFS4·3 months' vs 4·5 months) [45].

13.3.2 Second-Line Setting Versus Immune Checkpoint Inhibitors

Moving forward, other trials of Vinorelbine contained within the second-line setting have been examined, particularly with respect to immune checkpoint inhibitors (ICI), although outcomes have at times been contradictory. For instance, the PROMISE-meso trial was a 1:1 randomized Phase III trial designed to assess the efficacy of Pembrolizumab (an anti-PD1 inhibitor) versus institutional choice single-agent chemotherapy (Gemcitabine or Vinorelbine) in relapsed PM patients following first-line platinum-based chemotherapy [46]. This trial did not meet its primary endpoint and failed to demonstrate an improvement in OS for Pembrolizumab over single-agent chemotherapy among patients pretreated with platinum-based chemotherapy. Of note, in this trial, 83% of the patients (58 of 70 patients] in the chemotherapy arm of this trial received Vinorelbine [46].

In contrast, a separate real-time multi-center retrospective analysis of patients undergoing either second-line chemotherapy (Gemcitabine and/or Vinorelbine) or ICI therapy (Pembrolizumab or Nivolumab ± Ipilimumab), found an improved OS for ICI compared to chemotherapy in the second-line setting [47]. A limitation to this analysis however, is that there were no separate sub-analyses within the chemotherapy groups (48 Gemcitabine, 11 Vinorelbine, and 2 Gemcitabine +Vinorelbine), which limits the conclusions that can be drawn with respect to Vinorelbine versus ICI.

Metronomic oral dosing of Vinorelbine (MOV) is also an emerging possibility being investigated in the second-line setting in PM, as MOV relies on using a lower chemotherapy dose (typically one much less than the maximum tolerated dose), administered frequently to maintain a low concentration of the drugs in the plasma [48, 49]. This allows for the administration of less-toxic doses over prolonged periods of time. A mathematical model-based dosing strategy has been utilized in a Phase IA/IB trial of MOV in lung cancer (NSCLC and PM) [50, 51], and the latest data suggests that MOV does provide clinical benefit [52]. Unfortunately, it is hard to assess the true impact of this trial with respect to final outcomes in PM as the vast majority (i.e. 89%) of the patients were treated with MOV as their 3rd up to 10th line of treatment [52]. A Phase I trial of MOV combined with Durvalumab plus Tremelimumab (MOVIE-1) has been completed in patients with advanced solid tumors [53], and while PM was not included in this trial the results show that this combination is potentially possible in PM, and metronomic chemotherapy is increasingly being investigated alongside immunotherapy as a therapeutic strategy in many cancers [54].

Intriguingly, in this regard, treatment of PM cell lines with Vinorelbine has been shown to induce PD-L1 expression (a key target for several ICIs), suggesting that it may therefore be possible to prime patients prior to ICI. A recent in vitro study found that treating PM cells with Vinorelbine resulted in the induction of PD-L1 with no effect observed for cells treated with Pemetrexed [55]. However, this must be placed in context with a separate study also testing chemotherapy and ICI in preclinical cancer models for potential additive effects which found that Vinorelbine provided no additional benefit [56], and therefore further studies to investigate this possibility are warranted.

One additional important consideration concerning Vinorelbine versus ICI is the cost associated with each. A recent estimate found that the approximate cost for 24-week treatment with Vinorelbine is $515 [57], while recent analyses of ICI combinations such as Ipilimumab/Nivolumab exceeds the willingness-to-pay threshold from the perspective of US payers for the treatment of PM [58–61]. Therefore, a methodology such as "priming" tumors by pre-treatment with Vinorelbine to induce critical checkpoint targets such as PD-L1 may be an attractive approach to reduce costs associated with ICI and minimizing a blanket treatment therapy approach.

13.3.3 Biomarkers for Vinorelbine Sensitivity

Gender would appear to be a potential factor in outcomes to Vinorelbine therapy in PM as a recent study found that Vinorelbine emerged as the most advantageous treatment choice for female patients in the second-line setting [62]. However, a limitation in this analysis is that it represents a single-institute experience and studies involving multi-center outcomes will be required.

Are there any other potential biomarkers that can better stratify patients to receive Vinorelbine? In this regard, a study in 2010 by Sugarbaker and colleagues used *in vivo* chemosensitivity testing to assess the relative resistance of freshly cultured PM tissue explants to Cisplatin, Gemcitabine, and Vinorelbine [63]. On a basic level, a large number of patients had either extreme or intermediate drug resistance to Cisplatin (27%), Gemcitabine (31%), with the most common being to Vinorelbine (59%), while 11% of patients were resistant to all drugs. Intriguingly, no significant differences in resistance were observed between patients who had received neoadjuvant chemotherapy compared to those who had not. This study suggests that biomarkers capable of identifying patients who had either resistance or response to chemotherapy and in particular to Vinorelbine would be useful to stratify patients in the second or third-line setting.

Several studies have now identified potential biomarkers which could stratify patients more effectively. The mode of action of Vinorelbine is to inhibit microtubule dynamics resulting in cell division arrest. Given this mode of action, an early study identified TUBB3 a class III β tubulin frequently associated with drug resistance in cell lines as having predictive value in PM [64]. In this regard, this retrospective study was conducted on a cohort of patients treated with Cisplatin-Vinorelbine. In this same cohort, Zimling *et al.* had also examined the expression of Excision repair cross-complementation group one enzyme (ERCC1) a gene strongly associated with resistance to

Cisplatin and observed that low ERCC1 expression was also associated with prognosis [65]. A combined analysis of TUBB3/ERCC1 identified a subset of patients who were both ERCC1- and class III β-tubulin-negative and who experienced a significantly increased PFS and OS compared with patients who were positive for both markers. The median PFS was 6.7 months, and OS was 15.0 months in the double-positive group of patients, in contrast to a PFS of 15.3 months and an OS of 22.2 months in the group negative for both markers.

RRM1 is a subunit of Ribonucleotide Reductase an enzyme essential for DNA synthesis. Its overexpression is conventionally associated with resistance to Gemcitabine [66]. An analysis of a Phase III trial in NSCLC found that RRM1 expression was predictive for Vinorelbine sensitivity [67] and therefore its potential as a biomarker in Vinorelbine-treated PM was warranted. A subsequent study in the same cohort of Cisplatin-Vinorelbine treated patients found that loss of RRM1 expression was indeed associated with better OS [68].

BRCA1 expression has also been linked to Vinorelbine. An initial study indicated that loss of BRCA1 expression was associated with resistance to Vinorelbine in a PM cell line resistance model [69], and loss of BRCA1 expression was seen in 39% (56 of 144) PM patients examined [69], and an exploratory meta-analysis found suggestive evidence that higher BRCA1 expression is associated with a better ORR in patients treated with anti-microtubule agents (including Vinorelbine) [70]. However, the biomarker study which had identified ERCC1 and TUBB3 as candidate biomarkers had also looked at BRCA1 in their cohort of Cisplatin-Vinorelbine treated patients and did not find any correlation for BRCA1 expression and PFS or OS [64], and indeed when the VIM trial was analyzed for BRCA1 it found that loss of BRCA1 expression did not predict for resistance to Vinorelbine [44]. However, a further study of Vinorelbine-mediated resistance found that BRCA1 loss was associated with the depletion of a member of mitotic checkpoint complex, MAD2L [71] and subsequent analysis of BRCA1/MAD2L was examined in a small subset of patients who had received second-line treatment with Vinorelbine (n = 10). From this analysis, it was found that BRCA1/MAD2L1-negative patients (n = 6) had a worse median OS of 5.9 months versus 36.7 months for BRCA1/MAD2L1-positive patients [71].

It is now well established that BAP1 plays critical roles in mesothelioma. BAP1 or to give it its full name stands for BRCA1-associated Protein 1 therefore suggests that the BRCA complex may be a key complex in mesothelioma, and a retrospective response analysis of BAP1 expression from a subset of patients from the MSO1 chemotherapy trial found a small albeit, non-significant, OS disadvantage associated with nuclear BAP1 expression in tumors from patients treated with Vinorelbine [72]. Further linking BAP1 to previously identified biomarkers of Vinorelbine sensitivity/resistance, a recent study found that in PM cells, mutated BAP1 with loss of function is associated with the induction of resistance to Ribonucleotide Reductase inhibition [73].

Together these results confirm the potential of BRCA1/BAP1 complexes as either biomarkers or targets for understanding the mode(s) of action of Vinorelbine in PM and helping to unravel the potential mechanisms of resistance.

Moving into non-coding RNA (ncRNA), an in vitro study has found that loss of miR-15a, miR-16, and miR-34a appear to be indicators for acquired and intrinsic resistance to both Cisplatin or Vinorelbine in PM [74], and intriguingly an early study in nasopharyngeal cancer identified that BRCA1 was a target and regulated by both mir-15a and mir-16 [75]. As such moving forward, it would be interesting to assess these miRNAs in Vinorelbine-treated patient samples.

In conclusion, from the data arising it would appear that there are many markers emerging that are associated with the BRCA pathway, which could potentially stratify patients into treatment with Vinorelbine.

13.3.4 Ramucirumab

A preclinical rationale for targeting angiogenesis in PM has been identified, and the data from the Phase III trial of Bevacizumab (an anti-VEGF), which led to its approval for use in the first-line setting [35], supports this despite ongoing concerns in relation to cost [76, 77]. Early in vitro studies also identified that VEGFR-2/KDR were overexpressed in PM cell lines and tumor tissues [78, 79]. Targeting VEGFR2 has been explored in the second-line setting. One Phase II trial of nintedanib (a multi-tyrosine kinase inhibitor targeting VEGFR 1-3, PDFR α/β, FGFR 1-3, and Src-family members) given as a single agent in relapsed PM did not meet its primary endpoint based on PFS, with no responses to treatment [80]. A separate Phase III trial of nintedanib in combination with Pemetrexed and Cisplatin in chemotherapy naïve PM patients (LUME-Meso) also did not meet its primary endpoint of PFS [81]. However, a Phase II trial of Ramucirumab (an anti-VEGFR2 antibody) combined with Gemcitabine in the second-line setting significantly improved OS, with a median OS of 13·8 months in the Gemcitabine plus Ramucirumab group versus 7·5 months in the Gemcitabine plus placebo group [82], although questions remain as to the true benefit of this trial, mainly due to patient stratification [83]. Nevertheless, the latest ESMO guidelines for the management of PM Ramucirumab plus Gemcitabine is suggested as a treatment option for systemic therapy in the second line [15]. In the light of the concerns raised a properly controlled Phase III trial could perhaps be of benefit in this setting to resolve these outstanding issues and determine if this is valid second-line therapy in mesothelioma.

13.3.5 Gemcitabine

Gemcitabine has been trialed in the past for use in the front-line setting for mesothelioma, but current guidelines suggest that it should only be used as an alternative combination (Gemcitabine/Cisplatin) in patients who cannot receive Pemetrexed [30]. A separate prospective cohort study has recently been completed using low-dose Gemcitabine to determine the efficacy and safety of continuous infusion Gemcitabine-Cisplatin in chemotherapy naïve patients with unresectable PM, with a median OS was 16.16 months [84], and could be considered to be a cost-saving option when compared with other frequently used chemotherapy schemes moving forward.

In the second-line setting, a number of clinical trials have demonstrated that Gemcitabine should also be considered as a preferred agent for use in the second-line setting [39]. A more recent trial (NVALT19) has examined Gemcitabine for its utility as a maintenance drug in patients without disease progression after first-line chemotherapy. This Phase II trial examined if a switch to maintenance Gemcitabine was superior to best supportive care, and while PFS was shown to be significantly longer in the Gemcitabine arm, no OS benefit was achieved [85].

As alluded to in the previous section (13.3.4), there appears to be some benefit to the use of Gemcitabine in combination with Ramucirumab, although further trials will be required to validate this [15, 82, 83]. The existing data and potential for combining Gemcitabine with immunotherapies will be discussed in a later section.

13.4 TARGETED THERAPIES/NEW APPROACHES

13.4.1 Arginine Deprivation

Arginine is considered to be a semi-essential amino acid in the body, vital for many important cellular processes. Disruption of the arginine biosynthesis is common in cancer, resulting in an auxotrophic phenotype making arginine a crucial amino acid required for cancer cell survival [86]. The main mechanism for this disruption is often the loss of expression of a key gene called argininosuccinate synthase 1 (ASS1) [86, 87]. Loss of ASS1 was initially observed in PM cell lines, but subsequently its expression was also shown to be reduced or absent in 62% of n = 82 PM patients [88], suggesting that a large subset of patients may be dependent upon arginine. Experiments aimed at targeting arginine depletion confirmed anti-cancer activity in ASS1-negative but not positive cell lines [88] which led to the initiation of a Phase II clinical trial (the Arginine Deiminase and Mesothelioma (ADAM) study), using the arginine blocker ADI-PEG20, which was randomized 2:1 to arginine deprivation (ADI-PEG20, 36.8 mg/m^2, weekly intramuscular) plus best supportive care (BSC) or BSC alone [89]. The primary endpoint of the trial was PFS, measured from the randomization date to first progression or death from any cause, and ADI-PEG20 did provide a modest yet significant increase in PFS (median of 3.2 months in the ADI-PEG20 group vs 2.0 months in the BSC group). Following on from this a Phase I dose escalation study was conducted for an ADI-PEG20, Cisplatin, Pemetrexed to determine the recommended dose, safety, and tolerability of this combination for use in NSCLC and mesothelioma. No DLTs were observed and partial responses were observed in seven of nine patients (78%), including three with either sarcomatoid or biphasic PM [90]. These encouraging results lead to a further Phase I expansion study to trial this ADIPemCis at the recommended Phase II dose in 32 patients with ASS1-deficient PM [91], and the median PFS and OS were 5.6 and 10.1 months, respectively [91]. This has led to the currently ongoing randomized, double-blind, Phase 2/3 ATOMIC-Meso Phase study, which is limited to patients with unresectable biphasic or sarcomatoid histology, and naïve to chemotherapy or immunotherapy. In this trial n = 249 patients were randomized 1:1 to receive either the ADIPemCis combination versus Placebo PemCis given. Preliminary results of this trial indicate that the ADIPemCis combination provides a superior mOS with respect to SOC (9.3 months vs 7.7 months) [92].

13.4.2 Targeting PARP

Given the significant links between BRCA1 and BAP1 in mesothelioma, it has often been suggested that PM may therefore be sensitive to inhibitors of the poly (ADP-ribose) polymerase (PARP) pathway for which clear evidence exists for other cancers [93–95]. Preclinical data support the notion that mesotheliomas are sensitive to PARPi [96, 97].

Initial analysis in a small number of PM patients treated with PARPi did not see any responses [98]. However, several trials have now been completed using either BAP1, BRCA1, or both to stratify. In MIST1, a single-center, open-label, single-arm, Phase IIa trial eligible patients with cytoplasmic-BAP1-deficient or BRCA1-deficient PM (pleural or peritoneal or other primary localization) were given Rucaparib, and the primary outcome was disease control. The trial met its primary outcome with a disease control rate at 12 weeks of 58% [99]. A second single-center, nonrandomized, Phase 2 trial involving treating PM patients with Olaparib in the second-line setting. The primary objective of this trial was to determine the ORR on the basis of somatic or germline mutation status of DNA repair genes including BAP1. The results were inconclusive suggesting that Olaparib has limited activity in previously treated PM including patients with BAP1 mutations [100]. A third trial has opened as a prospective Phase II single-arm study that will examine aiming to investigate the safety and antitumor activity of the combination of Niraparib and Dostarlimab in patients with HRD-positive and PD-L1 ≥ 1% advanced NSCLC and/or pleural mesothelioma, with the primary endpoint of progression-free survival [101]. To our knowledge there are no preliminary data available from this trial.

13.4.3 Targeting CDK4/CDK6

CDK4/CDK6 have emerged as strong contenders for therapeutic intervention in mesothelioma, as loss of expression of CDKN2A, which encodes the cell-cycle regulator and cyclin-dependent kinase (CDK4 and CDK6 inhibitor p16ink4A) occur frequently in PM either through chromosomal copy number changes, germline variants, or through epigenetic inactivation [102–106]. Various in vitro studies have found that CDK4/CDK6 inhibitors have potential therapeutic benefits in mesotheliomas either as single agents [107] or to enhance the efficacy of existing chemotherapy [108]. Moreover, the sensitivity of PM to CDK4/CDK6 appears to require phosphorylation of CDK4, which was observed to occur in 80% of patient sample examined [109]. A single-arm open-label Phase II trial of a CDK4/CDK6 inhibitor (Abemaciclib) was conducted and met its primary endpoint, with a

12-week disease control rate of 54% [110], and while encouraging there are some serious concerns regarding the full outcomes [111]. More trials will be required to fully evaluate this possible therapy in mesothelioma.

13.4.4 Targeting EZH2

Enhancer of Zeste 2 (EZH2) was initially identified as being highly expressed in around 85% of PM and that pharmacological inhibition of EZH2 was associated with anti-proliferative and antitumor effects [112]. Subsequently it was found that loss of BAP1 was implicated in malignant transformation by EZH2 [113], and an immunohistochemical study in PM found that BAP1 loss and high EZH2 expression were observed in 17 (53%) and 22 (66%) PM cases, respectively, although the fraction cases which had BAP1-loss/EZH2-high was restricted to 31% [114]. The importance of this must be considered in the light of the earlier study which had found that loss of BAP1 made PM cells sensitive to pharmacologic intervention using EZH2 inhibitors [113]. An open-label single-arm Phase 2 study of the EZH2 inhibitor Tazemetostat was conducted in PM and failed in the second-line setting. The primary endpoint of the main element of the study was Disease Control rate (DCR) in patients with confirmed BAP1 loss at 12 weeks, which at the endpoint of the trial was assessed at 54% [115]. The study concluded that further biomarkers "*beyond BAP1 inactivation could help identify a subset of tumours that are most likely to derive prolonged benefit or shrinkage from this therapy*" [115]. Indeed, this may be critical as several new in vitro studies suggest that CDKN2A status may be important in this regard [116–118].

One area of concern regarding the potential use of EZH2 inhibitors in PM is their effects on the immune milieu in mesothelioma. In this regard a recent analysis found that PM patients with high EZH2 expression differ from those with low EZH2 expression in their tumor immune microenvironment, where high EZH2 expression is associated with reduced numbers of Natural Killer (NK) cells, Mast cells, and Th17 cells [119]. Moreover, in an animal model of mesothelioma, macrophages pretreated with an EZH2 inhibitor failed to control tumor growth of PM cells [120], while in vitro studies using 3D models found that tumor-associated macrophages (TAMs) can drive resistance to Tazemetostat [121].

13.5 IMMUNE CHECKPOINT INHIBITORS FOR MESOTHELIOMA

13.5.1 ICI in the First- and Second-Line Setting

It is within the first-line setting that ICI has had the most impact. Early results in Phase I/II trials proved promising [122, 123]. The completion of the Phase III Checkmate-743 trial demonstrated that a combination ICI therapy of Ipilimumab/Nivolumab in untreated, histologically confirmed unresectable PM resulted in significant improvements in OS versus standard-of-care Cisplatin-Pemetrexed chemotherapy [124, 125], leading to its approval in the US and Europe as a first-line therapy [126–128], and clinical practice guidelines for the use of ICI have been updated to include PM [129].

The path for inclusion of immune checkpoint inhibitors (ICI) in the second-line setting has not been as smooth. Initial trials using ICI were disappointing often with conflicting results. For instance, the PROMISE-meso trial was a Phase II trial investigating the efficacy of Pembrolizumab (an anti-PD-1) versus chemotherapy in patients who had progressed following platinum-based chemotherapy. This trial unfortunately did not find any improvement in either PFS or OS compared to chemotherapy [46]. In contrast, the CONFIRM trial assessed the efficacy of another anti-PD1 Nivolumab against chemotherapy, again in patients who had progressed following standard platinum-based chemotherapy, and in this instance median OS benefit was observed in the Nivolumab arm versus chemotherapy (median OS of 10·2 months vs 6·9 months) [130]. Nivolumab was also examined in the MERIT trial, a Phase II multi-center, open-label, uncontrolled, trial of patients within the second-line setting, which observed an OS of 17.3 months and resulted in Nivolumab being approved for salvage therapy in Japan [131]. Several studies have now examined data from within the real-world setting for Nivolumab, often with potentially conflicting outcomes. For instance, data from the Dutch expanded access program, suggests that in a real-world setting patients with recurrent pleural mesothelioma, Nivolumab did not provide the same benefits as observed in the above clinical trials with worse ORR and a median OS of only 6.7 months, although patients who had a good response as seen by radiological response had exceptional survival rates [132]. In contrast, a French multi-center retrospective real-world analysis of Nivolumab found a median OS of 12.8 months [133]. A separate study of retrospective real-life multi-center data examining outcomes for either Nivolumab or Ipilimumab plus Nivolumab found that treatments with ICI were associated with improved OS compared to chemotherapy in the second-line setting [47]. Other analyses have examined the real-world outcomes for other ICI and ICI combinations with similar mOS [134, 135]. One of the issues with respect to many of these real-world analyses is that they evaluate the use of ICI in the second-line setting but without comparison to other second-line chemotherapy such as Vinorelbine, and as such it is hard to make any definitive conclusions as to their true efficacy. Indeed, the one published attempt to assess this possibility found that ICIs did not show significant benefits over chemotherapy based on mOS [136].

Other ICI tested single agents in the second-line setting have not fared as well. The results of the DIADEM trial which examined the efficacy of Durvalumab (anti-PD-L1) in patients progressing platinum-Pemetrexed chemotherapy found that the treatment did not reach a meaningful clinical activity [137]. A separate study of another anti-PD-L1 (Avelumab) found a median OS of 10.7 months, however when stratified by PD-L1 positivity, a median OS of 20.2 months was observed for patients stratified by a cutoff of PD-L1 expression of 5% or greater [138].

13.5.2 Is There a Role for ICI + Chemotherapy in the Front-line Setting?

Given the excitement surrounding the approval of ICI for first-line therapy, it becomes imperative to see if there are any possibilities to combine both ICI and the current first-line chemotherapy. In this regard Phase II trials of Durvalumab and Cisplatin-Pemetrexed reported have promising clinical activity alongside an acceptable safety profile [139, 140], and have led to the development of an ongoing Phase III trial (DREAM3R) [141].

In a separate trial (IND227) using the same combination is running concurrently, and interim results were recently presented [142]. The results at cutoff when analyzed demonstrate a small but statistically significant increase in the mOS (17.3m for the ICI + Chemotherapy vs 16.1m for Chemo alone) [142].

A recent meta-analysis of several trials using chemo-immunotherapy combination(s) suggests that first-line chemo-immunotherapy achieves a 59% ORR and 92% DCR and may represent a novel new first-line approach for unresectable mesothelioma, but the authors acknowledge limitations with respect to this analysis [143]. These results suggest that much more will need to be resolved if an ICI-Chemotherapy combination will advance to become the standard of care for mesothelioma. Significant concerns have been raised regarding elements of the trial methodology and efficacy of most of the treatments in this section and will discussed in greater depth later on in this chapter.

13.5.3 Is There a Role for ICI + Chemotherapy in the Second-line Setting?

Data regarding the possibility of combining ICI + chemotherapy in the second-line setting is scarce. However, the PROMISE-trial was designed to assess ICI compared to either Vinorelbine or Gemcitabine, but allowed cross-over, and in this regard it is noteworthy that 63% of patients on chemotherapy crossed over to receive ICI [46]. To our knowledge, there are no other published studies assessing ICI + Chemotherapy in the second-line setting.

13.5.4 Is There a Role for ICI in the Neoadjuvant Setting Prior to Surgery?

There have been some studies of neoadjuvant chemotherapy prior to surgery in mesothelioma, often alongside radical radiotherapy in a tri-modality approach, and remains contentious [144–148].

Neoadjuvant treatments with ICIs are being tested within the setting of NSCLC [149, 150] and therefore is there an opportunity to use ICI within a neoadjuvant setting prior to surgery in mesothelioma? In 2021, the results of a trial of neoadjuvant Cisplatin-Pemetrexed plus Atezolizumab were reported [151]. This was a feasibility trial and met its prespecified criteria, with 21 patients completing neoadjuvant therapy. However, seven of these patients (33%) did not proceed to resection (2 toxicity, 4 disease progression, 1 death) [151].

In contrast, a second Phase II window of opportunity single-institute trial of ICI followed by surgery in patients with resectable malignant PM was also recently reported [152]. In this trial, 9 patients received monotherapy (Durvalumab) and 11 received combination (Durvalumab plus Ipilimumab) therapy. Seventeen of the 20 patients (85%) subsequently went on to receive planned thoracotomy. At the time of reporting those patients who received the combination ICI had longer median overall survival (not reached) compared with those receiving monotherapy (14.0 months) [152]. It is hard to make any definitive conclusions based on this trial as there were no comparators for surgery alone or for surgery plus neoadjuvant chemotherapy, but the results warrant further investigation in a larger controlled trial setting in a multi-institutional format.

13.5.5 Other ImmunoOncology Possibilities?

In addition to the current ICI targeting PD-1, PD-L1, and CTLA4, other immune checkpoint targets have been identified in PM (e.g. VISTA), and have been summarized elsewhere [122, 123, 153, 154]. As pharmaceutical companies are actively engaged in developing agents to target these, it will be interesting to see how many will have therapeutic use in mesothelioma.

There are also many other trials/investigations for other immunotherapy-based approaches in PM including trials examining the use of oncolytic viruses [155–157] and CAR-T based approaches [158–161].

13.5.6 Outstanding Issues Regarding Oncotherapy (ICI and Chemotherapy) in Mesothelioma

Despite the hype of ICI in PM one factor remains. Based on the results of the Checkmate-743 trial complete responses occurred in only 2% of patients [162]. In a manner similar to the uptake of Bevacizumab, the cost of treatment with ICIs is of concern to many clinicians and governmental regulatory bodies [58–61, 128, 163].

Moreover, there are emerging concerns regarding the significant toxicities associated with the use of ICIs. A recent meta-analysis of ICIs in advanced cancers other than melanoma found the following: [1] the Ipilimumab/Nivolumab combination was not associated with an improvement in OS over Nivolumab alone; [2] this combination was associated with significantly higher Grade 3/4 adverse events; and [3] this resulted in significantly higher treatment-related discontinuations [164], and this is reflected within the context of mesothelioma. For example, a single institutional experience of Nivolumab in three patients with sarcomatoid histology (a histological subtype associated with better outcomes for ICI) found significant side effects in 2/3 patients [165]. The Checkmate-743 trial reported discontinuation of treatment in 23% of patients along with 30% of patients experiencing > Grade 3 toxicities [142, 162]. In a similar manner the results of the IND227 trial examining the efficacy and safety of Pembrolizumab + Cisplatin + Pemetrexed in patients with PM also observed a significant degree of Grade3+ toxicities, again in the order of 30% [142]. More recent real-world assessments of the approved ICI combination/s have revealed significant toxicities [166, 167] and clinicians should therefore have a more cautious approach when using this combination particularly in frailer patients.

Aside from the general limitations with all comparisons of trials involving PM (heterogeneity of patient selection, different treatment dosing regimens etc.,) an area emerging that is causing concern regards the actual fragility inherent within many clinical trials of PM not only those using just ICI but also for the original trials underpinning current first-line chemotherapy [168–172]. Key to this is the issue of informative censoring which can introduce significant bias [173, 174], and make trial results uninterpretable [175]. Much more studies will therefore be required to truly advance ICI into the mainstream management of mesothelioma.

13.6 CONCLUSIONS

The modest impact of the standard and more recently proposed medical treatments for PM prompt the scientific community to push the current boundaries to overcome the substantial stall in patient outcomes that we are currently dealing with when treating patients with chemotherapy or ICI.

This impediment also hampers the combined treatment for this neoplasm i.e. combined medical and surgical approaches, due to the limitations and potential weaknesses of the medical pillars as described in this chapter, combined with the limited indications for surgery of mostly adequate for fit patients with limited disease and eligible for complete macroscopic resection [20].

In 20 years the treatment options available to the clinician treating PM have changed little. Some progress has been made with respect to the introduction of ICI, but patient survival prospects remain poor. There are many issues remaining to be resolved, which include the following:

- What are the options available for patients with BAP1 mutations or BAP1 cancer syndrome [176]?
- What is the role of surgery moving forward (MARS2 etc.) [177, 178], and is there a role for oncotherapy combined with surgery in the neoadjuvant or adjuvant setting [179, 180]?
- Is there a role for tumor-treating fields in the management of patient oncotherapy? [33, 181–184]?
- How do we resolve intra-tumoral heterogeneity (ITH) [183–186], and/or epigenetic intra-tumoral heterogeneity (epi-ITH) [189] in PM?
- Will CAR-T bring new outcomes to PM treatments [122, 158, 160, 161, 190, 191]?
- How should we approach the limitations imposed by fibrosis [190, 191] and hypoxia/ferroptosis [194–200] on drug delivery and immune cell infiltration in our approach to PM oncotherapy?

On this basis of all of these issues described, one cannot conclude anything at present other than that there is a critically unmet need to identify and develop bespoke approaches for oncotherapy-based approaches in the treatment of PM. Perhaps the next 20 years will provide some if not all of these answers, and dramatically improve both the options available for clinicians to treat patients with PM, and to further increase patient survival in the long term.

REFERENCES

1. Carbone M, Adusumilli PS, Alexander HR Jr., Baas P, Bardelli F, Bononi A, et al. Mesothelioma: Scientific clues for prevention, diagnosis, and therapy. *CA Cancer J Clin.* 2019;69(5):402–29.
2. Kocarnik JM, Compton K, Dean FE, Fu W, Gaw BL, Harvey JD, et al. Cancer incidence, mortality, years of life lost, years lived with disability, and disability-adjusted life years for 29 cancer groups from 2010 to 2019: A systematic analysis for the global burden of disease Study 2019. *JAMA Oncol.* 2022;8(3):420–44.
3. Baumann F, Ambrosi JP, Carbone M. Asbestos is not just asbestos: An unrecognised health hazard. *Lancet Oncol.* 2013;14(7):576–8.
4. Cabasag CJ, Vignat J, Ferlay J, Arndt V, Lemmens V, Praagman J, et al. The preventability of cancer in Europe: A quantitative assessment of avoidable cancer cases across 17 cancer sites and 38 countries in 2020. *Eur J Cancer.* 2022;177:15–24.

5. Bott M, Brevet M, Taylor BS, Shimizu S, Ito T, Wang L, et al. The nuclear deubiquitinase BAP1 is commonly inactivated by somatic mutations and 3p21.1 losses in malignant pleural mesothelioma. *Nat Genet.* 2011;43(7):668–72.
6. Testa JR, Cheung M, Pei J, Below JE, Tan Y, Sementino E, et al. Germline BAP1 mutations predispose to malignant mesothelioma. *Nat Genet.* 2011;43(10):1022–5.
7. Bononi A, Goto KG, Yoshikawa Y, Emi M, Pastorino S, et al. Heterozygous germline BLM mutations increase susceptibility to asbestos and mesothelioma. *Proc Natl Acad Sci U S A.* 2020;117(52):33466–73.
8. Carbone M, Ferris LK, Baumann F, Napolitano A, Lum CA, Flores EG, et al. BAP1 cancer syndrome: Malignant mesothelioma, uveal and cutaneous melanoma, and MBAITs. *J Transl Med.* 2012;10:179.
9. Carbone M, Harbour JW, Brugarolas J, Bononi A, Pagano I, Dey A, et al. Biological mechanisms and clinical significance of BAP1 mutations in human cancer. *Cancer Discov.* 2020;10(8):1103–20.
10. Alpert N, van Gerwen M, Taioli E. Epidemiology of mesothelioma in the 21(st) century in Europe and the United States, 40 years after restricted/banned asbestos use. *Transl Lung Cancer Res.* 2020;9(Supplement 1):S28–s38.
11. Chen T, Sun XM, Wu L. High time for complete ban on asbestos use in developing countries. *JAMA Oncol.* 2019;5(6):779–80.
12. Chimed-Ochir O, Rath EM, Kubo T, Yumiya Y, Lin RT, Furuya S, et al. Must countries shoulder the burden of mesothelioma to ban asbestos? A global assessment. *BMJ Glob Health.* 2022;7(12).
13. Bou-Samra P, Chang A, Azari F, Kennedy G, Segil A, Guo E, et al. Epidemiological, therapeutic, and survival trends in malignant pleural mesothelioma: A review of the national cancer database. *Cancer Med.* 2023;12(11):12208–20.
14. Zhu W, Liu J, Li Y, Shi Z, Wei S. Global, regional, and national trends in mesothelioma burden from 1990 to 2019 and the predictions for the next two decades. *SSM Popul Health.* 2023;23:101441.
15. Popat S, Baas P, Faivre-Finn C, Girard N, Nicholson AG, Nowak AK, et al. Malignant pleural mesothelioma: ESMO Clinical Practice Guidelines for diagnosis, treatment and follow-up(☆). *Ann Oncol.* 2022;33(2):129–42.
16. Opitz I, Bille A, Dafni U, Nackaerts K, Ampollini L, de Perrot M, et al. European epidemiology of pleural mesothelioma-real-life data from a joint analysis of the Mesoscape database of the European thoracic oncology platform and the European society of thoracic surgery mesothelioma database. *J Thorac Oncol.* 2023;18(9):1233–47.
17. Taioli E, Wolf A, Alpert N, Rosenthal D, Flores R. Malignant pleural mesothelioma characteristics and outcomes: A SEER-Medicare analysis. *J Surg Oncol.* 2023;128(1):134–41.
18. Taioli E, Wolf AS, Camacho-Rivera M, Kaufman A, Lee DS, Nicastri D, et al. Determinants of survival in malignant pleural mesothelioma: A surveillance, epidemiology, and end results (SEER) study of 14,228 patients. *PLoS One.* 2015;10(12):e0145039.
19. Wolf AS, Rosenthal A, Giroux DJ, Nowak AK, Bille A, de Perrot M, et al. The international association for the study of lung cancer pleural mesothelioma staging project: Updated modeling of prognostic factors in pleural mesothelioma. *J Thorac Oncol.* 2023.
20. Bölükbas S, Eberlein M, Kudelin N, Demes M, Stallmann S, Fisseler-Eckhoff A, et al. Factors predicting poor survival after lung-sparing radical pleurectomy of IMIG stage III malignant pleural mesothelioma. *Eur J Cardio Thorac Surg.* 2013;44(1):119–23.
21. Bueno R, Opitz I. Surgery in malignant pleural mesothelioma. *J Thorac Oncol.* 2018;13(11):1638–54.
22. Kindler HL, Ismaila N, Armato SG 3rd, Bueno R, Hesdorffer M, Jahan T, et al. Treatment of malignant pleural mesothelioma: American Society of Clinical Oncology clinical practice guideline. *J Clin Oncol.* 2018;36(13):1343–73.
23. Nowak AK, Jackson A, Sidhu C. Management of advanced pleural mesothelioma-at the crossroads. *JCO Oncol Pract.* 2022;18(2):116–24.
24. Rottenberg S, Disler C, Perego P. The rediscovery of platinum-based cancer therapy. *Nat Rev Cancer.* 2021;21(1):37–50.
25. Malakoti F, Targhazeh N, Abadifard E, Zarezadeh R, Samemaleki S, Asemi Z, et al. DNA repair and damage pathways in mesothelioma development and therapy. *Cancer Cell Int.* 2022;22(1):176.
26. van Meerbeeck JP, Gaafar R, Manegold C, Van Klaveren RJ, Van Marck EA, Vincent M, et al. Randomized phase III study of cisplatin with or without raltitrexed in patients with malignant pleural mesothelioma: An intergroup study of the European organisation for research and treatment of cancer lung cancer group and the national cancer institute of Canada. *J Clin Oncol.* 2005;23(28):6881–9.
27. Vogelzang NJ, Rusthoven JJ, Symanowski J, Denham C, Kaukel E, Ruffie P, et al. Phase III study of pemetrexed in combination with cisplatin versus cisplatin alone in patients with malignant pleural mesothelioma. *J Clin Oncol.* 2003;21(14):2636–44.

28. Vogelzang NJ, Rusthoven JJ, Symanowski J, Denham C, Kaukel E, Ruffie P, et al. Phase III study of pemetrexed in combination with cisplatin versus cisplatin alone in patients with malignant pleural mesothelioma. *J Clin Oncol.* 2023;41(12):2125–33.
29. Board PDQATE. *Malignant Mesothelioma Treatment (PDQ®): Health Professional Version. PDQ Cancer Information Summaries.* Bethesda, MD: National Cancer Institute, 2023. Available from: https://wwwncbinlmnihgov/books/NBK65983/.
30. Ettinger DS, Wood DE, Akerley W, Bazhenova LA, Borghaei H, Camidge DR, et al. NCCN guidelines insights: Malignant pleural mesothelioma, version 3.2016. *J Natl Compr Canc Netw.* 2016;14(7):825–36.
31. Nadal E, Bosch-Barrera J, Cedrés S, Coves J, García-Campelo R, Guirado M, et al. SEOM clinical guidelines for the treatment of malignant pleural mesothelioma (2020). *Clin Transl Oncol.* 2021;23(5):980–7.
32. Tsao AS, Lindwasser OW, Adjei AA, Adusumilli PS, Beyers ML, Blumenthal GM, et al. Current and future management of malignant mesothelioma: A consensus report from the National Cancer Institute thoracic malignancy steering committee, international association for the study of lung cancer, and mesothelioma applied research foundation. *J Thorac Oncol.* 2018;13(11):1655–67.
33. Wang Q, Xu C, Wang W, Zhang Y, Li Z, Song Z, et al. Chinese expert consensus on the diagnosis and treatment of malignant pleural mesothelioma. *Thorac Cancer.* 2023;14(26):2715–31.
34. Strizzi L, Catalano A, Vianale G, Orecchia S, Casalini A, Tassi G, et al. Vascular endothelial growth factor is an autocrine growth factor in human malignant mesothelioma. *J Pathol.* 2001;193(4):468–75.
35. Zalcman G, Mazieres J, Margery J, Greillier L, Audigier-Valette C, Moro-Sibilot D, et al. Bevacizumab for newly diagnosed pleural mesothelioma in the mesothelioma Avastin cisplatin pemetrexed Study (MAPS): A randomised, controlled, open-label, phase 3 trial. *Lancet.* 2016;387(10026):1405–14.
36. Tsao AS, Miao J, Wistuba II, Vogelzang NJ, Heymach JV, Fossella FV, et al. Phase II trial of Cediranib in combination with cisplatin and pemetrexed in chemotherapy-naïve patients with unresectable malignant pleural mesothelioma (SWOG S0905). *J Clin Oncol.* 2019;37(28):2537–47.
37. Borea F, Franczak MA, Garcia M, Perrino M, Cordua N, Smolenski RT, et al. Target therapy in malignant pleural mesothelioma: Hope or mirage? *Int J Mol Sci.* 2023;24(11).
38. Sørensen JB, Frank H, Palshof T. Cisplatin and vinorelbine first-line chemotherapy in non-resectable malignant pleural mesothelioma. *Br J Cancer.* 2008;99(1):44–50.
39. Zauderer MG, Kass SL, Woo K, Sima CS, Ginsberg MS, Krug LM. Vinorelbine and gemcitabine as second- or third-line therapy for malignant pleural mesothelioma. *Lung Cancer.* 2014;84(3):271–4.
40. Zucali PA, Perrino M, Lorenzi E, Ceresoli GL, De Vincenzo F, Simonelli M, et al. Vinorelbine in pemetrexed-pretreated patients with malignant pleural mesothelioma. *Lung Cancer.* 2014;84(3):265–70.
41. Toyokawa G, Takenoyama M, Hirai F, Toyozawa R, Inamasu E, Kojo M, et al. Gemcitabine and vinorelbine as second-line or beyond treatment in patients with malignant pleural mesothelioma pretreated with platinum plus pemetrexed chemotherapy. *Int J Clin Oncol.* 2014;19(4):601–6.
42. Banyal A, Tiwari S, Sharma A, Chanana I, Patel SKS, Kulshrestha S, et al. Vinca alkaloids as a potential cancer therapeutics: Recent update and future challenges. *3 Biotech.* 2023;13(6):211.
43. Ceresoli GL, Zucali PA. Vinca alkaloids in the therapeutic management of malignant pleural mesothelioma. *Cancer Treat Rev.* 2015;41(10):853–8.
44. Fennell DA, Porter C, Lester J, Danson S, Taylor P, Sheaff M, et al. Active symptom control with or without oral vinorelbine in patients with relapsed malignant pleural mesothelioma (VIM): A randomised, phase 2 trial. *EClinicalmedicine.* 2022;48:101432.
45. Kindler HL, Novello S, Bearz A, Ceresoli GL, Aerts J, Spicer J, et al. Anetumab ravtansine versus vinorelbine in patients with relapsed, mesothelin-positive malignant pleural mesothelioma (ARCS-M): A randomised, open-label phase 2 trial. *Lancet Oncol.* 2022;23(4):540–52.
46. Popat S, Curioni-Fontecedro A, Dafni U, Shah R, O'Brien M, Pope A, et al. A multicentre randomised phase III trial comparing pembrolizumab versus single-agent chemotherapy for advanced pre-treated malignant pleural mesothelioma: The European Thoracic Oncology Platform (ETOP 9–15) PROMISE-meso trial. *Ann Oncol.* 2020;31(12):1734–45.
47. Kim RY, Li Y, Marmarelis ME, Vachani A. Comparative effectiveness of second-line immune checkpoint inhibitor therapy versus chemotherapy for malignant pleural mesothelioma. *Lung Cancer.* 2021;159:107–10.
48. Cazzaniga ME, Cordani N, Capici S, Cogliati V, Riva F, Cerrito MG. Metronomic chemotherapy. *Cancers (Basel).* 2021;13(9).
49. André N, Tsai K, Carré M, Pasquier E. Metronomic Chemotherapy: Direct Targeting of Cancer Cells after all? *Trends Cancer.* 2017;3(5):319–25.
50. Barlesi F, Imbs DC, Tomasini P, Greillier L, Galloux M, Testot-Ferry A, et al. Mathematical modeling for Phase I cancer trials: A study of metronomic vinorelbine for advanced non-small cell lung cancer (NSCLC) and mesothelioma patients. *Oncotarget.* 2017;8(29):47161–6.

51. Elharrar X, Barbolosi D, Ciccolini J, Meille C, Faivre C, Lacarelle B, et al. A phase Ia/Ib clinical trial of metronomic chemotherapy based on a mathematical model of oral vinorelbine in metastatic non-small cell lung cancer and malignant pleural mesothelioma: Rationale and study protocol. *BMC Cancer.* 2016;16:278.
52. Barlesi F, Deyme L, Imbs DC, Cousin E, Barbolosi M, Bonnet S, et al. Revisiting metronomic vinorelbine with mathematical modelling: A Phase I trial in lung cancer. *Cancer Chemother Pharmacol.* 2022;90(2):149–60.
53. Vicier C, Isambert N, Cropet C, Hamimed M, Osanno L, Legrand F, et al. Movie: A phase I, open-label, multicenter study to evaluate the safety and tolerability of metronomic vinorelbine combined with durvalumab plus tremelimumab in patients with advanced solid tumors. *ESMO Open.* 2022;7(6):100646.
54. Muraro E, Vinante L, Fratta E, Bearz A, Höfler D, Steffan A, et al. Metronomic chemotherapy: Antitumor pathways and combination with immune checkpoint inhibitors. *Cancers (Basel).* 2023;15(9).
55. Terra S, Mansfield AS, Dong H, Peikert T, Roden AC. Temporal and spatial heterogeneity of programmed cell death 1-Ligand 1 expression in malignant mesothelioma. *Oncoimmunology.* 2017;6(11):e1356146.
56. Principe N, Aston WJ, Hope DE, Tilsed CM, Fisher SA, Boon L, et al. Comprehensive testing of chemotherapy and immune checkpoint blockade in preclinical cancer models identifies additive combinations. *Front Immunol.* 2022;13:872295.
57. Borrelli EP, McGladrigan CG. A review of pharmacologic management in the treatment of mesothelioma. *Curr Treat Options Oncol.* 2021;22(2):14.
58. Yang L, Cao X, Li N, Zheng B, Liu M, Cai H. Cost-effectiveness analysis of nivolumab plus ipilimumab versus chemotherapy as the first-line treatment for unresectable malignant pleural mesothelioma. *Ther Adv Med Oncol.* 2022;14:17588359221116604.
59. Ye ZM, Tang ZQ, Xu Z, Zhou Q, Li H. Cost-effectiveness of nivolumab plus ipilimumab as first-line treatment for American patients with unresectable malignant pleural mesothelioma. *Front Public Health.* 2022;10:947375.
60. Michaeli T, Jürges H, Michaeli DT. FDA approval, clinical trial evidence, efficacy, epidemiology, and price for non-orphan and ultra-rare, rare, and common orphan cancer drug indications: Cross sectional analysis. *BMJ.* 2023;381:e073242.
61. Michaeli DT, Michaeli T. Overall survival, progression-free survival, and tumor response benefit supporting initial US food and drug administration approval and indication extension of new cancer drugs, 2003–2021. *J Clin Oncol.* 2022;40(35):4095–106.
62. Saracino L, Bortolotto C, Tomaselli S, Fraolini E, Bosio M, Accordino G, et al. Integrating data from multidisciplinary management of malignant pleural mesothelioma: A cohort study. *BMC Cancer.* 2021;21(1):762.
63. Mujoomdar AA, Tilleman TR, Richards WG, Bueno R, Sugarbaker DJ. Prevalence of in vitro chemotherapeutic drug resistance in primary malignant pleural mesothelioma: result in a cohort of 203 resection specimens. *J Thorac Cardiovasc Surg.* 2010;140(2):352–55.
64. Zimling ZG, Sørensen JB, Gerds TA, Bech C, Andersen CB, Santoni-Rugiu E. A biomarker profile for predicting efficacy of cisplatin-vinorelbine therapy in malignant pleural mesothelioma. *Cancer Chemother Pharmacol.* 2012;70(5):743–54.
65. Zimling ZG, Sørensen JB, Gerds TA, Bech C, Andersen CB, Santoni-Rugiu E. Low ERCC1 expression in malignant pleural mesotheliomas treated with cisplatin and vinorelbine predicts prolonged progression-free survival. *J Thorac Oncol.* 2012;7(1):249–56.
66. Jordheim LP, Sève P, Trédan O, Dumontet C. The ribonucleotide reductase large subunit (RRM1) as a predictive factor in patients with cancer. *Lancet Oncol.* 2011;12(7):693–702.
67. Vilmar AC, Santoni-Rugiu E, Sorensen JB. Predictive impact of RRM1 protein expression on vinorelbine efficacy in NSCLC patients randomly assigned in a chemotherapy phase III trial. *Ann Oncol.* 2013;24(2):309–14.
68. Zimling ZG, Santoni-Rugiu E, Bech C, Sørensen JB. High RRM1 expression is associated with adverse outcome in patients with cisplatin/vinorelbine-treated malignant pleural mesothelioma. *Anticancer Res.* 2015;35(12):6731–8.
69. Busacca S, Sheaff M, Arthur K, Gray SG, O'Byrne KJ, Richard DJ, et al. BRCA1 is an essential mediator of vinorelbine-induced apoptosis in mesothelioma. *J Pathol.* 2012;227(2):200–8.
70. He Q, Zhang M, Zhang J, Zhong S, Liu Y, Shen J, et al. Predictive value of BRCA1 expression on the efficacy of chemotherapy based on anti-microtubule agents: A pooled analysis across different malignancies and agents. *Ann Transl Med.* 2016;4(6):110.
71. Busacca S, O'Regan L, Singh A, Sharkey AJ, Dawson AG, Dzialo J, et al. BRCA1/MAD2L1 deficiency disrupts the spindle assembly checkpoint to confer vinorelbine resistance in mesothelioma. *Mol Cancer Ther.* 2021;20(2):379–88.

72. Kumar N, Alrifai D, Kolluri KK, Sage EK, Ishii Y, Guppy N, et al. Retrospective response analysis of BAP1 expression to predict the clinical activity of systemic cytotoxic chemotherapy in mesothelioma. *Lung Cancer.* 2019;127:164–6.
73. Okonska A, Bühler S, Rao V, Ronner M, Blijlevens M, van der Meulen-Muileman IH, et al. Functional genomic screen in mesothelioma reveals that loss of function of BRCA1-associated protein 1 induces chemoresistance to ribonucleotide reductase inhibition. *Mol Cancer Ther.* 2020;19(2):552–63.
74. Williams M, Cheng YY, Phimmachanh M, Winata P, van Zandwijk N, Reid G. Tumour suppressor microRNAs contribute to drug resistance in malignant pleural mesothelioma by targeting anti-apoptotic pathways. *Cancer Drug Resist.* 2019;2(4):1193–206.
75. Zhu JY, Pfuhl T, Motsch N, Barth S, Nicholls J, Grässer F, et al. Identification of novel Epstein-Barr virus microRNA genes from nasopharyngeal carcinomas. *J Virol.* 2009;83(7):3333–41.
76. Barbier MC, Fengler A, Pardo E, Bhadhuri A, Meier N, Gautschi O. Cost effectiveness and budget impact of nivolumab plus ipilimumab versus platinum plus pemetrexed (with and Without bevacizumab) in patients with unresectable malignant pleural mesothelioma in Switzerland. *Pharmacoeconomics.* 2023.
77. Zhan M, Zheng H, Xu T, Yang Y, Li Q. Cost-effectiveness analysis of additional bevacizumab to pemetrexed plus cisplatin for malignant pleural mesothelioma based on the MAPS trial. *Lung Cancer.* 2017;110:1–6.
78. Loganathan S, Kanteti R, Siddiqui SS, El-Hashani E, Tretiakova M, Vigneswaran H, et al. Role of protein kinase C β and vascular endothelial growth factor receptor in malignant pleural mesothelioma: Therapeutic implications and the usefulness of Caenorhabditis elegans model organism. *J Carcinog.* 2011;10:4.
79. Miettinen M, Rikala MS, Rys J, Lasota J, Wang ZF. Vascular endothelial growth factor receptor 2 as a marker for malignant vascular tumors and mesothelioma: An immunohistochemical study of 262 vascular endothelial and 1640 nonvascular tumors. *Am J Surg Pathol.* 2012;36(4):629–39.
80. Wozniak AJ, Schneider B, Kalemkerian GP, Daly B, Chen W, Ventimiglia J, et al. Short report of a Phase II trial of nintedanib in recurrent malignant pleural mesothelioma (MPM). *Clin Lung Cancer.* 2023;24(6):563–7.
81. Scagliotti GV, Gaafar R, Nowak AK, Nakano T, van Meerbeeck J, Popat S, et al. Nintedanib in combination with pemetrexed and cisplatin for chemotherapy-naive patients with advanced malignant pleural mesothelioma (LUME-Meso): A double-blind, randomised, placebo-controlled phase 3 trial. *Lancet Respir Med.* 2019;7(7):569–80.
82. Pinto C, Zucali PA, Pagano M, Grosso F, Pasello G, Garassino MC, et al. Gemcitabine with or without ramucirumab as second-line treatment for malignant pleural mesothelioma (RAMES): A randomised, double-blind, placebo-controlled, phase 2 trial. *Lancet Oncol.* 2021;22(10):1438–47.
83. Porta C, Nardone V, Gray SG, Correale P, Mutti L. RAMES study: Is there really a role for VEGF inhibition in mesothelioma? *Lancet Oncol.* 2021;22(12):e532.
84. Arrieta O, Muñoz-Montaño W, Muñiz-Hernández S, Campos S, Catalán R, Soto-Molina H, et al. Efficacy, safety, and cost-minimization analysis of continuous infusion of low-dose gemcitabine plus cisplatin in patients with unresectable malignant pleural mesothelioma. *Front Oncol.* 2021;11:641975.
85. de Gooijer CJ, van der Noort V, Stigt JA, Baas P, Biesma B, Cornelissen R, et al. Switch-maintenance gemcitabine after first-line chemotherapy in patients with malignant mesothelioma (NVALT19): An investigator-initiated, randomised, open-label, phase 2 trial. *Lancet Respir Med.* 2021;9(6):585–92.
86. Chu YD, Lai MW, Yeh CT. Unlocking the potential of arginine deprivation therapy: Recent breakthroughs and promising future for cancer treatment. *Int J Mol Sci.* 2023;24(13).
87. Field GC, Pavlyk I, Szlosarek PW. Bench-to-bedside studies of arginine deprivation in cancer. *Molecules.* 2023;28(5).
88. Szlosarek PW, Klabatsa A, Pallaska A, Sheaff M, Smith P, Crook T, et al. In vivo loss of expression of argininosuccinate synthetase in malignant pleural mesothelioma is a biomarker for susceptibility to arginine depletion. *Clin Cancer Res.* 2006;12(23):7126–31.
89. Szlosarek PW, Steele JP, Nolan L, Gilligan D, Taylor P, Spicer J, et al. Arginine deprivation with pegylated arginine deiminase in patients with argininosuccinate synthetase 1-deficient malignant pleural mesothelioma: A randomized clinical trial. *JAMA Oncol.* 2017;3(1):58–66.
90. Beddowes E, Spicer J, Chan PY, Khadeir R, Corbacho JG, Repana D, et al. Phase 1 dose-escalation study of pegylated arginine deiminase, cisplatin, and pemetrexed in patients with argininosuccinate synthetase 1-deficient thoracic cancers. *J Clin Oncol.* 2017;35(16):1778–85.
91. Szlosarek PW, Phillips MM, Pavlyk I, Steele J, Shamash J, Spicer J *et al.*, Expansion phase 1 study of pegargiminase plus pemetrexed and cisplatin in patients with argininosuccinate synthetase 1-deficient mesothelioma: Safety, efficacy, and resistance mechanisms. *JTO Clin Res Rep.* 2020;1(4):100093.

92. Szlosarek PW, Creelan B, Sarkodie T, Nolan L, Taylor P, Olevsky O, et al. Abstract CT007: Phase 2–3 trial of pegargiminase plus chemotherapy versus placebo plus chemotherapy in patients with non-epithelioid pleural mesothelioma. *Cancer Res.* 2023;83(8):CT007-CT.
93. Herzog TJ, Vergote I, Gomella LG, Milenkova T, French T, Tonikian R, et al. Testing for homologous recombination repair or homologous recombination deficiency for poly (ADP-ribose) polymerase inhibitors: A current perspective. *Eur J Cancer.* 2023;179:136–46.
94. Guo M, Wang SM, The BRC. Aness landscape of cancer. *Cells.* 2022;11(23).
95. Fuso Nerini I, Roca E, Mannarino L, Grosso F, Frapolli R, D'Incalci M. Is DNA repair a potential target for effective therapies against malignant mesothelioma? *Cancer Treat Rev.* 2020;90:102101.
96. Rathkey D, Khanal M, Murai J, Zhang J, Sengupta M, Jiang Q, et al. Sensitivity of mesothelioma cells to PARP inhibitors is not dependent on BAP1 but is enhanced by temozolomide in cells with high-schlafen 11 and low-O6-methylguanine-DNA methyltransferase expression. *J Thorac Oncol.* 2020;15(5):843–59.
97. Parrotta R, Okonska A, Ronner M, Weder W, Stahel R, Penengo L, et al. A novel BRCA1-associated Protein-1 isoform affects response of mesothelioma cells to drugs impairing BRCA1-mediated DNA repair. *J Thorac Oncol.* 2017;12(8):1309–19.
98. Dudnik E, Bar J, Moore A, Gottfried T, Moskovitz M, Dudnik J, et al. BAP1-altered malignant pleural mesothelioma: Outcomes with chemotherapy, immune check-point inhibitors and poly(ADP-ribose) polymerase inhibitors. *Front Oncol.* 2021;11:603223.
99. Fennell DA, King A, Mohammed S, Branson A, Brookes C, Darlison L, et al. Rucaparib in patients with BAP1-deficient or BRCA1-deficient mesothelioma (MiST1): An open-label, single-arm, phase 2a clinical trial. *Lancet Respir Med.* 2021;9(6):593–600.
100. Ghafoor A, Mian I, Wagner C, Mallory Y, Agra MG, Morrow B, et al. Phase 2 study of olaparib in malignant mesothelioma and correlation of efficacy with germline or somatic mutations in BAP1 gene. *JTO Clin Res Rep.* 2021;2(10):100231.
101. Passiglia F, Bironzo P, Righi L, Listì A, Arizio F, Novello S, et al. A prospective phase II single-arm study of Niraparib plus Dostarlimab in patients with advanced non-small-cell lung cancer and/or malignant pleural mesothelioma, Positive for PD-L1 expression and germline or somatic mutations in the DNA repair genes: Rationale and study design. *Clin Lung Cancer.* 2021;22(1):e63–e66.
102. Hmeljak J, Sanchez-Vega F, Hoadley KA, Shih J, Stewart C, Heiman D, et al. Integrative molecular characterization of malignant pleural mesothelioma. *Cancer Discov.* 2018;8(12):1548–65.
103. Laure A, Rigutto A, Kirschner MB, Opitz L, Grob L, Opitz I, et al. Genomic and transcriptomic analyses of malignant pleural mesothelioma (MPM) samples reveal crucial insights for preclinical testing. *Cancers (Basel).* 2023;15(10).
104. Chen-Yost HI, Tjota MY, Gao G, Mitchell O, Kindler H, Segal J, et al. Characterizing the distribution of alterations in mesothelioma and their correlation to morphology. *Am J Clin Pathol.* 2023;160(3):238–46.
105. Belcaid L, Bertelsen B, Wadt K, Tuxen I, Spanggaard I, Højgaard M, et al. New pathogenic germline variants identified in mesothelioma. *Lung Cancer.* 2023;179:107172.
106. Wong L, Zhou J, Anderson D, Kratzke RA. Inactivation of p16INK4a expression in malignant mesothelioma by methylation. *Lung Cancer.* 2002;38(2):131–6.
107. Aliagas E, Alay A, Martínez-Iniesta M, Hernández-Madrigal M, Cordero D, Gausachs M, et al. Efficacy of CDK4/6 inhibitors in preclinical models of malignant pleural mesothelioma. *Br J Cancer.* 2021;125(10):1365–76.
108. Terenziani R, Galetti M, La Monica S, Fumarola C, Zoppi S, Alfieri R, et al. CDK4/6 inhibition enhances the efficacy of standard chemotherapy treatment in malignant pleural mesothelioma cells. *Cancers (Basel).* 2022;14(23):5925.
109. Paternot S, Raspé E, Meiller C, Tarabichi M, Assié JB, Libert F, et al. Preclinical evaluation of CDK4 phosphorylation predicts high sensitivity of pleural mesotheliomas to CDK4/6 inhibition. *Mol Oncol.* 2024;18(4):866–894.
110. Fennell DA, King A, Mohammed S, Greystoke A, Anthony S, Poile C, et al. Abemaciclib in patients with p16ink4A-deficient mesothelioma (MiST2): A single-arm, open-label, phase 2 trial. *Lancet Oncol.* 2022;23(3):374–81.
111. Nardone V, Porta C, Giannicola R, Correale P, Mutti L. Abemaciclib for malignant pleural mesothelioma. *Lancet Oncol.* 2022;23(6):e237.
112. Kemp CD, Rao M, Xi S, Inchauste S, Mani H, Fetsch P, et al. Polycomb repressor complex-2 is a novel target for mesothelioma therapy. *Clin Cancer Res.* 2012;18(1):77–90.
113. LaFave LM, Béguelin W, Koche R, Teater M, Spitzer B, Chramiec A, et al. Loss of BAP1 function leads to EZH2-dependent transformation. *Nat Med.* 2015;21(11):1344–9.

114. Shinozaki-Ushiku A, Ushiku T, Morita S, Anraku M, Nakajima J, Fukayama M. Diagnostic utility of BAP1 and EZH2 expression in malignant mesothelioma. *Histopathology.* 2017;70(5):722–33.
115. Zauderer MG, Szlosarek PW, Le Moulec S, Popat S, Taylor P, Planchard D, et al. EZH2 inhibitor tazemetostat in patients with relapsed or refractory, BAP1-inactivated malignant pleural mesothelioma: A multicentre, open-label, phase 2 study. *Lancet Oncol.* 2022;23(6):758–67.
116. Pinton G, Wang Z, Balzano C, Missaglia S, Tavian D, Boldorini R, et al. CDKN2A determines mesothelioma cell fate to EZH2 inhibition. *Front Oncol.* 2021;11:678447.
117. Kukuyan AM, Sementino E, Kadariya Y, Menges CW, Cheung M, Tan Y, et al. Inactivation of Bapl cooperates with losses of Nf2 and Cdkn2a to drive the development of pleural malignant mesothelioma in conditional mouse models. *Cancer Res.* 2019;79(16):4113–23.
118. Badhai J, Pandey GK, Song JY, Krijgsman O, Bhaskaran R, Chandrasekaran G, et al. Combined deletion of Bap1, Nf2, and Cdkn2ab causes rapid onset of malignant mesothelioma in mice. *J Exp Med.* 2020;217(6).
119. Fan K, Zhang CL, Zhang BH, Gao MQ, Sun YC. Analysis of the correlation between Zeste enhancer homolog 2 (EZH2) mRNA expression and the prognosis of mesothelioma patients and immune infiltration. *Sci Rep.* 2022;12(1):16583.
120. Hamaidia M, Gazon H, Hoyos C, Hoffmann GB, Louis R, Duysinx B, et al. Inhibition of EZH2 methyltransferase decreases immunoediting of mesothelioma cells by autologous macrophages through a PD-1-dependent mechanism. *JCI Insight.* 2019;4(18):e128474.
121. Mola S, Pinton G, Erreni M, Corazzari M, De Andrea M, Grolla AA, et al. Inhibition of the histone methyltransferase EZH2 enhances protumor monocyte recruitment in human mesothelioma spheroids. *Int J Mol Sci.* 2021;22(9): 4391.
122. Gray SG. Emerging avenues in immunotherapy for the management of malignant pleural mesothelioma. *BMC Pulm Med.* 2021;21(1):148.
123. Gray SG, Mutti L. Immunotherapy for mesothelioma: A critical review of current clinical trials and future perspectives. *Transl Lung Cancer Res.* 2020;9(Supplement 1):S100–s19.
124. Baas P, Scherpereel A, Nowak AK, Fujimoto N, Peters S, Tsao AS, et al. First-line nivolumab plus ipilimumab in unresectable malignant pleural mesothelioma (CheckMate 743): A multicentre, randomised, open-label, phase 3 trial. *Lancet.* 2021;397(10272):375–86.
125. Peters S, Scherpereel A, Cornelissen R, Oulkhouir Y, Greillier L, Kaplan MA, et al. First-line nivolumab plus ipilimumab versus chemotherapy in patients with unresectable malignant pleural mesothelioma: 3-year outcomes from CheckMate 743. *Ann Oncol.* 2022;33(5):488–99.
126. Nakajima EC, Vellanki PJ, Larkins E, Chatterjee S, Mishra-Kalyani PS, Bi Y, et al. FDA approval summary: Nivolumab in combination with ipilimumab for the treatment of unresectable malignant pleural mesothelioma. *Clin Cancer Res.* 2022;28(3):446–51.
127. Bristol Myers Squibb receives European commission approval for Opdivo (Nivolumab) plus Yervoy (Ipilimumab) as first-line treatment for unresectable malignant pleural mesothelioma. *News Release.* June 2, 2021. https://bit.ly/3fIXyw7. Accessed October 5, 2023. Press release;2021.
128. Adler AI, Slayen S, Stegenga H, Guo Y, Diaz R, Welton NJ, et al. NICE guidance on nivolumab plus ipilimumab for untreated, unresectable malignant pleural mesothelioma. *Lancet Respir Med.* 2022;10(10):e92–e93.
129. Govindan R, Aggarwal C, Antonia SJ, Davies M, Dubinett SM, Ferris A, et al. Society for Immunotherapy of Cancer (SITC) clinical practice guideline on immunotherapy for the treatment of lung cancer and mesothelioma. *J Immunother Cancer.* 2022; 10(5):e003956.
130. Fennell DA, Ewings S, Ottensmeier C, Califano R, Hanna GG, Hill K, et al. Nivolumab versus placebo in patients with relapsed malignant mesothelioma (CONFIRM): A multicentre, double-blind, randomised, phase 3 trial. *Lancet Oncol.* 2021;22(11):1530–40.
131. Fujimoto N, Okada M, Kijima T, Aoe K, Kato T, Nakagawa K, et al. Clinical efficacy and safety of nivolumab in Japanese patients with malignant pleural mesothelioma: 3-year results of the MERIT study. *JTO Clin Res Rep.* 2021;2(3):100135.
132. Cantini L, Belderbos RA, Gooijer CJ, Dumoulin DW, Cornelissen R, Baart S, et al. Nivolumab in pretreated malignant pleural mesothelioma: Real-world data from the Dutch expanded access program. *Transl Lung Cancer Res.* 2020;9(4):1169–79.
133. Assié JB, Crépin F, Grolleau E, Canellas A, Geier M, Grébert-Manuardi A, et al. Immune-checkpoint inhibitors for malignant pleural mesothelioma: A French, multicenter, retrospective real-world study. *Cancers (Basel).* 2022;14(6):1498.
134. Metaxas Y, Rivalland G, Mauti LA, Klingbiel D, Kao S, Schmid S, et al. Pembrolizumab as palliative immunotherapy in malignant pleural mesothelioma. *J Thorac Oncol.* 2018;13(11):1784–91.

135. Ahmadzada T, Cooper WA, Holmes M, Mahar A, Westman H, Gill AJ, et al. Retrospective evaluation of the use of pembrolizumab in malignant mesothelioma in a real-world Australian population. *JTO Clin Res Rep.* 2020;1(4):100075.
136. Guo X, Lin L, Zhu J. Immunotherapy vs. chemotherapy in subsequent treatment of malignant pleural mesothelioma: Which is better? *J Clin Med.* 2023;12(7):2531.
137. Canova S, Ceresoli GL, Grosso F, Zucali PA, Gelsomino F, Pasello G, et al. Final results of DIADEM, a phase II study to investigate the efficacy and safety of durvalumab in advanced pretreated malignant pleural mesothelioma. *ESMO Open.* 2022;7(6):100644.
138. Hassan R, Thomas A, Nemunaitis JJ, Patel MR, Bennouna J, Chen FL, et al. Efficacy and safety of Avelumab treatment in patients with advanced unresectable mesothelioma: Phase 1b results from the JAVELIN solid tumor trial. *JAMA Oncol.* 2019;5(3):351–7.
139. Forde PM, Anagnostou V, Sun Z, Dahlberg SE, Kindler HL, Niknafs N, et al. Durvalumab with platinum-pemetrexed for unresectable pleural mesothelioma: Survival, genomic and immunologic analyses from the phase 2 PrE0505 trial. *Nat Med.* 2021;27(11):1910–20.
140. Nowak AK, Lesterhuis WJ, Kok PS, Brown C, Hughes BG, Karikios DJ, et al. Durvalumab with first-line chemotherapy in previously untreated malignant pleural mesothelioma (DREAM): A multicentre, single-arm, phase 2 trial with a safety run-in. *Lancet Oncol.* 2020;21(9):1213–23.
141. Kok PS, Forde PM, Hughes B, Sun Z, Brown C, Ramalingam S, et al. Protocol of DREAM3R: DuRvalumab with chEmotherapy as first-line treAtment in advanced pleural mesothelioma-a phase 3 randomised trial. *BMJ, (Open)* 2022;12(1):e057663.
142. Chu QS, Piccirillo MC, Greillier L, Grosso F, Russo GL, Florescu M, et al. IND227 phase III (P3) study of cisplatin/pemetrexed (CP) with or without pembrolizumab (pembro) in patients (pts) with malignant pleural mesothelioma (PM): A CCTG, NCIN, and IFCT trial. *Journal of Clinical Oncology.* 2023;41(17_suppl):LBA8505-LBA.
143. Tagliamento M, Di Maio M, Remon J, Bironzo P, Genova C, Facchinetti F, et al. Meta-analysis on the combination of chemotherapy with programmed death-ligand 1 and programmed cell death Protein 1 blockade as first-line treatment for unresectable pleural mesothelioma. *J Thorac Oncol.* 2024;19(1):166–172.
144. Weder W, Stahel RA, Bernhard J, Bodis S, Vogt P, Ballabeni P, et al. Multicenter trial of neo-adjuvant chemotherapy followed by extrapleural pneumonectomy in malignant pleural mesothelioma. *Ann Oncol.* 2007;18(7):1196–202.
145. Stahel RA, Riesterer O, Xyrafas A, Opitz I, Beyeler M, Ochsenbein A, et al. Neoadjuvant chemotherapy and extrapleural pneumonectomy of malignant pleural mesothelioma with or without hemithoracic radiotherapy (SAKK 17/04): A randomised, international, multicentre phase 2 trial. *Lancet Oncol.* 2015;16(16):1651–8.
146. Thieke C, Nicolay NH, Sterzing F, Hoffmann H, Roeder F, Safi S, et al. Long-term results in malignant pleural mesothelioma treated with neoadjuvant chemotherapy, extrapleural pneumonectomy and intensity-modulated radiotherapy. *Radiat Oncol.* 2015;10:267.
147. Verma V, Ahern CA, Berlind CG, Lindsay WD, Grover S, Friedberg JS, et al. Treatment of malignant pleural mesothelioma with chemotherapy preceding versus after surgical resection. *J Thorac Cardiovasc Surg.* 2019;157(2):758–66.e1.
148. Voigt SL, Raman V, Jawitz OK, Bishawi M, Yang CJ, Tong BC, et al. The role of neoadjuvant chemotherapy in patients with resectable malignant pleural mesothelioma-an institutional and national analysis. *J Natl Cancer Inst.* 2020;112(11):1118–27.
149. Cascone T, Leung CH, Weissferdt A, Pataer A, Carter BW, Godoy MCB, et al. Neoadjuvant chemotherapy plus nivolumab with or without ipilimumab in operable non-small cell lung cancer: The phase 2 platform NEOSTAR trial. *Nat Med.* 2023;29(3):593–604.
150. Mountzios G, Remon J, Hendriks LEL, García-Campelo R, Rolfo C, Van Schil P, et al. Immune-checkpoint inhibition for resectable non-small-cell lung cancer - Opportunities and challenges. *Nat Rev Clin Oncol.* 2023;20(10):664–77.
151. Tsao A, Qian L, Cetnar J, Sepesi B, Gomez D, Wrangle J, et al. OA13.01 S1619 A trial of neoadjuvant cisplatin-pemetrexed with atezolizumab in combination and maintenance for resectable pleural mesothelioma. *J Thorac Oncol.* 2021;16(10):S870.
152. Lee HS, Jang HJ, Ramineni M, Wang DY, Ramos D, Choi JM, et al. A phase II window of opportunity study of neoadjuvant PD-L1 versus PD-L1 plus CTLA-4 blockade for patients with malignant pleural mesothelioma. *Clin Cancer Res.* 2023;29(3):548–59.
153. Nowak AK, Chin WL, Keam S, Cook A. Immune checkpoint inhibitor therapy for malignant pleural mesothelioma. *Lung Cancer.* 2021;162:162–8.

154. Perrino M, De Vincenzo F, Cordua N, Borea F, Aliprandi M, Santoro A, et al. Immunotherapy with immune checkpoint inhibitors and predictive biomarkers in malignant mesothelioma: Work still in progress. *Front Immunol.* 2023;14:1121557.
155. Ponce S, Cedrés S, Ricordel C, Isambert N, Viteri S, Herrera-Juarez M, et al. ONCOS-102 plus pemetrexed and platinum chemotherapy in malignant pleural mesothelioma: A randomized phase 2 study investigating clinical outcomes and the tumor microenvironment. *J Immunother Cancer.* 2023;11(9):e007552.
156. Chintala NK, Choe JK, McGee E, Bellis R, Saini JK, Banerjee S, et al. Correlative analysis from a phase I clinical trial of intrapleural administration of oncolytic vaccinia virus (Olvi-vec) in patients with malignant pleural mesothelioma. *Front Immunol.* 2023;14:1112960.
157. Frampton JE. Teserpaturev/G47Δ: First approval. *BioDrugs.* 2022;36(5):667–72.
158. Ding J, Guyette S, Schrand B, Geirut J, Horton H, Guo G, et al. Mesothelin-targeting T cells bearing a novel T cell receptor fusion construct (TRuC) exhibit potent antitumor efficacy against solid tumors. *Oncoimmunology.* 2023;12(1):2182058.
159. Quach HT, Skovgard MS, Villena-Vargas J, Bellis RY, Chintala NK, Amador-Molina A, et al. Tumor-targeted nonablative radiation promotes solid tumor CAR T-cell therapy efficacy. *Cancer Immunol Res.* 2023;11(10):1314–31.
160. Ghosn M, Cheema W, Zhu A, Livschitz J, Maybody M, Boas FE, et al. Image-guided interventional radiological delivery of chimeric antigen receptor (CAR) T cells for pleural malignancies in a phase I/II clinical trial. *Lung Cancer.* 2022;165:1–9.
161. Adusumilli PS, Zauderer MG, Rivière I, Solomon SB, Rusch VW, O'Cearbhaill RE, et al. A Phase I trial of regional mesothelin-targeted CAR T-cell therapy in patients with malignant pleural disease, in combination with the anti-PD-1 agent pembrolizumab. *Cancer Discov.* 2021;11(11):2748–63.
162. Ripley RT, Mansfield AS, Sepesi B, Bueno R, Burt BM. Checkpoint blockade in unresectable pleural mesothelioma: Event horizon for multimodal therapy. *J Thorac Cardiovasc Surg.* 2023;165(1):364–8.
163. Pass HI. Commentary: A chess game for mesothelioma treatment: Not checkmate yet! *J Thorac Cardiovasc Surg.* 2023;165(1):369–70.
164. Serritella AV, Shenoy NK. Nivolumab Plus ipilimumab vs nivolumab alone in advanced cancers other than melanoma: A meta-analysis. *JAMA Oncol.* 2023.
165. Hashimoto K, Ozasa H, Yoshizawa A, Yoshida H, Ogimoto T, Hosoya K, et al. Sarcomatoid malignant pleural mesothelioma treated with nivolumab: A case series. *Oncol Lett.* 2022;24(5):402.
166. McNamee N, Harvey C, GrayL, Khoo T, Lingam L, Zhang B, Nindra U, Yip PY, Pal A, Clay T, Arulananda S, Itchins M, Pavlakis N, Kao S, Bowyer S, Chin V, Warburton L, Pires da Silva I, John T, Solomon B, Alexander M, Nagrial A. Brief report: Real-world toxicity and survival of combination immunotherapy in pleural mesothelioma-RIOMeso. *J Thorac Oncol.* 2024;19(4):636–42.
167. Gray SG, Meirson T, Mutti L. Based on the real-world results from Australia, Immunotherapy is not a good option for patients wth mesothelioma. *J Thorac Oncol.* 2024;19(4):541–6.
168. Bomze D, Asher N, Hasan Ali O, Flatz L, Azoulay D, Markel G, et al. Survival-inferred fragility index of Phase 3 clinical trials evaluating immune checkpoint inhibitors. *JAMA Netw Open.* 2020;3(10):e2017675.
169. Bomze D, Azoulay D, Meirson T. Immunotherapy with programmed cell death 1 vs programmed cell death ligand 1 inhibitors in patients with cancer. *JAMA Oncol.* 2020;6(7):1114–5.
170. Pak K, Uno H, Kim DH, Tian L, Kane RC, Takeuchi M, et al. Interpretability of cancer clinical trial results using restricted mean survival time as an alternative to the hazard ratio. *JAMA Oncol.* 2017;3(12):1692–6.
171. Meirson T, Pentimalli F, Cerza F, Baglio G, Gray SG, Correale P, et al. Comparison of 3 randomized clinical trials of frontline therapies for malignant pleural mesothelioma. *JAMA Netw Open.* 2022;5(3):e221490.
172. Meirson T, Nardone V, Pentimalli F, Markel G, Bomze D, D'Apolito M, et al. Analysis of new treatments proposed for malignant pleural mesothelioma raises concerns about the conduction of clinical trials in oncology. *J Transl Med.* 2022;20(1):593.
173. Templeton AJ, Amir E, Tannock IF. Informative censoring - A neglected cause of bias in oncology trials. *Nat Rev Clin Oncol.* 2020;17(6):327–8.
174. Gilboa S, Pras Y, Mataraso A, Bomze D, Markel G, Meirson T. Informative censoring of surrogate endpoint data in phase 3 oncology trials. *Eur J Cancer.* 2021;153:190–202.
175. Olivier T, Haslam A, Prasad V. Omission of critical information from clinical trial reports-what to do about uninterpretable results. *JAMA Oncol.* 2023;9(4):459–60.
176. Carbone M, Pass HIG, Alexander HR Jr., Baas P, Baumann F, et al. Medical and surgical care of patients with mesothelioma and their relatives carrying germline BAP1 mutations. *J Thorac Oncol.* 2022;17(7):873–89.

177. Bou-Samra P, Chang A, Zhang K, Azari F, Kennedy G, Guo E, et al. Strategies to reduce morbidity following pleurectomy and decortication for malignant pleural mesothelioma. *Thorac Cancer.* 2023;14(27):2770–6.
178. Bilancia R, Nardini M, Waller DA. Extended pleurectomy decortication: The current role. *Transl Lung Cancer Res.* 2018;7(5):556–61.
179. Paajanen J, Jaklitsch MT, Bueno R. Contemporary issues in the surgical management of pleural mesothelioma. *J Surg Oncol.* 2023;127(2):343–54.
180. Klotz LV, Hoffmann H, Shah R, Eichhorn F, Gruenewald C, Bulut EL, et al. Multimodal therapy of epithelioid pleural mesothelioma: Improved survival by changing the surgical treatment approach. *Transl Lung Cancer Res.* 2022;11(11):2230–42.
181. Kutuk T, Walker JM, Ballo MT, Cameron RB, Alvarez JB, Chawla S, et al. Multi-institutional patterns of use of tumor-treating fields for patients with malignant pleural mesothelioma. *Curr Oncol.* 2023;30(6):5195–200.
182. Anadkat MJ, Lacouture M, Friedman A, Horne ZD, Jung J, Kaffenberger B, et al. Expert guidance on prophylaxis and treatment of dermatologic adverse events with tumor treating fields (TTFields) therapy in the thoracic region. *Front Oncol.* 2022;12:975473.
183. Mannarino L, Mirimao F, Panini N, Paracchini L, Marchini S, Beltrame L, et al. Tumor treating fields affect mesothelioma cell proliferation by exerting histotype-dependent cell cycle checkpoint activations and transcriptional modulations. *Cell Death Dis.* 2022;13(7):612.
184. Kutuk T, Appel H, Avendano MC, Albrecht F, Kaywin P, Ramos S, et al. Feasibility of tumor treating fields with pemetrexed and platinum-based chemotherapy for unresectable malignant pleural mesothelioma: Single-Center, real-world data. *Cancers (Basel).* 2022;14(8).
185. Di Stefano I, Alì G, Poma AM, Bruno R, Proietti A, Niccoli C, et al. New immunohistochemical markers for pleural mesothelioma subtyping. *Diagnostics (Basel).* 2023;13(18).
186. Meiller C, Montagne F, Hirsch TZ, Caruso S, de Wolf J, Bayard Q, et al. Multi-site tumor sampling highlights molecular intra-tumor heterogeneity in malignant pleural mesothelioma. *Genome Med.* 2021;13(1):113.
187. Cioce M, Sacconi A, Pass HI, Canino C, Strano S, Blandino G, et al. Insights into intra-tumoral heterogeneity: Transcriptional profiling of chemoresistant MPM cell subpopulations reveals involvement of NFkB and DNA repair pathways and contributes a prognostic signature. *Int J Mol Sci.* 2021;22(21).
188. Mangiante L, Alcala N, Sexton-Oates A, Di Genova A, Gonzalez-Perez A, Khandekar A, et al. Multiomic analysis of malignant pleural mesothelioma identifies molecular axes and specialized tumor profiles driving intertumor heterogeneity. *Nat Genet.* 2023;55(4):607–18.
189. Ushijima T, Clark SJ, Tan P. Mapping genomic and epigenomic evolution in cancer ecosystems. *Science.* 2021;373(6562):1474–9.
190. Rondon L, Fu R, Patel MR. Success of checkpoint blockade paves the way for novel immune therapy in malignant pleural mesothelioma. *Cancers (Basel).* 2023;15(11):2940.
191. Killock D. CAR T cells show promise in mesothelioma. *Nat Rev Clin Oncol.* 2021;18(9):541.
192. Perryman L, Gray SG. Fibrosis in mesothelioma: Potential role of lysyl oxidases. *Cancers (Basel).* 2022;14(4:981.
193. De Marco M, Del Papa N, Reppucci F, Iorio V, Basile A, Falco A, et al. BAG3 induces α-SMA expression in human fibroblasts and its over-expression correlates with poorer survival in fibrotic cancer patients. *J Cell Biochem.* 2022;123(1):91–101.
194. Bononi A, Wang Q, Zolondick AA, Bai F, Steele-Tanji M, Suarez JS, et al. BAP1 is a novel regulator of HIF-1α. *Proc Natl Acad Sci U S A.* 2023;120(4):e2217840120.
195. Gul K, Zaman N, Azam SS. Roxadustat and its failure: A comparative dynamic study. *J Mol Graph Model.l* 2023;120:108422.
196. Endoh D, Ishii K, Kohno K, Virgona N, Miyakoshi Y, Yano T, et al. Chemoresistance related to hypoxia adaptation in mesothelioma cells from tumor spheroids. *Exp Oncol.* 2022;44(2):121–5.
197. Li Petri G, El Hassouni B, Sciarrillo R, Funel N, Mantini G, Zeeuw van der Laan EA, et al. Impact of hypoxia on chemoresistance of mesothelioma mediated by the proton-coupled folate transporter, and preclinical activity of new anti-LDH-A compounds. *Br J Cancer.* 2020;123(4):644–56.
198. Li Z, Jiang L, Chew SH, Hirayama T, Sekido Y, Toyokuni S. Carbonic anhydrase 9 confers resistance to ferroptosis/apoptosis in malignant mesothelioma under hypoxia. *Redox Biol.* 2019;26:101297.
199. Felley-Bosco E, Gray SG. Mesothelioma driver genes, ferroptosis, and therapy. *Front Oncol.* 2019;9:1318.
200. Wu J, Minikes AM, Gao M, Bian H, Li Y, Stockwell BR, et al. Intercellular interaction dictates cancer cell ferroptosis via NF2-YAP signalling. *Nature.* 2019;572(7769):402–6.

14 Surgical Management of Mesothelioma

Sara Kryeziu, Harvey I. Pass, and Stephanie Chang

14.1 INTRODUCTION

Malignant pleural mesothelioma (MPM) is a rare and aggressive malignancy associated with exposure to asbestos that carries a poor prognosis. Though surgical intervention has a defined role in the diagnosis, staging, and palliation of patients with MPM, the exact role of surgery in the definitive treatment of MPM remains controversial due to lack of proven survival benefits in randomized trials. Additionally, only a limited subset of patients presenting with MPM are candidates for surgical resection. A definitive standard-of-care for MPM treatment has not been well defined; however, a multimodality approach, including surgery, systemic therapies, and radiotherapy (RT), has been shown to have superior outcomes compared with surgery alone. Furthermore, there is ongoing controversy regarding the optimal surgical procedure for the management of MPM.

14.2 PATIENT SELECTION FOR SURGERY

After the diagnosis of mesothelioma, typically confirmed through a thoracoscopic biopsy, patients must undergo a comprehensive staging work-up. This includes a computed tomography (CT) scan of the chest and upper abdomen and positron emitted tomography (PET)-CT scan to determine the extent of disease and resectability. Suspicious nodes identified on imaging are evaluated with endobronchial ultrasound-guided fine-needle aspiration or mediastinoscopy.[1] Surgical candidates must have good performance status and cardiopulmonary reserve. Laparoscopy may be performed to evaluate for intraabdominal metastases. Patients should be evaluated in high volume centers and in a multidisciplinary tumor board including medical oncology, surgery, and radiation oncology.[2] Surgical series demonstrate that histologic subtype, gender, and lymph node status affect survival, with the best outcomes in patients who have epithelial histology, are female, and have no lymph node involvement.[3, 4]

14.3 NON-PALLIATIVE SURGICAL APPROACHES

The optimal surgical approach for the resection of MPM has been controversial. There are two main non-palliative surgical approaches to MPM: extrapleural pneumonectomy (EPP) or (extended) pleurectomy/decortication (EPD). The goal of these operations is to achieve a macroscopic complete resection (MCR), which entails removing all visible and palpable disease within the hemithorax (R1 resection).[5] Achieving microscopically negative margins (R0) is not feasible in the majority of cases. Patients with MCR have overall survival (OS) comparative to those without.[4]

Extrapleural pneumonectomy (EPP) is a lung-sacrificing operation that involves total pleural resection, ipsilateral pneumonectomy, and resection of the pericardium and/or diaphragm en bloc, with reconstruction of the pericardium and/or diaphragm (Figure 14.1). Pleurectomy decortication (PD) is a lung-sparing operation that consists of resecting the entire pleura (parietal, visceral, mediastinal, and diaphragmatic) without the underlying lung. An extended PD (EPD) involves resection of the pericardium and diaphragm along with a P/D (Figure 14.2).

DOI: 10.1201/9781003431909-14

Advantages of EPP include being a highly standardized procedure, simplifying adjuvant radiation, and leaving behind less microscopic disease while disadvantages include higher morbidity and mortality and quality of life issues associated with pneumonectomy. Advantages of lung-sparing surgery include improved quality of life and the possibility of more physiologic reserve to tolerate more aggressive treatments while disadvantages include longer operative time, higher disease burden left behind, postoperative air leaks, challenges to adjuvant radiation, and lack of technique standardization.[6] Regarding EPD technique, there remains controversy regarding whether visually normal diaphragm and pericardium should be removed, the role of intraoperative frozen sections to assess areas that appear normal, and the extent of lymph node dissection.

Mortality following EPP has been reported to be 5–7% at 30 days or in-hospital and as high as 11% at 90 days postoperatively at high volume centers with complication rates as high as 45%.[7, 8]

However, data from the IASLC database suggest EPP may be associated with improved long-term OS in a highly select group of younger patients with epithelioid mesothelioma histological subtype and no lymph node metastases.[9] More recently the mortality rates for EPP have decreased to as low as 1–4% in high volume centers, however PD or EPD have been consistently associated with lower mortality and morbidity.[10, 11] EPP overall confers no survival benefit over PD/EPD, with patients tolerating EPD better.

14.4 MULTIMODAL THERAPY WITH CHEMOTHERAPY

Surgical resection alone for MPM does not confer a survival advantage, and should only perform in a setting of multimodal therapy along with systemic chemotherapy and/or RT. Protocols typically consist of induction chemotherapy followed by surgical resection and adjuvant radiation, though the timing of chemotherapy is still controversial. Neoadjuvant/adjuvant chemotherapy regimens include cisplatin and pemetrexed or cisplatin and gemcitabine.

14.4.1 MARS Trial

The Mesothelioma and Radical Surgery (MARS) trial, a prospective, randomized trial, attempted to evaluate the added benefit of surgical resection over chemotherapy alone and found that patients who underwent EPP had worse survival compared with a similar cohort of early-stage patients managed with chemotherapy (cisplatin plus gemcitabine) alone.[12] The MARS trial was criticized for being underpowered to achieve significance, randomizing only 50 patients. With increasing evidence demonstrating similar survival between EPP and EPD, but lower morbidity and improved quality of life with EPD, many thoracic surgeons have transitioned toward a lung-sparing approach with P/D or EPD for the resection of MPM. Studies have shown that survival outcomes improved in centers where the same surgeons transitioned from EPP toward EPD as the preferred surgical technique in the context of multimodal therapy.[12–14]

14.4.2 Surgery and Chemotherapy Versus Chemotherapy Alone: MARS 2 Trial

14.4.2.1 Study Design

The most recent study evaluating the efficacy of surgery and adjuvant treatment versus medical management alone is the MARS 2 trial. MARS 2 is a multicenter, randomized phase III trial compared patients randomized to EPD and chemotherapy with patients randomized to chemotherapy alone, with the primary endpoint of overall survival. Secondary outcomes were progression-free survival, safety, health-related quality of life, and cost effectiveness. Inclusion criteria included tissue-confirmed mesothelioma, disease limited to one hemithorax, patient deemed surgically resectable, a performance status 0––1, and no end-organ failure. They underwent two cycles of platinum-based chemotherapy and pemtrexed, followed by repeat chest CT. If the patients remained resectable, they were randomized to EPD follow by up to four cycles of platinum-based chemotherapy and pemtrexed versus up to four cycles of chemotherapy without surgery.

14.4.2.2 Patient Demographics and Treatment

A total of 169 patients were randomized to surgery, with 14 patients withdrawing after randomization; 166 patients were randomized to no surgery, with 11 patients withdrawing after randomization. In both arms, 86% of patients had epithelioid mesothelioma. The clinical T, N, and M stages were similar between both groups. In the surgical arm, 89% underwent EPD and 8% underwent PD. On pathologic examination, only 3.2% had a no residual tumor (R0), with 80.9% having microscopic residual tumor (R1), and 15.9% having macroscopic residual tumor (R2). Mortality was 3.8% at 30 days and 8.9% at 90 days. When evaluating the total number of chemotherapy cycles, only 59.8% of patients in the surgery arm completed three cycles and 39.1% completed all six cycles. This was substantially lower than the no-surgery arm with 92.8% completing three cycles and 56% completing six cycles. Furthermore, less patients in the surgery arm received immunotherapy (21.9% surgery vs 38.6% in no surgery).

14.4.4.3 Outcomes

Between 0 and 42 months, the group that received chemotherapy alone had higher OS (HR = 1.28 [1.02,1.60] p = 0.03). After 42 months, there was no significant difference in OS (HR = 0.48 [0.18, 1.29] p = 0.15). There was no difference in progression-free survival (PFS) between the two groups (HR=0.90 [0.72,1.11]). Patients who underwent EPD and chemotherapy had no overall benefit in PFS or OS, more serious adverse events, and poorer quality of life compared to those who received chemotherapy alone.[15, 16]

14.4.3 Neoadjuvant Versus Adjuvant Chemotherapy: EORTC 1205

The use of induction therapy for patients with early-stage disease (Stage I/II) has decreased in centers in the United States, and there is a question of whether there is a difference between preoperative induction therapy compared with postoperative adjuvant therapy. EORTC 1205 is a multicenter, randomized phase II trial that sought to determine the optimal sequence of surgery and chemotherapy. The surgical intervention employed in this trial was EPD. The study randomized patients between upfront surgery, followed by three cycles of chemotherapy (cisplatin plus pemetrexed) (n = 34) and deferred surgery), following neoadjuvant chemotherapy (if no progression (n = 35) in early-stage MPM, irrespective of histological subtype.[17] The primary endpoint of the trial was the successful completion of multimodality treatment defined as completing two cycles of chemotherapy plus surgical intervention and being alive without progressive disease and without persistent grade III–IV treatment-related adverse events within 20 weeks. Secondary endpoints included PFS, OS, operative morbidity and mortality, toxicity and safety.

Overall surgical mortality was 1.7%; however, there was a high incidence of overall complications (>75%), and serious adverse events (30.4%). At 2 years, there was no statistically significant difference in OS in the upfront surgery group (56.6% [36.0–72.8]) compared with the deferred surgery group (63.1% [44.1–77.1]) or in PFS (22.8% [9.5–39.5] versus 29.8% [15.3–45.8]). These results suggest that multimodal therapy with EPD is feasible with a low mortality rate and there is no major difference when it is combined with neoadjuvant chemotherapy compared with adjuvant chemotherapy.

14.4.4 Role of Surgery in Mesothelioma

While the results of MARS 2 trials suggest that chemotherapy without surgical intervention results in better outcomes, cross-trial comparison to EORTC 1205 demonstrates some discrepancies that should be further scrutinized. Both studies were randomized trials in Europe with accrual during the same time period, with significant differences in survival for patients undergoing EPD. The presented MARS 2 data shows an overall survival of roughly 50% at 2 years for the no-surgery group and 40% for the surgery group[15] However, the EORTC 1205 has a 2-year survival of 59% among all patients in the cohort[17], all of whom underwent EPD and received chemotherapy, suggesting that multimodality treatment with surgery has a survival benefit compared to the no-surgery arm in MARS 2. This difference is likely due to poor surgical outcomes in the MARS 2 trial, with an 8.9% 90-day mortality – a rate that is nearly double other large institutional data reporting a 4.6% 90-day mortality.[4] Once additional granular data is available for both trials, further analysis is necessary to determine the exact role for surgical resection in the treatment of resectable mesothelioma.

14.5 INDUCTION WITH IMMUNE CHECKPOINT BLOCKADE

Over the last decade, immunotherapy has arisen as a viable systemic treatment for multiple malignancies including MPM. Due to the successful results as salvage therapy in patients with unresectable MPM, immune checkpoint blockade (ICB) against programmed cell death-1(PD-1)/programmed cell death-ligand 1 (PD-L1) with durvalumab alone or in combination with blockade against CTL-associated antigen-4 (CTLA-4) with tremelimumab has been evaluated in the neoadjuvant setting. A phase II, window-of-opportunity, trial randomized patients with early-stage, resectable epithelioid or non-epithelioid MPM to neoadjuvant durvalumab (n = 9), durvalumab plus tremelimumab (n = 11), or no ICB (n = 4), followed by surgery (EPP or EPD) in 3–6 weeks. Tumor biopsies were taken prior to ICB via thoracoscopy at the time of staging and post-ICB at the time of surgical resection. The study found that a single cycle of neoadjuvant durvalumab and tremelimumab lead to a pathologic response (>20% tumor regression) in 35% of MPM tumors with a major pathologic response (≤10% residual viable tumor) rate of 12%. Additionally, tertiary lymphoid structures (TLS), aggregates of lymphocytes and antigen-presenting cells that aid in the development of antitumor immune responses, were seen in MPM tumors. These TLS and peripheral immune compartments were enriched with CD57+ memory T cells while the bone marrow was depleted, indicating that ICB mobilizes specialized subsets of circulating CD57-expressing memory CD8 and CD4 T cells from the bone marrow for their recruitment into tumor TLSs. Patients treated with combination ICB had longer OS and DFS (P = 0.040 and P = 0.009) compared with those treated with monotherapy. Median OS and DFS were 14.0 and 8.4 months in the monotherapy group, respectively, and not yet reached in the combination group at 34.1 months after randomization.[18]

Another phase II trial was designed to evaluate whether neoadjuvant atezolizumab (PD-L1 inhibition) in combination with pemetrexed and cisplatin, followed by resection, and maintenance atezolizumab in patients with resectable MPM would increase OS. Patients underwent neoadjuvant therapy with four cycles of cisplatin and pemetrexed plus atezolimumab followed by surgical resection, EPP or EPD, and 1 year of maintenance atezolizumab. At the time of the presentation in September 2021, median progression-free survival was 18 months, overall survival at 30 months was approximately 60%, and safety criteria were met.[19]

14.6 SURGERY FOR MESOTHELIOMA AFTER RADIATION THERAPY (SMART) PROTOCOL

A novel approach to the management of mesothelioma consists of an accelerated course of high-dose intensity-modulated radiotherapy (IMRT) to the hemithorax followed by EPP soon after to mitigate the risk of radiation pneumonitis. The rationale behind the SMART protocol was to optimize the delivery of radiation to the whole tumor bed with a shorter treatment plan, limit the risk of spillage during surgery, and to stimulate the immune response.[20] With the SMART protocol, patients received 25 Gy in five daily fractions over one week to the entire ipsilateral hemithorax with a concomitant 5 Gy boost to high-risk areas followed by EPP within 1 week. The results of the

SMART trial demonstrated a 5-year cumulative incidence of local recurrence of 17 (20.1% [95% CI 11.4–28.8]) and distant recurrence of 62 (63.3% [52·3–74·4]) with a median OS of 24.4 months (95% CI 18.5–31.1) and median disease-free survival of 18 months (95% CI 12.6–21.7). Thirty-day and 90-day mortality in SMART trial were 1% and 3%, respectively. In comparison, the phase II trial by de Perrot et al. also reported an operative mortality of 1.6% suggesting that with appropriate patient selection, radiotherapy and EPP may yield good results.[20–22]

14.7 RADIATION AFTER LUNG-SPARING RESECTION

Conventional postoperative radiation with external-beam RT to the ipsilateral hemithorax has been used as part of multimodality treatment to decrease the risk of local and regional failure. With the increase in EPD, institutions began to use postoperative hemithoracic pleural IMRT (Intensity-modulated pleural radiation therapy [IMPRINT]) for a more precise application to minimize the risk of radiotoxicity to the lung. A retrospective study from MSKCC analyzed 209 patients who received P/D and adjuvant RT either with conventional techniques or IMPRINT. OS was significantly higher after IMPRINT (median 20.2 vs 12.3 months, $p = 0.001$) but there was no statistically significant difference in PFS between the two groups. IMPRINT was associated with higher rates of fatigue and cough compared with conventional RT, but lower rates of esophagitis and pneumonitis.[23]

14.8 PLEURAL-DIRECTED ADJUNCTS

Intraoperative hyperthermic lavage with chemotherapy drugs, including cisplatin, doxorubicin, mitomycin C, gemcitabine, or providone-iodine, during EPP or EPD has been evaluated in phase I/II trials with data suggesting there is may be some benefit in extending interval to recurrence but there have been no randomized trials.[24–26] Other intraoperative strategies include the use of photodynamic therapy, which entails administering a photosensitizing agent along with laser light applied to the thoracic cavity, the application of cisplatin-fibrin gel directly to the surface of the thoracic cavity, and intracavitary infusion. Other preclinical studies are evaluating other pleural-directed adjuncts including expansile nanoparticles and hydrogel nanocomposite.[27]

14.9 PALLIATIVE SURGICAL APPROACHES

Patients with poor performance status and/or cardiopulmonary reserve who are not candidates for EPP or EPD or those with advanced disease may still be considered for palliative surgery. Palliative procedures include partial pleurectomy, video-assisted thoracoscopic surgery (VATS) with pleurodesis, or indwelling pleural catheter placement, all of which aim to control recurrent effusions or re-expand a partial trapped lung. MesoVATS compared partial pleurectomy with talc pleurodesis in patients with mesothelioma and pleural effusion and concluded that partial pleurectomy did not improve survival, although it found that patients in the better prognostic group had improved HRQoL after 6 months.[28] The MesoTRAP trial is a feasibility, multicenter, randomized controlled clinical trial evaluating the role of VATS with pleurodesis compared with indwelling pleural catheter placement in patients with trapped lung and pleural effusions.[29]

REFERENCES

1. Kindler HL, Ismaila N, Armato SG, et al. Treatment of malignant pleural mesothelioma: American society of clinical oncology clinical practice guideline. *J Clin Oncol.* 2018;36(13):1343–1373.
2. Verma V, Ahern CA, Berlind CG, et al. Facility volume and postoperative outcomes for malignant pleural mesothelioma: A national cancer data base analysis. *Lung Cancer.* 2018;120:7–13.
3. Taioli E, Wolf AS, Camacho-Rivera M, et al. Determinants of survival in malignant pleural mesothelioma: A surveillance, epidemiology, and end results (SEER) study of 14, 228 patients. *PLOS ONE.* 2015;10(12):e0145039.

4. Lapidot M, Gill RR, Mazzola E, et al. Pleurectomy decortication in the treatment of malignant pleural mesothelioma. *Ann Surg.* 2022;275(6):1212–1220.
5. Popat S, Baas P, Faivre-Finn C, et al. Malignant pleural mesothelioma: ESMO Clinical Practice Guidelines for diagnosis, treatment and follow-up☆up☆. *Ann Oncol.* 2022;33(2):129–142.
6. Friedberg JS, Culligan MJ, Tsao AS, et al. A proposed system toward standardizing surgical-based treatments for malignant pleural mesothelioma, from the joint national cancer institute-international association for the study of lung cancer-mesothelioma applied research foundation taskforce. *J Thorac Oncol.* 2019;14(8):1343–1353.
7. Flores RM, Pass HI, Seshan VE, et al. Extrapleural pneumonectomy versus pleurectomy/decortication in the surgical management of malignant pleural mesothelioma: Results in 663 patients. *J Thorac Cardiovasc Surg.* 2008;135(3).
8. Sugarbaker DJ, Richards WG, Bueno R. Extrapleural pneumonectomy in the treatment of epithelioid malignant pleural mesothelioma: Novel prognostic implications of combined N1 and N2 nodal involvement based on experience in 529 patients. *Ann Surg.* 2014;260(4):577–582.
9. Rusch VW, Giroux D, Kennedy C, et al. Initial analysis of the international association for the study of lung cancer mesothelioma database. *J Thorac Oncol.* 2012;7(11):1631–1639.
10. Tsao AS, Pass HI, Rimner A, Mansfield AS. Special series: Thoracic oncology: current and future therapy review articles new era for malignant pleural mesothelioma: Updates on therapeutic options. *J Clin Oncol.* 2022;40(6):681–692.
11. Zhou N, Rice DC, Tsao AS, et al. Extrapleural pneumonectomy versus pleurectomy/decortication for malignant pleural mesothelioma. *Ann Thorac Surg.* 2022;113(1):200–208.
12. Treasure T, Lang-Lazdunski L, Waller D, et al. Extra-pleural pneumonectomy versus no extra-pleural pneumonectomy for patients with malignant pleural mesothelioma: Clinical outcomes of the Mesothelioma and Radical Surgery (MARS) randomised feasibility study. *Lancet Oncol.* 2011;12(8):763–772.
13. Nakamura A, Hashimoto M, Matsumoto S, Kondo N, Kijima T, Hasegawa S. Outcomes of conversion to extrapleural pneumonectomy from pleurectomy/decortication for malignant pleural mesothelioma. *Semin Thorac Cardiovasc Surg.* 2021;33(3):873–881.
14. Klotz LV, Hoffmann H, Shah R, et al. Multimodal therapy of epithelioid pleural mesothelioma: Improved survival by changing the surgical treatment approach. *Transl Lung Cancer Res.* 2022;11(11):2230–2242.
15. Lim E, Darlison L, Edwards J, et al. Mesothelioma and Radical Surgery 2 (MARS 2): protocol for a multicentre randomised trial comparing (extended) pleurectomy decortication versus no (extended) pleurectomy decortication for patients with malignant pleural mesothelioma On behalf of MARS 2 Trialists. *BMJ Open.* 2020;10(9):e038892.
16. Lim E, Waller D, Lau K et al. MARS 2: A multicentre randomised trial comparing (extended) pleurectomy decortication versus no radical surgery for mesothelioma, 2023. https://cattendee.abstractsonline.com/meeting/10925/presentation/2751.
17. Raskin J, Surmont V, Cornelissen R, Baas P, van Schil PEY, van Meerbeeck JP. A randomized phase II study of pleurectomy/decortication preceded or followed by (neo-)adjuvant chemotherapy in patients with early stage malignant pleural mesothelioma (EORTC 1205). *Transl Lung Cancer Res.* 2018;7(5):593–598.
18. Lee H-S, Jang H-J, Ramineni M, et al. A Phase II window of opportunity study of neoadjuvant PD-L1 versus PD-L1 plus CTLA-4 blockade for patients with malignant pleural mesothelioma. *Clin Cancer Res.* 2023;29(3):548–559.
19. Tsao A, Qian L, Cetnar J et al. S1619: A trial of neoadjuvant cisplatin-pemetrexed with atezolizumab in combination and maintenance for resectable pleural mesothelioma. *J Thorac Oncol.* 2021;16(10):S870.
20. De Perrot M, Feld R, Leighl NB, et al. Accelerated hemithoracic radiation followed by extrapleural pneumonectomy for malignant pleural mesothelioma. *J Thorac Cardiovasc Surg.* 2016;151(2):468–475.
21. Cho BCJ, Feld R, Leighl N, et al. A feasibility study evaluating surgery for mesothelioma after radiation therapy: The "SMART" approach for resectable malignant pleural mesothelioma. *J Thorac Oncol.* 2014;9(3):397–402.
22. Cho BCJ, Donahoe L, Bradbury PA, et al. Surgery for malignant pleural mesothelioma after radiotherapy (SMART): Final results from a single-centre, phase 2 trial. *Lancet Oncol.* 2021;22(2):190–197.
23. Shaikh F, Zauderer MG, Von Reibnitz D, et al. Improved outcomes with modern lung-sparing trimodality therapy in patients with malignant pleural mesothelioma. *J Thorac Oncol.* 2017;12(6):993–1000.
24. Burt BM, Richards WG, Lee HS, et al. A Phase I trial of surgical resection and intraoperative hyperthermic cisplatin and gemcitabine for pleural mesothelioma. *J Thorac Oncol.* 2018;13(9):1400–1409.

25. Sugarbaker DJ, Gill RR, Yeap BY, et al. Hyperthermic intraoperative pleural cisplatin chemotherapy extends interval to recurrence and survival among low-risk patients with malignant pleural mesothelioma undergoing surgical macroscopic complete resection. *J Thorac Cardiovasc Surg.* 2013;145(4):955–963.
26. Richards WG, Zellos L, Bueno R, et al. Phase I to II study of pleurectomy/decortication and intraoperative intracavitary hyperthermic cisplatin lavage for mesothelioma. *J Clin Oncol.* 2006;24(10):1561–1567.
27. Choi AY, Singh A, Wang D, Pittala K, Hoang CD. Current state of pleural-directed adjuncts against malignant pleural mesothelioma. *Front Oncol.* 2022;12:886430.
28. Rintoul RC, Ritchie AJ, Edwards JG, et al. Efficacy and cost of video-assisted thoracoscopic partial pleurectomy versus talc pleurodesis in patients with malignant pleural mesothelioma (MesoVATS): An open-label, randomised, controlled trial. *Lancet.* 2014;384(9948):1118–1127.
29. Matthews C, Freeman C, Sharples LD, et al. MesoTRAP: A feasibility study that includes a pilot clinical trial comparing video-assisted thoracoscopic partial pleurectomy decortication with indwelling pleural catheter in patients with trapped lung due to malignant pleural mesothelioma designed to a. *BMJ Open Respir Res.* 2019;6(1):e000368.

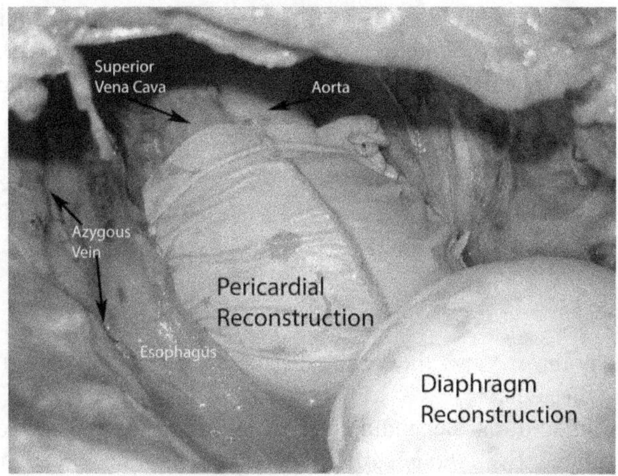

FIGURE 14.1 Thoracotomy view of completed right-sided extrapleural pneumonectomy. The pleura, lung, diaphragm, and pericardium have been surgically removed. A Gortex™ patch is used to reconstruct the diaphragm, and bovine pericardium used as a pericardial substitute. Although no visible disease is seen, the majority of these resections leave microscopic disease behind necessitating some sort of adjuvant therapy.

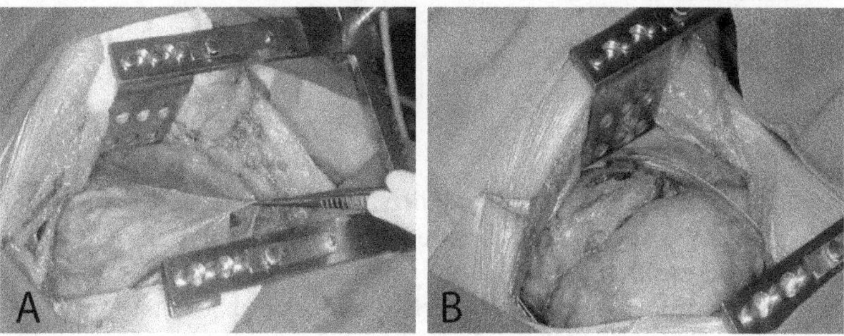

FIGURE 14.2 Right-sided pleurectomy decortication for early-stage mesothelioma. A.The visceral pleural (held by the forceps) is carefully dissected from the lung B. The completed decortication revealing the fissure between the middle and the lower lobe which has also had removal of the visceral pleura, sparing all lobes.

15 Asbestos-Related Cancers

Sara Ricciardi, Delia Giovanniello, and Giuseppe Cardillo

15.1 INTRODUCTION

Asbestos is frequently defined "the hidden killer" as its microscopic, tasteless, and odorless fibers can be associated to several cancers.

In 1977, the International Agency for Research on Cancer (IARC) classified asbestos as a Group 1 carcinogen, with several cancers directly associated with asbestos exposure, primarily thoracic neoplasms including lung cancer [1, 2]. It is well recognized that asbestos, either through professional or environmental exposure, is the main cause of mesothelioma. In 2020, the International Agency for Research on Cancer (IARC) reported 30,870 new cases diagnosed worldwide, and 26,278 deaths [3].

Moreover, in 2009, IARC stated that epidemiological studies provide sufficient evidence that asbestos is also associated with larynx and ovarian cancer, as well as limited evidence that it is associated with colorectal, pharyngeal, and gastric cancer [4].

15.1.1 Asbestos Fibers

From a public health point of view, the term asbestos suggests the concept of fibrous minerals responsible for several diseases.

Asbestos has several definitions depending on the setting, with regulatory definitions categorizing minerals to be regulated. Even though all asbestos fibers have been recognized as carcinogenic agents, uncertainty arises regarding which fibers should be regulated, and the regulatory health agencies regulate only the six commercial varieties of asbestos.

Those six different fibrous minerals are:

- Chrysotile (white asbestos)
- Amosite (brown asbestos)
- Crocidolite (blue asbestos)
- Tremolite
- Anthophyllite
- Actinolite

Based on the statement that only commercial utilization can cause an extensive human exposure, only those six fibers are regulated because they were the only mineral fibers commercially employed when regulations were presented.

Asbestos has been used in construction materials, such as insulation, roofing, and tiles, as well as in automotive parts, textiles, and other industrial applications. While asbestos was highly valued for its properties, it has also been linked to severe health risks, particularly the development of asbestos-related cancers.

All commercial asbestos fiber types, including amphibole anthophyllite and chrysotile, have been implicated in causing lung cancer. Crocidolite and amosite are considered particularly potent, with chrysotile also having a role, especially in the chrysotile textile industry [5].

The common asbestos-related nonmalignant diseases are [6, 7]:

DOI: 10.1201/9781003431909-15

1. Pleural effusion – usually unilateral, but may be bilateral and occasionally subside.
2. Diffuse pleural thickening – that can cause a severe restrictive ventilatory impairment.
3. Pleural plaques – discrete areas of fibrous tissue limited to the parietal pleura.
4. Round atelectasis – much less frequent than circumscribed plaques or diffuse pleural fibrosis. Can be determined by a low-grade inflammatory pleural reaction at one site, which evolves in a compression of the underlying lung and bronchial occlusion.
5. Asbestosis – occurs in case of high asbestos exposure. It is characterized by cough, dyspnea, basilar rales inspiration, and digital clubbing.

15.1.2 Environmental Asbestos Exposure

Rubino et al. in 1968, analyzing subjects who lived in the neighborhood of the Balangero Chrysotile mine in the Province of Turin, northern Italy, showed records on pleural plaque prevalence in nonoccupationally exposed individuals [8]. Moreover, Thomson and Graves in 1966 published an article showing the presence of asbestos bodies in more than 25% of the lungs of 500 subjects at autopsy in Miami, Florida [9]. Donna et al. reported an even higher prevalence in Italian subjects in 1968 [10].

In 1990, at the New York conference on asbestos the term “third wave of asbestos disease” was coined to cover the effects of outdoor pollution in urban/extra-urban areas [11]. Asbestos not yet removed may cause the release of airborne fibers in external and internal environments. Furthermore, friable asbestos-insulating materials can be present in the environment. The sources of environmental asbestos exposure can involve outdoor exposure such as the neighborhood of industrial use of asbestos, fibers from natural sources (outcrops, soils, deposits), and indoor exposure, such as whitewashing with a fibrous mineral [12].

The problem of airborne spreading of fibers from materials that contain asbestos persists, especially during standard maintenance interventions or natural degradation. Fibrous minerals, contained in many geological formations, are not dangerous unless weathering or crushing emits them [13]. Moreover, lands created from the erosion of these rocks could also contain mineral macroscopic fibers, which can disintegrate into microfibrils that are emitted into the environment.

Therefore, individuals are exposed to these fibers when human actions (quarrying, mining, roadwork) or natural events (earthquake, volcanic eruption) produce dust [12, 13].

The six regulated mineral fibers are not the only mineral fibers that are carcinogenic. A well-known example is the zeolite erionite. This fibrous material has been discovered in houses and roads built from volcanic stones in some Cappadocia villages, where a malignant mesothelioma epidemic was registered [14]. In vitro and in vivo experiments confirmed that erionite fibers are genotoxic and more carcinogenic than asbestos [15].

Environmental exposure may affect categories not encompassed in the conventional list of at-risk occupations. Moreover, because environmental exposure is hard to establish, exposure associated with the environment is probably underestimated [16].

The WHO document on air quality is a useful instrument, even though this text cannot be considered as an absolute reference for each category [17].

Occurrence in air [17]:

1. Rural areas (remote from asbestos emission sources): below 100 F/m^3
2. Urban areas: general levels may vary from below 100 to 1,000 F/m^3
3. Near various emission sources the following figures have been measured as yearly averages:
   a. Downwind from an asbestos-cement plant at 300 m: 2,200 F/m^3
      - at 700m: 800 F/m^3
      - at 1,000 m: 600 F/m^3
   b. At a street crossing with heavy traffic, 900 F/m^3
   c. On an express-way, up to 3,300 F/m^3

4. Indoor air:
   a. In buildings without specific asbestos sources, concentrations are generally below 1,000 F/m^3
   b. In buildings with friable asbestos, concentrations vary irregularly; usually less than 1,000 F*/m^3 are found, but in some cases, exposure reaches 10,000 F*/m^3

Note: * fibers counted with an optical microscope.

Currently there is a very low exposure due to the environmental asbestos pollution, however it is not simple to assess if the occupational/environmental exposure before banning may play a role in a future mesothelioma and asbestos-related cancers epidemic.

15.1.3 Association Versus Causation

In epidemiology, the terms "association" and "causation" are crucial concepts used to describe the relationships between variables, particularly when studying the causes and effects of diseases in populations. These terms help epidemiologists to draw conclusions about whether a particular exposure or factor is responsible for a specific health outcome.

Association refers to a statistical relationship or correlation between two or more variables. It means that there is a connection or a pattern observed between an exposure (such as a risk factor) and an outcome (such as a disease), but it does not imply that one variable causes the other.

Causation, on the other hand, goes beyond association and implies a cause-and-effect relationship. It means that changes in one variable directly lead to changes in another, and the first variable is responsible for the occurrence of the second.

The attribution of causation needs reasonable medical certainty on a probability basis that the agent (asbestos) has caused or contributed significantly to the disease. The probability that asbestos exposure has had a substantial contribution increases when the exposure increases. Cumulative exposure, on a probability basis, should therefore be considered the key criterion for the attribution of a substantial contribution by asbestos to cancer risk.

15.2 LUNG CANCER

The first international expert meeting on "Asbestos, asbestosis, and cancer" took place in Helsinki in 1997. A multidisciplinary panel of experts analyzed disorders associated with asbestos, in order to agree on the criteria for diagnosis and attribution of cancer to asbestos [18].

A cumulative asbestos exposure of 25 fiber-years is the level considered to be associated with an estimated doubling of lung cancer relative risk to a nonexposed person.

The Helsinki Criteria for asbestos-related lung cancers have been widely accepted and used for several years, either for diagnosis or compensation. However, these criteria have been highly controversial with several revisions and they are still an ongoing debate.

According to Helsinki Criteria, because of the high incidence of lung cancer in the general population, it is not possible to establish in accurate deterministic terms that asbestos is the causative factor for a single patient, even when asbestosis is present. For cohorts exposed at a cumulative exposure of 25 fiber-years or with a comparable occupational history, the relative risk is almost doubled, even if, at this level, asbestosis may or may not be present or detectable. For this reason, in the absence of radiologically diagnosed asbestosis, the heavy exposure is considered sufficient to increase the risk of lung cancer. Cumulative exposure lower than 25 fiber-years is also associated with an increasing risk of lung cancer, but to a lesser extent.

Hence, lung cancer is epidemiologically considered to be associated with asbestos exposure rather than directly caused by asbestos. Asbestos exposure has been consistently linked to a higher incidence of lung cancer among individuals with a history of exposure, particularly among those who were heavily exposed to asbestos fibers and who also smoked. Smoking is the most significant risk factor for lung cancer, and it synergistically increases the risk when combined with asbestos exposure. Other factors, such as genetic predisposition, exposure to other carcinogens, and environmental factors, also play a role in the development of lung cancer [19].

The presence of asbestosis, diagnosed clinically, radiologically (including HRCT), or histologically is an indicator of high exposure and can be used to attribute a substantial causal or contributory role to asbestos for an associated lung cancer.

15.2.1 Criteria for Attribution of Lung Cancers to Asbestos Exposure

There has to be objective medical evidence of exposure to asbestos which includes in order of reliability at least one of the following: lung content analyses demonstrating higher than background levels of asbestos and or a diagnosis of asbestosis, bilateral pleural plaques, a presence of ferruginous bodies detected histologically, or at least a credible professional history of asbestos exposure. Of note, people who have been exposed to asbestos usually have all these findings.

A set of criteria modified from the original Helsinki Criteria has been proposed in 2011 [20]

Asbestos exposure with a minimum latency interval of 10 years

AND

For current smokers:

A no disputed or majority clinical-radiologic or histologic diagnosis of asbestosis.

OR

The occurrence of asbestosis among other workers in the same workforce carrying out similar work for similar durations of time and at similar times.

OR

A no disputed/majority estimate of cumulative exposure to asbestos of 25 fiber/years or more for mixed-fiber, end-use exposure to asbestos.

For amphibole-only (amosite or crocidolite) exposures, a no disputed estimated cumulative exposure of 20 or 25 fiber/years, and 25 fiber/years for asbestos textile workers.

For chrysotile-only exposures, and exposure to friction products, 200 fiber/years, and for other chrysotile-only exposure, 100 fiber- years.

This is based on the estimated relative potency of 1:4 amphibole: chrysotile [21].

OR

At least 5 years of asbestos exposure before 1975, or 5–10 years after 1975, for asbestos textile workers, asbestos insulation workers including work in power stations, railways workshops, shipbuilding and others in close proximity to such work, especially when it was carried out in confined and poorly ventilated workplaces, or a duration of one year for work that involved consistent or frequent spraying of asbestos insulation.

OR

For never-smokers or those who had ceased smoking 30 years or more before the diagnosis of lung cancer; cumulative exposure amounting to 5- fiber/years, or exposure amounting to 1/3 of the durations for work set forth in the preceding paragraph.

OR

A concentration of asbestos bodies or uncoated amphibole fibers at or in excess of the 5th percentile count in cases of asbestosis for the same laboratory (for fibers of the same length) for mixed-fiber end-use exposures.

Because chrysotile fibers are cleared from lung more rapidly than amphibole, fiber assays should not be used for chrysotile-only exposures; instead, the occupational history should be substituted.

Those criteria are designed mainly for statutory compensation where smoking is not to be considered.

Those criteria cannot properly reflect the complex biological reality in individual lung cancer. For this reason, a revised criteria that also takes genetic susceptibility into account is mandatory.

15.2.2 The Problem Dimensions

Lung cancer remains a leading cause of cancer mortality worldwide, with a significant portion (10% to 15%) of cases attributed to occupational exposures to lung carcinogens [21–25].

Asbestos is a major occupational carcinogen and a leading cause of occupational lung cancer deaths globally. It accounted for approximately 30% of occupational lung cancer deaths in 2015, with higher proportions in specific countries [26].

Despite the attention given to mesothelioma, asbestos-related lung cancer is more common, making up at least twice as many cases [27, 28].

15.2.3 Historical Background

This historical account delves into the early recognition of a concerning link between asbestosis and lung cancer. It begins with anecdotal autopsy reports in the mid-1930s that hinted at the connection [29–33]. In 1938, significant evidence emerged from three German papers and an Austrian review, shedding light on the association between asbestosis and lung cancer [34].

Nordmann and Sorge, pivotal figures in this narrative, labeled this phenomenon as the "occupational cancer of asbestos workers" and estimated that approximately 12% of asbestosis patients could develop lung cancer [35, 36]. Their groundbreaking research involved inducing lung tumors in mice by exposing them to chrysotile asbestos, as detailed in Proctor's book *The Nazi War on Cancer*. This research had profound consequences, leading the German government in 1943 to officially recognize lung cancer associated with any degree of asbestosis as a compensable disease [34].

This discovery was later revisited by Doll, who meticulously followed up on 113 men with prolonged asbestos exposure, spanning at least two decades [37]. He compared their mortality rates with those expected from the general male population. Shockingly, 39 deaths occurred in this group, far exceeding the anticipated 15.4 deaths. The surplus was primarily attributed to lung cancer, with 11 cases against the expected 0.8, along with respiratory and cardiovascular diseases linked to asbestosis. Notably, all lung cancer cases were histologically confirmed and closely associated with the presence of asbestosis. Men employed for 20 or more years faced a staggering tenfold higher risk compared to the general population, with the risk diminishing as exposure to dusty conditions decreased over time.

Doll's research underscored the significance of Merewether's 1949 observation, which revealed a high prevalence of lung cancer in asbestosis cases (13.2%), significantly contrasting with the lower rate in silicosis cases (1.3%). Gloyne's analogous findings further strengthened this argument, with a 14.1% incidence of lung cancer in asbestosis autopsy cases compared to 6.9% in silicosis cases [33, 38].

This historical account sheds light on pivotal moments in understanding the correlation between asbestos exposure, asbestosis, and the development of lung cancer, providing critical insights into occupational health and safety.

15.2.4 Smoking

The interaction between asbestos exposure and smoking is complex, with some debate over the strength of this interaction. The prevailing view is that smoking and asbestos exposure have a synergistic effect on lung cancer risk.

A study focused on insulation workers in North America found that asbestos exposure alone increased lung cancer mortality among non-smokers, even in the absence of asbestosis on chest x-rays. Smoking without asbestos exposure also contributed to a higher risk of lung cancer. The joint effect of smoking and asbestos exposure was additive, and for asbestosis, it was supra-additive. Lung cancer mortality decreased significantly within 10 years of smoking cessation [38].

A comprehensive study of UK asbestos workers confirmed a multiplicative interaction between tobacco and asbestos exposure in relation to lung cancer risk. It also found an increased risk of lung cancer in never-smoking asbestos workers compared to the never-smoking general population and observed a substantial reduction in lung cancer risk with smoking cessation [39].

A large pooled analysis of case-referent studies in Europe and Canada found that asbestos exposure had a more-than-additive effect on lung cancer risk in females and showed a dose–response relationship in males [40].

A study by Karjalainen and colleagues examined the association between lung asbestos fiber burden and lung cancer risk. It found that higher asbestos fiber concentrations were associated with an elevated risk of lung cancer, even when cases of asbestosis and minor fibrosis were excluded. The study suggested a trend of increasing risk with higher fiber concentrations [41].

Created with Biorender.com

15.2.5 Pathophysiology

Extensive research over the past few decades has shed light on the mechanisms underlying fiber-induced lung cancer, with a focus on asbestos.

Current consensus views indicate that asbestos plays a role in both the initiation and proliferation phases of tumor development [42].

Fiber-induced carcinogenesis is thought to involve multiple stages, possibly resulting from fiber-induced genetic or epigenetic alterations, altered cell proliferation, disrupted apoptosis regulation, and chronic inflammation.

Asbestos exposure contributes to tumor development at all stages [43]. Asbestos fibers may increase the uptake and metabolism of carcinogens in cigarette smoke by lung cells.

Several mechanisms have been proposed as possible reasons for the synergy between cigarette smoking and asbestos:

a) Cigarette smoke may promote the penetration of asbestos fibers into bronchial walls [44].
b) Benzopyrene and other carcinogens contained in cigarette can be adsorbed onto asbestos fibers and subsequently delivered at high concentrations into cells [45].
c) Cigarette smoke may impede the clearance of asbestos from the lungs. An increased concentration of asbestos fibers in the bronchi of smokers compared to that of non-smokers, especially for short fibers, has been reported [46]. The relationship between fibers and cellular processes is stochastic, meaning that the probability of fiber–cell interaction depends on factors like the number of fibers and cells present [42].
d) Free fatty acids contained in cigarette may translocate iron into cell membranes, with enhancement of cell sensitivity to oxidants such as active oxygen species [43].
e) Gulino et al. mention a proposed mechanism involving asbestos-induced epithelial-to-mesenchymal transition (EMT) mediated through the transforming growth factor (TGF) β pathway, which could link asbestosis, lung cancer, and mesothelioma pathogenesis [22].

While some genetic markers show associations with asbestos exposure, there is currently no definitive genetic test that can distinguish asbestos-caused lung carcinomas from those unrelated to asbestos with certainty. More research and prospective studies are needed to explore the potential utility of genetic biomarkers in this context.

15.2.6 Screening

Low-dose chest CT (LDCT) screening has been shown to reduce lung cancer mortality in high-risk populations, as demonstrated by the National Lung Screening Trial (NLST) and the Dutch–Belgian Nederlands–Leuvens Longkanker Screenings Onderzoek (NELSON) trial [47, 48].

Screening eligibility criteria have primarily relied on age and smoking history, with limited consideration of other risk factors. Some lung cancer risk prediction models incorporate a broader set of risk factors, including occupational exposures like asbestos.

Studies have shown that certain risk prediction models outperform traditional eligibility criteria in terms of sensitivity and reducing lung cancer deaths.

While the use of risk prediction models for lung cancer screening has gained acceptance in Europe, the United States has generally retained simpler eligibility criteria based on age and smoking history.

The application of risk prediction models for lung cancer screening remains an area of debate and research, including optimizing models, cost-effectiveness, integrating biomarkers, determining screening intervals, and implementing screening programs effectively [49].

Prospective studies are needed to further evaluate the performance of risk prediction models in identifying individuals at high risk for lung cancer.

More than 20 lung cancer risk prediction models have been developed based on larger datasets, including the Prostate, Lung, Colorectal, and Ovarian Cancer Screening Trial (PLCO) and the Liverpool Lung Project (LLP) models [50].

These models aim to improve the accuracy of identifying individuals at risk of lung cancer by considering a wide range of risk factors beyond age and smoking.

Unlike clinical trials such as the NLST and NELSON, which primarily relied on age and smoking history, these risk prediction models incorporate a more comprehensive set of risk factors. These include gender, race, body mass index (BMI), intensity and duration of smoking, years since smoking cessation, presence of chronic lung diseases (especially chronic obstructive pulmonary disease or COPD), personal and family history of cancer, education level, and asbestos exposure.

Notably, among these models, only a few, such as the LLP and Bach models, include asbestos exposure as a risk factor. Asbestos exposure is treated as a binary variable (yes/no) in these models, despite its known association with lung cancer.

Some studies, like the one conducted by Ten Haaf, compared the performance of these risk prediction models with traditional criteria like those used in NLST. The results showed that several risk prediction models had higher sensitivity in detecting lung cancer incidence and mortality compared to the traditional criteria [51].

The US Preventive Services Task Force (USPSTF) considered the use of these risk prediction models when making recommendations for lung cancer screening. They found that risk prediction models offered better outcomes in terms of reducing lung cancer deaths and minimizing false positive tests compared to using age and smoking history alone [52].

The article highlights that in Europe, there is a more favorable attitude toward using lung cancer risk prediction models, particularly the PLCOm2012 and LLPv2 models. These models have been incorporated into lung cancer screening programs in the United Kingdom, potentially improving the accuracy of identifying individuals at risk [53].

As Markowitz et al. suggest, the focus should be on practical aspects of implementing LDCT screening, such as identifying at-risk workers, organizing and funding screening programs, educating individuals about screening benefits, and promoting awareness of occupational lung cancer risk factors in healthcare decision-making. The recommended approach involves screening workers aged 50 and older who have a history of at least 5 years of asbestos exposure and either a history of smoking (including specific criteria related to pack-years and quitting duration) or other lung cancer risk factors. Workers with intense but less than 5 years of asbestos exposure should also be considered for LDCT screening. There is still uncertainty regarding LDCT screening for asbestos-exposed non-smokers without other risk factors, emphasizing the need for further research and analysis [50].

15.3 LARYNGEAL CANCER

In 2012, the Committee on Asbestos [54] stated that there is a dose–response relationship between laryngeal cancer and asbestos exposure.

The asbestos-induced pathogenesis of laryngeal cancer may be the same as that of lung cancer, for the following reasons:

a) The larynx is a direct path for asbestos fibers as the lungs.
b) Asbestos fibers are accumulated in the larynx, as happened in the lungs, causing inflammation and damage.
c) The larynx is constituted by squamous cells as the lungs.
d) Laryngeal cancer, in approximately 90% of cases, is a squamous cell carcinoma, results from squamous metaplasia and dysplasia caused by exposure to various substances.

The majority of laryngeal cancers are attributed to the combined use of tobacco and excessive alcohol consumption, along with human papillomavirus (HPV) infection. Occupational exposure to certain substances is also a known risk factor. Risk factors for these cancers include wood dust exposure and nickel refining, with additional risk observed in leather workers, those exposed to hexavalent chromium, and textile workers exposed to cotton dust [55–58]. In countries that recognize laryngeal cancer as an occupational disease, its approval standards are the same as the criteria for lung cancer.

The potential association between asbestos exposure and laryngeal cancer has remained a subject of debate, with most reports on this topic based on older studies [59, 60].

To address this ongoing debate, Goldenberg et al. conducted a systematic review to examine the literature from 2000 to 2016 to assess the potential connection between asbestos and laryngeal cancer [61].

Among the five case-control studies included in the review, the odds ratios reported varied. Three studies considered smoking and alcohol exposure when determining odds ratios but did not find a significant correlation between asbestos exposure and laryngeal cancer. Two studies that did not account for smoking and alcohol exposure produced conflicting results, with only one suggesting a correlation with asbestos.

The ten cohort studies also presented diverse results. Some accounted for smoking and alcohol exposure and reported elevated risks of laryngeal cancer with asbestos exposure, while others did not find such an association. They concluded that confounding factors, varying study results, and a lack of mechanistic understanding contribute and will contribute to the ongoing debate [61].

Furthermore, a systematic search of electronic databases was conducted to identify relevant studies that investigated the relationship between occupational asbestos exposure and laryngeal cancer. The primary outcome measure for this meta-analysis was the standardized mortality rate (SMR), along with its associated 95% confidence interval (CI).

The meta-analysis revealed a statistically significant increase in the standardized mortality rate (SMR) for laryngeal cancer among individuals exposed to asbestos (SMR 1.69, 95% CI 1.45–1.97, $P < 0.001$). Also, the analysis identified specific factors that were associated with larger effect estimates, including cohorts predominantly consisting of male subjects, studies conducted in Europe and Oceania, employment in mining and textile industries, exposure to crocidolite asbestos, extended study follow-up periods exceeding 25 years, and SMR values for lung cancer exceeding 2.0 [62].

15.4 OVARIAN CANCER

Unlike the well-established link between asbestos exposure and lung cancer, mesothelioma, and other respiratory diseases, the evidence connecting asbestos exposure to ovarian cancer is less clear.

Some studies have suggested that asbestos fibers could theoretically reach the ovaries through the bloodstream after inhalation or ingestion. This has led to the hypothesis that asbestos fibers might contribute to the development of ovarian cancer [63, 64].

Several epidemiological studies have attempted to investigate this potential association, but the results have been mixed [65].

The difficulty in establishing a clear link may be due, in part, to the fact that ovarian cancer is a complex disease with multiple risk factors, including genetic factors, hormone use, reproductive history, and more. These confounding factors can make it challenging to isolate the specific impact of asbestos exposure.

Unlike lung cancer, where occupational exposure to asbestos is a well-known risk factor, the exposure levels and mechanisms for asbestos-related ovarian cancer are less defined. Occupational exposure to asbestos is less common among women compared to men, which further complicates the analysis.

Asbestos has been correlated to ovarian cancer since 1960, when Mr. Keal, an English physician, believed an increased incidence in women exposed to asbestos in occupational settings [66].

This connection recently returned to the limelight as Johnson & Johnson removed all baby powder products from North American markets because of thousands of claims by women affected by ovarian cancer who appealed that those were caused by asbestos. Supporting these claims is the declaration that baby powder talc could have contained asbestos [67–70].

Talc was also contained in several products other than baby powder, such as condoms, female diaphragms, birth control pills, and crayons [71].

Several observational studies connected the cosmetic perineal application of talc and ovarian cancer [72, 73].

However, a recently published large prospective study failed to find a higher rate of ovarian cancer in women who utilized perineal talc [74].

The IARC monograph contained a revision of the evidence connecting both asbestos and talc with ovarian cancer. In this book, considering the link between talc and ovarian cancer, just limited evidence of a connection was reported [75].

Many are the challenges in distinguishing between serous neoplasms of the peritoneum, such as ovarian cancer, and malignant mesothelioma using histology due to their similar morphology.

From a biological perspective, gene expression profiling and the analysis of key signaling components have been employed to investigate the similarities and differences between malignant mesothelioma and ovarian cancer.

For example, Davidson et al. used high throughput gene expression profiling to identify 189 distinct genes that were differentially expressed between ovarian cancer and malignant mesothelioma. Among these markers, they found MUC4, a transmembrane mucin that is upregulated in ovarian cancer effusions compared to primary carcinomas and solid metastases [76].

Another study validated the expression of tenascin-X, which showed increased expression in malignant mesothelioma effusions compared to ovarian/peritoneal serous carcinoma effusions. In contrast, tenascin-X was found to be absent in ovarian carcinoma biopsies, suggesting its potential utility in differential diagnosis [77].

Yuan et al. also demonstrated differential expression of folate receptor genes (FOL1 and FOL3) in serous effusions to distinguish between breast and ovarian origin and malignant mesothelioma [78].

These studies represent biomarker-guided investigations that help differentiate between seemingly similar diseases. They establish a workflow for identifying unique biomarkers and validating their potential diagnostic value.

However, the development of model systems that faithfully recapitulate the disease process is also crucial for a deeper understanding of these diseases.

Cheng et al. developed an intraperitoneal tumor model expressing mesothelin protein and producing ascites fluid, providing a controlled system for studying these diseases' characteristics and responses under various conditions. Notably, this model exhibited high levels of mesothelin expression, a characteristic shared by many ovarian cancers and malignant mesotheliomas. They also established a correlation between serum and ascites mesothelin levels and tumor burden in mice carrying these tumor cells [79].

Saito et al. discuss various aspects related to asbestos-related diseases (ARD-T) and asbestos consumption in Brazil, comparing mortality rates for ARD-T, lung cancer, and ovarian cancer in municipalities with high asbestos consumption (H-ASB) and other Brazilian municipalities. They highlighted that age-standardized mortality rates for pooled ARD-T, lung cancer, and ovarian cancer were notably higher in 29 municipalities with a history of high asbestos use compared to the rest of the country during the specified time frame. Asbestos-related health effects were not limited to occupational settings. The text suggests that environmental exposure to asbestos, such as dust emissions from nearby plants or domestic asbestos from water containers and roofing tiles, may contribute to mesothelioma incidence in women [80].

Furthermore, the clinical perspective and characteristics can be compared to evaluate the potential connection between ovarian cancer and malignant mesothelioma. These characteristics include their different etiologies, clinical and pathological findings, staging, surgical and chemotherapeutic approaches, and outcomes of treatment. While mesothelioma is definitively linked to asbestos exposure, there is limited evidence supporting a similar association between asbestos exposure and ovarian cancer. Despite this difference in etiology, both diseases exhibit similar disease progression patterns and clinical behaviors, making a comparison between ovarian cancer and mesothelioma more relevant than comparing either to benign pleural diseases.

Both diseases have non-specific symptoms, and there are no standardized screening guidelines for either. While ovarian cancer exclusively affects women, mesothelioma affects both genders, with a male predominance linked to occupational asbestos exposure. Clinical similarities include their propensity to spread like a sheet of tumor, leading to the production of ascites or pleural fluid. Both tumors tend to infiltrate tissue planes and surrounding structures without hematogenous metastasis, often causing symptoms due to external compression of adjacent structures.

Similarly, primary pleural mesothelioma or ovarian carcinoma metastatic to the chest presents with pleural tumor implants and pleural effusion, compressing the underlying lung. Biopsy is essential for distinguishing between these diseases, relying on specific markers to make an accurate diagnosis.

While distinguishing mesothelioma from adenocarcinoma histologically has historically been challenging, recent advances in immunohistochemical stains using marker panels have improved accuracy. Immunohistochemical staining can also provide insights into the biological behavior of these tumors.

Ovarian carcinoma can be subclassified into various subtypes, including papillary serous cystadenocarcinoma, adenocarcinoma, endometrioid tumor, mucinous carcinoma, clear cell carcinoma, and less common subtypes.

Surgery by oophorectomy is curative for early-stage ovarian cancer, whereas there is no accepted curative procedure for mesothelioma.

Cytoreductive procedures include pleurectomy/decortication and extrapleural pneumonectomy for mesothelioma, while peritonectomy with or without the resection of solid abdominal viscera is performed for ovarian carcinoma.

Response to cisplatin has been observed via intravenous and intrathoracic or intraabdominal administration, though results vary. Most experts advocate for a multimodal approach combining surgery, chemotherapy, and/or radiotherapy.

Survival rates for ovarian cancer vary based on stage, with 10-year survival ranging from 84% in stage IA to 11% in stage IIIC, while mesothelioma has a 5-year survival rate of under 15% for all stages [81].

15.5 RENAL CANCER

Kidney cancer is a significant health issue, with varying incidence rates worldwide, and several risk factors including genetics, lifestyle factors (smoking, obesity, hypertension), and environmental agents (solvents, pesticides, dust, diesel, etc.).

The association between asbestos exposure and kidney cancer remains controversial, prompting the need for an updated systematic review and meta-analysis of relevant studies.

Zunarelli et al. conducted a systematic review and meta-analysis of cohort studies focusing on workers exposed to asbestos in various industries. The study aimed to update previous research and included studies from 2001 to May 2020. The majority of cohorts were predominantly male and from Europe, with chrysotile asbestos being the main type of asbestos fiber. Pooled results showed a relative risk (RR) of 1.14 (95% CI 1.04–1.29) for kidney cancer mortality, with limited evidence of heterogeneity. The summary RR for cancer incidence was 0.98 (95% CI 0.79–1.22), and there was no evidence of heterogeneity. The authors concluded that the study's results showed no significant association between occupational asbestos exposure and kidney cancer. The limitations of the study included a small number of cancer incidence studies, potential survival bias in mortality studies, and low accuracy of cause-of-death data [82].

15.6 PROSTATE CANCER

The correlation between prostate cancer and asbestos exposure is a subject of ongoing research and debate in the scientific community.

Asbestos fibers can cause inflammation, oxidative stress, and genetic alterations in the body, which are factors that can contribute to cancer development. However, the specific mechanisms involved in prostate cancer are not well-established.

Research has explored whether the mode of asbestos exposure (respiratory inhalation vs. oral ingestion) plays a role in the development of prostate cancer.

Dutheil et al. findings suggest that respiratory inhalation of asbestos may be associated with an increased risk of prostate cancer, while oral ingestion of asbestos-contaminated water did not show statistical significance. This distinction is essential because it aligns with the well-established understanding of asbestos's lung and pleural toxicity. The carcinogenic mechanisms of asbestos exposure in prostate cancer involve oxidative stress, chronic inflammation, genetic and epigenetic alterations, cellular toxicity, and fibrosis [83].

There may be geographic variations in the relationship between asbestos exposure and prostate cancer. Dutheil et al.'s study also found that the risk of prostate cancer associated with asbestos exposure remained prevalent in Europe. This implies that European regions had a notable correlation between asbestos exposure and prostate cancer risk. The study hints that the differences in geographical findings may be related to a lack of epidemiologic monitoring surveillance in certain regions. Inadequate monitoring and data collection may lead to variations in the detection and reporting [84, 85].

On the other hand, Godono et al. conducted a systematic review and meta-analysis, providing evidence that men with occupational asbestos exposure do not appear to have a significantly increased risk of prostate cancer incidence and mortality compared to the general population. However, certain temporal and geographical variables, such as employment after 1960 and specific regions, were associated with slightly higher standardized incidence ratios (SIRs) or standardized mortality ratios (SMRs). Additionally, the study emphasizes the impact of methodological quality on the results, highlighting the need for well-designed research in this area. Overall, the findings suggest that the relationship between asbestos exposure and prostate cancer risk is not straightforward and may vary based on specific factors [86].

15.7 CONCLUSION

Asbestos, the "Hidden Killer," is not only responsible for death related to malignant mesothelioma. It is already well known that asbestos exposure is associated with several other cancers, with the most important in terms of frequency and mortality, lung cancer. However, while mesothelioma is definitively linked to asbestos exposure, there are still controversies in terms of diagnosis and compensation of asbestos-related lung cancer. Moreover, limited evidence supports the association between asbestos exposure and prostate, renal and ovarian cancer. Nevertheless, modifications in the type of exposure, which has changed from being mainly occupational to environmental, have made it more complex to establish whether there is an association between previous exposure and disease. Systematic studies are required to establish the health impact of asbestos exposure, even in future years, considering the long latency of asbestos-related malignancies and given that asbestos consumption in many municipalities hasn't been discontinued until recently.

REFERENCES

1. Asbestos, *IARC Monographs on the Evaluation of Carcinogenic Risk of Chemicals to Man Volume 14*, 1977.Lyon.
2. Kamp DW, Asbestos-induced lung diseases: An update. *Transl. Res.* 2009 Apr;153(4):143–152.
3. Mesothelioma Fact Sheet, *Cancer Today*, 2020. https://gco.iarc.fr/today/fact-sheets-cancers.
4. Straif K, Benbrahim-Tallaa L, Baan R, et al., A review of human carcinogens—Part C: Metals, arsenic, dusts, and fibres. *Lancet Oncol.* 2009;10(5):453–454.
5. Baumann F, Ambrosi JP, Carbone M, Asbestos is not just asbestos: An unrecognised health hazard. *Lancet Oncol.* 2013 Jun;14(7):576–578.
6. Cugell DW, Kamp DW, Asbestos and the pleura: A review. *Chest* 2004;125(3):1103–1117.
7. Roggli VL, Gibbs AR, Attanoos R, et al., Pathology of asbestosis- an update of the diagnostic criteria. Report of the asbestosis committee of the College of American Pathologists and Pulmonary Pathology Society. *Arch. Pathol. Lab. Med. Times* 2010;134(3):462–480.
8. Rubino GF, Concina E, Scansetti G, et al., Ricerca nella popolazione delle placche pleuriche calcifiche come segno radiologico di esposizione all'asbesto (crisotilo). Atti del Convegno di Studi sulla Patologia da Asbesto. Torino: 21 Giugno 1968:63–76.
9. Thomson JG, Graves WM Jr, Asbestos as an urban air contaminant. *Arch. Pathol.* 1966;81(5):458–464.
10. Donna A, Corpuscoli dell'asbestosi nel polmone umano reperiti nel comune materiale autoptico. Atti del Convegno di Studi sulla Patologia da Asbesto. Torino: 21 Giugno 1968:49–61.
11. Landrigan PJ, The third wave of asbestos disease: Exposure to asbestos in place: Public health control. *Ann. N. Y. Acad. Sci.* 1991;643:xv–xvi.
12. Baumann F, Buck B, Metcalf R, et al., The presence of asbestos in the natural environment is likely related to mesothelioma in young individuals and women in Southern Nevada. *J. Thorac. Oncol.* 2015;10(5):731–737.
13. Wylie AG, Candela PA, Methodologies for determining the sources, characteristics, distribution and abundance of asbestiform and non-asbestestiform amphibole and serpentine in ambient air and water. *J. Toxicol. Environ. Health* 2015 Part B 18:1–42.
14. Carbone M, Emri S, Dogan AU, et al., A Mesothelioma epidemic in Cappadocia: Scientific developments and unexpected social outcomes. *Nat. Rev. Cancer* 2007;7(2):147–154.
15. Fraire AE, Greenberg SD, Spjut HJ, et al., Effect of erionite on the pleural mesothelium of the Fisher 344 rat. *Chest* 1997;111(5):1375–1380.
16. Lacourt A, Gramond C, Rolland P, et al., Occupational and non-occupational attributable risk of asbestos exposure for malignant pleural mesothelioma. *Thorax* 2014;69(6):532–539.
17. WHO, *Regional Office for Europe. Air Quality Guidelines for Europe*, 2nd ed. Bilthoven, Netherlands: WHO Regional Publications, 2000.
18. Tossavainen A, Asbestos, asbestosis, and cancer: The Helsinki criteria for diagnosis and attribution. Consensus Report. *Scand. J. Work Environ. Health* 1997;23(4):311–316.
19. Klebe S, Leigh J, Henderson DW, et al., Asbestos, smoking and lung cancer: An update. *Int. J. Environ. Res. Public Health* 2019 Dec 30;17(1):258.
20. Henderson DW, Leigh J, Asbestos and carcinoma of the lung. In *Asbestos: Risk Assessment, Epidemiology and Health Effects*, 2nd ed., Dodson RF, Hammar SP, Eds. Boca Raton, FL: CRC Press/Taylor&Francis, 2011.
21. Van der Bij S, Koffijberg H, Lenters V, et al., Lung cancer risk at low cumulative asbestos exposure: Meta-regression of the exposure-response relationship. *Cancer Causes Control* 2013;24(1):1–12.
22. Gulino GR, Polimeni M, Prato M, et al., Effects of chrysotile exposure in human bronchial epithelial cells: Insights into the pathogenic mechanisms of asbestos-related diseases. *Environ. Health Perspect.* 2016;124(6):776–784.
23. Markowitz SM, Dickens B, Screening for occupational lung cancer: An unprecedented opportunity. *Clin. Chest Med.* 2020;41(4):723–737.

24. Driscoll T, Nelson DI, Steenland K, et al., The global burden of disease due to occupational carcinogens. *Am. J. Ind. Med.* 2005;48(6):419–431.
25. Boffetta P, Autier P, Boniol M, et al., An estimate of cancers attributable to occupational exposures in France. *J. Occup. Environ. Med.* 2010;52(4):399–406.
26. Brown T, Darnton A, Fortunato L, et al., British occupational cancer burden study group occupational cancer in Britain: Respiratory cancer sites: Larynx, lung and mesothelioma. *Br. J. Cancer* 2012;107(Suppl. 1):S56–S70.
27. Global Burden of Disease, Risk factors collaborators global, regional, and national comparative risk assessment of 79 behavioural, environmental and occupational, and metabolic risks or clusters of risks, 1990–2015: A systematic analysis for the global burden of disease study 2015. *Lancet* 2015;388:1659–1724.
28. Furuya S, Chimed-Ochir O, Takahashi K, et al., Global asbestos disaster. *Int. J. Environ. Res. Public Health* 2018;15(5):1000.
29. Lemen RA, *Asbestos Exposure among Seamen and Shipyard Workers.* Washington, DC: Committee on Merchant Marine and Fisheries, Subcommittee on Coast Guard and Navigation; United States. House of Representatives, 1980.
30. Lynch KM, Smith WA, Pulmonary asbestosis III: Carcinoma of lung in asbesto-silicosis. *Am. J. Cancer* 1935;24(1):56–64.
31. Gloyne SR, Two cases of squamous carcinoma of the lung occurring in asbestosis. *Tubercle* 1935;17(1):5–10.
32. Egbert DS, Geiger AJ, Pulmonary asbestosis and carcinoma. Report of a case with necropsy findings. *Am. Rev. Tuberc.* 1936;34:143–150.
33. Gloyne SR, A case of oat cell carcinoma of the lung occurring in asbestosis. *Tubercle* 1936;18(3):100–101.
34. Proctor RN, *The Nazi War on Cancer.* Princeton, NJ: Princeton University Press, 1999, pp. 73–119.
35. Nordmann M, Sorge A, Lungenkrebs durch Asbeststaub im Tierversuch. *Z. Krebsforsch.* 1941;51(2):170.
36. Enterline PE, Changing attitudes and opinions regarding asbestos and cancer 1934–1965. *Am. J. Ind. Med.* 1991;20(5):685–700.
37. Doll R, Mortality from lung cancer in asbestos workers. *Br. J. Ind. Med.* 1955;12(2):81–86.
38. Markowitz SB, Levin SM, Miller A, et al., Asbestos, asbestosis, smoking, and lung cancer. New findings from the North American insulator cohort. *Am. J. Respir. Crit. Care Med.* 2013;188(1):90–96.
39. Frost G, Darnton A, Harding AH, The effect of smoking on the risk of lung cancer mortality for asbestos workers in Great Britain (1971–2005). *Ann. Occup. Hyg.* 2011;55(3):239–247.
40. Olsson AC, Vermeulen R, Schuz J, et al., Exposure-response analyses of asbestos and lung cancer subtypes in a pooled analysis of case-control studies. *Epidemiology* 2017;28(2):288–299.
41. Karjalainen A, Anttila S, Vanhala E, et al., Asbestos exposure and the risk of lung cancer in a general urban population. *Scand. J. Work Environ. Health* 1994;20(4):243–250.
42. Arsenic, Metals, Fibres and Dust, *International Agency for Research on Cancer (IARC) Monographs.* Lyon, France: International Agency for Research on Cancer, 2012.
43. Keeling B, Hobson J, Churg A, Effects of cigarette smoke on epithelial uptake of non-asbestos mineral particles in tracheal organ culture. *Am. J. Respir. Cell Mol. Biol.* 1993;9(3):335–340.
44. Nelson HH, Kelsey KT, The molecular epidemiology of asbestos and tobacco in lung cancer. *Oncogene* 2002;21(48):7284–7288.
45. Churg A, Stevens B, Enhanced retention of asbestos fibers in the airways of human smokers. *Am. J. Respir. Crit. Care Med.* 1995;151(5):1409–1413.
46. Bach PB, Kattan MW, Thornquist MD, Kris MG, Tate RC, Barnett MJ, et al., Variations in lung cancer risk among smokers. *J. Natl Cancer Inst.* 2003;95(6):470–478.
47. de Koning HJ, van der Aalst CM, de Jong PA, et al., Reduced lung-cancer mortality with volume CT screening in a randomized trial. *N. Engl. J. Med.* 2020;382(6):503–513.
48. National Lung Screening Trial Research Team, Aberle DR, Adams AM, Berg CD, et al., Reduced lung-cancer mortality with low-dose computed tomographic screening. *N. Engl. J. Med.* 2011;365(5):395–409.
49. Oudkerk M, Liu S, Heuvelmans MA, et al., Lung cancer LDCT screening and mortality reduction—Evidence, pitfalls and future perspectives. *Nat. Rev. Clin. Oncol.* 2021;18(3):135–151.
50. Markowitz SB, Lung cancer screening in asbestos-exposed populations. *Int. J. Environ. Res. Public Health* 2022 Feb 25;19(5):2688.
51. Ten Haaf K, Jeon J, Tammemägi MC, et al., Risk prediction models for selection of lung cancer screening candidates: A retrospective validation study. *PLoS Med.* 2017;14(4):e1002277.
52. Krist AH, Davidson KW, Mangione CM, Barry MJ, Cabana M, Caughey AB, Davis EM, Donahue KE, Doubeni CA, Kubik M, Landefeld CS, Li L, Ogedegbe G, Owens DK, Pbert L, Silverstein M,

Stevermer J, Tseng CW, Wong JB, Screening for Lung Cancer: US Preventive Services Task Force Recommendation Statement . JAMA. 2021 Mar 9;325(10):962–970. doi: 10.1001/jama.2021.1117. PMID: 33687470.

53. *Recognition of an Industrial Accident Due to Asbestos.* Ministry of Health, Labour and Welfare. Japan, 2012. https://www.jisha.or.jp/english/topics/202307_19.html
54. Carvalho AL, Nishimoto IN, Califano JA, et al., Trends in incidence and prognosis for head and neck cancer in the United States: A site-specific analysis of the seer database. *Int. J. Cancer* 2005;114(5):806–816.
55. Awan KH, Effects of tobacco use on oral health - An overview. *Ann. Dent.* 2011;18(1):18–23.
56. Paget-Bailly S, Cyr D, Luce D, Occupational exposures to asbestos, polycyclic aromatic hydrocarbons and solvents, and cancers of the oral cavity and pharynx: A quantitative literature review. *Int. Arch. Occup. Environ. Health* 2012;85(4):341–351.
57. Clin B, Gramond C, Thaon I, et al., Head and neck cancer and asbestos exposure. *Occup. Environ. Med.* 2022 Oct;79(10):690–696.
58. Kamp DW, Asbestos-induced lung diseases: An update. *Transl. Res.* 2009 Apr;153(4):143–152.
59. Sen D, Working with asbestos and the possible health risks. *Occup. Med. (Lond.)* 2015 Jan;65(1):6–14.
60. Ries LAG, Melbert D, Krapcho M, et al., *SEER Cancer Statistics Review, 1975–2005. Surveillance, Epidemiology, and End Results Program, National Cancer Institute,* National Institutes of Health. http://seer.cancer.gov/archive/csr/1975_2005/.
61. Ferster APO, Schubart J, Kim Y, et al., Association between laryngeal cancer and asbestos exposure: A systematic review. *JAMA Otolaryngol. Head Neck Surg.* 2017 Apr 1;143(4):409–416.
62. Peng W, Mi J, Jiang Y, Asbestos exposure and laryngeal cancer mortality. *Laryngoscope* 2016;126(5):1169–1174.
63. Reid A, Heyworth J, de Klerk N, et al., The mortality of women exposed environmentally and domestically to blue asbestos at Wittenoom, Western Australia. *Occup. Environ. Med.* 2008;65(11):743–749.
64. Rai AJ, Flores RM, Association of malignant mesothelioma and asbestos related conditions with ovarian cancer: Shared biomarkers and a possible etiological link? *Clin. Chem. Lab. Med.* 2011 Jan;49(1):5–7.
65. Slomovitz B, de Haydu C, Taub M, et al., Asbestos and ovarian cancer: Examining the historical evidence. *Int. J. Gynecol. Cancer Off. J. Int. Gynecol. Cancer Soc.* 2021;31(1):122–128.
66. KEAL EE, Asbestosis and abdominal neoplasms. *Lancet* 1960;2(7162):1211–1216.
67. Dyer O, Jury awards $4.7bn damages against Johnson & Johnson in talcum cancer case. *BMJ* 2018;362:k3135.
68. Hall v. Johnson & Johnson, Civil Action No.: 18–1833 (FLW) (D.N.J. Dec. 27, 2019).
69. Hsu T, Rabin RC, Johnson & Johnson to end talc-based baby powder sales in North America. *The New York Times,* 2020. https://www.nytimes.com/2020/05/19/business/johnsonbaby-powder-sales-stopped.html.
70. Dyer O, Johnson & Johnson recalls its baby powder after FDA finds asbestos in sample. *BMJ* 2019;367:l6118.
71. Longo DL, Young RC, Cosmetic talc and ovarian cancer. *Lancet* 1979;2(8138):349–351.
72. Cramer DW, Welch WR, Scully RE, et al., Ovarian cancer and talc: A case-control study. *Cancer* 1982;50(2):372–376.
73. Huncharek M, Muscat J, Perineal talc use and ovarian cancer risk: A case study of scientific standards in environmental epidemiology. *Eur. J. Cancer Prev.* 2011;20(6):501–507.
74. O'Brien KM, Tworoger SS, Harris HR, et al., Association of powder use in the genital area with risk of ovarian cancer. *JAMA* 2020;323(1):49–59.
75. Black C, Dioxide T, IARC monographs on the evaluation of carcinogenic risks to humans. https://monographs.iarc.fr/ wp-content/uploads/2018/06/mono93.pdf.
76. Davidson B, Baekelandt M, Shih IeM. MUC4 is upregulated in ovarian carcinoma effusions and differentiates carcinoma cells from mesothelial cells. *Diagn. Cytopathol.* 2007;35(12):756–760.
77. Yuan Y, Nymoen DA, Stavnes HT, et al., Tenascin-X is a novel diagnostic marker of malignant mesothelioma. *Am. J. Surg. Pathol.* 2009;33(11):1673–1682.
78. Yuan Y, Nymoen DA, Dong HP, et al., Expression of the folate receptor genes FOLR1 and FOLR3 differentiates ovarian carcinoma from breast carcinoma and malignant mesothelioma in serous effusions. *Hum. Pathol.* 2009;40(10):1453–1460.
79. Cheng WF, Hung CF, Chai CY, et al., Generation and characterization of an ascitogenic mesothe- lin-expressing tumor model. *Cancer* 2007;110(2):420–431.
80. Saito CA, Bussacos MA, Salvi L, et al., Sex-specific mortality from asbestos-related diseases, lung and ovarian cancer in municipalities with high asbestos consumption, brazil, 2000–2017. *Int. J. Environ. Res. Public Health* 2022 Mar 19;19(6):3656.

81. https://www.cancer.org/cancer/types/ovarian-cancer/detection-diagnosis-staging/survival-rates.html.
82. Zunarelli C, Godono A, Visci G, et al., Occupational exposure to asbestos and risk of kidney cancer: An updated meta-analysis. *Eur. J. Epidemiol.* 2021 Sep;36(9):927–936.
83. Dutheil F, Zaragoza-Civale L, Pereira B, et al., Prostate cancer and asbestos: A systematic review and meta-analysis. *Per. M. J* 2020;24:19.086.
84. Subramanian V, Madhavan N, Asbestos problem in India. *Lung Cancer* 2005 Jul;49(Suppl. 1):S9–S12.
85. Le GV, Takahashi K, Park E-K, et al., Asbestos use and asbestos-related diseases in Asia: Past, present and future. *Respirology* 2011 Jul;16(5):767–775.
86. Godono A, Clari M, Franco N, et al., The association between occupational asbestos exposure with the risk of incidence and mortality from prostate cancer: A systematic review and meta-analysis. *Prostate Cancer Prostatic Dis.* 2022 Apr;25(4):604–614.

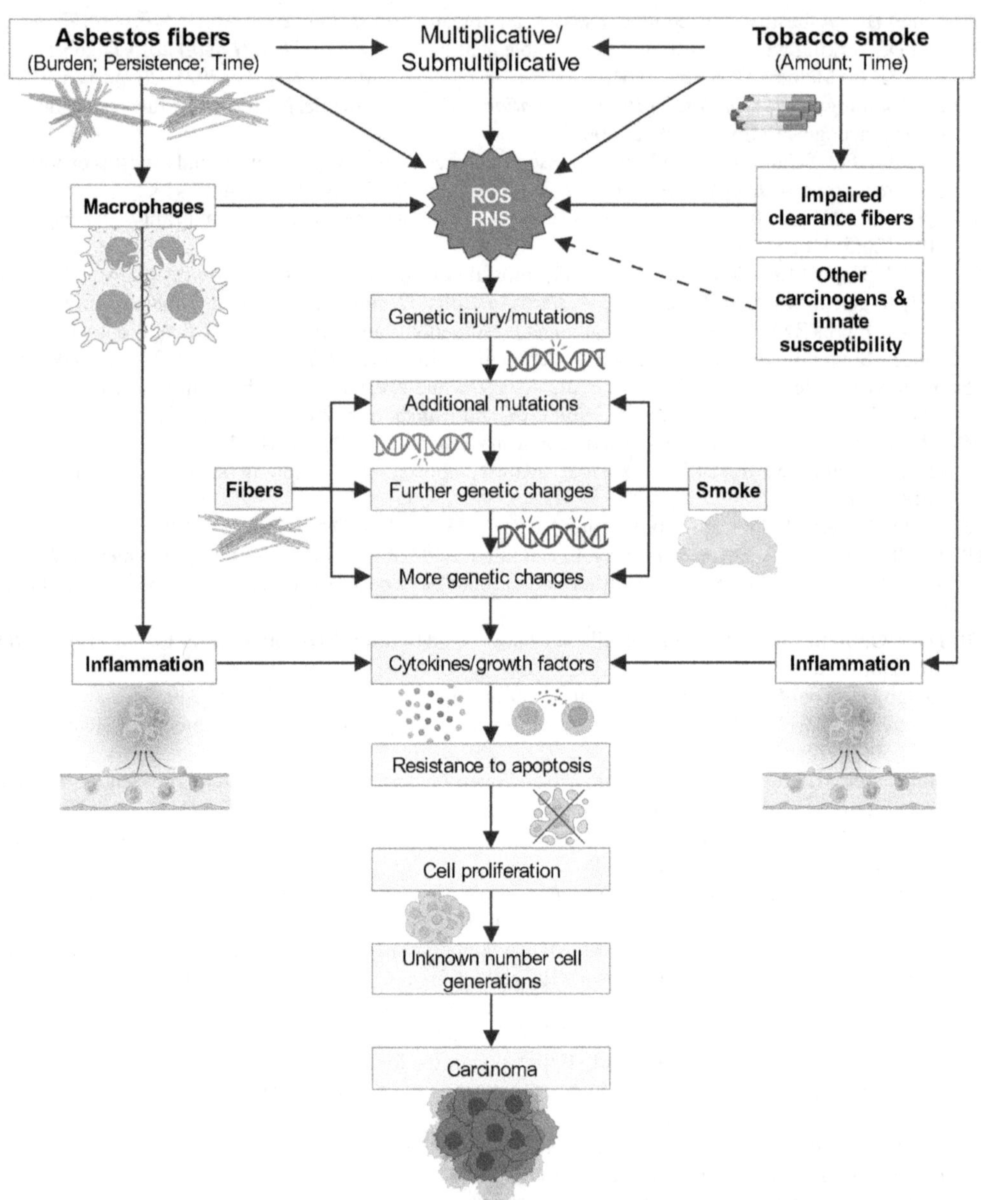

FIGURE 15.1

16 Asbestos Litigation and Trust Funds in the United States

Alan Brayton, Ellen Tenenbaum, and Craig Zimmerman

16.1 INTRODUCTION

Asbestos personal injury litigation in the United States is the world's first, largest, and longest-running mass tort. The first strict products liability asbestos case, *Tomplait*, was filed in Texas in December 1966. In the almost 60 years since, more than 1 million asbestos personal injury claims have been filed against over 10,000 different defendants in every state and federal court of general jurisdiction in the United States. More than 100 companies have gone into bankruptcy citing asbestos personal injury litigation as a principal cause. In connection with federal legislation considered during the mid-2000s, several experts then estimated the total cost of asbestos litigation in the United States, including legal expenses, would be between $250 billion and $300 billion: there is every reason, now 20 years later, to believe these estimates were low.

An asbestos personal injury claim includes any attempt to obtain compensation based upon an individual's assertion that he or she (or the decedent, in a wrongful death case), was exposed to some form of asbestos[1] released from one or more products for which one or more defendant businesses is legally responsible, and that this exposure either caused or significantly contributed to a bodily injury.[2] Such claims are asserted against asbestos product manufacturers and distributors, contractors, and others who installed or disturbed those products, as well as against the owners and operators of worksites at which asbestos products were present and used (a/k/a "premises" cases). Historically, most claimants asserted occupational exposures in heavy industrial, construction, or shipbuilding settings. In more recent years, a higher percentage of claimants have based their claims on nonoccupational exposures, such as exposures during home remodeling or "shade-tree" automotive brake changes, as well as "take home" exposure from parents or other relatives. The injuries claimants allege almost always fit into one of four categories: (a) a type of diffuse malignant mesothelioma (i.e. pleural, peritoneal, tunica vaginalis, or pericardial); (b) lung cancer; (c) another cancer linked to asbestos (e.g. kidney); or (d) a nonmalignant asbestos-related condition, ranging from severe asbestosis to asymptomatic scarring of the lungs (pleural plaques).

In the United States today, asbestos claimants can pursue compensation through either or both of two tracks.[3] A claimant can file a lawsuit in federal or state court, naming as defendants the entities the claimant contends are legally liable for his or her injury. This track is the litigation or "tort system" track. In addition, depending upon the nature of the alleged exposures and the entities that may be liable for them, a claimant may pursue compensation from one or more of the approximately 60 operating trusts which have been established through bankruptcy proceedings since the first trust – the Manville Personal Injury Settlement Trust ("Manville Trust") – was established in 1988. This is the "trust system" track. The tort and the trust system tracks for claim compensation are *not* mutually exclusive: a claimant may pursue claims against defendants through a lawsuit in the tort system and seek additional recovery by filing claims against various trusts, simultaneously or sequentially.

At the outset, it is important to acknowledge at least two points. The foundational factual predicate for asbestos litigation as a mass tort is that millions of workers and others were, in fact, exposed to asbestos products and, for many years, provided no warning of the potential risks arising from exposure. And, each individual's asbestos claim is important to the claimant and his or her family,

DOI: 10.1201/9781003431909-16

presents facts unique to the claimant, and deserves to be resolved in a manner that comports with due and fair process to the claimant and the defendants. With that said, the number of asbestos claims filed in the tort system has frequently overwhelmed judicial and private party resources, often for years at a time. As discussed more fully below, from the mid-1990s to the mid-2000s, tens of thousands of new asbestos lawsuits were filed each year.[4] Not surprisingly, then, those involved in asbestos litigation frequently think and speak of claims in the aggregate and observe trends based upon these aggregations.

The contours of asbestos litigation have changed dramatically since 2007. Today, far fewer claims are filed in the tort system: however, these claims – primarily filed by those diagnosed with cancer – have much greater individual resolution value (a claim's value in settlement or at trial). Although there is no definitive or official count of the number of claims filed each year, the best current estimate available is that there are approximately 3,550 new asbestos tort cases filed each year, of which approximately 1,859 allege mesothelioma and another 1,251, lung cancer.[5]

This chapter discusses the following:

- The evolution of asbestos claims in the tort system, from the legal developments which made such claims possible starting in the mid-1960s through the litigation's more recent transition to focus on cases involving mesothelioma and lung cancer;.
- The nature of asbestos claims in the tort system today, as well as the types of case management approaches adopted by the courts most active in the litigation, which, in turn, have a significant impact on how litigated claims are resolved.
- A discussion of the similarities and differences between asbestos litigation and "talc" litigation, which is, depending on one's point of view, either identical to or a close cousin to asbestos litigation.[6]
- The anatomy and representative progress of a hypothetical asbestos claim in the tort system.
- The evolution of asbestos bankruptcy trusts and the conditions necessary for their establishment.
- An overview of how such trusts operate and how claims are evaluated and compensated.
- Some of the current and most controversial strategies and issues impacting asbestos claims and litigation.

Finally, the reader should know that practically every issue – factual and legal – that touches in any way on asbestos litigation or trusts is heavily contested, normally by skilled and zealous advocates passionately committed to their point of view (or to the points of view of their clients). Your authors' objective is to provide as useful and *neutral* a presentation of the asbestos litigation and trust landscape as we can. To the extent it appears we have taken sides on a currently contested issue, that was not our intent.

16.2 HISTORICAL DEVELOPMENT OF THE LITIGATION THROUGH 2007

16.2.1 Before the Beginning (to 1966)

Before the mid-1960s, individuals injured by defective products in the United States normally had little recourse against the manufacturers of the offending products. This was because claims for compensation for such injuries were limited to traditional causes of action at common law. Throughout the nineteenth century and the first 60 years of the twentieth century, an injured party's claims based upon a defective product were largely limited to claims for negligence and/or for breach of an implied warranty of fitness.

These common law causes of action created substantial barriers to an injured party's recovery in a product injury situation. They were largely developed before mass production and distribution and were ill-suited to handle claims arising from goods sold into a national economy. Negligence – a tort claim – required a claimant to prove that a manufacturer's conduct fell below the reasonable standard of care (i.e. what an objectively reasonable manufacturer would have done in the same circumstances). Before the advent of modern discovery practice (discussed further below), a claimant had little hope of learning what the manufacturer had done in terms of care or diligence concerning product safety, much less being able to prove the manufacturer's conduct was culpable. Even after discovery became available, proving that a manufacturer acted negligently was a prohibitive burden for most plaintiffs.

Breach of warranty claims were even more limited. Because breach of warranty claims are contract claims (i.e. the common law governing agreements), such claims were normally subject to contract defenses, including lack of privity (i.e. that the claimant was a "stranger" to the sale of the product, meaning not the buyer). Even in those jurisdictions where the privity requirement was relaxed or eliminated, recovery on breach of warranty claims was often foreclosed or limited by other defenses.

The lack of a meaningful common law remedy for accident victims was a particular focus of several judges, legal academics, and leading tort lawyers throughout the 1940s and 1950s, especially as the number of automobile fatalities increased dramatically. In the early 1960s, two separate state supreme courts – in New Jersey and in California – changed some of their requirements for common law claims, to make claims by accident victims against product manufacturers more viable.[7] Most importantly, in 1964, the American Law Institute (ALI)[8] adopted and, in 1965, published the Restatement Second of Torts ("Second Restatement").

The Second Restatement included two principles that made products' liability claims (like asbestos personal injury claims), possible:

- Section 402A of the Second Restatement provides that a manufacturer (or distributor) is strictly liable for physical harm arising from a product defect which makes the product unreasonably dangerous to the user or consumer. A product can be "defective" due to a defect in its manufacture or design, or because the warnings provided by the manufacturer are absent or inadequate. Whether a product is "unreasonably dangerous," per the Second Restatement, is to be gauged based upon the expectations of an objectively reasonable, informed consumer.[9]
- Section 431 of the Second Restatement provides that an actor is liable for physical harm to another if their action (or inaction, where action was required), was a substantial factor in bringing about the harm. The actor's conduct need not be either a necessary or independently sufficient cause: the conduct need only be adjudged by a jury to have contributed "substantially" to the claimant's harm.[10]

Section 402A's strict liability provision was a significant innovation in the common law, not just a "restatement" of existing common law. It was an innovation, however, whose time had plainly come: almost every US jurisdiction adopted some version of 402A's strict products' liability by the early 1970s. Section 431's "substantial factor" causation standard was more rooted in existing law because many jurisdictions had already adopted standards for proving causation when multiple torts were involved. However, the Second Restatement's formulation of the standard as "substantial factor" (and not a more rigorous standard), was influential in leading many jurisdictions to modify their own causation standards to clarify that plaintiffs could demonstrate harm from multiple tortfeasors.

The nature and timing of these changes in the law set the stage for asbestos personal injury litigation in the United States. At precisely the same time that Dr Selikoff and his Mount Sinai colleagues' work linking asbestos exposure to an epidemic of disease was gaining national attention in the mid-1960s, the common law in many jurisdictions was changing to allow claimants to pursue claims based upon the harmful nature of the products at issue, without regard to the reasonableness of the asbestos producer's conduct. Under Section 402A, a plaintiff could sue an asbestos products manufacturer based on the allegation that its product was unreasonably dangerous, due to its design or the lack of a warning: the plaintiff *did not* need to prove that the manufacturer had been negligent. Equally important, Section 431's "substantial factor" test opened the way for a plaintiff to allege that many different asbestos exposures contributed to his or her illness, without the obligation to prove that each exposure was necessary or sufficient, by itself, to cause the plaintiff's illness.

16.2.2 The Early Years of Litigation (1966-1982)

In 1966, Claude Tomplait filed the first asbestos strict products liability lawsuit in Beaumont, Texas.[11] Tomplait, a career insulator, had severe asbestosis. Tomplait alleged that asbestos insulation exposures at 26 different job sites caused his asbestosis and sought recovery from 11 asbestos suppliers and asbestos insulation manufacturers. After a one-week trial, the jury returned a verdict for the defendants.

In 1969, Tomplait's lawyer, Ward Stephenson, filed a similar lawsuit on behalf of one of Tomplait's co-workers, Clarence Borel. Like Tomplait, Borel was a career insulator diagnosed with severe asbestosis and his lawsuit identified a number of different job sites at which he alleged exposure to insulation manufactured by a number of different companies. Like Tomplait, Borel asserted claims in strict liability for defective products, including claims based on the manufacturers' failure to warn of the potential health effects of working with asbestos insulation. Unlike Tomplait, Borel won at trial.

In a comprehensive, landmark decision, *Borel v. Fibreboard Paper Prod. Corp.*,[12] the United States Court of Appeals for the Fifth Circuit affirmed the trial court's judgment for Borel. The court's opinion outlined Borel's work history as an insulator, starting in the 1930s, and then provided a somewhat detailed recitation of when information about the hazards of asbestos in the workplace became available to the public health community. In light of this evidence, the Fifth Circuit panel concluded that the trial court did not err in submitting Borel's failure to warn claims to the jury, nor was the jury's verdict holding defendants liable for such failure reversible. With regard to defendants' challenge to Borel's showing of causation arising from multiple exposures at various sites to various products contributing to his cumulative exposure and illness, the *Borel* court held:

> In the instant case, it is impossible, as a practical matter, to determine with absolute certainty which particular exposure to asbestos dust resulted in injury to Borel. It is undisputed, however, that Borel contracted asbestosis from inhaling asbestos dust and that he was exposed to the products of all the defendants on many occasions. It was also established that the effect of exposure to asbestos dust is cumulative; that is, each exposure may result in an additional separate injury. We think, therefore, that on the basis of strong circumstantial evidence the jury could find that each defendant was the cause in fact of some injury to Borel.[13]

The *Borel* decision had a profound impact, both because of its substance and because of its timing. The substance of the decision – affirming the liability of key asbestos defendants for their failure to warn in light of public health information available as early as the 1930s and agreeing that cumulative causation could be acceptable – sent a powerful signal to the legal community nationally that asbestosis personal injury claims were viable. Moreover, the *Borel* decision was issued in late 1973, at a time when the ubiquitous use of asbestos and its potential health hazards were receiving a great deal of public attention.[14] Not surprisingly, a good many similar lawsuits were filed around the country in the years immediately following *Borel.* By 1978, an estimated 1,000 such claims had been filed.[15]

Although many suits were filed in the 1970s, asbestos defendants were often successful at trial arguing that they could not have appreciated the hazards of working with asbestos until the 1960s. Defendants' trial success began to change in the late 1970s. Evidence discovered by plaintiffs in various cases produced a host of revelations about asbestos manufacturers' conduct, both alone and in concert, which undermined their defenses and prejudiced them in jurors' eyes. For instance, a

Johns-Manville Corp. ("JM") plant manager acknowledged in deposition that it was company policy for decades (and well into the 1970s), to *not* tell employees of physical changes to their lungs caused by asbestos exposure when these findings were revealed by annual company-mandated physicals. Philip Carey Manufacturing Co., a significant asbestos insulation manufacturer, hired a nationally recognized occupational health expert to evaluate the risks of its asbestos products in the early 1960s: the company fired the expert immediately after he warned the company it could be sued by workers harmed by its products.[16]

Even more damning was evidence demonstrating that supposedly competing manufacturers had collaborated to suppress public health information about asbestos. Correspondence from the 1930s and 1940s to and from Sumner Simpson, the long-time Chair of Raybestos-Manhattan, concerning asbestos was discovered. The "Sumner Simpson papers" contained letters between Simpson and Vandiver Brown, JM's General Counsel, on the topic of suppressing asbestos health information.[17] In addition, Simpson's papers included exchanges from about the same time with the editors of "Asbestos," a widely read trade publication, in which Simpson urged the magazine to not publish information on asbestosis: the magazine complied. Finally, the papers included evidence of a set of animal studies concerning the health effects of asbestos, commissioned by six companies and conducted at Saranac Laboratories in New York. Related documents revealed that the sponsoring companies – all leading manufacturers of asbestos products – retained significant control over what results from the study, if any, would be made public. When the study results were finally published – *18 years* after the studies were first commissioned – the companies exercised that control. For instance, all references to potential links between asbestos and cancer which might be drawn from the study data were removed.[18]

As a result of these and other revelations, plaintiffs in many jurisdictions were able to proceed on negligence claims and were permitted to add claims for conspiracy and fraud, in addition to strict products' liability. These additional claims allowed plaintiffs to introduce evidence of defendants' knowledge and conduct, and plaintiffs could often pursue punitive, as well as compensatory, damages.[19] Asbestos defendants increasingly lost at trial and the amounts of the verdicts against them increased as well.

JM was the dominant supplier of raw asbestos and asbestos products in and to the United States for decades. Consequently, JM was named as a defendant in the vast majority of lawsuits filed. In August 1982, JM commenced bankruptcy proceedings in the Eastern District of New York. JM filed for bankruptcy protection notwithstanding its significant financial wherewithal because, it said, although it had already resolved 4,000 asbestos claims, there were still approximately 16,000 pending lawsuits and an unknown number of future asbestos injury claims, with total liability estimates exceeding $2B.[20]

16.2.3 Ending One Wave and Beginning a Second (1982–2001)

The JM bankruptcy was not the first asbestos bankruptcy filed,[21] but it was the most significant. Given JM's dominance of the US asbestos market, it was implicated in almost every asbestos claim filed. When JM commenced its bankruptcy reorganization case (also known as "Chapter 11"), every asbestos plaintiff also became a bankruptcy claimant. Moreover, the JM bankruptcy posed a number of new and unresolved questions, such as whether bankruptcy protection is available to a debtor which is not in immediate financial distress but faces overwhelming prospective toxic tort liability, and how to address – if at all – claims that had not yet accrued and may not accrue for decades.[22] As discussed below, how the court and parties in the JM Chapter 11 approached and resolved these novel issues established the template for all future asbestos bankruptcies.

More immediately, because all litigation against debtors in bankruptcy is automatically stayed, the JM Chapter 11 filing removed one of the most important defendants from the tort system. JM's exit – and the potential that other significant defendants would do the same – led plaintiffs and their counsel to look more broadly at other potential sources of asbestos exposure and other potentially liable parties. Thus, for instance, asbestos textile manufacturers were increasingly named as defendants, as were manufacturers of various noninsulation asbestos products used in shipbuilding and industrial settings, such as packing and gaskets. This cycle – the exit or diminution of one type of defendant leading to the seeming focus by plaintiffs and plaintiffs' counsel on a different set of asbestos-containing products or different industries, often referred to as "waves" – is a recurring and ongoing feature of asbestos litigation in the United States. It started in response to JM's exit from the tort system: it continues to this day. One successful asbestos plaintiffs' counsel is widely quoted as having described asbestos litigation as an "endless search for a solvent bystander."[23]

From its inception through at least the mid-2000s, asbestos litigation principally concerned workplace exposures. Claimants were largely identified with and by their job sites. Heavy industrial facilities (e.g. chemical plants and steel mills), shipyards, power plants, and refineries were commonly the job sites at issue. State and federal courts in jurisdictions where such industries concentrated became dockets of choice for new lawsuits, for instance: Cleveland and Pittsburgh (steel mills and other heavy industry); Boston, Baltimore, Norfolk, VA, San Francisco, and Oakland (shipyards); New York City (power plants); and, Texas and Mississippi (petrochemical plants and refineries), to name just a few. The widespread use of asbestos products at those types of facilities created an enormous volume of discrete exposures, connected back to a broad array of defendant manufacturers and suppliers. Organizations with close connections with workers at those facilities – especially labor unions – established programs to assist workers in identifying exposure and retaining counsel. Finally, the predominant injury alleged was nonmalignant lung scarring, because asbestos scarring could be evidenced by chest x-rays even in the absence of significant impairment of pulmonary function. The number of potential claimants was enormous. Many filed claims. The judicial system was overwhelmed with tens of thousands of new lawsuits, starting in the 1980s.

As new claims flooded the courts, those involved in asbestos litigation experimented with new approaches to managing litigation at volume. Courts in many jurisdictions consolidated all their asbestos cases onto a single "docket," managed by one or two dedicated "asbestos" judges in accordance with court-imposed or plaintiff/defense bar-negotiated procedural orders. For instance, all asbestos claims filed in state court in and around New York City were (and still are) assigned to a single judge for pretrial proceedings and litigated in accordance with the procedures established in the New York City Asbestos Litigation (NYCAL) case management order. After many years of refusing to do so, the Judicial Panel on Multi-District Litigation created MDL No. 875 in 1991, assigned to a federal trial court judge in Philadelphia. All asbestos personal injury and wrongful death cases then pending in the federal courts (and all such claims filed thereafter) were transferred to MDL No. 875 for pretrial coordination. Approximately 26,000 cases were initially transferred.[24]

From late 1991 through approximately 1999, certain plaintiffs' counsel and the most active defendants (organized as the "Center for Conflict Resolution" or "CCR") used the critical mass generated by the creation of the MDL to make a concerted effort to find a "global resolution" to asbestos litigation through a federal class action. A "class action" is a procedure by which one or a handful of individual plaintiffs sue defendants as representatives of all potential claimants similarly situated vis-à-vis the claims at issue. Whether the proposed class treatment can be approved (or, "certified"), depends upon the nature of the relief plaintiffs seek, the degree to which the proposed class representative's claims and interests are truly representative of those of other class members, and, finally, whether the claims asserted are fairly subject to single universal resolution. Class certification is often denied because individual issues predominate over collective issues. If class treatment is certified by a court, however, the result of the case binds all members of the class.

In 1994, the parties agreed upon a proposed class action settlement, the overall effect of which would have been to resolve most pending and almost all future asbestos personal injury claims. The trial court certified the class and approved the settlement in 1994, but the intermediate appellate court reversed and rejected it in 1996.[25] In *Amchem Prods. Inc. v. Windsor*, 521 U.S. 591 (1997), the United States Supreme Court held that the settlement, as presented, could not satisfy federal class action certification requirements. The Court's discussion of the specific problems presented by the settlement strongly suggested that there was no class action vehicle which could work as a global settlement. Two years later, an attempt to obtain a class settlement to resolve all claims against just a single defendant was also rejected by the Supreme Court, in *Ortiz v. Fibreboard Corp.*, 527 U.S. 815 (1999) (class action when only a "limited fund" is available *not* proper where funds are limited only by virtue of the parties' agreement and allocation scheme is inadequate given conflicting interests among putative class members). By the end of the 1990s, then, any hope for a global solution through the judiciary outside of bankruptcy was essentially extinguished.

While these efforts were ongoing at the federal level, cases continued to be filed and litigated in state courts. Many of these claims were the result of an increasing number of "mass screenings." In general, some organizations (a law firm or union) would arrange to have a mobile radiology unit set up in a location – a union hall, for instance – near a worksite or worksites for a day or several days and publicize its availability in advance to workers at those sites. Such units could take x-rays of 100s of workers per day. A small core of radiologists certified as B-readers[26] would then review the x-rays and frequently diagnose the minimum radiographic result necessary to support a claim. Mass screening events were typically associated with one or more law firms willing to file lawsuits on each worker's behalf. Many of the mass screenings took place in southern states: Texas and Mississippi were favored venues for mass screening claim filings. As a result of mass screenings, the volume of new asbestos claims filings went up dramatically. It is estimated that the number of lawsuits filed doubled from 100,000 to 200,000 between 1990 and 2000: approximately 90,000 new claims were filed in 2001 alone.[27] Although exact estimates were and are impossible, it appears that well over half of the newly filed claims were filed by plaintiffs with no then-present impairment of pulmonary function.[28]

When JM and others commenced bankruptcy proceedings in the 1980s, the parties relied on the bankruptcy courts' general equitable powers to provide permanent relief. In 1988, the JM plan of reorganization was confirmed, establishing the Manville Trust to liquidate all current and future asbestos claims, and a channeling injunction was issued, making the trust the exclusive remedy available to any Manville claimant. There were, however, serious questions as to whether a bankruptcy court had sufficient legal authority to do what the JM court had done. To settle those questions and to provide others with the bankruptcy option JM had pursued, Congress enacted 11 U.S.C. δ 524(g)–(h) in 1994. As discussed in greater detail below, δ 524(g) permits a debtor in bankruptcy to resolve its existing and *future* asbestos liabilities through the establishment of a trust to pay those claims, and the issuance of a channeling injunction, which requires all asbestos claims against the debtor (and other related entities) to be brought to the trust alone for resolution.[29]

16.2.4 Bankruptcies, Failed Legislation, and "Tort Reform" (2001–2006)

Considering the number of new claims being filed and the absence of any foreseeable "global resolution," a number of prominent asbestos defendants went into bankruptcy between 2000 and 2004. Insulation manufacturers (e.g. W.R. Grace,[30] Owens-Corning, Pittsburgh-Corning), refractory manufacturers (e.g. Halliburton, A.P. Green, NARCO), boiler makers (e.g. Babcock & Wilcox), and others involved in heavy industry (e.g. Combustion Engineering), all sought bankruptcy protection with an eye toward a δ 524(g) result. In almost every case, the companies claimed they were financially distressed only or primarily because of the overwhelming number of pending and future asbestos claims. For instance, when North American Refractories Company (a small, mostly regional refractories manufacturer) commenced its bankruptcy in early 2002, it had approximately 115,000 open asbestos claims.

History repeated itself. As the most-often named defendants exited the litigation into bankruptcy and, ultimately, to the trust system, plaintiffs identified and pursued many new defendants. For instance, both automobile and automotive brake manufacturers became more frequent targets.[31] So did the makers of asbestos-containing construction products, including joint compound (used with drywall at most construction sites), plaster/stucco, wall texture, and acoustic ceiling. Many of these claimants did have some occupational exposure as a mechanic or from construction experience. However, in a break with the past, an increasing percentage of claims were brought based upon "do-it yourself" or "at home" nonoccupational work involving over-the-counter asbestos-containing products.

There had been calls on Congress for many years to "fix" the asbestos litigation crisis,[32] though proposed asbestos litigation reform legislation made almost no progress before 2003. By then, however, the high number of filings and the succession of bankruptcies by large and otherwise seemingly healthy corporations created an environment in which a nationwide legislative solution appeared both necessary and politically viable. From 2003 through early 2006, legislation to establish a nationwide trust for asbestos claim compensation made significant progress in the United States Senate. As proposed, the government-administered trust would have been funded primarily by mandated contributions from asbestos defendants and insurers in a total amount of over $140B, to be distributed to asbestos claimants over time as their exclusive remedy, applying claims criteria akin to those already in use by the various asbestos bankruptcy trusts.[33] The proposal which made the most progress was S.B. 852, the "Fairness in Asbestos Injury Resolution Act of 2005" or FAIR Act. Notwithstanding intense lobbying for passage by a number of parties from both sides of the litigation, the FAIR Act fell one vote short of passing a procedural hurdle in February 2006 and, thereafter, stalled entirely. No asbestos litigation reform legislation proposed in Congress since the FAIR Act has come as close to passage. No comprehensive reform legislation is, as of this writing, expected anytime soon.

The high number of new case filings in the late 1990s and early 2000s aggravated the crisis in many state courts. No court system is designed to manage tens of thousands of new toxic tort cases each year. Many of these cases were filed by individuals with no present serious functional impairment – just an allegation of asbestos exposure and a report from a certified B-reader of radiographic findings related to prior asbestos exposure. Many of the cases that alleged minimal current injuries alleged a fear of developing cancer and the need for medical monitoring to assess the progression of disease and early detection of malignancy. Most jurisdictions at that time did not have mechanisms in place to prioritize cases based upon plaintiff's alleged physical condition – so in states like Texas and Mississippi, where most of these claims were filed, the cases of unimpaired plaintiffs frequently clogged the courts and delayed the progress of other plaintiffs with more significant conditions.

State courts in crisis and the intense attention created by the Senate's consideration of asbestos litigation reform legislation, together, created enormous pressure to find solutions. Added to this mix were assertions that many of the mass screenings produced claims that were meritless and/or fraudulent. In June 2005, Judge Janis Jack of the US District Court for the Southern District of Texas issued a scathing 249-page opinion in the *silica* litigation MDL, dismissing thousands of claims.[34] Judge Jack's opinion focused on abuses in the "mass screening" process, which produced thousands of meritless silicosis and asbestosis claims, and on the "sharp practices" of some plaintiffs' firms involved, which cavalierly filed claims without regard for merit in an attempt to maximize leverage and potential recovery. In particular, Judge Jack recounted the diagnostic practices of a small group of certified B-readers, who appeared to conduct pro forma x-ray reviews for the sole purpose of making a legally actionable diagnosis without regard to the minimum attention required by any reasonable medical standard of care. Judge Jack's opinion led to Congressional hearings on the "mass screening" practice (in connection with the FAIR Act), which further discredited the practice,[35] and to a number of asbestos bankruptcy trusts barring any reliance by claimants on reports generated by the identified B-readers.[36]

Each of the state courts or individual jurisdictions with significant asbestos litigation took some action to clear their dockets and prioritize claims of those alleging a more serious current injury, such as mesothelioma and lung cancer. The Texas legislature, for instance, assigned all new asbestos cases filed in the state to a single judge for pretrial coordination and barred nonmalignant cases from proceeding beyond filing a complaint in the absence of medical proof of physical impairment.[37] Florida also adopted minimum medical claims criteria, which deferred claims by unimpaired plaintiffs.[38] In Mississippi, the state Supreme Court held that joining hundreds of claims together in a single action without detailed claims information – as was the practice with many unimpaired claims – was improper[39] and enforced new venue rules which significantly disadvantaged filings by out-of-state plaintiffs (effectively ending and unwinding mass filings in the state). Courts in other jurisdictions – NYCAL, Philadelphia, and Madison County for example – adopted case management regimes which assigned nonmalignant cases to deferred or inactive dockets, permitting such claims to move beyond their initial filing only after the claimant produced evidence of sufficient physical impairment.[40]

16.3 CURRENT STATE OF ASBESTOS CLAIMS IN THE TORT SYSTEM (2007 FORWARD)

This history set the stage for and informs the operation of the asbestos personal injury claim systems – tort and trust – in the United States today:

- There is no realistic expectation that either Congress or the judicial branch will provide any comprehensive asbestos litigation solution, like that proposed in the FAIR Act or by the class action settlement in *Amchem*. An asbestos defendant who wants to end the uncertainty associated with litigation and achieve a permanent resolution of all claims has very few options. One alternative is bankruptcy and a § 524(g) trust. A significant number of defendants have pursued that option. The only other option typically involves a comprehensive divestiture of the liabilities often with a corporate reorganization. In either scenario, the cost to the defendant is likely to approximate the total estimated cost of litigating and resolving claims over the life of the liability (i.e. total costs for the next 25–45 years).
- Every jurisdiction in which asbestos claims are litigated has some rule, express or de facto, which prioritizes cases involving plaintiffs alleging mesothelioma, lung cancer, another cancer, and severe asbestosis – frequently prioritized in that order.[41] In part as a result of the rules and reforms adopted deferring the majority of nonmalignant claims, there are no longer mass filings in the tort system alleging asbestos exposure but no impairment. The number of new tort system claims filed nationwide has dropped from a high of approximately 90,000 in 2001 to approximately 3,550 in 2022: the vast majority of claims now filed in the tort system allege the claimant has mesothelioma or lung cancer.
- The general evidentiary case for liability at trial (e.g. knowledge of asbestos hazards over time) is well-rehearsed by both the plaintiff and defense bar, as is each side's respective position with regard to broader issues such as legal duty and causation. This is not to say these issues are settled: they are not. Each of the plaintiff and defense bar has distinct views on these issues and those positions clash in practically every case. It is to say, however, that asbestos trial practice has matured to the point where the most important issues at trial tend to be: (a) factual issues focused on the individual parties involved, plaintiff, and defendants; (b) legal issues that either plaintiffs or defendants believe are open to favorable change through appeal in that jurisdiction; or, (c) in particular cases, the admissibility and meaning of cutting-edge scientific findings (e.g. genetic causation). For these reasons, most courts treat asbestos personal injury cases as among their most complex cases pending trial.
- The wave of bankruptcy cases filed in the 2000–2004 period by the most frequently named asbestos defendants concluded with the establishment of individual trusts to pay asbestos claims, and the issuance of channeling injunctions requiring claims against the parties protected by those injunctions to be pursued exclusively against the trusts. This means at least two things. First, the companies most substantially responsible for the use of raw asbestos and asbestos insulation in the United States are no longer in the tort system. Defendants

> today tend to be businesses which used asbestos in a narrower range of products and/or have succeeded to businesses that sold asbestos-containing products. Second, there are approximately 60 operating asbestos bankruptcy trusts from which claimants can recover, currently holding total assets estimated at $30 billion.

This changed litigation landscape dove-tailed well with ongoing changes in the pool of potential plaintiffs. The industrial use of asbestos in the United States declined significantly throughout the late 1970s and early 1980s. For instance, the US Navy stopped using asbestos products on new ships in 1980 and removed a significant amount of asbestos from its fleet by 1985. Similarly, most industries that had used asbestos heavily found alternatives by the early 1980s and often, earlier. The most intense occupational asbestos exposures – i.e. those likely to cause asbestosis – were at least 25 to 30 years or more in the past by the mid-2000s. The generation of workers which had had the heaviest occupational exposure to asbestos was declining and younger generations did not and would not have comparable exposures. In short, the number of individuals with significant workplace exposure was and is shrinking.

Unlike other asbestos-related diseases, causation attribution in mesothelioma cases arguably does not depend upon intense or prolonged exposure to asbestos. There is consensus that mesothelioma is a dose-related disease: however, medical science has not established a threshold exposure below which there is no observable risk of disease. Moreover, because the causative dose at issue is to some degree "cumulative," expert witnesses testifying in the tort system have been permitted to attribute mesothelioma causation, in part, to what might otherwise be viewed as minimal or nominal asbestos exposures (e.g. a handful of at-home automotive brake changes, a single home remodeling project using asbestos-containing joint compound). Because the standard for legal causation in most jurisdictions is "substantial factor" – permitting almost any contribution to cumulative dose to be considered by juries – such minimal or nominal exposures have led to defendant liability.

A significant and largely contemporaneous broader cultural change has also impacted the tort and trust systems: how most claimants learn they might have compensable claims. Before the mid to late 2000s, claimants were largely identified through their job sites or trades, and frequently through their unions. Even in nonunion situations, most plaintiff recruiting efforts focused on industrial facilities or shipyards. More recently, by virtue of advertising, the internet, and relationships cultivated between plaintiff firms and diagnosing physicians, claimants increasingly learn about their potential legal claim as a result of their diagnosis. In other words, once diagnosed with mesothelioma, a patient (or their family) looking for information about the disease will inevitably be made aware, through one channel or another, of the availability of legal representation. Any person who has watched commercial television in the United States in the past 10–15 years will be familiar with the near-ubiquitous advertising by a number of plaintiff firms directed at persons diagnosed with mesothelioma and lung cancer. Anyone who searches "asbestos" or "mesothelioma" on the internet will get dozens of plaintiff law firm websites as their response.[42]

The typical plaintiff with mesothelioma making a tort claim today, therefore, is different from the typical mesothelioma plaintiff of 25 years ago. Circa 2000, such a plaintiff most likely had occupational exposures either at or from a heavy industrial or shipbuilding site: the principal issues in the case revolved around which products he or she had been exposed to. Today, a plaintiff with mesothelioma is unlikely to have had as much, if any, occupational asbestos exposure, but instead alleges some combination of minimal workplace exposure (e.g. asbestos abatement at the office), exposures from avocational activities (e.g. at-home brake changes), and/or "take home" or "bystander" exposure to asbestos from parents or older relatives who did have heavy workplace exposures when the claimant was a child. Product identification remains a key issue in such cases, but causation – i.e. was the exposure of a nature sufficient to contribute to causing disease – is ordinarily a focal point.

The nature of the claimant's disease and their credible history of asbestos exposure will often dictate which of the two compensation tracks, tort or trust, their claim will take and how it will proceed. In general, claimants diagnosed with mesothelioma who had any plausible asbestos exposures associated with companies that have not been through bankruptcy will file claims in the tort system. To a lesser degree, claimants with little or no smoking history and diagnosed with lung or another asbestos-related cancer may do the same. These tort claimants will likely also assert claims against various bankruptcy trusts, either contemporaneously with or subsequent to the resolution of their tort claims. Claimants whose exposure is limited entirely to products for which bankruptcy trusts are responsible, as well as those with nominal impairment, will generally pursue compensation only through the trusts.

A significant driver for many plaintiffs and their counsel for whether to pursue claims in the tort system is economics. Litigation is both time-consuming and potentially expensive for plaintiffs and their lawyers. Mesothelioma claims *can* (but do not always) garner significant judgments at trial. Over time, the amounts awarded by juries to mesothelioma plaintiffs have significantly increased, with some awards well in excess of $10 million. As a consequence, such claims often command significant (albeit lesser) sums in settlement from defendants who perceive a judgment risk. A lung cancer or other cancer case, with the right facts, can likewise result in a significant verdict, and, therefore, can generate a substantial settlement. The potential returns in these cases may make litigation a worthwhile investment. Other claims, however, are likely to produce far less return in litigation and, in the absence of especially efficient plaintiffs' counsel, will cost the claimant and counsel more in prosecuting the case than they are likely to recover.

By contrast, as reflected below in the discussion regarding trust claims processing, asserting a claim against a bankruptcy trust is neither time-consuming nor cost prohibitive. Preparation of the claim material requires only a moderate investment of time and effort by claimants and their counsel and most trusts do not charge filing or processing fees. There is little downside to making claims against a trust when a claimant is able to potentially satisfy the trust's claims criteria. Although the amounts recovered from any single trust are typically less than settlements in the tort system, the aggregate recovery from all trusts against which a claimant might file can be significant.

16.3.1 Tort System Causes of Action and Defenses

A plaintiff initiates an asbestos personal injury lawsuit, like any lawsuit, with the filing of a "complaint." The function of a complaint is to put the defendants on notice of the basic facts underlying the plaintiff's claims and the specific legal causes of action the plaintiff asserts entitles him or her to recovery. The content of asbestos complaints will vary greatly from jurisdiction to jurisdiction and is, in many jurisdictions, dictated by rules adopted specifically for asbestos litigation. So, for instance, individual plaintiffs file long-form, more detailed complaints in Madison County, Illinois: in NYCAL, plaintiffs file a short-form complaint, largely devoid of facts, together with an information sheet intended to provide sufficient plaintiff-specific information to allow the court and defendants to preliminarily assess a plaintiff's claims.

There is a laundry list of possible causes of action a plaintiff can assert and many assert them all, depending upon local practice. Negligence (e.g. negligent design, negligent failure to warn), breach of warranty, fraud, and conspiracy claims are common. In almost every jurisdiction, however, plaintiffs assert and proceed to trial primarily on theories based upon strict products' liability. In most jurisdictions, to recover on strict products' liability claims, a plaintiff at trial must prove by a preponderance of the evidence that:

- The product at issue was "defective" at the time it was placed in the stream of commerce by the defendant (a manufacturer or distributor). In asbestos cases, two types of "defects" can be at issue: design defect and failure to (adequately) warn. "Design defect" requirements vary from state to state, but the most common tests are: (a) whether the product created a risk of harm that an objectively reasonable consumer would not anticipate arising out of the product's ordinary use or foreseeable misuse (the "consumer expectations" test)[43]: or, (b) the risk of harm created by the design exceeded the utility of the product, when taking into account the availability of reasonable alternative designs (the "risk/utility" test).[44] In a failure to warn case, a manufacturer is liable if it fails to warn (or to adequately warn) against a known or reasonably foreseeable risk that would not be obvious to a reasonable consumer. Because manufacturers did not place *any* warnings on asbestos-containing products until the late 1960s, failure to warn claims predominated early in the history of asbestos litigation. Most manufacturers did put warnings on their asbestos-containing products by the mid- to late 1970s, so what is now frequently at issue is whether the manufacturer's warning was adequate. In addition, design defect claims have become more important: in other words, plaintiffs often contend that the product at issue was defectively designed *because* it contained asbestos.

- The risk of harm created by the defect was known or reasonably foreseeable to the defendant based upon the ordinary use or foreseeable misuse of its product. Since *Borel*, asbestos manufacturers and distributors have been held to the standard of experts. In most jurisdictions, this means any manufacturer who used asbestos in its products is chargeable with whatever health information was in the published literature (anywhere) at the time the product was sold.
- The defect caused or was a "substantial factor" in causing injury to the plaintiff.
- The plaintiff does, in fact, suffer from the injury that he or she alleges, arising from his or her exposure to the defendant's product.

Although strict products' liability claims are most common, plaintiffs additionally pursue negligence claims in many jurisdictions. The principal difference between a strict liability claim and a negligence claim is that the former focuses on the nature of the product, whereas the latter claim focuses on the defendant's conduct. In many jurisdictions, it is the negligence claim which makes the defendant's alleged past misconduct relevant and admissible and which may support an award of punitive damages in jurisdictions where such damages are allowed.

Defendants generally have a range of responses they can deploy in opposition to plaintiff's complaint. The most common of these are:

- Product identification: defendant contends that the plaintiff is mistaken about exposure to its product or, alternatively, that the product to which plaintiff alleges exposure did not contain asbestos.
- Causation: defendant contends that the alleged exposure to its product could not have contributed to plaintiff's injury, because of the nature of the asbestos in its product (e.g. processed chrysotile), the nature of the alleged exposure (e.g. insufficient duration and/or intensity), or both. Causation is discussed in greater detail in the hypothetical below.
- Diagnosis: defendant contends that the plaintiff (or decedent, in wrongful death cases) does not have the disease he or she alleges or that the disease at issue was not caused by asbestos exposure. Thus, for instance, individuals diagnosed with well-differentiated papillary mesothelioma have pursued asbestos claims, notwithstanding the absence of evidence linking this benign condition to asbestos exposure. The fact that the condition shares the name "mesothelioma" with diffuse malignant mesothelioma is often enough, by itself, for the plaintiff to seek some recovery.

Once the plaintiff has filed his/her complaint and the defendants have responded, the parties move into the "discovery" phase – the period of time for all sides to seek information from each other and third parties, including expert witnesses, and to develop the evidence they will each present at trial. Discovery – again, as illustrated in the hypothetical below – is the most time-consuming, labor-intensive, and lengthy phase of any litigation. The scope of permissible discovery, the obligation to provide complete and accurate discovery responses, and the manner and means of conducting discovery are all governed by court rules. There are court rules governing discovery in all civil cases:

in most jurisdictions with active asbestos dockets, these rules have been modified for asbestos cases by courts through comprehensive case management orders.

16.3.2 Jurisdictions: Differing Case Management Approaches

The rules and process by which courts move cases from the filing of plaintiff's complaint through discovery to trial are generally referred to as "case management." Every court with any significant asbestos docket has adopted some form of case management regime specific to these cases. The regimes vary widely from jurisdiction to jurisdiction and frequently have unique or differing requirements that are the outgrowth of that jurisdiction's own particular history in attempting to manage its asbestos litigation crisis. In many jurisdictions – like NYCAL – expertise in the local asbestos case management process can be akin to a distinct professional specialty.

Case management regimes when compared, however, do fall along an identifiable spectrum defined by the degree to which a jury trial in any given case is probable and, therefore, anticipated by the court and parties. At one end of this spectrum are jurisdictions, such as Madison County, that have case management regimes that heavily incentivize and depend upon the pretrial settlement of all or almost all cases filed. At the other end of the spectrum are jurisdictions, such as Alameda County, California (Oakland), that have case management regimes in which the expectation of all parties is that a case is more likely to need to go to trial to be resolved. Other case management regimes can be placed along the range between these two extremes: Texas, for instance, with its centralized pretrial procedures that increase the opportunities for pretrial resolution and narrow the opportunities for getting to trial, is closer to Madison County; NYCAL, Philadelphia, and Florida, for instance, are closer to Alameda.

Where a plaintiff's case is filed, therefore, will have a significant impact on the case's likely outcome. Madison County has been the most active jurisdiction in terms of new mesothelioma cases filed for some years: for example, of the 1,859 new mesothelioma cases filed in 2022, 832 were filed in Madison County. It is expected that all of these cases will be resolved through settlement, without the need for trial, at some point during the discovery or final pretrial phases. It is rare for Madison County to have even one asbestos jury trial go to verdict in a year.[45] By contrast, only 57 mesothelioma cases were filed in Alameda County in 2022, but a number of mesothelioma cases start trial and go to verdict in that jurisdiction every year.

16.3.3 The Emergence of "Talc" Litigation (2009 into the future)

Talc has been mined and milled for many uses, both industrial and commercial, since at least the late nineteenth century. Very early on in talc's use, it was understood that at least some deposits used to obtain industrial-grade talc were intermingled with asbestos, including amphibole asbestos.[46] Miners and millers of industrial talc have always been among the claimants involved in asbestos personal injury litigation. In such cases, one key issue has been whether the talc deposits to which the plaintiff alleges exposure were, in fact, among those contaminated with asbestos and, if so, with what type and at what concentration.

Whether and the degree to which talc used for consumer or cosmetic purposes has been contaminated with asbestos, however, is a much more controversial topic. Although talc has many consumer uses, talcum powder is principally associated with baby powder, which was sold in the United States for approximately 120 years. A number of companies were involved in mining, milling, and distributing cosmetic grade talcum powder, including Johnson & Johnson (whose name was for many years synonymous with "baby powder").

A *detailed* history of the controversy concerning whether baby powder contained fibrous asbestos or the same minerals in nonfibrous form, what hazards those minerals posed, and what baby powder producers and distributors knew or should have disclosed about asbestos in their products, is beyond the scope of this chapter.[47] However, a brief summary will help put the current situation in context. In the late 1960s and early 1970s, research by Dr Selikoff's group at Mt. Sinai indicated that the then-marketed baby powder contained some small percentage of asbestos.[48] The federal Food & Drug Administration (FDA), in response, began to consider adopting a testing and content standard for asbestos in baby powder. Seeking to preempt FDA action, the cosmetics industry, through its trade association (with the involvement of Johnson & Johnson management), adopted a testing standard for asbestos in talc that appeared to satisfy the FDA regulators then in place. The FDA did not proceed with or adopt a talcum powder standard: instead, the industry applied its testing protocol to demonstrate that baby powder was "asbestos-free," and the status quo was largely maintained from the early days of asbestos litigation (the mid-1970s) through approximately 2009. However, there were criticisms of the industry testing standard at the time it was adopted as not sufficiently sensitive to detect amphibole asbestos in concentrations of concern and not capable of identifying chrysotile asbestos at any protective detection level. These criticisms persisted throughout the decades and have become more robust over the past 15 years as the litigation over these issues has intensified.

From the mid-1970s through approximately 2009, cosmetic talc suppliers were only rarely named in asbestos litigation. In 2009, plaintiff Deane Berg sued Johnson & Johnson in the federal court in South Dakota, alleging that her use of Johnson & Johnson baby powder had caused her ovarian cancer. The *Berg* case went to trial in 2013, resulting in a plaintiff verdict, but the jury awarded no damages. Over the course of the next few years, Johnson & Johnson was largely successful in litigation, either winning at trial or on appeal in most of its cases. Eventually, however, it suffered some very widely reported trial defeats (especially in St. Louis), including a $72 million verdict in the *Fox* case in 2016 and a $4.69 billion award to 22 plaintiffs in the *Ingham* case in 2018.[49] The notoriety of these results and a nationwide push by certain plaintiffs' firms generated thousands of plaintiffs with ovarian cancer who had used baby powder and alleged that use contributed to the onset of their disease. As of October 2021, Johnson & Johnson had approximately 38,000 ovarian cancer claims pending.[50]

It is important to note a significant change in the substance of the ovarian cancer causation case presented by plaintiffs over time. In early cases, such as *Berg*, the plaintiff contended that talc itself (as opposed to asbestos fibers in talc), caused her cancer. In *Ingham* (tried in 2018) and later cases, the plaintiffs have more often contended that it was the "asbestos" in talc that caused ovarian cancer. Although there is little scientific evidence that talc, alone, can contribute to cancer, there is obviously an established body of evidence that asbestos causes cancer.

Given the view of certain plaintiffs' experts that mesothelioma can be caused by only a minimal asbestos exposure, individuals diagnosed with mesothelioma in recent years have also pursued "talc" claims against talcum powder manufacturers and distributors. Johnson & Johnson was named as a defendant in less than two dozen mesothelioma claims over the course of the first 36 years of asbestos litigation. Between 2017 and October 2021, it was named as a defendant in 1,345 cases.[51]

Through October 2021, Johnson & Johnson was the predominant (but far from the only) defendant named in talc litigation. It largely took the position that it would not settle cases and tried a significant number to verdict, with results indicated above. In October 2021, Johnson & Johnson pursued a strategy, more fully discussed below, of executing a corporate divisive merger under Texas law and having one of the corporate entities created by the demerger – LTL Management LLC – file for Chapter 11 bankruptcy protection and pursue a § 524(g) trust resolution of all talc claims. As of this writing, litigation arising from this Johnson & Johnson strategy is ongoing in federal court: talc claims continue to be pursued separately against all defendants in state and federal courts throughout the country.

16.3.4 Hypothetical Asbestos Case: Process and Issues

A walk-through a hypothetical case illustrates many of the dynamics in play in current asbestos cases in the tort system. We choose a hybrid "trial" jurisdiction, meaning one that treats asbestos cases like other civil cases seeking monetary damages, with certain special case management procedures. As noted above, some jurisdictions have asbestos case management procedures that serve to incentivize defendants to undertake large group settlements, some have case management procedures that streamline the process of litigating cases and prioritizing cases for trial, and some dockets (frequently those with fewer numbers of asbestos cases) treat cases like any other individual civil case seeking monetary damages. Our hybrid jurisdiction provides that a living plaintiff diagnosed with mesothelioma may seek an expedited trial date, thus accelerating all case deadlines and litigation of the case.[52]

In this hypothetical, the plaintiff, Ron Hammond, is a living 58-year-old man who has been diagnosed with peritoneal mesothelioma. The plaintiff's diagnosing physician advises him that peritoneal mesothelioma is caused by asbestos exposure, but Ron has no knowledge of having been exposed to asbestos. Through online research, Ron contacts a national law firm, which acts as a clearinghouse to help him find an appropriate lawyer. Ron is referred to a plaintiff law firm with significant experience assisting individuals in developing their cases to seek damages for alleged asbestos-related injuries. This law firm has deep trial experience in numerous jurisdictions, with several of its trial lawyers claiming some of the largest jury awards ever in asbestos cases. The law firm files Ron's case in one of those high-jury-award jurisdictions, though Ron does not live there (known as "forum-shopping") and seeks an expedited trial date.

16.3.4.1 Plaintiff Complaint and Defendant Answer

Based on the law firm's exposure investigation, Ron files a complaint against two companies that manufactured joint compound, two boiler companies, and four companies that manufactured or distributed asbestos-containing brake linings. This is somewhat unusual as complaints in many jurisdictions name in excess of 40 defendants who may be in some measure responsible for a plaintiff's injuries. Ron's complaint alleges that his exposure occurred as a result of asbestos brought home on the clothing of his father, Andy, and grandfather, Martin, who lived with his family when he was a child. Martin was an auto mechanic who changed brakes regularly. Andy was a construction worker on mostly commercial and industrial worksites: he assists his son's law firm by identifying construction-related products he worked with or around that contained asbestos. Martin, with Andy, also did brake changes on the side for family and friends ("shade-tree" brake work). As a child, Ron was sometimes nearby during the shade-tree brake work. Martin is deceased and Andy, who is 84 years old, has end-stage renal disease, so is frequently fatigued and sometimes confused.

The claims Ron asserts in his complaint include strict liability failure to warn, negligent failure to warn, breach of warranty, and conspiracy. The jurisdiction where Ron's case is filed allows for both strict liability and negligence claims (many allow only strict liability claims or require the plaintiff to choose between proceeding on negligence or strict liability, but not both). This can be a benefit for a plaintiff as the negligence claim provides an opportunity to focus on the conduct of the defendant, not just the nature of the product. Juries can find the defendant "bad behavior" narratives compelling.

In this typical scenario, each defendant files a responsive pleading either admitting or denying factual allegations in the complaint and asserting affirmative defenses. Defenses typically asserted include challenges to product identification and causation (through denial of factual allegations), and certain legal (affirmative) defenses. Legal defenses such as challenges based on statute of limitations or lack of the court's jurisdiction over the defendant are common. Though not in play in the hypothetical *Hammond* case, there are also certain defendant or product-specific defenses that can be available, such as a government contractor defense (immunity based on producing the product at issue as specified and required by the federal government) or, in some jurisdictions, the "bare metal" defense (no duty to warn imposed on manufacturer of non-asbestos product that required the use of another manufacturer's asbestos-containing component to function in its intended manner). A complex legal defense that is relevant to Hammond's claims is that a defendant had no legal duty to the plaintiff for a "take-home" exposure.[53] This issue is treated differently in different jurisdictions: in some, a "take-home" duty is firmly established, in others a "take-home" duty is imposed only for the time period after which courts have determined a defendant "should have known" of a potential "take-home" risk. Thus, the time period of the plaintiff's exposure can be critical in a "limited take home duty" jurisdiction; the *Hammond* case is venued in such a jurisdiction.

All defendants in the *Hammond* case assert that they had no legal duty to the plaintiff for "take-home" exposures that resulted from the work of the plaintiff's grandfather and father. All defendants also deny all factual allegations associated with Ron's exposure and product identification, and further deny that any exposure to their products caused his disease.

16.3.4.2 Discovery

The discovery phase of a case involves the court-mandated exchange of information and documents related to the case and occurs in connection with specific court rules concerning the timing and the scope of discovery allowed. Asbestos cases typically include a fact discovery period and an expert discovery period. Each stage is time-limited by court deadlines. In fact discovery, a plaintiff, and defendant must each respond to written questions concerning case facts posed to each other (interrogatories), produce to each other pertinent documents requested, and then depose witnesses under oath concerning relevant factual information. Similarly, in most (but not all) jurisdictions, the parties may serve interrogatories related to experts and expert opinions and may depose those experts after they serve reports that elucidate their expert opinions.

Fact discovery is the opportunity each side has to develop their factual side of the case: thus, the plaintiff seeks to explore, substantiate, and bolster product allegations such as product composition, expected use, and dates of manufacture and distribution. The plaintiff also seeks support for the circumstances under which he/she claims exposure to the asbestos-containing products. Conversely, defendants seek to raise questions about and undermine plaintiff exposure allegations. So, in the *Hammond* case, the plaintiff's counsel seeks to expedite the deposition of Andy, Ron's father, who is in poor health, to preserve his recollections of his own work and that of Martin, his father, as Andy may be the only source of such information given the passage of time. At deposition, defendants explore whether Andy is competent to testify given his age and illness, whether he or Martin have living co-workers or other family members who can corroborate or dispute Ron's and Andy's allegations, whether there is any evidence of other exposures, the extent to which Andy's and Martin's work with asbestos-containing products pre-dated Ron's birth, the frequency of such exposures over time (when did they end, were they infrequent after Ron was born), and so on.

There are often disputes concerning the scope of discovery allowed, and the parties commonly resort to the court to resolve those disputes. For example, in the hypothetical, the plaintiff firm seeks broad written and document discovery into the type of asbestos used by each defendant, the full range of the types of the defendant's products that incorporated asbestos, and the duration of the defendant's use of asbestos in products, seeking to expand Ron's alleged exposure. Each defendant, however, seeks to limit the plaintiff's discovery to facts around the defendant's use of asbestos in the specific product/products to which Ron alleges exposure and to thoroughly explore, define, and thus limit his exposure. How the court resolves these issues varies: the allowable scope of discovery differs from jurisdiction to jurisdiction and, sometimes, from court to court within a single jurisdiction. Disputes that arise routinely in deposition include the scope issues noted above, as well as a deposing lawyer questioning the witness on topics not included in the deposition notice or perceived harassment of the witness. Plaintiff complaints can also include the failure of a corporate or company witness to have knowledge and be able to testify about appropriate topics. The fact discovery process is often highly contested and fraught with opportunities and risks that may shift the strength of a case for the plaintiff and defendant.

In fact discovery in the *Hammond* case, the parties learn that there are no living co-workers of Martin who might be able to provide or contradict product identification, or elaborate on potential alternative exposures. Andy, however, testifies in deposition that Martin did mechanic work at a General Motors dealership for some years in the 1960s and 1970s, implicating Delco (GM-branded replacement brakes), and that he and Martin used only two brands of brakes for "shade-tree" brake work from the 1960s to the 1980s. Andy, struggling with his memory and poor health, is unable to remember any specific brand of joint compound he worked with, though he knows he used it from the late 1950s to at least the 1980s. He does name two boiler manufacturers whose boilers he assisted in installing and then tearing out in the early 1970s, at three or four industrial facilities. Based on historic product information available to the plaintiff's law firm, the plaintiff can show that the boilers were manufactured with insulation that contained asbestos in the 1950s to the 1960s.

At his deposition, Andy also names two companies that manufactured insulation he installed at several industrial facilities during their initial construction, during the 1950s and through the 1960s. Since these manufacturers went out of business and dissolved long ago with no successors, there is no legal recourse against them. However, defendants will argue at trial that this alternative "take home" exposure in the 1960s is the actual cause of Ron's disease, because the insulation products contained a more dangerous type of asbestos.

16.3.4.3 Experts

Expert witnesses participate in asbestos cases to address a myriad of mostly causation-related scientific issues, though they may also address disease diagnosis when it is in question. Both the plaintiff and defendants bring experts to trial to testify about their competing and contrary opinions. There are differing standards for admissibility of expert testimony at trial across jurisdictions. In most jurisdictions, the standards can be summarized as: the expert's opinion is admissible if it is reliable and grounded in accepted scientific methodology and is also helpful to the jury, meaning relevant to the case issues. The applicable legal evidentiary standards are different from the rigors applied in the world of scientific research and academia.

The range of subject matter covered by expert witnesses in asbestos cases can be wide: pathology, epidemiology, molecular biology, genetics, material science, state-of-the-art, historical product type and use, and more. In our hypothetical, the plaintiff's counsel discloses only three experts (molecular biology, pathology, and material science), and defendants disclose several more, which is typical. Defending against causation arguments is difficult for defendants. The level of public awareness of the disease risk associated with "asbestos" generally is high due to an extensive litigation history, regulatory treatment of asbestos including workplace protections, and pervasive attorney advertising.[54] Most potential jurors have a much vaguer understanding of the nuances of critical causation issues, however. Defendants, to make their case, must educate jurors on such issues, including different asbestos fiber types used and their impact on the human body, the importance of the quantum, frequency, and duration of exposure, and other potential causes of disease.

Each party in a lawsuit must disclose experts to other parties by a date set by the court, and in many jurisdictions, must serve expert reports that explain the entirety of the experts' opinions and the bases for those opinions. In expert discovery, parties may serve on one another the same types of discovery used in fact discovery: interrogatories, document requests, and (in most jurisdictions) notices of deposition. Through these tools, parties explore the nature and scope of expert opinions, expert bias and expert credibility. The goal of expert discovery is generally to develop tools to challenge the admissibility of experts and their opinions, or to use in trial to undermine the credibility of the testifying expert and the merits of his or her opinions.

In asbestos litigation, it is common for the same experts to appear again and again. Thus, Ron Hammond is likely to use experts with whom his law firm has established relationships so his trial counsel knows exactly what each expert's opinions will be and how strong he or she will be testifying in deposition and at trial. The same is true of most experts retained by defense firms. This phenomenon makes asbestos case experts particularly susceptible to arguments that they are not offering independent professional opinions but are acting as advocates for a particular side of the causation debate. Bias arguments can be compelling for jurors and can sway case outcomes.

16.3.4.4 The Causation Debate

Causation is the most hotly contested issue in present-day asbestos cases. To understand the basics of the causation debate, it is necessary to have a brief tutorial on asbestos fiber types.[55] "Asbestos" is a family of minerals with certain mineralogical characteristics, only some of which were used commercially (amosite, crocidolite, and chrysotile). Notwithstanding their common "family" association, the commercially used types of asbestos have different physical and chemical traits and toxicological potencies, thus different risks of causing disease. Early asbestos litigation grew out of the use of asbestos in shipyards and heavy industrial plants, on-board ships, and by insulators. Most of those products contained amosite and/or crocidolite, among the more potent types of asbestos known as amphiboles.

It is widely (but not exclusively) believed that amphibole asbestos types were and are the primary cause of mesothelioma, and this has given rise to the "chrysotile defense" utilized by some defendants whose products contained only chrysotile asbestos.[56] After the wave of asbestos bankruptcies in 2000–2004, it was no longer possible to sue most of the companies responsible for putting amphibole asbestos into the stream of commerce in the United States. In the intervening years, plaintiffs have targeted products containing chrysotile asbestos, and many plaintiffs have had low-dose exposures associated with nonoccupational work. Most causation experts testifying for plaintiffs are of the opinion that all fiber types cause disease[57] and that mesothelioma is a "signature disease" for asbestos exposure, meaning that if an individual has mesothelioma, the individual must have had some causative asbestos exposure even if it is unknown or minimal. Moreover, many plaintiff experts believe and will testify that "every fiber counts," meaning all exposures, no matter how minimal, contributed to causing plaintiff's disease and should support liability. Defendants responsible for chrysotile-containing products – and the experts they retain – are of the opinion that low-dose and intermittent chrysotile asbestos exposures do not cause asbestos-related diseases, including mesothelioma.

Many defense experts will testify that there is substantial support in the scientific literature for the opinion that low-dose and intermittent chrysotile exposure does not result in the sustained biological impact that leads to disease, claiming that a critical factor is the body's ability to clear chrysotile fibers fairly rapidly, limiting the biopersistence of these fibers and thus the chronic inflammation associated with the development of mesothelioma.[58] They cite medical and scientific articles reporting, for instance, "[o]ur data suggest that fiber biopersistence is one of the main differences between the carcinogenicities of crocidolite and chrysotile … support[ing] the notion that only continuous exposure to chrysotile is able to maintain the processes that may lead to [malignant mesothelioma] over a prolonged time span."[59] Plaintiff experts hotly contest these contentions, citing medical and scientific articles that arrive at a different conclusion, and assert: "It has been generally accepted, that like other asbestos types, chrysotile fibers are capable of inducing human malignant mesothelioma,"[60] and, the "associations of … mesothelioma mortality with cumulative exposure to chrysotile asbestos fibers, as well as with the duration of exposure and time since exposure, support the conclusion that chrysotile causes mesothelioma."[61]

Putting aside the long-running and strident debate about asbestos fiber types and their biological impact, there is substantial acceptance that there are causes of mesothelioma other than asbestos, such as other fibrous minerals (e.g. erionite), therapeutic radiation, and chronic inflammation. Moreover, genetic factors may predispose individuals to the development of mesothelioma and other asbestos-related disease[62] and some mesotheliomas may be spontaneous or naturally occurring in individuals with no demonstrated history of exposure to asbestos.[63] In these last circumstances, the issue of "demonstrating" history to a sufficient quantum of exposure is another disputed area, with some defense experts opining that radiographic evidence of exposure is necessary to conclude there was any potentially causative exposure.

The *Hammond* case implicates yet another significant causation issue: that of peritoneal as opposed to pleural mesothelioma. Peritoneal mesothelioma arises in the lining of the abdominal cavity, while pleural mesothelioma impacts the lining of the chest cavity and lungs. Some scientific literature reflects that a much smaller percentage of peritoneal mesotheliomas as compared to pleural mesotheliomas have been associated with asbestos exposure, and that peritoneal mesothelioma is seen only with significant industrial amphibole asbestos exposures.[64] Plaintiff experts, however, frequently dispute this distinction, making the peritoneal mesothelioma causation question another battleground in cases involving that disease.

Developments in scientific understanding of how mesothelioma develops in the human body have offered dramatic insights into causation issues in recent years. Various disciplines – including epidemiology, pathology, molecular biology, and genetics – have all contributed meaningfully to a better understanding of these issues. Cutting-edge science does and will continue to profoundly impact causation debates in litigation. Grappling with these complex issues and applying these concepts to particular exposure situations can be extraordinarily challenging for parties, courts, and especially, for juries. Research will continue to focus on the issues, however, and – the hope is eventually – provide definitive scientific answers to the causation debate, as well as effective and life-saving methods for early detection and treatment of mesothelioma.[65]

16.3.4.5 Settlement

A plaintiff's and defendant's evaluations of settlement prospects and settlement value are based on many of the same issues: the risk and magnitude of a potential plaintiff jury verdict (or for the plaintiff, the risk of a defense verdict), the magnitude of likely litigation costs (which can be particularly expensive in jurisdictions without streamlined docket procedures), the trial capabilities and track record of plaintiff's and defendants' trial counsel, the law of the jurisdiction and, after it is chosen, the composition of the jury. Jury dynamics are a science and art unto themselves, so the final make-up of a jury can dramatically alter a plaintiff's or defendant's assessment of trial risk. In addition, analysis of the presence and strength of viable appellate issues impacts settlement decisions.

There are a few settlement factors peculiar to one side or the other. A plaintiff cares about the timing of ultimate resolution: any positive trial outcome – meaning a substantial jury award for the plaintiff's injuries or death – will likely be subject to appeal. The road to payment on the judgment a court enters on a jury award can be lengthy (typically measured in years rather than months). A settlement, however, will be paid in weeks or a few months at most. Defendants consider what impact a particular settlement might have on its relationship with and the expectations of the plaintiff firm in the future (given that they are likely to encounter each other routinely in asbestos cases).

Settlement discussions can occur at almost any stage of a case, depending on the plaintiff and defense lawyer approaches to negotiations. Each side wants to strategically use timing and the posture of the case to advance their positions. Frequently, plaintiff lawyers do not provide settlement demands, a first step in the process, until the case is sufficiently well developed for them to assess its strength and potential verdict value; defendants similarly cannot value a case for settlement until the case is sufficiently well developed, though when that happens can depend very much on the idiosyncrasies of the particular case.

16.3.4.6 Pre-trial and Trial

In the final pre-trial phase of an asbestos case, the plaintiff and defendants seek the court's guidance to narrow the legal issues and the evidence in play in a case, with a strategic eye to improving their positions at trial. Pursuant to deadlines set by the court, they may submit motions asking the court to rule on both dispositive legal issues and evidentiary issues before the trial commences.

In the *Hammond* case, the plaintiff's counsel submits a motion asking the court to exclude the testimony of defense experts who opine that chrysotile-containing products do not cause disease, alleging that the testimony is insufficiently based on reliable scientific evidence generated in conformance with acceptable scientific methodologies. The joint compound defendants seek dismissal through a motion for summary judgment, since there is no product identification of their products. Other defendants seek summary judgment, asking the court to disallow the plaintiff's negligence claims based on the argument that they have no duty for "take-home" exposures. Defendants also submit motions asking the court to exclude the testimony of plaintiff experts to the extent they rely on the opinion that asbestos is a signature disease for asbestos exposure, as not reliable science and as an attempt to achieve an improper avoidance of the plaintiff's burden of proof. Both sides submit numerous *motions in limine* (MILs) seeking to exclude certain factual evidence based on many theories, and the court must wade through and rule on these motions. Hammond's MILs include one seeking to exclude evidence of asbestos exposures to the extent that there is allegedly insufficient evidence of the exposure (no specific evidence of the company that manufactured insulation used by the plaintiff's father).

Trial courts ordinarily have broad discretion over what evidence will be presented to the jury and what evidence should be excluded. Due to the burden imposed by ruling on so many motions, courts often address all MILs in a single pre-trial hearing and frequently "split the baby," ruling for and against parties in ways that do not substantially alter their positions in the case.

The court in the *Hammond* case dismisses the joint compound defendants, and partially grants the defendant motion on duty for "take-home" exposure, to the extent that alleged exposure pre-dated 1972, when the court holds that defendants should have become aware of take-home exposure risks. The court denies expert challenges posed by both sides, ruling that the credibility of the expert and his or her opinions are issues for the jury's consideration, not to be addressed as a matter of law. Similarly, the court does not exclude any factual evidence. Importantly for defendants, the court denies plaintiff's MIL to exclude alternative exposure evidence (the insulation exposure). Given the expedited and thus limited discovery period, defendants do not have much opportunity to develop specifics on the insulation exposures but can rely on an expert for the opinion that all insulation for the uses identified by Andy contained amphibole asbestos during the relevant years.

Asbestos trials typically last 2–3 weeks, but depending on what constraints the court imposes, can be considerably longer. Initially, counsel for each party, starting with the plaintiff, will present its opening statement. As in all civil trials, the party with the burden of proof (here, the plaintiff), puts on his/her case first, offering witness testimony and documentary evidence for the jury's consideration. After the plaintiff rests his/her case, the defendants make and the court rules on motions for a directed verdict based on arguments that the plaintiff did not, as a matter of law, prove its case by a preponderance of the evidence. Such motions are rarely granted but are typically required to develop a robust record to be utilized on appeal. Defendants then have the opportunity to offer their evidence to the court and jury. After the close of evidence, either or both parties may move for a directed verdict arguing that based on the evidence presented at trial, either the plaintiff or the defendant has not produced evidence on which a jury could find in their favor. If granted, the case is over. If not, the court, with input from the parties, decides how to structure and word the jury instructions and the verdict form (the documents that the jury will use to guide their deliberations and decision-making). Finally, the parties present closing arguments to the jury, the judge instructs the jury on the law applicable to the case, and the jury retires to deliberate.

In the *Hammond* case, after a two-week trial and nearly three days of deliberations, the jury awards Ron Hammond $21.15 million in compensatory damages, but no punitive damages, against all viable defendants in the case, as well as attributing 30% responsibility for the verdict to the "alternative exposure" insulation companies. So, the outcomes of Ron's claims against those alleged to be responsible for his disease are: (1) 0% allocated to joint compound defendants dismissed on summary judgment due to no product identification; (2) allocations of 20% and 15% of the $21.15 million verdict against two brake companies for which Andy provided solid product identification, and 0% for two brake companies with weak product identification; (3) 25% against the boiler company with the strongest product identification and greater amount of use by Andy (thus greater exposure to Ron), and 10% against the boiler company with less exposure; and (4) 30% against two insulation manufacturers (not recoverable since companies long defunct). The jury did not attribute fault to General Motors/Delco brakes in the tort action, because as a nonparty bankrupt entity, it did not appear on the verdict form; however, the plaintiff may submit a claim in the General Motors Asbestos Trust (created out of GM 2009 bankruptcy filing).[66] Assuming a jury finds causation, these results are typical and somewhat predictable, even given the variations in so many factors in play in asbestos cases.

16.3.4.7 Appeal

In almost every state, the losing party at trial may challenge its loss on appeal to a higher court as a matter of right. During the trial of a case, the parties must work to preserve and bolster their appellate records, meaning they seek to support all dispositive motions with well-articulated and complete rationales, pay attention to what evidence does and does not get formally admitted, object in a timely fashion to the admission of key evidence, object and make motions for a mistrial in the face of egregious behavior on the part of opposing counsel (such as his/her failure to abide by the court's earlier rulings), and more. After a verdict, the parties may submit posttrial motions to the trial court identifying for the court's reconsideration points of error asserted during the trial and seeking relief. For example, our hypothetical plaintiff submits a posttrial motion renewing his arguments concerning the court's admission of the alternative exposure insulation evidence, and the defendants submit posttrial motions renewing arguments about the court's admission of expert testimony by the plaintiff, among other issues. When the court denies all posttrial motions and enters judgment on the verdict, it starts the clock for appeal.

Settlement discussions are common during this period. Plaintiffs are frequently individuals or families with significant medical expenses, a devastating disease and eventual loss of life, and difficult family dynamics to deal with. While approaches vary, plaintiffs often value closure and finality in asbestos litigation, and have a desire to avoid appeals. Thus, the financial ability of one or more large corporate defendants to appeal a judgment can be a significant advantage in post-judgment settlement negotiations. On the other hand, the existence of the substantial jury award pressures defendants to desire to settle for a more moderate amount. Moreover, the relief afforded by appeal is often a retrial, which results in substantial additional litigation costs and delays closure for all parties. In our hypothetical, plaintiff and all defendants settle during this post-judgment period before the appeal deadline, for a total of $6.75 million in damages to the plaintiff (roughly 46% of the recoverable verdict).

This hypothetical is necessarily cursory; however, it serves to demonstrate that asbestos cases in 2024 are very complex. Significant resources are expended both prosecuting and defending such cases. For this reason, it is not surprising that the tort system today is largely concerned with those claims with the greatest potential value in litigation, whereas the trust system receives and resolves a broader volume and range of claims. The wisdom of use of the tort system as the means to resolve such disputes has been questioned many times, as observed in the historical discussion above.

16.4 THE TRUST SYSTEM

In the United States, individuals and business entities imminently overwhelmed by debt or otherwise insolvent may seek to resolve their indebtedness through bankruptcy. Bankruptcy is a subject matter committed to federal law and is governed by the federal Bankruptcy Code, codified as Title 11 of the United States Code. The Bankruptcy Code offers two paths to organizations in bankruptcy. One avenue is through a liquidation of the company under Chapter 7 of the Bankruptcy Code, through which the company ceases to exist. The second avenue is a reorganization under Chapter 11 of the Code. Filing a Chapter 11 case stays all civil lawsuits and other actions against the debtor during the bankruptcy and allows companies to continue to operate while they work out a plan to restructure and repay their debts, often over an extended period of time.

16.4.1 Chapter 11 and § 524(g)

As discussed above, Johns-Manville Corporation (JM) was the largest manufacturer, distributor, and installer of asbestos-containing products in the United States, and as such was one of the most significant defendants in the burgeoning asbestos litigation. JM was also one of the first companies to avail itself of the protection of the Bankruptcy Code, electing in 1982 to seek reorganization under Chapter 11. The bankruptcy filing stayed all litigation against JM while the company struggled to come up with a way to deal with the thousands of pending lawsuits and a mechanism for dealing with future claims. During this time, the company continued to operate as a debtor in possession.

JM came out of bankruptcy in 1988 as a result of a plan that created the Manville Personal Injury Settlement Trust. All of JM's asbestos liabilities were transferred to the Manville Trust, and the newly reorganized company, Manville Corporation, was protected from all current and future liability for asbestos-related claims. This protection was accomplished through a channeling injunction that precluded future claims against the reorganized debtor while directing all claims to the trust. The Manville Trust was funded with approximately $2.5 billion of the financial assets of JM, which included a majority share of the stock of the company and available insurance.

It was anticipated that there would be up to 100,000 claims, and that the trust would resolve and process these claims and pay claimants 100% of the value of their claims. It soon became clear that the number of future claims had been seriously underestimated, and concerns that the funds in the trust would be exhausted before all claimants were paid led many claimants to avail themselves of provisions that allowed them to sue the trust. As a result, by 1992 in excess of 190,000 claimants had filed claims or initiated litigation, and the trust itself was insolvent. This led to a settlement in 1995 that altered both the financial arrangement with the reorganized Manville as well as implemented revised claims processing procedures designed to curb the flood of litigation that had caused the insolvency of the trust.

As discussed above, in 1994, Congress amended § 524 of the Bankruptcy Code to address the myriad problems caused by the impact of escalating asbestos litigation and the resulting bankruptcies of multiple companies by creating a statutory framework specifically for dealing with asbestos bankruptcies. Learning from the experience of Manville and other early bankruptcies, § 524(g) provides that companies facing significant asbestos liabilities can avail themselves of a channeling injunction as part of a Chapter 11 reorganization that protects them from all current and future asbestos liabilities. This is accomplished by funding a trust to pay all the debtor's current and future asbestos claims that meets all of the requirements of § 524(g). These requirements include a determination by the bankruptcy court that the debtor is likely to be subject to substantial future demands as a result of asbestos-related claims, that the magnitude and timing of such claims cannot be determined, and that the pursuit of such demands outside the context of the plan is likely to threaten the plan's purpose to deal equitably with existing claims and future demands. The section requires that the trust be funded by securities or debt from the debtor, that the trust own or have a right to own a majority share of the stock of the debtor or specified related entities, and that the trust use its assets or income to pay asbestos-related present and future claims. Additional conditions to approval require that the trust treat both present and future claimants in a substantially similar manner and that the bankruptcy plan and resulting trust be approved by a vote of 75% of current claimants in number and 2/3 of current claims in terms of value. As part of the proceedings to issue the channeling injunction that shields the debtor from asbestos liabilities, the court is required to appoint a legal representative to protect the interests of future claimants, commonly called a future claimants' representative (FCR). Only after all the requirements of § 524(g) are met and the entire reorganization plan approved by the bankruptcy court, will the new bankruptcy trust be established, and the reorganized company leave bankruptcy and resume normal business operations.

16.4.2 Bankruptcy Trust Administration

Asbestos trusts created pursuant to § 524(g) of the Bankruptcy Code exist for the purpose of assuming a debtor's asbestos-related liabilities and using the trust's assets to equitably compensate both current and future claimants suffering from asbestos-related diseases. Each trust is governed by a Trust Agreement (TA), which establishes the trust and creates the operational framework for the trust and how it is administered, and by Trust Distribution Procedures (TDP), which describe procedures for the filing, evaluation, and payment of claims. The operative provisions of the TA and TDP are negotiated as part of the bankruptcy process and approved by the bankruptcy court as part of the plan of reorganization confirmation process. The key players involved in the administration of the trusts include the Trustees, the Trust Advisory Committee (TAC), and the Future Claims Representative (FCR).

The trusts are managed by Trustees who are approved by the bankruptcy court. They are responsible for the day-to-day operations of the trusts, hiring and supervising necessary support personnel, managing the investments of the trust, filing taxes, filing annual reports to the supervising bankruptcy court, and hiring legal counsel and other outside professionals to advise them. Their obligation is to manage the trust for the benefit of present and future claimant beneficiaries, to ensure that both present and future claimants are treated equitably and that their claims are valued in a substantially similar manner. There is often a tension between the interests of current claimants, who desire rapid compensation and payment of the full value of their claims, and unknown future claimants, whose interests are focused on preserving trust assets to ensure the assets are adequate to satisfy future claims. In order to protect both interest groups, the role of representing the interests of current claimants resides with the TAC, while the FCR represents the interests of future claimants.

The TACs usually consist of five to nine attorneys who individually represent some of the thousands of individuals who have already been diagnosed with an asbestos-related disease, the present claimants. They advocate for, and have a fiduciary duty to, all current trust beneficiaries, not just the claimants they may individually represent. Often members of the TAC are drawn from the law firms representing the largest number of claimants.

The FCR, a position statutorily required by § 524(g), is charged with protecting the rights of future trust beneficiaries. These beneficiaries include individuals who may have been diagnosed with an asbestos-related disease but who are not represented by counsel and have not yet filed a claim, and individuals who have been exposed to asbestos and have not yet been diagnosed with an asbestos-related disease but are at risk of developing asbestos-related disease in the future.

Both the TAC and the FCR act as advisors to the Trustees on trust administration and issues facing the trusts and their consent must normally be obtained to any significant changes in the TA or TDP, which might include changes in the disease levels compensated by the trusts, changes in the payment percentage, or changes in the claims payment ratio all of which are discussed herein. Disputes between the Trustees, the TAC, and the FCR that cannot be resolved internally revert to the supervising bankruptcy court for resolution.

16.4.3 Claims Processing

The way that claims are processed will vary from trust to trust. Some trusts process their claims "in house" with their own staff of claims processors and attorneys, while most trusts employ an outside firm to process the claims. However, whoever does the processing must follow the Trust Distribution Procedures (TDPs) established during the Chapter 11 case and approved by the bankruptcy court. The TDP not only sets forth the procedures and requirements for filing the claim, but also the manner in which the claims will be reviewed, the way that claims will be valued, the manner in which claims will be liquidated and paid, and a process to resolve any disputes that might arise between a claimant and a trust on either the validity or value of a claim.

Each trust develops its own claim form to elicit the information necessary to evaluate its claims. This form typically not only requires biographical information about the claimant, but also information necessary to determine the nature and extent of any asbestos-related disease from which the claimant suffers, and the nature and extent of exposure to asbestos or asbestos-containing products for which the trust, substituting itself for the debtor, is responsible. The trusts use electronic claim filing, although provision is also made to file hard copy claims to accommodate any claimant who may not have access to file electronic claims.

To facilitate the valuation of claims, most trusts recognize and define disease levels. This assists the trust in treating similarly situated claimants equitably and provides a framework for placing values on claims based on the severity of the disease. The most common disease categories used by trusts include:

- Mesothelioma (Level VIII)
- Lung Cancer, with evidence of bilateral asbestos-related nonmalignant disease (Level VII)
- Lung Cancer without evidence of bilateral nonmalignant asbestos-related disease (Level VI)
- Other defined asbestos-related cancers with evidence of bilateral asbestos-related nonmalignant disease (Level V)
- Severe Asbestosis (Level IV)
- Asbestosis/pleural disease with resulting pulmonary impairment (Level III)
- Asbestosis/pleural disease without significant pulmonary impairment (Level II)
- Other asbestos-related disease (Level I)

These disease levels, and their specific diagnostic criteria vary slightly from trust to trust, but all use basically the same framework for evaluating the nature and extent of the asbestos-related disease at issue.

Within each disease category, there are additional medical and exposure requirements that must be met to qualify the claim. In every instance, there must be sufficient latency (time from first exposure to manifestation/diagnosis) for the development of the disease. For mesothelioma and other levels involving malignancies, confirmation by a board-certified pathologist is often required. For Level III to Level VII, a physician from an appropriate medical specialty is also required to establish that asbestos exposure was a significant contributing factor to causing the claimed disease. For nonmalignant diseases, most trusts require a diagnosis from a physician with an appropriate medical specialty who has examined the claimant. For nonmalignant cases where the claimant is deceased, pathological evidence or other evidence of extensive asbestos-related disease is often required to substantiate the claim. Pulmonary function testing is normally required for Level III and Level IV claims, and this testing must demonstrate a reduction of 20–25% below normal predicted levels of lung function, in a pattern consistent with asbestos-related lung disease as opposed to findings more commonly seen from smoking.

In addition to the medical requirements, the trusts also evaluate exposure to asbestos-containing products or conduct for which the debtor is responsible. To qualify for a claim for any individual trust, it is not sufficient to simply demonstrate a diagnosis of an asbestos-related disease. There must be some connection between the claimant's disease and the products or conduct of the debtor. The extent of such exposure, normally defined by length of exposure, often varies by disease level with mesothelioma requiring relatively brief exposures. Other diseases often require at least six months of exposure to a debtor's products or conduct, and a total of five years of exposure to asbestos from all sources, in order to meet minimum exposure requirements. This exposure can be demonstrated through sworn testimony, declarations or affidavits, employment records, invoices or any other reliable evidence.

Claims processed under expedited review are typically liquidated by offering values specified in the TDP, called scheduled values. These scheduled values vary by disease level and in some instances the nature of the exposure, with the more severe diseases and exposures receiving higher scheduled values. Trusts publish criteria for the medical evidence and exposure history that are necessary to qualify for expedited review as well as the documentation that must be submitted to the trust to support the claim. If a claimant is able to sufficiently document the claim and meet the criteria, the trusts presume the claim is valid and proceed with review and further processing.

Claims processed under individual review have the goal of being valued at the historical value of similar claims in the tort system, different from and typically higher than the scheduled values.

Trusts consider valuation factors such as age, severity of disease, marital status, number of dependents, economic loss and noneconomic damages, nature and extent of exposure to the debtor's products, the jurisdiction where the underlying case would have been filed and the verdict or settlement history of the claimant's law firm. In most instances, the specific "formula" for evaluating and weighing these valuation factors is not disclosed. This approach has been criticized from time to time for lack of transparency, and not adequately dealing with changing tort system values in different jurisdictions over time, changing composition of law firms, and how to deal with new firms handling cases that have no verdict or settlement history.

The exceptions to this lack of transparency are four trusts based in Reno, Nevada, including the Western Asbestos Settlement Trust, the Thorpe Insulation Settlement Trust, the J.T. Thorpe Settlement Trust, and the Plant Asbestos Settlement Trust. These four trusts value all claims using a fully disclosed case valuation matrix (CVM). The CVM reflects base-case values derived from historical settlement data, establishes criteria for the base-case value for each disease level, and then makes specified adjustments to the base-case value based on multiple factors including age, whether living or deceased, marital status, other dependents, loss of earnings, medical expenses, duration and intensity of exposure, and for some diseases, smoking history. The CVM is designed to yield average values equivalent to tort system values for similar claims. Monetary values and monetary factors are adjusted for inflation annually. Claimants can calculate the value of their claims using the CVM.

For many trusts, if a claim does not meet the specified medical or exposure requirements, there is a provision allowing individual review of claims that are otherwise cognizable in the tort system, sometimes with limitations on the value such claims can be paid. Individual review can also be used to address claimants who feel the facts of their claim warrant a higher-than-average claim value.

For all trusts, once a claim is approved and liquidated, it is placed in a queue for payment based on first in, first out or FIFO. While every trust would like to pay each claimant the full liquidated value of the claim immediately, a variety of factors make this virtually impossible. While at any time the number of existing claims is known and quantifiable, the number of future claims can only be estimated and is very uncertain. Experience with trusts over the last 40 years is that in most instances there have been more claims than were forecast when the trusts were established. In virtually every trust, the assets of the trust are limited and fixed. Since the mandate of the trusts is to treat all present and future claimants substantially the same, if the number of future claimants is underestimated, current claimants will be overpaid, and funds will be depleted before all future claimants are paid, resulting in underpayment of future claimants violating the trust's mandate.

To deal with this problem, and the reality that many trusts were never funded sufficiently by the debtor's estate to pay the liquidated value to all claimants, trust agreements and Trust Distribution Procedures (TDP) allow the Trustees, with the consent of the TAC and FCR, to obtain estimates of the value of existing and projected future claims and compare that value to the available assets of the trust, to determine what percentage of liquidated value the trust can pay current claimants and have sufficient funds to pay that percentage of liquidated value to all future claimants. This pro rata reduction is often referred to as the payment percentage. Once the payment percentage is determined, it is applied to the liquidated value to determine the payment that a claimant will receive.

Payment percentages are highly variable across multiple trusts, ranging from just over 1% to over 50%. Experience over the last 40 years has been that the payment percentage for most trusts has been decreased from the initial payment percentage paid by the trusts, due almost entirely to the trusts experiencing far more claims than were projected.

Other mechanisms designed to preserve assets for future claimants include the imposition of a maximum annual payment (MAP) a trust can make each year. The MAP is determined based on projected future claims and is periodically reevaluated. It basically controls the flow or rate of claims payments, but not the percentage of liquidated value that is paid. If a trust hits its MAP in any given year, further payments are suspended, and individuals in the payment queue who have not been paid will be placed at the beginning of the queue for the following year. This can result in delays in payments to some claimants but works to try to ensure that the trust's funds will not be prematurely depleted. A trust that consistently hits the MAP, or experiences excessively long waits in the payment queue, often must face the unpleasant task of considering a reduction in its payment percentage.

Another device designed to preserve assets for the most seriously injured claimants and used by some trusts is a claims payment ratio. This ratio sets limits on the proportion of the MAP that can be used to pay nonmalignant claimants. Although the ratio varies from 10% to 30% allocated to nonmalignant claims, it is designed to ensure that the largest percentage of available funds go to the most severely injured claimants. Much like the MAP, it restricts the flow rate on nonmalignant claims, and potentially could delay payments to nonmalignant claimants. Adopted during an era when there was a proliferation of filing of nonmalignant claims, recent experience with reduced filings of nonmalignant claims has made it essentially a nonissue with very few trusts experiencing claimants' payments being delayed due to the ratio.

16.4.4 Bankruptcy Trusts Today

Today there are over 100 companies that have filed for bankruptcy as a result of asbestos-related liabilities and there are approximately 60 bankruptcy trusts that are currently accepting and paying claims. Additional companies have filed for bankruptcy protection under Chapter 11 and are currently in bankruptcy: these companies may emerge with §524(g) trusts in the future. These proceedings often take many years to resolve. To date, bankruptcy trusts have paid in excess of $25 billion to claimants and it is estimated that current asbestos trusts have remaining assets in excess of $30 billion dollars. Payments from asbestos bankruptcy trusts comprise a significant portion of the compensation available to victims of asbestos-related disease as most companies responsible for their exposure have filed for bankruptcy protection and are not available in the tort system. Whether or not an individual will be eligible to be compensated by any given bankruptcy trust will be a function of the nature of the exposure and the trust's responsibility for that exposure, and the nature of the disease from which they suffer. Most claimants will qualify for claims against 20–30 trusts. The other source of compensation remains litigation in the tort system against solvent companies responsible for the claimant's exposure to asbestos.

16.5 EMERGING ISSUES AND STRATEGIES

Asbestos litigation in the tort and trust systems has been a continual process of evolution and innovation. Today is no different in this regard. This section briefly identifies three issues – two relating to defendant attempts at individual global resolution and the third, dealing with the practicalities of contingency fee litigation – that are drawing the attention and energies of the bench and bar. These issues are the "Texas-Two-Step," the divestiture of liabilities, and litigation funding.

At this juncture, asbestos personal injury liabilities are "legacy" liabilities for business defendants: these are not liabilities that arise out of current business operations. Moreover, such liabilities are frequently materially detrimental to a business' bottom line, given contingent liability reserve requirements and the constant balance sheet impact of the annual cost of the litigation. Finally, such liabilities in the tort system are perceived by business managers as unpredictable, because the risk of a very large jury award is at least theoretically at issue in many cases. As a consequence, almost every defendant would like to resolve all of its asbestos personal injury liabilities – present and future – once and for all. As discussed above, a company in serious imminent financial distress can pursue Chapter 11 relief and seek a § 524(g) trust. However, for successful companies for which asbestos litigation does not pose an imminent or existential threat, a Chapter 11 proceeding may not be a practical option.

In the recent past, two strategies have emerged for a business entity to seek resolution without, itself, going through a Chapter 11 proceeding. One strategy has come to be called the "Texas Two-Step"; the other is the divestiture of liabilities.

16.5.1 The Texas Two-Step

The "Texas Two-Step" bankruptcy strategy is largely untested and remains controversial. The strategy depends upon a transaction uniquely permitted by Texas corporate law (the source of the strategy's nickname). Every state's corporate law permits two separate corporations to merge, joining all of their separate assets and liabilities into a single surviving entity. Texas, however, permits a single corporation to engage in a "divisive merger," by which it divides itself into two (or more) entities, allocating assets and liabilities as between the two surviving entities and, at least initially, binding the rest of the world to that allocation.

The Texas Two-Step process involves establishing a Texas company, merging an existing non-Texas company with asbestos liabilities into that entity, then using the Texas divisive merger law to split off the liabilities into a new company while retaining the assets in a separate company. While the divisive merger was initially designed to facilitate normal divisions and spin-offs, when the divisive merger is combined with the Bankruptcy Code and, particularly § 524(g), it potentially allows solvent companies to shield their assets from litigants while ridding themselves of their asbestos liabilities.

Although Texas divisive mergers have been available since 1989, they have not been widely used. The first use of the Texas Two-Step was in 2017, when Georgia Pacific assigned its asbestos liabilities to a new entity named Bestwall through a divisive merger, which was followed by Bestwall declaring bankruptcy three months later. Georgia Pacific's example was followed in 2019 by Saint Gobain, which spun off its asbestos liabilities for their subsidiary Certainteed into DBMP (a non-operating company with no employees and limited assets), through a divisive merger, followed by DBMP filing bankruptcy three months later. In 2020, Trane Technologies used a divisive merger to put its asbestos liabilities into Aldrich Pump and Murray Boiler (again both nonoperating companies with few assets). These entities sought bankruptcy court protection seven weeks later. All of these Chapter 11 cases are ongoing as of this writing. To date, neither the federal appellate courts nor the Supreme Court of the United States has addressed whether the Texas Two-Step strategy can survive appellate review.

The largest, and perhaps the most controversial use of the technique occurred in 2021 when Johnson & Johnson created LTL Management LLC, assigning its liabilities related to talc litigation to this company using a divisive merger. In this instance, unlike prior Texas Two-Step bankruptcies, significant assets were also transferred to LTL Management LLC. LTL Management declared bankruptcy within a week.

The Bankruptcy Code requires that debtors must act in "good faith," a term of art, when they initiate their bankruptcy cases. Although the bankruptcy court initially decided that LTL Management's bankruptcy filing was made in good faith, on appeal the United States Court of Appeals for the Third Circuit disagreed, concluding that the bankruptcy filing was not in good faith because the debtor was too financially sound and did not have sufficient financial distress to justify a bankruptcy filing.[67] Consequently, LTL Management's first Chapter 11 was dismissed. On the same day the first Chapter 11 was dismissed, LTL Management filed a second bankruptcy petition and asserted that a proposed global settlement agreement, together with modifications to its funding agreement with Johnson & Johnson, made its new Chapter 11 filing proper. The bankruptcy court dismissed this second case as well.[68] As of this writing, this bankruptcy proceeding is on-going.

All of these cases raise significant issues surrounding whether a solvent company is able to shed its asbestos liabilities using the Texas Two-Step, including whether bankruptcies filed after a divisive merger can satisfy the Bankruptcy Code's "good faith" requirement, and whether, when dealing with solvent companies not in financial distress, the entire Texas Two-Step process can be characterized as a "fraudulent transfer" and, therefore, undone. These issues and others will likely occupy the courts at all levels for many years to come.

16.5.2 Divestiture of Liabilities

As noted above, bankruptcy protection as a means to manage asbestos liabilities and achieve finality may not be available to some companies and, even if the Texas Two-Step is ultimately feasible for more companies, it may not be desirable for a host of reasons (e.g. reputational impact, time delays, costs of implementation, and complexities such as triggering renegotiation or notification under numerous loan agreements or other contracts). Conceptually, in its simplest form, an alternative is to divest an entity or entities that hold legacy asbestos liabilities along with sufficient assets to pay them for the life of the liability; this is a potentially quicker, less-complicated and less-expensive option than bankruptcy to achieve finality.[69] This is both an old and a new strategy: the transactional and structuring tools are those of traditional corporate transactions, and those appropriate to a particular situation depend on where the liabilities currently reside and the overall goals of the transaction. The "new" aspect includes the goal of taking legacy asbestos liabilities off the balance sheet of the divesting company or parent, and achieving true finality in the transfer of the liabilities. There may be other goals associated with the transaction as well, such as the transfer of an operating business or its assets, that inform the structure and process chosen for the transaction.

The value of assets transferred to cover the divested liabilities must be at least commensurate with a reliable future life-of-the-liability forecast that is based on sufficiently stable historical experience to capture potential future variability. The total assets generally cover both estimated future costs of liability and defense. The company acquiring the liabilities and assets to cover them, and its affiliates or partners, generally will have expertise in managing the resolution of asbestos claims, collecting outstanding insurance reimbursements, and potentially managing any operational assets.

Critical factors for an effective transfer of asbestos liabilities in these transactions are that the value of assets included with the liabilities must be sufficiently robust; the transaction must be at arm's length and for fair consideration; and the entity to be transferred must be solvent and adequately capitalized immediately prior to the transaction. It is for these reasons that the future liability estimate must be stable and methodologically sound. These and other protections are necessary to avoid any clawback of the transaction or any viable claim of fraudulent conveyance. There are numerous examples of such transactions in recent years.[70]

16.5.3 Litigation Funding

Litigation funding is the practice where a third-party unrelated to the lawsuit provides funds for litigation, usually in return for a portion of any financial recovery from the litigation. This practice can allow plaintiffs, who would otherwise not have the financial resources to pursue a lawsuit, to do so, providing greater access to justice. Although often used to pay attorney fees and costs in personal injury and products' liability cases, it can also be used by companies in commercial litigation as a valuable tool for managing the costs and risks of litigation, or for providing working capital during legal proceedings. In asbestos litigation and other mass torts, litigation funding totaling millions of dollars has been used, for instance, to fund advertising campaigns to assist firms in acquiring new cases.

One of the benefits of litigation funding is that it can serve to level the playing field between underresourced plaintiffs and well-resourced defendants. In most instances, this funding is nonrecourse and the funder assumes the risk of an unsuccessful lawsuit, only being compensated if the plaintiff recovers. One leading legal scholar and authority on the industry has described the development of litigation funding as "the most important civil justice development of this era."[71]

While litigation funding has many virtues and benefits, it is not without potential disadvantages. Of course, lenders/investors face the prospect of losing all their investments if the lawsuit is not successful. Such arrangements have also been criticized as being expensive, with some litigation finance companies being accused of charging exorbitant fees. Other critics have expressed concern that litigation financing might tend to encourage frivolous lawsuits or allow undue influence by non-lawyers in the practice of law. Along these same lines, concerns have been raised that where financing arrangements cover a number of cases – as opposed to a single case – potential conflicts of interest may be created between the individual plaintiff and plaintiff's counsel, with regard to the resolution of that individual's case.

To address these concerns, many jurisdictions have adopted rules regarding litigation funding, or issued ethics opinions outlining a lawyer's responsibility to fully inform clients of the risks and benefits of such funding, to exercise independent professional judgment when advising a client, and to ensure that the litigation funding agreement will not interfere with the lawyer–client relationship or compromise the quality and soundness of advice offered to a client. When used in compliance with all ethical standards, litigation funding provides a powerful tool to enhance access to justice.

16.6 CONCLUSION

As this history shows, parties impacted by asbestos disease and asbestos litigation have for upwards of 50 years sought the means to compensate individuals harmed by asbestos exposure in the most efficient and fair means possible, running into numerous roadblocks: some legal, such as the failure of class action efforts; some political, such as the failure of federal legislation; some practical, such as the liquidation of many companies unable to reorganize with § 524(g) protection, to name a few. There have been some successes: in connection with reforms focused on streamlining and providing court processes that provide those with asbestos-related disease with relief and compensation and at the same time seek to maximize resources for future claimants; and in connection with the Trust System, with the same goals. Companies today involved in asbestos litigation continue to seek solutions that allow them to operate into the future without the overhang of substantial legacy liabilities, while funding entities whose purpose is to compensate claimants, such as trusts and "divestiture of liability" entities. While no system for compensation, whether tort or trust system, can fully remedy the history of asbestos use, exposure, and health impacts, especially largely fatal pleural mesothelioma, there is at this juncture the prospect that dramatic developments in scientific understanding of mesothelioma in the last decade and increased collaboration among scientists focused on the disease will provide hope for victims, beyond just compensation.

ACKNOWLEDGMENTS

The authors would like to acknowledge the review and critical input provided by Peter J. Neeson of Rawle & Henderson LLP, and Michael J. Angelides of Simmons Hanly Conroy LLP, as well as the comments provided by unidentified reviewers. The final chapter benefited substantially from these contributions, and we are very grateful for the time and careful thought each of our reviewers invested in this effort.

NOTES

1. As discussed in Chapters 1 and 2, *supra* pp. 1–2, 23, "asbestos" is a commercial term which refers to all or any one of six naturally occurring minerals (amosite, crocidolite, chrysotile, tremolite, actinolite, and anthophyllite) when they manifest in fiber form (defined as a 5:1 aspect ratio). Three forms of "asbestos" – chrysotile (white), amosite (brown), and crocidolite (blue) – were the asbestos fiber types principally in commercial use in the United States until the late twentieth century. As discussed below, in connection with talc litigation, these minerals can also appear in non-asbestos form (meaning not as fibers but as fragments).

2. The term "asbestos litigation" can also include claims for compensation brought by property owners, who assert that the presence or use of asbestos on their property has injured the property, reduced its value, and/or required costly remediation. Although a significant source of litigation at one time, the volume of such claims has greatly diminished with the passage of time. Property damage claims are not discussed in this chapter.
3. In some states, claimants may also pursue worker compensation claims, asserting their employers' liability for an asbestos-related workplace injury. Asbestos claims made in the worker compensation system have historically been treated much like other workplace injury claims.
4. To put this volume of case filings in perspective: because the average asbestos case takes 2-3 weeks to try to a jury verdict, it would take 100 judges and approximately 120,000 jurors 38.5 years to try 10,000 claims, if none of the cases settled and the judges handled no other cases.
5. KCIC, "Asbestos Litigation: 2022 Year in Review," available at www.kcic.com.
6. "Talc" claims, like asbestos claims, involve allegations that the claimant developed a disease – typically mesothelioma or ovarian cancer – as a result of his or her use of or exposure to cosmetic talc. Talc is a naturally occurring mineral, deposits of which can be "contaminated" with other minerals, including asbestos like amosite and chrysotile. "Contaminants" can appear in talc deposits in asbestos and nonasbestos form.
7. *Henningsen v. Bloomfield Motors, Inc.*, 161 A.2d 69 (NJ 1960)(expanding breach of implied warranty claims and permitting such claims to be asserted notwithstanding express disclaimers in a contract); *Greenman v. Yuba Power Prods., Inc.*, 377 P.2d 897 (CA 1963)(adopting strict products liability).
8. The ALI is an organization of select judges, legal academics, and lawyers, the purpose of which is to: (a) study developments in the common law of all U.S. jurisdictions by defined topic; (b) identify and synthesize the principles that are evidenced in that case law; and (c) debate, articulate, adopt, and publish those principles, in "restatements of law," for use by the bench and bar. The ALI's restatements in various subject matters, including tort law, have been and continue to be influential.
9. Restatement (Second) of Torts, § 402A (1965).
10. *Id.*, § 431.
11. Sherman EF, "The Evolution of Asbestos Litigation," *Tulane L. Rev* 2014;88:1021, 1024: *see also* Brodeur, Paul, *Outrageous Misconduct: The Asbestos Industry on Trial* (Pantheon Books, 1985).
12. 493 F.2d 1076 (5th Cir., 1973), *cert. denied* 419 U.S. 869 (1974).
13. *Id.* at 1094.
14. For instance, the Occupational Safety & Health Act, creating the federal Occupational Safety & Health Administration ("OSHA"), was enacted in 1970. Among OSHA's first regulations was one establishing a maximum standard for workplace exposure to asbestos, which went into effect in 1972. Throughout the 1970's and 1980's, OSHA routinely revisited and lowered this maximum exposure standard.
15. Richards B, "New Data on Asbestos Indicates Cover-up of Effects on Workers," *Washington Post*, November 12, 1978.
16. *Id.*
17. *Id.*
18. *Id.*: *see also Jones v. Pneumo Abex LLC,* 160 N.E.3d 881, 891 (IL 2019) (Kilbride, J., dissent) (discussing the history and controversy surrounding the editing and publication of the Saranac study results).
19. See e.g. *Johns Manville Prods. Corp. v. Superior Court*, 612 P.2d 940 (CA 1980)(former Manville worker may pursue claims for intentional harm, notwithstanding worker compensation bar).
20. *In re Johns-Manville Corp*, 60 B.R. 842 (S.D.NY 1986): Schmidt WE, "Manville Asserts U.S. Must Share Costs of Asbestos Damage Claims," *NewYork Times*, August 28, 1982.
21. UNR Industries, the company responsible for manufacturing UNARCO asbestos insulation, had filed for bankruptcy two months earlier, in June 1982.
22. Asbestos disease, especially mesothelioma, has a very long latency period, with disease frequently manifesting 20–70 years following exposure. In most jurisdictions, a claimant's legal cause of action does not accrue – become actionable – until the claimant manifests some physical change which can be characterized as an injury.
23. Schwartz V, Behrens M, "Asbestos Litigation: The Endless Search for a Solvent Bystander," *Widener L.J* 2013–2014;23:59.
24. MDL No. 875 remained active from 1991 through approximately 2019. During that 28 years, more than 186,000 cases were transferred to it for pretrial coordination. Hon. Eduardo Robreno J, "MDL 875: Past, Present, and Future" presentation (6/12/2009, as amended 11/10/2016), available at www.paed.uscourts.gov/documents2/mdl/mdl875About.
25. *Georgine v. Amchem Prods., Inc.*, 83 F.3d 610 (3rd Cir. 1996). Notwithstanding that the subsequent US Supreme Court decision was captioned *Amchem Products, Inc. v. Windsor*, most people refer to this effort as the *Georgine* settlement.

26. The National Institute for Occupational Safety and Health (NIOSH) runs a program to certify radiologists as proficient in the application of the International Labor Organization (ILO) system for classification of radiographs of pneumoconiosis, of which asbestosis is one type. Radiologists certified by NIOSH are referred to as "certified B-readers."
27. Berenson A, "A Surge in Asbestos Suits, Many By Healthy Plaintiffs," *New York Times*, April 10, 2002.
28. Carroll SJ, et al., *Asbestos Litigation*, pp. 75–76 (Rand Corporation, 2005), available at www.rand.org.
29. 11 U.S.C. § 524(g) made a trust and channeling injunction solution available to debtors prospectively. 11 U.S.C. § 524(h) blessed the trusts and channeling injunctions already approved at that time by various bankruptcy courts, eliminating any uncertainty about the long-term legal viability of those trusts.
30. W.R. Grace ("Grace") commenced its Chapter 11 case in 2001 and had a large number of asbestos cases pending around the country. Separately, Grace was also principally responsible for vermiculite mining and milling operations in Libby, Montana, a business it acquired in 1963 and operated through 1990 to make its very popular Zonolite insulation. The vermiculite mined in Libby was, however, contaminated with tremolite and actinolite (forms of amphibole asbestos). Grace's operations allegedly created widespread contamination and harm, including personal injury, throughout Libby, and in connection with the transportation of vermiculite to plants, and the manufacturing and use of Zonolite insulation. The Libby situation garnered a significant amount of attention from the U.S. EPA and media, given the number of indivduals (in the thousands), impacted. Grace addressed the vermiculite related personal injury claims in its reorganization plan. The Libby claimants claims against other defendants – like Grace's worker compensation insurer – continue as of this writing. *See*, Robbins J, "Ex-Worker Wins $36.5 Million from Company That Hid Asbestos Damage," *New York Times*, February 25, 2022.
31. From the 1920s through well into the 1990s, almost all automotive brakes were manufactured using processed chrysotile asbestos as a principal raw material.
32. Report of the Judicial Conference Ad Hoc Committee on Asbestos Litigation (1991) (the report's first recommendation was to urge the judiciary to urge Congress to act).
33. Congressional Research Service, RS22081, "S.B. 852: The Fairness in Asbestos Injury Resolution (FAIR) Act of 2005," 2006.
34. *In re Silica Products Liability Litigation,* 398 F.Supp.2d 563 (SD Tex. 2005).
35. *See,* "The Silicosis Story: Mass Tort Screening and the Public Health," Hearings before the Subcommittee of Oversight and Investigations of the Committee on Energy and Commerce, House of Representatives, 109th Congress (3/2006-7-2006), available at www.access.gpo.gov/congress/house, Serial No. 109–124.
36. Creswell J, "Testing for Silicosis Comes Under Scrutiny in Congress," *New York Times*, March 8, 2006.
37. Texas Civil Practice and Remedies Codes, Chapter 90, §§ 90.001-90.012. Some years later, Texas moved all asbestos cases – new and previously pending – to the intrastate coordination judge.
38. 2012 Florida Statutes, Chapter 774, §§774.001-008, 774.201–209.
39. *Harold's Auto Parts, Inc. v. Mangialardi,* 889 So.2d 493 (MS 2004).
40. Courts in many, though not all, of these tort reform jurisdictions either prohibited or imposed limitations on punitive damages in asbestos cases, again seeking fairness and equity for all claimants against a finite pool of defendant resources. *See* Behrens MA, Silverman C, "Punitive Damages in Asbestos Personal Injury Litigation," *Rutgers J Law & Pub Pol* 2011;8(1):50, 51.
41. There are a few jurisdictions, such as California and Michigan, that permit minimally impaired nonmalignant claims to proceed through the litigation process. In those jurisdictions, such claims are typically placed on a longer-term track and allocated fewer court resources.
42. Google auctions the right to be among the first responses to specific keyword searches to the highest bidders. According to a study by the international consulting firm Kantar, "mesothelioma" was by far the most expensive keyword on Google in 2009. Kantar's subsequent study of the most expensive Google keywords during the period 2014–2018 found that 67 of the 100 most expensive search terms were related to asbestos litigation, primarily connected to mesothelioma. Kantar, "The Most Expensive Keywords on Google," available at www.kantar.com/inspiration/advertising-media/the-most-expensive-keywords-on-google.
43. Restatement (Second) of Torts, § 402A (1965).
44. Restatement (Third) Torts: Products Liability, § 2 (1998).
45. KCIC, "Asbestos Litigation: 2022 Year in Review."
46. The International Agency for Research on Cancer (IARC), identified talc *with* asbestos or asbestiform minerals as a Group 1 human carcinogen very early on in its work. However, IARC, in later evaluating talc *without* asbestos or asbestiform minerals, concluded that there was insufficient evidence from which to classify asbestos free talc as a human carcinogen (although it noted that such talc may be implicated in ovarian cancer). IARC Monographs, "Carbon Black, Titanium Dioxide, and Talc," IARC (2010), ISBN 978-92-8321593-6.

47. For a more detailed narrative of this history from the defendant's perspective, *see In re LTL Management LLC,* Case No. 21-39589 (JCW), United States Bankruptcy Court, Western District of North Carolina, "Informational Brief of LTL Management LLC.," ("LTL Informational Brief"), available at www.document.epiq11.com (LTL's informational brief at the start of its first Chapter 11 case). For a more detailed narrative of this history from plaintiff experts' perspective, *see* Bird T, et al., "A Review of the Talc Industry's Influence on Federal Regulation and Scientific Standards for Asbestos in Talc," *New Solut.* 2021 Aug;31(2):152–169, doi: 10.1177/1048291121996645
48. Lawrence S, "Asbestos in Talcum? FDA to test." *New York Post*, 13 August 1971.
49. LTL Informational Brief, pp. 2–3, 46–49.
50. *Id.*, p. 124.
51. *Id.*, pp. 124–126.
52. A typical civil case might take two years or more from case filing to trial. Accelerated asbestos cases involving terminally ill plaintiffs can, depending on the jurisdiction, take only 120 days to trial or some interim date intended to allow the plaintiff to have his/her day in court while still living. These compressed deadlines are challenging for all parties, especially defendants with limited time to learn what they need to know about the case and to prepare for trial.
53. E.g., *Georgia-Pacific, LLC v. Farrar*, 432 Md. 532 (MD Ct App, 2013) (no duty to warn prior to 1972 adoption of OSHA regulations governing asbestos due to infeasibility of effective warning and questions about foreseeability of harm).
54. The legal burden of proof in most civil cases rests on the plaintiff to prove his or her contentions as more likely than not to be true (the preponderance of the evidence standard). Defendants are frequently in the position of needing to show that public perceptions of asbestos risk and causation are inaccurate and oversimplified. This scenario results in a de facto shifting of the burden of proof.
55. *See* Chapter 1 and fn 2 of this Chapter for a further discussion of this issue; *see also* Bernstein DM, "The Effects of Short Fiber Chrysotile and Amphibole Asbestos," *Crit Rev Tox* 2022;52:2–90, https://doi.org/10.1080/10408444.2022.2056430; Paustenbach D, Brew D, Ligas S, Heywood J, "A Critical Review of the 2020 EPA Risk Assessment for Chrysotile and Its Many Shortcomings," *Crit Rev Tox* 2021;51(6):509–539, 511, https://doi.org/10.1080/10408444.2021.1968337.
56. E.g. Mossman BT, "Mechanisms of Asbestos Carcinogenesis and Toxicity: The Amphibole Hypothesis Revisited," *B J of Indus Med* 1993;50:673 ("the prevalence of mesothelioma varies considerably according to fiber type"); Gibbs AR, Attanoos RL, "Non-Asbestos Related Diffuse Malignant Mesothelioma", in Advances in Surgical Pathology: Mesothelioma (Attanoos RL, Allen TC eds. 2014) ("overwhelming epidemiological and mineralogic evidence showing amphiboles as the cause of the vast majority of diffuse malignant mesothelioma in men"); *see also* Darnton L, "Quantitative Assessment of Mesothelioma and Lung Cancer Risk Based on Phase Contrast Microscopy (PCM) Estimates of Fibre Exposure: An Update of 2000 Asbestos Cohort Data," *Environ Res* 2023;230:114753:1, https://doi/org/10/1016/j.envres.2022.114753; Gilham C, Rake C, Burdett G, Nicholson AG, Davison L, Franchini A, Carpenter J, Hodgson J, Darnton A, Peto J, "Pleural Mesothelioma and Lung Cancer Risks in Relation to Occupational History and Asbestos Lung Burden," *Occup Environ Med* 2016;73:290–299, 296, http://dx.doi.org/10.1136/oemed-2015-103479.
57. E.g. Lemen RA, "Letter to the Editor on Chrysotile Asbestos and Mesothelioma," *Environ Hlth Persp* 2010;118: 7–A282, http://doi:10.1289/ehp.1002446 ("science has not changed its opinion that all forms of asbestos, including chrysotile, cause mesothelioma"); Loomis D, Richardson DB, Elliott L, "Quantitative Relationships of Exposure to Chrysotile Asbestos and Mesothelioma Mortality," *Am J Ind Med* 2019;62:471, 476, http://doi:10.1002/ajim.22985.
58. E.g. Bernstein, "The Effects of Short Fiber Chrysotile and Amphibole Asbestos," 93–94; Mossman, "Mechanisms of Asbestos Carcinogenesis and Toxicity," 675; *see also* Gilham, *et al.*, "Pleural Mesothelioma and Lung Cancer Risks," 296; Paustenbach, *et al.,* "A Critical Review of the 2020 EPA Risk Assessment," 511.
59. Qi F, Okimoto G, Jube S, Napolitano A, Pass HI, Laczko R, DeMay RM, Khan G, Tiirikainen M, Rinaudo C, Croce A, Yang H, Gaudino G, Carbone M, "Continuous Exposure to Chrysotile Can Cause Transformation of Human Mesothelial Cells via HMGB1 and TNF-a Signaling," *Am J Pathol* 2013;183:1654, 1665, http://dx.doi.org/10.1016/j.ajpath.2013.07.029.
60. E.g. Suzuki Y, Yuen SR, "Asbestos Fibers Contributing to the Induction of Human Malignant Mesothelioma," *Ann NY Acad Sci* 2002;982:160–176, 173, https://oi.org/10.1111/j.1749-6632-2002.tb04931.x.
61. Loomis, *et al.,* "Quantitative Relationships of Exposure," 476.

62. E.g. Roggli VL, et al., "Chronological Trends in the Causation of Malignant Mesothelioma: Fiber Burden Analysis of 619 Cases Over Four Decades," *Environ Res* 2023;230:114530, 1–7, https://doi.org/10.1016/j.envres.2022.114530; Attanoos RL, Churg A, Galateau-Salle F, Gibbs AR, Roggli VL, "Malignant Mesothelioma and Its Non-Asbestos Causes," *Arch Pathol Lab Med* 2018;142:753–760, http://doi:10.5858/arpa.2017-0365-RA ("It is clear that not all mesotheliomas are related to asbestos exposure", and elaborating on other causes); Moolgavkar S, Chang ET, Leubeck EG, "Multistage Carcinogenesis: Impact of Age, Genetic, and Environmental Factors on the Incidence of Malignant Mesothelioma," *Environ Res* 2023;230:114582,1–6, https://doi.org/10.1016/j.envres.2022.114582.
63. E.g. Attanoos, *et al.,* "Malignant Mesothelioma and Its Non-Asbestos Causes," 756–757; Gibbs AR, "Spontaneous/Idiopathic Diffuse Malignant Mesothelioma", in Advances in Surgical Pathology: Mesothelioma (Attanoos RL, Allen TC eds, 2014).
64. E.g. Attanoos RL, *et al.*, "Malignant Mesothelioma and Its Non-Asbestos Causes," 753, 757.
65. See e.g. Carbone M, Adusumilli PS, Alexander, Jr. HR, Baas P, Bardelli F, Bononi A, Bueno R, Felley-Bosco E, Galateau-Salle F, Jablons D, Mansfield AS, Minaai M, dePerrot M, Pesavento P, Rusch V, Severson DT, Taioli E, Tsao A, Woodard G, Yang H, Zauderer MG, Pass HI, "Mesothelioma: Scientific Clues for Prevention, Diagnosis, and Therapy," *CA Cancer J Clin* 2019;69:402–429, 402, https://doi:10.3322/caac.21572 ("Multidisciplinary international collaboration will be necessary to improve prevention, early detection and treatment.")
66. Whether a nonparty can appear on a verdict form varies from jurisdiction to jurisdiction.
67. *In re LTL Management LLC,* 58 F.4th 738 (3rd Cir. 2023).
68. *In re LTL Management LLC*, 652 B.R. 433 (USBC NJ 2023).
69. *See* https://fararecovery.com for more information on the variety, scope, and characteristics of such transactions.
70. E.g. https://www.businesswire.com/news/home/20220812005385/en/Crane-Holdings-Co.-Announces-Transaction-to-Divest-Legacy-Asbestos-Liabilities; https://www.bloomberg.com/press-releases/2021-07-01/itt-announces-sale-of-subsidiary-holding-legacy-liabilities-to-delticus-an-affiliate-of-warburg-pincus; https://spx.gcs-web.com/news-releases/news-release-details/spx-technologies-divests-legacy-asbestos-liabilities.
71. Steinitz M, "Follow the Money? A Proposed Approach for Disclosure of Litigation Finance Arrangements," *U.C. Davis Law Rev* 2019;53:1073.

Index

Note: Page locators followed by 'n' refer to notes.

B

D

E

F

G

H

Q

R

U

V

W

X

Y

Z

For Product Safety Concerns and Information please contact our EU representative GPSR@taylorandfrancis.com
Taylor & Francis Verlag GmbH, Kaufingerstraße 24, 80331 München, Germany

www.ingramcontent.com/pod-product-compliance
Lightning Source LLC
LaVergne TN
LVHW081313110826
845149LV00006B/1496

* 9 7 8 1 0 3 2 5 5 7 1 7 5 *